Ventilatory Support for Chronic Respiratory Failure

LUNG BIOLOGY IN HEALTH AND DISEASE

Executive Editor

Claude Lenfant
Former Director, National Heart, Lung, and Blood Institute
National Institutes of Health
Bethesda, Maryland

1. Immunologic and Infectious Reactions in the Lung, *edited by C. H. Kirkpatrick and H. Y. Reynolds*
2. The Biochemical Basis of Pulmonary Function, *edited by R. G. Crystal*
3. Bioengineering Aspects of the Lung, *edited by J. B. West*
4. Metabolic Functions of the Lung, *edited by Y. S. Bakhle and J. R. Vane*
5. Respiratory Defense Mechanisms (in two parts), *edited by J. D. Brain, D. F. Proctor, and L. M. Reid*
6. Development of the Lung, *edited by W. A. Hodson*
7. Lung Water and Solute Exchange, *edited by N. C. Staub*
8. Extrapulmonary Manifestations of Respiratory Disease, *edited by E. D. Robin*
9. Chronic Obstructive Pulmonary Disease, *edited by T. L. Petty*
10. Pathogenesis and Therapy of Lung Cancer, *edited by C. C. Harris*
11. Genetic Determinants of Pulmonary Disease, *edited by S. D. Litwin*
12. The Lung in the Transition Between Health and Disease, *edited by P. T. Macklem and S. Permutt*
13. Evolution of Respiratory Processes: A Comparative Approach, *edited by S. C. Wood and C. Lenfant*
14. Pulmonary Vascular Diseases, *edited by K. M. Moser*
15. Physiology and Pharmacology of the Airways, *edited by J. A. Nadel*
16. Diagnostic Techniques in Pulmonary Disease (in two parts), *edited by M. A. Sackner*
17. Regulation of Breathing (in two parts), *edited by T. F. Hornbein*
18. Occupational Lung Diseases: Research Approaches and Methods, *edited by H. Weill and M. Turner-Warwick*
19. Immunopharmacology of the Lung, *edited by H. H. Newball*
20. Sarcoidosis and Other Granulomatous Diseases of the Lung, *edited by B. L. Fanburg*
21. Sleep and Breathing, *edited by N. A. Saunders and C. E. Sullivan*
22. *Pneumocystis carinii* Pneumonia: Pathogenesis, Diagnosis, and Treatment, *edited by L. S. Young*
23. Pulmonary Nuclear Medicine: Techniques in Diagnosis of Lung Disease, *edited by H. L. Atkins*

24. Acute Respiratory Failure, *edited by W. M. Zapol and K. J. Falke*
25. Gas Mixing and Distribution in the Lung, *edited by L. A. Engel and M. Paiva*
26. High-Frequency Ventilation in Intensive Care and During Surgery, *edited by G. Carlon and W. S. Howland*
27. Pulmonary Development: Transition from Intrauterine to Extrauterine Life, *edited by G. H. Nelson*
28. Chronic Obstructive Pulmonary Disease: Second Edition, *edited by T. L. Petty*
29. The Thorax (in two parts), *edited by C. Roussos and P. T. Macklem*
30. The Pleura in Health and Disease, *edited by J. Chrétien, J. Bignon, and A. Hirsch*
31. Drug Therapy for Asthma: Research and Clinical Practice, *edited by J. W. Jenne and S. Murphy*
32. Pulmonary Endothelium in Health and Disease, *edited by U. S. Ryan*
33. The Airways: Neural Control in Health and Disease, *edited by M. A. Kaliner and P. J. Barnes*
34. Pathophysiology and Treatment of Inhalation Injuries, *edited by J. Loke*
35. Respiratory Function of the Upper Airway, *edited by O. P. Mathew and G. Sant'Ambrogio*
36. Chronic Obstructive Pulmonary Disease: A Behavioral Perspective, *edited by A. J. McSweeny and I. Grant*
37. Biology of Lung Cancer: Diagnosis and Treatment, *edited by S. T. Rosen, J. L. Mulshine, F. Cuttitta, and P. G. Abrams*
38. Pulmonary Vascular Physiology and Pathophysiology, *edited by E. K. Weir and J. T. Reeves*
39. Comparative Pulmonary Physiology: Current Concepts, *edited by S. C. Wood*
40. Respiratory Physiology: An Analytical Approach, *edited by H. K. Chang and M. Paiva*
41. Lung Cell Biology, *edited by D. Massaro*
42. Heart–Lung Interactions in Health and Disease, *edited by S. M. Scharf and S. S. Cassidy*
43. Clinical Epidemiology of Chronic Obstructive Pulmonary Disease, *edited by M. J. Hensley and N. A. Saunders*
44. Surgical Pathology of Lung Neoplasms, *edited by A. M. Marchevsky*
45. The Lung in Rheumatic Diseases, *edited by G. W. Cannon and G. A. Zimmerman*
46. Diagnostic Imaging of the Lung, *edited by C. E. Putman*
47. Models of Lung Disease: Microscopy and Structural Methods, *edited by J. Gil*
48. Electron Microscopy of the Lung, *edited by D. E. Schraufnagel*
49. Asthma: Its Pathology and Treatment, *edited by M. A. Kaliner, P. J. Barnes, and C. G. A. Persson*
50. Acute Respiratory Failure: Second Edition, *edited by W. M. Zapol and F. Lemaire*
51. Lung Disease in the Tropics, *edited by O. P. Sharma*
52. Exercise: Pulmonary Physiology and Pathophysiology, *edited by B. J. Whipp and K. Wasserman*

53. Developmental Neurobiology of Breathing, *edited by G. G. Haddad and J. P. Farber*
54. Mediators of Pulmonary Inflammation, *edited by M. A. Bray and W. H. Anderson*
55. The Airway Epithelium, *edited by S. G. Farmer and D. Hay*
56. Physiological Adaptations in Vertebrates: Respiration, Circulation, and Metabolism, *edited by S. C. Wood, R. E. Weber, A. R. Hargens, and R. W. Millard*
57. The Bronchial Circulation, *edited by J. Butler*
58. Lung Cancer Differentiation: Implications for Diagnosis and Treatment, *edited by S. D. Bernal and P. J. Hesketh*
59. Pulmonary Complications of Systemic Disease, *edited by J. F. Murray*
60. Lung Vascular Injury: Molecular and Cellular Response, *edited by A. Johnson and T. J. Ferro*
61. Cytokines of the Lung, *edited by J. Kelley*
62. The Mast Cell in Health and Disease, *edited by M. A. Kaliner and D. D. Metcalfe*
63. Pulmonary Disease in the Elderly Patient, *edited by D. A. Mahler*
64. Cystic Fibrosis, *edited by P. B. Davis*
65. Signal Transduction in Lung Cells, *edited by J. S. Brody, D. M. Center, and V. A. Tkachuk*
66. Tuberculosis: A Comprehensive International Approach, *edited by L. B. Reichman and E. S. Hershfield*
67. Pharmacology of the Respiratory Tract: Experimental and Clinical Research, *edited by K. F. Chung and P. J. Barnes*
68. Prevention of Respiratory Diseases, *edited by A. Hirsch, M. Goldberg, J.-P. Martin, and R. Masse*
69. *Pneumocystis carinii* Pneumonia: Second Edition, *edited by P. D. Walzer*
70. Fluid and Solute Transport in the Airspaces of the Lungs, *edited by R. M. Effros and H. K. Chang*
71. Sleep and Breathing: Second Edition, *edited by N. A. Saunders and C. E. Sullivan*
72. Airway Secretion: Physiological Bases for the Control of Mucous Hypersecretion, *edited by T. Takishima and S. Shimura*
73. Sarcoidosis and Other Granulomatous Disorders, *edited by D. G. James*
74. Epidemiology of Lung Cancer, *edited by J. M. Samet*
75. Pulmonary Embolism, *edited by M. Morpurgo*
76. Sports and Exercise Medicine, *edited by S. C. Wood and R. C. Roach*
77. Endotoxin and the Lungs, *edited by K. L. Brigham*
78. The Mesothelial Cell and Mesothelioma, *edited by M.-C. Jaurand and J. Bignon*
79. Regulation of Breathing: Second Edition, *edited by J. A. Dempsey and A. I. Pack*
80. Pulmonary Fibrosis, *edited by S. Hin. Phan and R. S. Thrall*
81. Long-Term Oxygen Therapy: Scientific Basis and Clinical Application, *edited by W. J. O'Donohue, Jr.*
82. Ventral Brainstem Mechanisms and Control of Respiration and Blood Pressure, *edited by C. O. Trouth, R. M. Millis, H. F. Kiwull-Schöne, and M. E. Schläfke*

83. A History of Breathing Physiology, *edited by D. F. Proctor*
84. Surfactant Therapy for Lung Disease, *edited by B. Robertson and H. W. Taeusch*
85. The Thorax: Second Edition, Revised and Expanded (in three parts), *edited by C. Roussos*
86. Severe Asthma: Pathogenesis and Clinical Management, *edited by S. J. Szefler and D. Y. M. Leung*
87. *Mycobacterium avium*–Complex Infection: Progress in Research and Treatment, *edited by J. A. Korvick and C. A. Benson*
88. Alpha 1–Antitrypsin Deficiency: Biology • Pathogenesis • Clinical Manifestations • Therapy, *edited by R. G. Crystal*
89. Adhesion Molecules and the Lung, *edited by P. A. Ward and J. C. Fantone*
90. Respiratory Sensation, *edited by L. Adams and A. Guz*
91. Pulmonary Rehabilitation, *edited by A. P. Fishman*
92. Acute Respiratory Failure in Chronic Obstructive Pulmonary Disease, *edited by J.-P. Derenne, W. A. Whitelaw, and T. Similowski*
93. Environmental Impact on the Airways: From Injury to Repair, *edited by J. Chrétien and D. Dusser*
94. Inhalation Aerosols: Physical and Biological Basis for Therapy, *edited by A. J. Hickey*
95. Tissue Oxygen Deprivation: From Molecular to Integrated Function, *edited by G. G. Haddad and G. Lister*
96. The Genetics of Asthma, *edited by S. B. Liggett and D. A. Meyers*
97. Inhaled Glucocorticoids in Asthma: Mechanisms and Clinical Actions, *edited by R. P. Schleimer, W. W. Busse, and P. M. O'Byrne*
98. Nitric Oxide and the Lung, *edited by W. M. Zapol and K. D. Bloch*
99. Primary Pulmonary Hypertension, *edited by L. J. Rubin and S. Rich*
100. Lung Growth and Development, *edited by J. A. McDonald*
101. Parasitic Lung Diseases, *edited by A. A. F. Mahmoud*
102. Lung Macrophages and Dendritic Cells in Health and Disease, *edited by M. F. Lipscomb and S. W. Russell*
103. Pulmonary and Cardiac Imaging, *edited by C. Chiles and C. E. Putman*
104. Gene Therapy for Diseases of the Lung, *edited by K. L. Brigham*
105. Oxygen, Gene Expression, and Cellular Function, *edited by L. Biadasz Clerch and D. J. Massaro*
106. Beta$_2$-Agonists in Asthma Treatment, *edited by R. Pauwels and P. M. O'Byrne*
107. Inhalation Delivery of Therapeutic Peptides and Proteins, *edited by A. L. Adjei and P. K. Gupta*
108. Asthma in the Elderly, *edited by R. A. Barbee and J. W. Bloom*
109. Treatment of the Hospitalized Cystic Fibrosis Patient, *edited by D. M. Orenstein and R. C. Stern*
110. Asthma and Immunological Diseases in Pregnancy and Early Infancy, *edited by M. Schatz, R. S. Zeiger, and H. N. Claman*
111. Dyspnea, *edited by D. A. Mahler*
112. Proinflammatory and Antiinflammatory Peptides, *edited by S. I. Said*
113. Self-Management of Asthma, *edited by H. Kotses and A. Harver*

114. Eicosanoids, Aspirin, and Asthma, *edited by A. Szczeklik, R. J. Gryglewski, and J. R. Vane*
115. Fatal Asthma, *edited by A. L. Sheffer*
116. Pulmonary Edema, *edited by M. A. Matthay and D. H. Ingbar*
117. Inflammatory Mechanisms in Asthma, *edited by S. T. Holgate and W. W. Busse*
118. Physiological Basis of Ventilatory Support, *edited by J. J. Marini and A. S. Slutsky*
119. Human Immunodeficiency Virus and the Lung, *edited by M. J. Rosen and J. M. Beck*
120. Five-Lipoxygenase Products in Asthma, *edited by J. M. Drazen, S.-E. Dahlén, and T. H. Lee*
121. Complexity in Structure and Function of the Lung, *edited by M. P. Hlastala and H. T. Robertson*
122. Biology of Lung Cancer, *edited by M. A. Kane and P. A. Bunn, Jr.*
123. Rhinitis: Mechanisms and Management, *edited by R. M. Naclerio, S. R. Durham, and N. Mygind*
124. Lung Tumors: Fundamental Biology and Clinical Management, *edited by C. Brambilla and E. Brambilla*
125. Interleukin-5: From Molecule to Drug Target for Asthma, *edited by C. J. Sanderson*
126. Pediatric Asthma, *edited by S. Murphy and H. W. Kelly*
127. Viral Infections of the Respiratory Tract, *edited by R. Dolin and P. F. Wright*
128. Air Pollutants and the Respiratory Tract, *edited by D. L. Swift and W. M. Foster*
129. Gastroesophageal Reflux Disease and Airway Disease, *edited by M. R. Stein*
130. Exercise-Induced Asthma, *edited by E. R. McFadden, Jr.*
131. LAM and Other Diseases Characterized by Smooth Muscle Proliferation, *edited by J. Moss*
132. The Lung at Depth, *edited by C. E. G. Lundgren and J. N. Miller*
133. Regulation of Sleep and Circadian Rhythms, *edited by F. W. Turek and P. C. Zee*
134. Anticholinergic Agents in the Upper and Lower Airways, *edited by S. L. Spector*
135. Control of Breathing in Health and Disease, *edited by M. D. Altose and Y. Kawakami*
136. Immunotherapy in Asthma, *edited by J. Bousquet and H. Yssel*
137. Chronic Lung Disease in Early Infancy, *edited by R. D. Bland and J. J. Coalson*
138. Asthma's Impact on Society: The Social and Economic Burden, *edited by K. B. Weiss, A. S. Buist, and S. D. Sullivan*
139. New and Exploratory Therapeutic Agents for Asthma, *edited by M. Yeadon and Z. Diamant*
140. Multimodality Treatment of Lung Cancer, *edited by A. T. Skarin*
141. Cytokines in Pulmonary Disease: Infection and Inflammation, *edited by S. Nelson and T. R. Martin*
142. Diagnostic Pulmonary Pathology, *edited by P. T. Cagle*

143. Particle–Lung Interactions, *edited by P. Gehr and J. Heyder*
144. Tuberculosis: A Comprehensive International Approach, Second Edition, Revised and Expanded, *edited by L. B. Reichman and E. S. Hershfield*
145. Combination Therapy for Asthma and Chronic Obstructive Pulmonary Disease, *edited by R. J. Martin and M. Kraft*
146. Sleep Apnea: Implications in Cardiovascular and Cerebrovascular Disease, *edited by T. D. Bradley and J. S. Floras*
147. Sleep and Breathing in Children: A Developmental Approach, *edited by G. M. Loughlin, J. L. Carroll, and C. L. Marcus*
148. Pulmonary and Peripheral Gas Exchange in Health and Disease, *edited by J. Roca, R. Rodriguez-Roisin, and P. D. Wagner*
149. Lung Surfactants: Basic Science and Clinical Applications, *R. H. Notter*
150. Nosocomial Pneumonia, *edited by W. R. Jarvis*
151. Fetal Origins of Cardiovascular and Lung Disease, *edited by David J. P. Barker*
152. Long-Term Mechanical Ventilation, *edited by N. S. Hill*
153. Environmental Asthma, *edited by R. K. Bush*
154. Asthma and Respiratory Infections, *edited by D. P. Skoner*
155. Airway Remodeling, *edited by P. H. Howarth, J. W. Wilson, J. Bousquet, S. Rak, and R. A. Pauwels*
156. Genetic Models in Cardiorespiratory Biology, *edited by G. G. Haddad and T. Xu*
157. Respiratory-Circulatory Interactions in Health and Disease, *edited by S. M. Scharf, M. R. Pinsky, and S. Magder*
158. Ventilator Management Strategies for Critical Care, *edited by N. S. Hill and M. M. Levy*
159. Severe Asthma: Pathogenesis and Clinical Management, Second Edition, Revised and Expanded, *edited by S. J. Szefler and D. Y. M. Leung*
160. Gravity and the Lung: Lessons from Microgravity, *edited by G. K. Prisk, M. Paiva, and J. B. West*
161. High Altitude: An Exploration of Human Adaptation, *edited by T. F. Hornbein and R. B. Schoene*
162. Drug Delivery to the Lung, *edited by H. Bisgaard, C. O'Callaghan, and G. C. Smaldone*
163. Inhaled Steroids in Asthma: Optimizing Effects in the Airways, *edited by R. P. Schleimer, P. M. O'Byrne, S. J. Szefler, and R. Brattsand*
164. IgE and Anti-IgE Therapy in Asthma and Allergic Disease, *edited by R. B. Fick, Jr., and P. M. Jardieu*
165. Clinical Management of Chronic Obstructive Pulmonary Disease, *edited by T. Similowski, W. A. Whitelaw, and J.-P. Derenne*
166. Sleep Apnea: Pathogenesis, Diagnosis, and Treatment, *edited by A. I. Pack*
167. Biotherapeutic Approaches to Asthma, *edited by J. Agosti and A. L. Sheffer*
168. Proteoglycans in Lung Disease, *edited by H. G. Garg, P. J. Roughley, and C. A. Hales*
169. Gene Therapy in Lung Disease, *edited by S. M. Albelda*
170. Disease Markers in Exhaled Breath, *edited by N. Marczin, S. A. Kharitonov, M. H. Yacoub, and P. J. Barnes*

171. Sleep-Related Breathing Disorders: Experimental Models and Therapeutic Potential, *edited by D. W. Carley and M. Radulovacki*
172. Chemokines in the Lung, *edited by R. M. Strieter, S. L. Kunkel, and T. J. Standiford*
173. Respiratory Control and Disorders in the Newborn, *edited by O. P. Mathew*
174. The Immunological Basis of Asthma, *edited by B. N. Lambrecht, H. C. Hoogsteden, and Z. Diamant*
175. Oxygen Sensing: Responses and Adaptation to Hypoxia, *edited by S. Lahiri, G. L. Semenza, and N. R. Prabhakar*
176. Non-Neoplastic Advanced Lung Disease, *edited by J. R. Maurer*
177. Therapeutic Targets in Airway Inflammation, *edited by N. T. Eissa and D. P. Huston*
178. Respiratory Infections in Allergy and Asthma, *edited by S. L. Johnston and N. G. Papadopoulos*
179. Acute Respiratory Distress Syndrome, *edited by M. A. Matthay*
180. Venous Thromboembolism, *edited by J. E. Dalen*
181. Upper and Lower Respiratory Disease, *edited by J. Corren, A. Togias, and J. Bousquet*
182. Pharmacotherapy in Chronic Obstructive Pulmonary Disease, *edited by B. R. Celli*
183. Acute Exacerbations of Chronic Obstructive Pulmonary Disease, *edited by N. M. Siafakas, N. R. Anthonisen, and D. Georgopoulos*
184. Lung Volume Reduction Surgery for Emphysema, *edited by H. E. Fessler, J. J. Reilly, Jr., and D. J. Sugarbaker*
185. Idiopathic Pulmonary Fibrosis, *edited by J. P. Lynch III*
186. Pleural Disease, *edited by D. Bouros*
187. Oxygen/Nitrogen Radicals: Lung Injury and Disease, *edited by V. Vallyathan, V. Castranova, and X. Shi*
188. Therapy for Mucus-Clearance Disorders, *edited by B. K. Rubin and C. P. van der Schans*
189. Interventional Pulmonary Medicine, *edited by J. F. Beamis, Jr., P. N. Mathur, and A. C. Mehta*
190. Lung Development and Regeneration, *edited by D. J. Massaro, G. Massaro, and P. Chambon*
191. Long-Term Intervention in Chronic Obstructive Pulmonary Disease, *edited by R. Pauwels, D. S. Postma, and S. T. Weiss*
192. Sleep Deprivation: Basic Science, Physiology, and Behavior, *edited by Clete A. Kushida*
193. Sleep Deprivation: Clinical Issues, Pharmacology, and Sleep Loss Effects, *edited by Clete A. Kushida*
194. Pneumocystis Pneumonia: Third Edition, Revised and Expanded, *edited by P. D. Walzer and M. Cushion*
195. Asthma Prevention, *edited by William W. Busse and Robert F. Lemanske, Jr.*
196. Lung Injury: Mechanisms, Pathophysiology, and Therapy, *edited by Robert H. Notter, Jacob Finkelstein, and Bruce Holm*

197. Ion Channels in the Pulmonary Vasculature, *edited by Jason X.-J. Yuan*
198. Chronic Obstructive Pulmonary Disease: Cellular and Molecular Mechanisms, *edited by Peter J. Barnes*
199. Pediatric Nasal and Sinus Disorders, *edited by Tania Sih and Peter A. R. Clement*
200. Functional Lung Imaging, *edited by David Lipson and Edwin van Beek*
201. Lung Surfactant Function and Disorder, *edited by Kaushik Nag*
202. Pharmacology and Pathophysiology of the Control of Breathing, *edited by Denham S. Ward, Albert Dahan and Luc J. Teppema*
203. Molecular Imaging of the Lungs, *edited by Daniel Schuster and Timothy Blackwell*
204. Air Pollutants and the Respiratory Tract: Second Edition, *edited by W. Michael Foster and Daniel L. Costa*
205. Acute and Chronic Cough, *edited by Anthony E. Redington and Alyn H. Morice*
206. Severe Pneumonia, *edited by Michael S. Niederman*
207. Monitoring Asthma, *edited by Peter G. Gibson*
208. Dyspnea: Mechanisms, Measurement, and Management, Second Edition, *edited by Donald A. Mahler and Denis E. O'Donnell*
209. Childhood Asthma, *edited by Stanley J. Szefler and Søren Pedersen*
210. Sarcoidosis, *edited by Robert Baughman*
211. Tropical Lung Disease, Second Edition, *edited by Om Sharma*
212. Pharmacotherapy of Asthma, *edited by James T. Li*
213. Practical Pulmonary and Critical Care Medicine: Respiratory Failure, *edited by Zab Mosenifar and Guy W. Soo Hoo*
214. Practical Pulmonary and Critical Care Medicine: Disease Management, *edited by Zab Mosenifar and Guy W. Soo Hoo*
215. Ventilator-Induced Lung Injury, *edited by Didier Dreyfuss, Georges Saumon, and Rolf D. Hubmayr*
216. Bronchial Vascular Remodeling In Asthma and COPD, *edited by Aili Lazaar*
217. Lung and Heart–Lung Transplantation, *edited by Joseph P. Lynch III and David J. Ross*
218. Genetics of Asthma and Chronic Obstructive Pulmonary Disease, *edited by Dirkje S. Postma and Scott T. Weiss*
219. *Reichman and Hershfield's* Tuberculosis: A Comprehensive, International Approach, Third Edition (in two parts), *edited by Mario C. Raviglione*
220. Narcolepsy and Hypersomnia, *edited by Claudio Bassetti, Michel Billiard, and Emmanuel Mignot*
221. Inhalation Aerosols: Physical and Biological Basis for Therapy, Second Edition, *edited by Anthony J. Hickey*
222. Clinical Management of Chronic Obstructive Pulmonary Disease, Second Edition, *edited by Stephen I. Rennard, Roberto Rodriguez-Roisin, Gérard Huchon, and Nicolas Roche*
223. Sleep in Children, Second Edition: Developmental Changes in Sleep Patterns, *edited by Carole L. Marcus, John L. Carroll, David F. Donnelly, and Gerald M. Loughlin*

224. Sleep and Breathing in Children, Second Edition: Developmental Changes in Breathing During Sleep, *edited by Carole L. Marcus, John L. Carroll, David F. Donnelly, and Gerald M. Loughlin*
225. Ventilatory Support for Chronic Respiratory Failure, *edited by Nicolino Ambrosino and Roger S. Goldstein*

The opinions expressed in these volumes do not necessarily represent the views of the National Institutes of Health.

Ventilatory Support for Chronic Respiratory Failure

Edited by
Nicolino Ambrosino
University Hospital Pisa
Pulmonary Rehabilitation and Weaning Center
Volterra, Italy
Roger S. Goldstein
West Park Healthcare Centre
University of Toronto
Toronto, Ontario, Canada

informa
healthcare
New York London

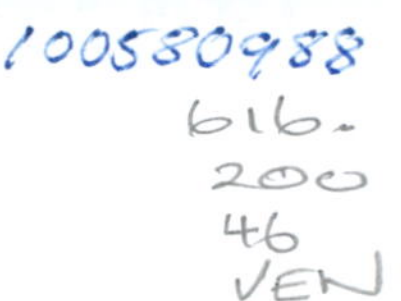

Informa Healthcare USA, Inc.
52 Vanderbilt Avenue
New York, NY 10017

Printed in the United States of America on acid-free paper
10 9 8 7 6 5 4 3 2 1

International Standard Book Number-10: 0-8493-8498-2 (Hardcover)
International Standard Book Number-13: 978-0-8493-8498-1 (Hardcover)

Library of Congress Cataloging-in-Publication Data

Ventilatory support for chronic respiratory failure/edited by Nicolino Ambrosino, Roger S. Goldstein.
p. ; cm. — (Lung biology in health and disease ; v. 225)
Includes bibliographical references and index.
ISBN-13: 978-0-8493-8498-1 (hb : alk. paper)
ISBN-10: 0-8493-8498-2 (hb : alk. paper) 1. Respiratory insufficiency—Treatment. 2. Respirators (Medical equipment) 3. Artificial respiration. I. Ambrosino, N. (Nicolino), 1948- II. Goldstein, Roger. III. Series.
[DNLM: 1. Respiratory Insufficiency—therapy. 2. Chronic Disease—therapy. 3. Respiration, Artificial. W1 LU62 v. 225 2008/WF 145 V4655 2008]

RC776.R4V457 2008
612.2—dc22

2007041965

For Corporate Sales and Reprint Permissions call 212-520-2700 or write to: Sales Department, 52 Vanderbilt Avenue, 16th floor, New York, NY 10017.

Visit the Informa Web site at
www.informa.com

and the Informa Healthcare Web site at
www.informahealthcare.com

Introduction

The concept of ventilatory support is not new. It has been reported that BC Egyptians and Greeks described the theories of respiration. The Old Testament (800 BC) tells us that the Prophet Elisha induced mouth to mouth pressure breathing in a dying child! Much later, in the sixteenth century Theophrastus Bombastus von Hohenheim, or the "Famoso Doctor" Paracelsus, also known as the "wandering spirit," used the fire bellows of the time as devices for assisted ventilation: they were connected to the patients by a tube inserted in the mouth. In the following centuries, medical pioneers such as Vesalius, Hooke, Fathergill, and Hunter, among others, continued to advance the concept of ventilatory support, while others in the engineering field developed devices to expand its application.

However, it is the Scandinavian polio epidemics of the 1950s that gave rise to a new era of mechanical ventilation defined by the realization that many patients could benefit from it. This was coupled with the emergence of blood gas analysis and of a new medical discipline, that is, Respiratory Intensive Care. The description of the adult respiratory distress syndrome by Ashbaugh et al. in 1967, and the many studies thereafter on the treatment of this syndrome and related conditions led to an ever increasing use of mechanical ventilation with IPPV during the next 40 years, primarily to treat respiratory failure resulting from acute situations.

Meanwhile, years of productive research have demonstrated that patients with chronic respiratory insufficiency can also benefit from mechanical ventilation. As the Preface of this volume mentions "their survival as well as their health status" may be dependent on long-term ventilatory support. The ever increasing incidence and prevalence of chronic respiratory disease suggests that the use of ventilatory support will markedly increase. However, the techniques and strategies to use it, and when and where (non-intensive care unit, or home), are very different from treating the respiratory failure resulting from acute conditions and in patients with structurally near normal lungs.

This new volume of the series of monographs Lung Biology in Health and Disease edited by Nico Ambrosino and Roger Goldstein is truly a "how to" apply and monitor ventilatory support in patients with chronic respiratory failure treated in an ICU, in the hospital, or at home. It is really a "must read" for health professionals who care for such patients. The editors have called upon experts from many countries to contribute the many subjects presented in this volume. As a result, perspectives from different countries and cultures are considered.

The ultimate goal of this series of monographs is to contribute to better care of the many patients worldwide with chronic respiratory diseases: this is just the goal of this volume! I am grateful to the editors and authors for the opportunity to present such an important and timely contribution.

Claude Lenfant, M.D.
Gaithersburg, Maryland, U.S.A.

Foreword

As our understanding of respiratory failure has deepened, and as the technical aspects of life support have advanced, increasing numbers of patients now survive acute critical illness but are unable to regain complete independence from ventilatory support. Patients with progressive ventilatory insufficiency due to neuromuscular disease or another chronic condition may experience both physiologic benefit and improved quality of life through the institution of part- or full-time mechanical support of ventilation, either invasive or noninvasive. For these and other patients with chronic respiratory failure, ventilatory support has become an established therapy, whose evidence base and practical application have expanded dramatically during the last 20 years. This book perfectly combines both the science and the art of long-term mechanical ventilation, bringing key research findings along with the wisdom of vast experience to the bedside in the care of patients with chronic respiratory failure. It is a remarkable achievement.

To appreciate the pathophysiology of respiratory failure, and to appropriately tailor therapy to the needs of the individual patient, the different components of the illness must be understood and assessed. The degree to which oxygenation, ventilation, airway protection, and secretion clearance are impaired, and what measures are required to manage each of them, are important determinants of where and by whom a particular patient may be cared for. They determine, for example, whether invasive or noninvasive ventilation will be more appropriate for that patient, how likely it is that the patient can be managed successfully at home, and how much external support in the form of equipment and personnel will be required.

Caring for the patient with chronic respiratory failure involves other considerations as well. General physical conditioning and peripheral muscle training, nutritional support, and attention to personal and psychological needs are only some of the important nonrespiratory areas if long-term outcomes are to be optimal. In addition, the perspectives of the patient himself or herself, as well as those of family members and others most closely involved in that person's ongoing daily care, are vital to successful overall management.

While the needs of individual patients vary, the array of resources and professional skills that must be available for optimal management is consistent regardless of the particular health care system in which those patients are cared for. Respiratory care for patients with chronic respiratory failure is a multidisciplinary, team enterprise whose members may vary by region, practice setting, or job title, but whose purposes and needs remain the same. The management team may be under the overall direction of a pulmonologist, rehabilitation specialist, or other physician, and may include respiratory therapists, nurses, or physical therapists in varying combination; the apparatus and supplies used for ventilatory support, airway care, and monitoring may be different, provided and maintained through different systems and approaches; how ancillary services and consultation are accessed may vary. Despite these differences, however, all patients receiving ventilatory support for chronic respiratory failure need access to state-of-the-art care provided in the context of best information and up-to-date resources.

This book thoroughly covers all aspects of its subject. After reviewing the pathophysiology and manifestations of chronic respiratory failure and the available approaches to mechanical ventilation, it considers the various aspects of weaning, including how to optimize the likelihood of success and to determine whether complete liberation from ventilatory support is appropriate for a given individual. It takes the patient from the intensive care unit, through the various specialized institutional facilities that may exist in different areas, into the community and the patient's home. The rationale, evidence, and practical application of different specialized interventions and the components of rehabilitation are covered in detail. Thorough discussion is provided about the personnel involved in long-term mechanical ventilation—their different roles, how they should be trained, and how they work together as a team in meeting the needs of the patient. Separate chapters address available devices and techniques and their optimal application in individual cases, as well as the use of pharmacological agents and the management of secretions. The important topics of quality of life, legal and ethical issues, and end-of-life care are covered in detail. In addition, separate chapters discuss the special circumstances and needs of patients with different underlying or complicating conditions, and different causes of chronic respiratory failure.

Professors Ambrosino and Goldstein have done a masterful job of bringing all this together. The author list—76 authorities in 13 countries who represent every relevant profession and specialty—is essentially a "Who's Who" of the most respected investigators and clinicians in the field. The book has been conceived and organized so that every aspect is addressed. Clinicians involved in the care of patients with chronic respiratory failure will find here a complete, practical, accessible resource, regardless of their practice setting or the health care system in which they work.

David J. Pierson, M.D.
Pulmonary and Critical Care Medicine
University of Washington
Seattle, Washington, U.S.A.

Preface

Chronic respiratory failure (CRF) is a global issue as, increasingly, patients with both obstructive and restrictive conditions survive longer. In parallel, the intensive care unit (ICU) has enabled major advances in the management of patients with respiratory failure, attributable to acute respiratory and non respiratory conditions. Therefore, an increasing number of patients with chronic respiratory insufficiency become dependent for their survival as well as their health status, on long term mechanical ventilation. Home mechanical ventilation (HMV) is becoming an increasingly relevant option for patients with CRF, encouraged by; the introduction of noninvasive positive pressure ventilation (NIPPV), the recognition of the many different diagnostic categories of patients who can benefit from this approach and the pressures on institutions worldwide, to reduce healthcare costs by reducing in-patient hospitalization. As the population ages, we can expect this issue to increase in importance, challenging society as well as all levels of the healthcare system.

This book, is designed to address the growing need for information on long term ventilation in CRF. It is structured in nine parts, beginning with introductory chapters on chronic respiratory failure as a global problem, broad principles of acute and chronic ventilation and the prevalence of the major diagnostic categories. The text then moves from the difficult to wean ICU patient, to the newer concept of rehabilitation in the ICU, long-term ventilation in the non ICU settings in hospital and the community to special respiratory and non respiratory considerations of this population. The last three sections provide insights into CRF among different patient groups, perspectives on long-term ventilation by the healthcare professionals, the patient and the family care givers and finally worldwide approaches, encompassing Europe, North and South America and Asia.

The editors and authors hope that this text will assist healthcare professionals interested in this area, by providing an overview of the clinical, economic and ethical challenges to the healthcare system, posed by those requiring long-term ventilation. In this way, it may assist healthcare professionals in addressing the various exciting challenges of caring for this population.

Nicolino Ambrosino
Roger S. Goldstein

Contributors

Nicolino Ambrosino Pulmonary and Respiratory Intensive Care Unit-University Hospital Pisa, Italy and Pulmonary Rehabilitation and Weaning Center, Auxilium Vitae, Volterra (PI), Italy

Monica Avendano West Park Healthcare Centre, Toronto, Ontario, Canada

John R. Bach University of Medicine and Dentistry of New Jersey–The New Jersey Medical School, Newark, New Jersey, U.S.A.

Rita F. Bonczek Hospital for Special Care, New Britain, Connecticut, U.S.A.

Dina Brooks West Park Healthcare Centre, University of Toronto, Toronto, Ontario, Canada

P. M. A. Calverley Department of Medicine, Clinical Sciences Centre, University Hospital Aintree, Liverpool, U.K.

Annalisa Carlucci Pulmonary Rehabilitation and Respiratory Intensive Care, Fondazione S. Maugeri-IRCCS, Pavia, Italy

Laura Carrozzi University Hospital of Pisa, Pisa, Italy

Pamela A. Cazzolli The ALS/Neuromuscular Education Project, Canton, Ohio, U.S.A.

Bartolome R. Celli Caritas St. Elizabeth's Medical Center, Tufts University School of Medicine, Boston, Massachusetts, U.S.A.

Enrico M. Clini University of Modena, Modena, and Ospedale Villa Pineta, Pavullo (MO), Italy

Gerard J. Criner Temple University School of Medicine, Philadelphia, Pennsylvania, U.S.A.

Antoine Cuvelier Pulmonary Department and Respiratory Intensive Care Unit, Rouen University Hospital, Rouen, France

Lori Davis West Park Healthcare Centre, Toronto, Ontario, Canada

Marc Decramer University Hospitals Leuven and Katholieke Universiteit Leuven, Leuven, Belgium

Eduardo Luis De Vito Universidad de Buenos Aires, Buenos Aires, Argentina

Miguel Divo Caritas St. Elizabeth's Medical Center, Tufts University School of Medicine, Boston, Massachusetts, U.S.A.

Claudio F. Donner Mondo Medico, Multidisciplinary and Rehabilitation Outpatient Clinic, Borgomanero, Novara, Italy

Mark W. Elliott St. James's University Hospital, Leeds, U.K.

Scott K. Epstein Tufts University School of Medicine, Boston, Massachusetts, U.S.A.

Joan Escarrabill Hospital Universitari de Bellvitge, L'Hospitalet de Llobregat, Barcelona, Spain

Brigitte Fauroux Pediatric Pulmonary and INSERM UMR S719 AP-HP, Hopital Armand Trousseau and Université Pierre et Marie Curie, Paris, France

Miquel Ferrer Servei de Pneumologia, Institut Clínic del Tòrax, Hospital Clínic, Institut d'Investigacions Biomèdiques August Pi I Sunyer (IDIBAPS), CibeRes (CB06/06/0028), University of Barcelona, Barcelona, Spain

Debbie Field Lane Fox Respiratory Intensive Care Unit, St. Thomas' Hospital, London, U.K.

Pamela Frigerio Azienda Ospedaliera Niguarda Ca' Granda, Milano, Italy

Elizabeth Gartner West Park Healthcare Centre, Toronto, Ontario, Canada

Barbara Gibson West Park Healthcare Centre, University of Toronto, Toronto, Ontario, Canada

Allen Goldberg American College of Chest Physicians, Northbrook, Illinois, U.S.A.

James Goldring Royal Free and University College Medical School, London, U.K.

Roger S. Goldstein West Park Healthcare Centre, University of Toronto, Toronto, Ontario, Canada

Miguel R. Gonçalves Pulmonary Medicine Department, Intensive Care and Emergency Department, University Hospital S. João, Porto, Portugal

M. Gorini Respiratory Intensive Care and Thoracic Physiopathology Unit, Careggi University Hospital, Firenze, Italy

Rik Gosselink University Hospitals Leuven and Katholieke Universiteit Leuven, Leuven, Belgium

Inderjit Hansra Tufts-New England Medical Center, Boston, Massachusetts, U.S.A.

Rachel Heft West Park Healthcare Centre, Toronto, Ontario, Canada

Nicholas S. Hill Tufts-New England Medical Center, Boston and New England Sinai Hospital, Stoughton, Massachusetts, U.S.A.

Christina Hurtado West Park Healthcare Centre, Toronto, Ontario, Canada

Hideki Ishihara Osaka Prefectural Medical Center for Respiratory and Allergic Diseases, Osaka, Japan

Yuka Ishikawa National Yakumo Hospital, Yakumo, Hokkaido, Japan

Sharon Jankey West Park Healthcare Centre, Toronto, Ontario, Canada

Victor Kim Temple University School of Medicine, Philadelphia, Pennsylvania, U.S.A.

Shih-Chi Ku Department of Internal Medicine, National Taiwan University Hospital, Taipei, Taiwan

Franco Laghi Loyola University of Chicago Stritch School of Medicine and Edward Hines, Jr. Veterans Administration Hospital, Maywood, Illinois, U.S.A.

Gerhard Laier-Groeneveld Evangelisches und Johanniterkrankenhaus Oberhausen, Medizinische Klinik II, Lungen-und Bronchialheilkunde, Oberhausen, Germany

Allison Lane-Reticker University of Connecticut Health Center, Hartford, Connecticut, U.S.A.

Patrick Leger Laboratoire du sommeil, Service de Pneumologie, Centre Hospitalier Lyon Sud, France

Susan Sortor Leger ResMed Europe, Parc Technologique de Lyon, France

Frédéric Lofaso Physiology Department and INSERM 841 AP-HP, Hopital Raymond Poincaré and Université Versailles Saint-Quentin en Yvelines, Garches, France

Neil R. MacIntyre Duke University Medical Center, Durham, North Carolina, U.S.A.

Barry Make University of Colorado School of Medicine, Denver, Colorado, U.S.A.

Douglas A. McKim University of Ottawa, Ottawa, Ontario, Canada

Jean-François Muir Pulmonary Department and Respiratory Intensive Care Unit, Rouen University Hospital, Rouen, France

Paolo Navalesi Intensive Care Unit, Università del Piemonte Orientale "A. Avogadro", Azienda Ospedaliera "Maggiore della Carità", Novara, Italy

Pauleen Pratt Critical Care and Chronic Ventilation Service, University Hospitals of Leicester, NHS Trust, Leicester, U.K.

Jane Reardon Hartford Hospital, Hartford, Connecticut, U.S.A.

Cathy Relf West Park Healthcare Centre, Toronto, Ontario, Canada

J. Afonso Rocha Hospital da Senhora da Oliveira-Guimaraes, Guimaraes, Portugal

Carolyn L. Rochester Yale University School of Medicine, New Haven and VA Connecticut Healthcare System, West Haven, Connecticut, U.S.A.

Paul J. Scalise University of Connecticut Medical School, Farmington, Connecticut, U.S.A.

Bernd Schönhofer Hospital Oststadt-Heidehaus, Hannover Area Hospital, Hannover, Germany

Suzanne Scinto West Park Healthcare Centre, Toronto, Ontario, Canada

Anita K. Simonds Royal Brompton Hospital, London, U.K.

Katsunori Tatara National Yakumo Hospital, Yakumo, Hokkaido, Japan

Antoni Torres Servei de Pneumologia, Institut Clínic del Tòrax, Hospital Clínic, Institut d'Investigacions Biomèdiques August Pi I Sunyer (IDIBAPS), CibeRes (CB06/06/0028), University of Barcelona, Barcelona, Spain

Ludovico Trianni University of Modena, Modena, and Ospedale Villa Pineta, Pavullo (MO), Italy

Thierry Troosters* University Hospitals Leuven and Katholieke Universiteit Leuven, Leuven, Belgium

Douglas Turner Critical Care and Chronic Ventilation Service, University Hospitals of Leicester, NHS Trust, Leicester, U.K.

Mauricio Valencia Servei de Pneumologia, Institut Clínic del Tòrax, Hospital Clínic, Institut d'Investigacions Biomèdiques August Pi I Sunyer (IDIBAPS), CibeRes (CB06/06/0028), University of Barcelona, Barcelona, Spain

Andrea Vianello Respiratory Pathophysiology Unit, University Hospital, Padova, Italy

Michele Vitacca Fondazione S. Maugeri, IRCCS, Lumezzane (BS), Italy

John J. Votto University of Connecticut Medical School, Farmington, Connecticut, U.S.A.

Chong-Jen Yu Department of Internal Medicine, National Taiwan University Hospital, Taipei, Taiwan

Jadwiga Wedzicha Royal Free and University College Medical School, London, U.K.

Alex White Tufts-New England Medical Center, Boston and New England Sinai Hospital, Stoughton, Massachusetts, U.S.A.

Peter J. Wijkstra University Medical Centre Groningen, Groningen, The Netherlands

João C. Winck Serviço de Pneumologia, Faculdade de Medicina do Porto, Portugal

---

*Post-doctoral Fellow of FWO-Vlaanderen.

Contents

1
Chronic Respiratory Failure

P. M. A. CALVERLEY
Department of Medicine, Clinical Sciences Centre,
University Hospital Aintree, Liverpool, U.K.

M. GORINI
Respiratory Intensive Care and Thoracic Physiopathology Unit,
Careggi University Hospital, Firenze, Italy

I. Definition

The term respiratory failure describes a condition in which the respiratory system fails in one or both of its principal gas exchange functions: oxygenation and elimination of carbon dioxide. In clinical practice it is conventionally defined as an arterial oxygen tension (Pa_{O_2}) <60 mmHg, an arterial carbon dioxide tension (Pa_{CO_2}) >45 mmHg, or both, while breathing air. It is important to emphasize that respiratory failure is a laboratory diagnosis and that there is no absolute definition of the levels of arterial Pa_{O_2} and Pa_{CO_2} that indicate respiratory failure: the cutoff levels serve as a general guide, and their significance depends on the history and clinical assessment of patients.

These threshold values are empirically derived estimates of the point at which bulk transport of gases to and from the tissues may become compromised. Thus, 60 mmHg approximates to the inflection point on the normal oxyhemoglobin dissociation curve when small changes in Pa_{O_2} produce large changes in hemoglobin saturation. Similarly, once the Pa_{CO_2} rises above 45 mmHg for any period, the normal blood-buffering capacity will be exceeded and the pH will fall. Unlike hypoxemia, which cannot be physiologically compensated for, renal compensation for CO_2 retention is possible and occurs over a two- to three-day period during which the pH returns to normal (chronic ventilatory failure). The risks of impaired tissue oxygenation are mitigated by acute increases in cardiac output and more chronically by adaptations in the concentrations of 2,3-diphosphoglycerate, which affects the position of the dissociation curve and an increase in the hemoglobin concentration. This secondary polycythemia preserves the oxygen content of arterial blood at a cost in terms of blood viscosity and an increased tendency to thrombosis.

II. Classification

The two principal components of the respiratory system are the lung, which participates in gas exchange, and a muscular pump, which ventilates the lungs (1,2). The ventilatory pump consists of the chest wall (rib cage and abdomen), including the muscles that displace this structure and thereby inflate and deflate the lung, together with the ventilatory control circuits in the central nervous system, and the pathways that connect controllers with respiratory muscles (spinal and peripheral nerves) provide a self-regulating feedback mechanism that maintains blood gas homeostasis.

Respiratory failure may be classified as hypoxemic (type I) or hypercapnic (type II or ventilatory failure) (3), either of which may be acute and chronic. Hypoxemic respiratory failure is due to failure of the lungs, caused by acute (cardiogenic pulmonary edema, pneumonia, acute respiratory distress syndrome) or chronic (emphysema, interstitial lung disorders) diseases (Tables 1 and 2). It is characterized by hypoxemia with normocapnia or hypocapnia. In these conditions central respiratory drive is high and there is sufficient alveolar ventilation (VA) to eliminate CO_2 and prevent hypercapnia.

Hypercapnic respiratory failure is due to failure of the ventilatory pump caused by acute (drug overdose, acute neuromuscular diseases) or chronic (chest wall abnormalities, chronic neuromuscular diseases) disorders. It is characterized by alveolar hypoventilation, which leads to hypercapnia with coexistent, usually mild, hypoxemia. The central drive may be globally reduced with the fall in Pao_2 resulting from the increase in alveolar CO_2. More commonly, the drive remains high, but the mechanical load on the respiratory system is too great or the capacity of the muscles too low to ensure efficient CO_2 elimination (Fig. 1).

In individual patients, however, both types of respiratory failure may coexist, as one respiratory problem leads to another with a cascade of interaction (3). For example, patients with cardiogenic pulmonary edema or status asthmaticus first develop hypoxemia due to lung failure; if the disease persists or progresses, pump failure and hypercapnia appear because of several mechanisms (increased work of breathing, reduced oxygen delivery, hyperinflation).

Respiratory failure can develop over minutes to hours (acute respiratory failure) or over several days or longer (chronic respiratory failure). The distinction between acute and

Table 1 Causes of Chronic Hypoxemia with Normal or Low $Paco_2$

Obstructive ventilatory disorders
COPD
Chronic asthma
Mixed ventilatory disorders
Bronchiectasis
Sequelae of tuberculosis
Interstitial lung disorders
Idiopathic pulmonary fibrosis
Pneumoconiosis
Sarcoidosis
Extrinsic allergic alveolitis
Pulmonary vascular diseases
Pulmonary vascular hypertension
Chronic pulmonary thrombosis
Arteriovenous malformations
Nonpulmonary diseases
Severe heart failure
Hepatopulmonary syndrome

Abbreviations: $Paco_2$, arterial carbon dioxide pressure; COPD, chronic obstructive pulmonary disease.

Table 2 Causes of Chronic Hypoxemia with Hypercapnia

Causes
Pulmonary diseases
Obstructive ventilatory disorders
COPD
Mixed ventilatory disorders
Bronchiectasis
Sequelae of tuberculosis
Nonpulmonary diseases
Dysfunction of respiratory centers
Primary alveolar hypoventilation
Obesity hypoventilation syndrome
Depressant drugs
Myxoedema
Lesion of brainstem
Neuromuscular diseases
Poliomyelitis
Amyotrophic lateral sclerosis
Myasthenia gravis
Muscular dystrophies, polymyositis
Chest wall deformities
Kyphoscoliosis
Ankylosing spondylitis
Chest trauma
Thoracoplasty
Pleural thickening
Obstruction of upper respiratory tract

Abbreviation: COPD, chronic obstructive pulmonary disease.

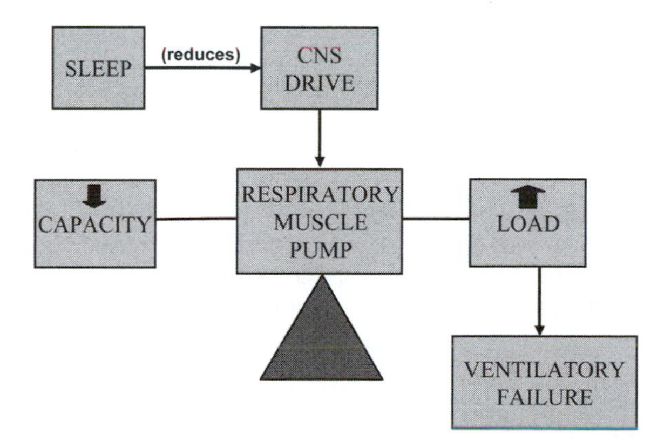

Figure 1 Schematic representation of the balance of forces on the respiratory pump. *Source*: Courtesy of J. Moxham.

chronic hypoxemic respiratory failure cannot readily be made on the basis of arterial blood gases. The presence of clinical markers of chronic hypoxemia (polycythemia or cor pulmonale) suggests a long-standing disorder. Acute hypercapnic respiratory failure is characterized by hypercapnia with respiratory acidosis (pH < 7.35), whereas in chronic hypercapnic respiratory failure there is time for renal compensation with increase in bicarbonate concentration. Therefore, the pH usually is normal or only slightly decreased.

III. Pathophysiology of Chronic Respiratory Failure

A. Hypoxemic Respiratory Failure

The pathophysiological mechanisms that account for the hypoxemia observed in a wide variety of diseases are ventilation/perfusion (V/Q) mismatch, shunt, diffusion impairment, and alveolar hypoventilation (4,5). In some areas of the world, living at high altitude further compromises oxygen delivery, and lesser degrees of disease severity can produce clinically alarming degrees of hypoxemia. In most cases of oxygenation failure in patients living at or close to the sea level, V/Q mismatch and varying degrees of right to left shunting are the major causes of hypoxemia. V/Q mismatch develops when there are lung regions with low ventilation relative to their perfusion (low V/Q units), as occurs in chronic obstructive pulmonary disease (COPD) and interstitial lung diseases. An intrapulmonary or intracardiac shunt causes deoxygenated mixed venous blood to bypass ventilated alveoli and results in venous admixture. This condition can occur in patients with arteriovenous malformations but is also seen in intensive care unit (ICU) practice when an acute increase in pulmonary artery pressure can lead to a patent foramen ovale's reopening with a major effect on Pao_2. Diffusion impairment contributes to hypoxemia in conditions characterized by a combination of widened alveolocapillary distance and shortened pulmonary capillary transit time, such as extensive destruction and fibrosis of pulmonary parenchyma, especially when cardiac output is high (as during exercise).

In the absence of underlying lung disease, hypoxemia due to alveolar hypoventilation is associated with normal alveolar-arterial oxygen difference; in contrast, the other three mechanisms are characterized by a widening of alveolar-arterial oxygen gradient, resulting in severe hypoxemia. Hypoxemia due to V/Q mismatch, diffusion impairment, and alveolar hypoventilation can be corrected by administering a low concentration of inspired oxygen, whereas hypoxemia due to shunt cannot be corrected even with a high concentration of inspired oxygen (4,5).

B. Hypercapnic Respiratory Failure

For a given level of CO_2 production (Vco_2), hypercapnic respiratory failure results only from an inadequate VA. A simple equation describes these relationships quantitatively under steady state conditions:

$$Paco_2 = K\frac{Vco_2}{VA}$$

where K is the respiratory exchange ratio.

Since VA = minute ventilation (VE) – dead-space ventilation (VD), this equation can be expressed as

$$Paco_2 = K\frac{Vco_2}{VE - VD}$$

or

$$Paco_2 = K\frac{Vco_2}{VT\,Fr(1 - VD/VT)}$$

where VT is the tidal volume and Fr is the respiratory frequency (2).

From these equations, it follows that VA decreases and so $Paco_2$ increases when VE decreases. Likewise, when VE and VD remain unchanged but VT decreases and respiratory frequency (RF) increases (rapid shallow breathing), $Paco_2$ increases. Patients adopt a rapid shallow breathing pattern to minimize respiratory work per breath, but this form of compensatory behavior can be deleterious to gas exchange and is a major factor producing chronic hypercapnic respiratory failure in patients with COPD and neuromuscular disorders (6–10).

The function of the ventilatory pump is critically dependent on three factors: the respiratory workload, the respiratory muscle strength, and the ventilatory drive (Fig. 1). Chronic hypercapnic respiratory failure can result from one or more of these abnormalities: inadequate ventilatory drive, excessive respiratory load, and inadequate inspiratory muscle strength.

Ventilatory Drive

Reduction in the output of the respiratory centers to respiratory muscles leads to reduced VA and to CO_2 retention. Although this is the least common of the major causes of ventilatory failure, it can contribute to exacerbation of ventilatory failure resulting from other causes. Acute failure of ventilatory drive most often results from overdoses of sedative or narcotic drugs, especially opiates and benzodiazepines. In patients with other causes of ventilatory pump failure, metabolic alkalosis or administration of excessive oxygen can contribute to reduction in VA and exacerbate hypercapnia. Myxedema due to hypothyroidism (11) and idiopathic congenital central hypoventilation syndrome, in which chemoresponsiveness is reduced or absent when asleep (12), are two conditions characterized by inadequate ventilatory drive that result in chronic hypercapnia. Much more commonly, the onset of normal sleep is accompanied by a reduction in ventilatory responsiveness and a small increase in $Paco_2$. This reduction in the central drive and in respiratory muscle tone is important when other causes of respiratory failure are only just being compensated for by the waking drive to breathe.

Respiratory Load

During spontaneous breathing the inspiratory muscles must generate sufficient force to overcome the elastic and resistive load of the respiratory system. The pressure developed by the inspiratory muscles per breath (Pi) is increased if the elastic (decreased compliance of the lungs or the chest wall) or resistive (airway obstruction) load is increased. Furthermore, in patients with hyperinflation of the chest wall (see below), a substantial effort must be made by the inspiratory muscles to overcome intrinsic positive end-expiratory alveolar pressure (PEEPi) before any inspiratory airflow can occur (13,14). This threshold load can account for a significant proportion of the respiratory workload in patients with COPD during acute exacerbations or during the weaning process from mechanical ventilation (15). If the pressure required for breathing (PI) becomes greater than 60% of maximum inspiratory pressure (MIP), the load cannot be sustained indefinitely and inspiratory muscles are at risk of fatigue (16). Bellemare and Grassino also observed that the Pi/MIP that can be sustained indefinitely decreases when Ti/Ttot increases and that the product of Pi/MIP and Ti/Ttot (the "tension-time index") is related to the endurance time (17). When the tension-time index becomes greater than a critical value (0.15 for the diaphragm), there is risk of inspiratory muscle fatigue and pump failure (17).

Respiratory Muscle Strength

The maximum pressure-generating capacity of inspiratory muscles can be impaired by several causes (Table 3). Like all skeletal muscles, the strength of respiratory muscles depends on the length-tension relationship (18). Hyperinflation reduces inspiratory muscle strength by shortening the inspiratory muscles, especially the diaphragm, below their optimum force-producing length (18,19). Neuromuscular disorders can affect respiratory muscles; among patients without intrinsic pulmonary or chest wall disease, chronic hypercapnic respiratory failure usually occurs when the respiratory muscle strength falls below 30% of the predicted value (20). Muscle wasting due to malnutrition does not spare respiratory muscles (21). Several metabolic factors can also reduce the strength of otherwise normal respiratory muscles. Hypercapnia and hypoxemia have been reported to reduce diaphragmatic strength (22) and the endurance of inspiratory muscles (23). Corticosteroid treatment (24), hypocalcemia (25), hypophosphatemia (26), hypokalemia, and hypomagnesemia (27) may be additional contributory factors acting in concert with malnutrition to promote generalized respiratory muscle weakness in patients with chronic respiratory diseases.

Table 3 Causes of Reduced Respiratory Muscle Strength

Neuromuscular disorders
Hyperinflation
Malnutrition
Electrolyte disorders
Hypophosfatemia
Hypomagnesemia
Hypocalcemia
Hypokalemia
Hypoxemia
Hypercapnia
Drugs
Corticosteroids
Aminoglycoside antibiotics
Disuse
Controlled mechanical ventilation

IV. Some Specific Diseases Associated with Respiratory Failure

A. COPD

Abnormalities of gas exchange are infrequent in COPD at rest before the forced expiratory volume in the first second (FEV_1) has fallen to 50% of the predicted value or less. Thereafter, hypoxemia becomes increasingly more frequent, as lung mechanics worsen. The additional worsening of lung mechanics that accompanies an exacerbation can merit acute oxygen therapy, the characteristic increase in static lung volumes being accompanied by lower VA/Q units. These changes resolve slowly during recovery, but Pao_2 can improve enough for domiciliary oxygen to be no longer needed. Inappropriately, severe hypoxemia in an exacerbating COPD patient raises the possibility of coincident pathology, such as cardiogenic pulmonary edema or acute pulmonary embolization, which is now more readily diagnosed with a computed tomographic (CT) pulmonary angiogram. Acute increases in low VA/Q units cause hypercapnia and worsening acidosis, which predicts both an increased mortality and the need for ventilatory support.

Although chronic hypercapnic respiratory failure is a common and important event in patients with severe COPD (28), the mechanisms leading to its occurrence are not completely understood. There is a considerable variability in the relationship of $Paco_2$ to indices of airway obstruction or V/Q mismatch (29,30), suggesting that factors other than lung pathology may be relevant. Neural drive assessed by measuring mouth occlusion pressure (6,7) or electromyographic activity of diaphragm (7) has been found to be higher in both eucapnic and hypercapnic patients with COPD than in normals. Given the increase in VD/VT ratio that characterizes COPD, normocapnia can be maintained only by increasing VE to a sufficiently high level. Mechanical constraint to breathing can, however, cause problems in maintaining a sufficiently high level of ventilation in patients with COPD. On the one hand, the load placed on the inspiratory muscles is increased because of high airflow resistance, reduced dynamic compliance, and presence of dynamic hyperinflation with PEEPi. On the other hand, the pressure-generating ability of respiratory muscles can be impaired because of hyperinflation, malnutrition, drug therapy, and electrolytes abnormalities (31). Bégin and Grassino (8) have shown in a large group of COPD patients that the probability of developing hypercapnia increases with the severity of airway obstruction, obesity, and inspiratory muscle weakness. When the load placed on the respiratory muscle pump becomes excessive in relation to its capacity, patients may avoid respiratory muscle fatigue and pump failure by modifying the breathing pattern. A reduction in VT could allow COPD patients to reduce PI relative to inspiratory muscle strength, thus minimizing respiratory effort and dyspnea, and avoiding fatigue (32). In line with this hypothesis a more rapid and shallower pattern of breathing has frequently been observed in hypercapnic than in eucapnic COPD patients (6,7,33–35). More recently, it has been shown that in stable COPD patients with severe airflow obstruction there was a significant association between hypercapnia and both shallow breathing and inspiratory muscle weakness, these variables explaining more than 70% of variance in $Paco_2$ (9). In this study VT was related directly to Ti, indicating that a small VT is primarily the consequence of alteration in respiratory timing (9).

The mechanisms leading to alteration in respiratory timing in patients with COPD have not yet been clearly defined. In line with the concept that the perception of inspiratory effort and dyspnea is closely linked to the PI relative to inspiratory muscle strength (36), it is possible that reduction in Ti and VT involves an integrated response of the respiratory system to the perception of breathlessness. Studies showing an inverse relationship between Ti and PI relative to inspiratory muscle strength, and a significant association of the severity of dyspnea with both the increase in PI and the decrease in Ti, support the above hypothesis (9). In conclusion, it seems evident that patients with COPD alter the pattern of breathing in an attempt to optimize the performance of respiratory muscles, to reduce breathlessness, and to prevent fatigue. The rapid shallow breathing however reduces VA and increases $Paco_2$.

B. Restrictive Disorders

Neuromuscular Diseases

Ventilatory failure, often in association with pneumonia, is a frequent cause of death in many neuromuscular disorders. Severe weakness of the respiratory muscles produces a restrictive pattern with decrease in vital capacity and total lung capacity, whereas functional residual capacity generally tends to be low and the residual volume is within normal limits (37,38). Hypercapnia is likely when respiratory muscle strength falls to 30% of the predicted value (20). Chronic respiratory failure in patients with subacute or chronic neuromuscular diseases is not simply due to the direct effect of weakness of respiratory muscles leading to inability to inflate the lungs and alveolar hypoventilation. A variety of additional factors play a role, including alteration in the mechanical properties of the lung (37,38) and the chest wall (39), respiratory abnormalities during sleep (40–45), and inability to cough (46). Abnormalities during sleep, including frequent arousals, decreased rapid eye movement sleep, hypoventilation, and hypoxemia, are common in patients with neuromuscular diseases (40–45), particularly in those with severe diaphragmatic weakness (42,45). These abnormalities usually precede and probably contribute to daytime ventilatory failure (40,43,44). The effectiveness of cough is reduced in patients with neuromuscular diseases because of both inspiratory and expiratory muscle weakness. Inspiratory muscle weakness affects the inspiratory phase of cough and expiratory muscle weakness reduces the cough-induced dynamic compression and hence the linear velocity of airflow through the large intrathoracic airways (46). As a result the clearance of secretions is defective in these patients, thus contributing to the high prevalence of bronchopulmonary infections. Finally, in patients with neuromuscular diseases, chronic hypercapnic respiratory failure is associated with rapid shallow breathing leading to alveolar hypoventilation (10), probably as a result of afferent signals in weakened respiratory muscles, intrapulmonary receptors, or both (10,47).

Thoracic Deformity

In patients with kyphoscoliosis the severity is quantified by measuring the angle between the upper and lower portions of the spinal curve (Cobb angle). When this angle exceeds 100° (severe scoliosis), the vital capacity falls below 50% of the predicted value (48). A major factor in the pathophysiology of chronic respiratory failure in patients with kyphoscoliosis is the decrease in the compliance of the chest wall and lungs (49,50). In severe scoliosis the compliance of the chest wall may be about 25% of the predicted value.

Furthermore, the spinal deformity causes inefficient coupling between the respiratory muscles and the chest wall, with reduction in the maximum pressure-generating capacity of inspiratory and expiratory muscles (49,51). The imbalance between the increased elastic load and the reduced capacity of respiratory muscles elicits a rapid and shallow pattern of breathing (52). Although this breathing pattern does have the advantage of minimizing the work of breathing, it causes alveolar hypoventilation. Like patients with neuromuscular disorders, patients with kyphoscoliosis develop sleep-disordered breathing, especially during rapid eye movement sleep (53).

Obesity Hypoventilation Syndrome

The obesity hypoventilation syndrome (OHS) was originally described in 1955 in subjects with severe obesity, chronic hypercapnic respiratory failure, polycythemia, hypersomnolence, and right ventricular failure (54). The pathogenesis of OHS is certainly multifactorial in nature and not fully understood. Abnormalities of chest wall mechanics with increased work of breathing, reduction in inspiratory muscle strength, hypoventilation during sleep, and abnormalities in ventilatory control with blunting of both hypercapnic and hypoxic ventilatory responsiveness could explain chronic hypoventilation in these patients (55). Clinically, it is important to distinguish this condition from obstructive sleep apnea (OSA) with overlap. OSA is a common condition, often a result of obesity, and when it coexists with significant airflow obstruction or chronic heart failure, hypoxemia with CO_2 retention can occur. Marked daytime somnolence is characteristic of these patients, and they do well with continuous positive airway pressure rather than ventilatory support, often correcting their gas exchange abnormality as their hypersomnolence resolves.

References

1. Roussos C. Ventilatory failure and respiratory muscles. In: Roussos C, Macklem PT, eds. The Thorax. New York: Marcel Dekker, 1985:884–888.
2. Roussos C, Koutsoukou A. Respiratory failure. Eur Respir J 2003; 22(suppl 47):3S–14S.
3. Fishman AP, Hansen-Flashen J. Acute respiratory failure: introduction. In: Fishman AP, ed. Pulmonary Diseases and Disorders. 2nd ed. New York: McGraw-Hill, 1988:2185–2188.
4. West JB. Pulmonary pathophysiology: the essentials. Baltimore, Maryland: William & Wilkins, 1982.
5. Hall JB, Schmidt GA, Wood LD. Acute hypoxemic respiratory failure. In: Murray JF, Nadel JA, eds. Textbook of Respiratory Medicine. Philadelphia: Saunders, 2000:2413–2442.
6. Sorli J, Grassino A, Lorange G, et al. Control of breathing in patients with chronic obstructive pulmonary disease. Clin Sci Mol Med 1978; 54(3):295–304.
7. Gorini M, Spinelli A, Ginnani R, et al. Neural respiratory drive and neuromuscular coupling in patients with chronic obstructive pulmonary disease. Chest 1990; 98(5):1179–1186.
8. Begin P, Grassino A. Inspiratory muscle dysfunction and chronic hypercapnia in chronic obstructive pulmonary disease. Am Rev Respir Dis 1991; 143:905–912.
9. Gorini M, Misuri J, Corrado A, et al. Breathing pattern and carbon dioxide retention in severe chronic obstructive pulmonary disease. Thorax 1996; 51:677–683.
10. Misuri G, Lanini B, Gigliotti F, et al. Mechanism of CO_2 retention in patients with neuromuscular disease. Chest 2000; 117:447–453.
11. Zwillich CW, Pierson DJ, Hofeldt FD, et al. Ventilatory control in mixedema and hypothyroidism. New Engl J Med 1975; 292:662–667.

12. ATS guidelines: Idiopathic congenital central hypoventilation syndrome: diagnosis and management. Am J Respir Crit Care Med 1999; 160:368–375.
13. Pepe PE, Marini JJ. Occult positive end-expiratory pressure in mechanically ventilated patients with airflow obstruction: the auto-PEEP effect. Am Rev Respir Dis 1982; 126:166–170.
14. Haluszka J, Chartrand DA, Grassino AE, et al. Intrinsic PEEP and arterial Pco_2 in stable patients with chronic obstructive pulmonary disease. Am Rev Respir Dis 1990; 141:1194–1197.
15. Appendini L, Purro A, Patessio A, et al. Partitioning of inspiratory muscle workload and pressure assistance in ventilator-dependent COPD patients. Am J Respir Crit Care Med 1996; 154:1301–1309.
16. Roussos C, Fixley D, Gross D, et al. Fatigue of the respiratory muscles and their synergistic behavior. J Appl Physiol 1979; 46:897–904.
17. Bellemare F, Grassino A. Effects of pressure and timing of contraction on human diaphragm fatigue. J Appl Physiol 1982; 53:1190–1195.
18. Braun NMT, Arora NS, Rochester DF. Force-length relationship of the normal human diaphragm. J Appl Physiol 1982; 53:405–412.
19. Similowski T, Yan S, Gauthier AP, et al. Contractile properties of the human diaphragm during chronic hyperinflation. N Eng J Med 1991; 325:917–923.
20. Braun NMT, Arora NS, Rochester DF. Respiratory muscle and pulmonary function in polymiositis and other proximal myopathies. Thorax 1983; 38:616–623.
21. Arora NS, Rochester DF. Respiratory muscle strength and maximal voluntary ventilation in patients in undernourished patients. Am Rev Respir Dis 1982; 126:5–8.
22. Juan G, Calverley P, Talamo C, et al. Effect of carbon dioxide on diaphragmatic function in human beings. N Engl J Med 1984; 310:874–879.
23. Jardim J, Farkas G, Prefaut C, et al. The failing inspiratory muscles under normoxic and hypoxic conditions. Am Rev Respir Dis 1981; 124:274–279.
24. Decramer M, Lacquet LM, Fagard R, et al. Corticosteroids contribute to muscle weakness in chronic airflow obstruction. Am J Respir Dis 1994; 150:11–16.
25. Aubier M, Viires N, Piquet J, et al. Effects of hypocalcemia on diaphragm strength generation. J Appl Physiol 1985; 58:2054–2061.
26. Aubier M, Murciano D, Lecocguic Y, et al. Effects of hypophosphatemia on diaphragmatic contractility in patients with acute respiratory failure. N Engl J Med 1985; 313:420–424.
27. Molloy DW, Dhingra S, Solven F, et al. Hypomagnesemia and respiratory muscle power. Am Rev Respir Dis 1984; 129:497–498.
28. Calverley PMA. Respiratory failure in chronic obstructive pulmonary disease. Eur Respir J 2003; 22(suppl 47):26–30.
29. Lane DJ, Howell JBL, Giblin B. Relation between airways obstruction and CO_2 tension in chronic obstructive airways disease. Br Med J 1968; 3:707–709.
30. West JB. Causes of carbon dioxide retention in lung disease. N Engl J Med 1971; 284: 1232–1236.
31. De Troyer A. Respiratory muscle function in chronic obstructive pulmonary disease. In: Casaburi R, Petty YL, eds. Principles and Practice of Pulmonary Rehabilitation. Philadephia: WB Saunders Company, 1993:33–49.
32. Rochester D. Respiratory muscle weakness, pattern of breathing, and CO_2 retention in chronic obstructive pulmonary disease. Am Rev Respir Dis 1991; 143:901–903.
33. Parot S, Saunier C, Gautier H, et al. Breathing pattern in patients with chronic obstructive lung disease. Am Rev Respir Dis 1980; 121:985–991.
34. Javaheri S, Blum J, Kazemi H. Pattern of breathing and carbon dioxide retention in chronic obstructive lung disease. Am J Med 1981; 71:228–234.
35. Loveridge B, West P, Kriger MH, et al. Alteration in breathing pattern with progression of chronic obstructive pulmonary disease. Am Rev Respir Dis 1986; 134:930–934.
36. Killian KJ, Jones NL. Respiratory muscles and dyspnoea. Clin Chest Med 1988; 9:237–248.

37. De Troyer A, Borenstein S, Cordier R. Analysis of lung volume restriction in patients with respiratory muscle weakness. Thorax 1980; 35:603–610.
38. Gibson GJ, Pride NB, Newsom Davis J, et al. Pulmonary mechanics in patients with respiratory muscle weakness. Am Rev Respir Dis 1977; 115:389–395.
39. Estenne M, Heilporn A, Delhez L, et al. Chest wall stiffness in patients with chronic respiratory muscle weakness. Am Rev Respir Dis 1983; 128:1002–1007.
40. Smith PE, Calverley PM, Edwards RH. Hypoxemia during sleep in Duchenne muscular dystrophy. Am Rev Respir Dis 1988; 137:884–888.
41. Arnulf I, Similowski T, Salachas F, et al. Sleep disorders and diaphragmatic function in patients with amyotrophic lateral sclerosis. Am J Respir Crit Care Med 2000; 161:849–856.
42. White JE, Drinnan MJ, Smithson AJ, et al. Respiratory muscle activity and oxygenation during sleep in patients with muscle weakness. Eur Respir J 1995; 8:807–814.
43. Hukins CA, Hillman DR. Daytime predictors of sleep hypoventilation in Duchenne muscular dystrophy. Am J Respir Crit Care Med 2000; 161:166–170.
44. Labanowski M, Schmidt-Nowara W, Guilleminault C. Sleep and neuromuscular disease: frequency of sleep-disordered breathing in a neuromuscular disease clinic population. Neurology 1996; 47:1173–1180.
45. Bourke SC, Gibson GJ. Sleep and breathing in neuromuscular disease. Eur Respir J 2002; 19:1194–1201.
46. De Troyer A, Estenne M. The respiratory system in neuromuscular disorders. In: Roussos C, ed. The Thorax. 2nd ed. New York: Marcel Dekker, 1995 (part C):2177–2212.
47. Brack T, Jubran A, Tobin MJ. Dyspnea and decreased variability of breathing in patients with restrictive lung disease. Am J Respir Crit Care Med 2002; 165(9):1260–1264.
48. Kearon C, Viviani GR, Kirkley A, et al. Factors determining pulmonary function in adolescent idiopathic thoracic scoliosis. Am Rev Respir Dis 1993; 148:288–294.
49. Cooper DM, Rojas JV, Mellins RB, et al. Respiratory mechanics in adolescents with idiopathic scoliosis. Am Rev Respir Dis 1984; 130:16–22.
50. Estenne M, Derom E, De Troyer A. Neck and abdominal muscle activity in patients with severe thoracic scoliosis. Am J Respir Crit Care Med 1998; 158:452–457.
51. Lisboa C, Moreno R, Fava M, et al. Inspiratory muscle function in patients with severe kyphoscoliosis. Am Rev Respir Dis 1985; 132:48–52.
52. Ramonatxo M, Milic-Emili J, Prefaut C. Breathing pattern and load compensatory responses in young scoliotic patients. Eur Respir J 1988; 1:421–427.
53. Ellis E, Grunstein R, Chan S, et al. Noninvasive ventilatory support durino sleep improves respiratory failure in kyphoscoliosis. Chest 1988; 94:811–815.
54. Achincloss JH, Cook E, Renzetti AD. Clinical and physiological aspects of a case of polycythemia and alveolar hypoventilation. J Clin Invest 1955; 34:1537–1545.
55. Teichtahl H. The obesity-hypoventilation syndrome revisited. Chest 2001; 120:336–339.

2
Principles of Positive Pressure Mechanical Ventilatory Support

NEIL R. MACINTYRE
Duke University Medical Center, Durham, North Carolina, U.S.A.

I. Introduction

Positive pressure mechanical ventilation (PPMV) uses positive pressure tidal breaths to either totally or partially affect O_2 and CO_2 transport between the environment and the alveolar spaces. Positive pressure is also used to maintain alveolar patency during expiration. The desired effect of PPMV is to maintain appropriate levels of Po_2 and Pco_2 in arterial blood while properly unloading the ventilatory muscles. Although a life-support technology, PPMV can also be harmful if used inappropriately. The discussion that follows, describes the principles of PPMV, its physiologic effects, the complications that can occur, and recent innovations.

II. Positive Pressure Mechanical Ventilator Design Features

A. Positive Pressure Breath Controller

Most PPMV devices utilize piston systems or controllers of high-pressure sources to drive gas flow (1–3). Tidal breaths can either be controlled entirely by the ventilator or be interactive with patient efforts. Pneumatic, electronic, or microprocessor systems provide for various breath types, which can be classified by what initiates the breath (trigger variable), what controls gas delivery during the breath (target or limit variable), and what terminates the breath (cycle variable) (4). Trigger variables are either patient effort (detected by the ventilator as a pressure or flow change) or a set machine timer. Target or limit variables are a set flow or a set inspiratory pressure. Cycle variables are a set volume, an inspiratory time, or a flow rate. Figure 1 uses this classification scheme to describe the five most common breath types on the current generation of mechanical ventilators.

B. Mode Controller

The availability and delivery logic of different breath types define the "mode" of mechanical ventilation (3,4). The mode controller provides a combination of breaths, according to algorithms and feedback data (Table 1). Newer designs incorporate advanced

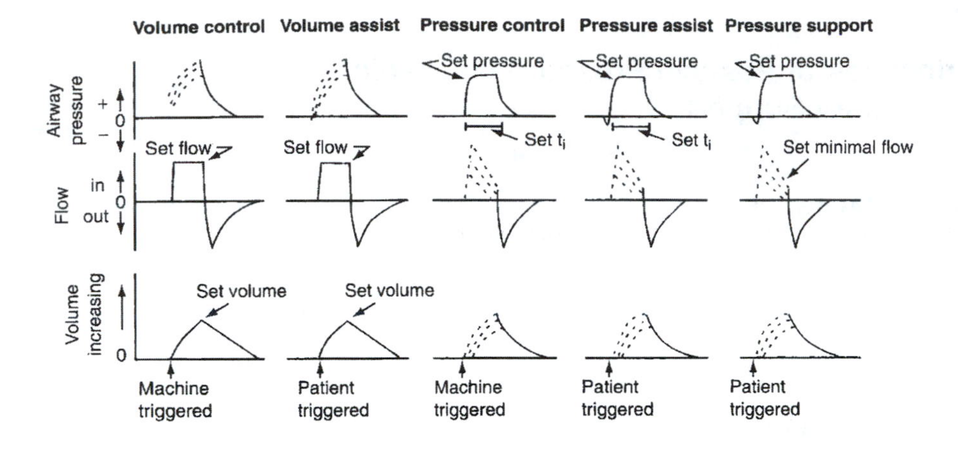

Figure 1 Airway pressure, flow and volume tracings, over time, depicting the five basic breaths available in most modern ventilators. Breaths are classified by their trigger, target/limit, and cycle variables. *Abbreviation*: t_i, inspiratory time. *Source*: From Ref. 74.

monitoring and feedback functions to allow for continuous adjustments in mode algorithms, as the patient's condition changes (4–6).

C. Subsystems

These include flow- or pressure-based effort sensors, gas blenders, humidifiers, and expiratory pressure generators. Mechanical ventilators also have an array of monitors and alarm systems.

Table 1 Breath Types Available on Common Modes of Mechanical Ventilation

		VC	VA	PC[a]	PA[a]	PS[a]	PR	Sp
Volume assist control		X	X					
Pressure assist control				X	X			
Volume SIMV	X	X			X		X	
Pressure SIMV			X	X	X		X	
Pressure support						X		
Airway pressure release						X	X	X

In addition to the five "basic" breaths shown in Figure 1, this table includes the Pressure Relief breath (PR, a pressure-targeted breath that allows spontaneous breathing during the inflation phase) and spontaneous unassisted/unsupported breaths (Sp).

[a]Some ventilators offer a volume guarantee feedback option (pressure-regulated volume control and volume assist).

Abbreviations: VC, volume control; VA, volume assist; PC, pressure control; PA, pressure assist; PS, pressure support; PR, pressure release; Sp, spontaneous unassisted; SIMV, synchronized intermittent mandatory ventilation.

III. Physiologic Effects of PPMV

A. Ventilation and Respiratory System Mechanics

Equation of Motion

Lung inflation occurs when pressure and flow, applied at the airway opening, interact with the respiratory system compliance—lung and chest wall, and airway resistance—to effect gas flow (7,8). The interactions of pressure, flow, and volume can be expressed by the simplified equation of motion:

$$\text{Driving pressure} = (\text{flow} \times \text{resistance}) + (\text{volume}/\text{system compliance})$$

In the ventilated patient, this relationship is expressed as

$$\Delta\text{PAO} = (\text{V}' \times \text{R}) + (\text{VT}/\text{CRS})$$

where ΔPAO is the change in pressure above baseline at the airway opening; V′ is the flow into the patient's lungs; R is the resistance of circuit, artificial airway, and natural airways; VT is the tidal volume; and CRS is the respiratory system compliance.

By performing an inspiratory hold at end inspiration the components of ΔPAO required for flow and for respiratory system distension can be separated. Specifically, when $\text{V}' = 0$ at end inspiration, ΔPAO is referred to as a "plateau" pressure and reflects the static respiratory system compliance (CRS = VT/ΔPAOplateau). Adding ΔPAO to the baseline pressure gives the total respiratory system distending pressure at end inspiration (ΔPAO-plateau + baseline pressure = PAOplateau). Calculating the difference in ΔPAO during flow and during no-flow (the "peak to plateau difference") allows for a calculation of inspiratory airway resistance ($R = \Delta\text{PAOpeak} - \Delta\text{PAOplateau}/\text{V}'$).

Separating chest wall and lung compliances (CCW and CL, respectively) during a passive machine-controlled positive pressure breath requires esophageal pressure (Pes) to approximate pleural pressure. The inspiratory change in Pes (ΔPes) can be used in the following calculations: CCW = VT/ΔPes and CL = VT/(ΔPAO−ΔPes). In clinical practice, because CCW usually is quite high and ΔPes is quite low, ΔPAOplateau and PAO-plateau are often taken as approximations of the lung distending pressure. However, in situations where CCW is reduced, such as obesity, anasarca, ascites, and surgical dressings, a stiff chest wall can have a significant effect on ΔPAOplateau and PAOplateau and should be considered when assessing lung stretch.

Intrinsic Positive End-Expiratory Pressure and the Ventilatory Pattern

Although the ventilator can supply positive end-expiratory pressure (PEEP), it can also develop within the alveoli because of either inadequate expiratory time or collapsed airways during expiration (or both). Often called "intrinsic PEEP" or "air trapping," it depends on three factors: minute ventilation, the expiratory time fraction, and the respiratory systems expiratory time constant (the product of resistance and compliance) (9). As minute ventilation increases, the expiratory time fraction decreases, and the time constant lengthens, the potential for intrinsic PEEP to develop increases (9).

The development of intrinsic PEEP will have different effects on pressure-targeted versus flow- or volume-targeted ventilation. In flow- or volume-targeted ventilation, the constant delivered volume in the setting of a rising intrinsic PEEP will increase both the

PAOpeak and the end-inspiratory PAOplateau. In contrast, in pressure-targeted ventilation, the set PAO limit coupled with a rising intrinsic PEEP level will decrease ΔPAO and the delivered VT.

In the passive patient, intrinsic PEEP can be assessed in two ways. First, when an inadequate expiratory time is producing intrinsic PEEP, analysis of the flow graphic will show that expiratory flow has not returned to zero before the next breath is given. Second, intrinsic PEEP in alveolar units that have patent airways can be quantified during a prolonged expiratory hold maneuver that permits equilibration of the intrinsic PEEP throughout the ventilator circuitry (10).

B. Alveolar Recruitment and Gas Exchange

Lung disease produces severe ventilation-perfusion (V/Q) mismatching (11,12). In many diseases, collapsed alveoli can be recruited during a positive-pressure breath (12–16). Three specific techniques to optimize this recruitment are the application of PEEP, the use of recruitment maneuvers, and prolongation of the inspiratory time.

PEEP

PEEP is defined as an elevation of transpulmonary pressures at the end of expiration (17). It prevents alveoli from “de-recruiting” during expiration, which is beneficial, as recruited alveoli improve V/Q matching and gas exchange (12–14), patent alveoli are not exposed to the risk of injury from the stress of repeated opening and closing (17,18), and recruited alveoli prevent surfactant breakdown, thus improving CL (19).

PEEP can also be detrimental, as a tidal breath delivered on top of the baseline PEEP will raise end-inspiratory pressure (7,8). Since alveolar injury is heterogeneous, appropriate PEEP for one region may be suboptimal in one or excessive in another (12–16). Optimizing PEEP is a balance between recruiting alveoli in diseased regions without overdistending already recruited alveoli in healthier regions. PEEP also raises intrathoracic pressure, which can compromise cardiac filling in susceptible patients (20).

Recruitment Maneuvers

Recruitment maneuvers are based on the concept that alveolar recruitment occurs throughout a positive-pressure inflation—all the way to the total lung capacity (TLC) (21). In practice, they are performed using sustained inflations of 30–40 cmH_2O for up to two minutes (21,22). An alternative approach is to use frequent “sigh breaths” that briefly take the lung to near TLC (22,23). The duration of recruitment depends on an appropriate setting of PEEP to prevent subsequent de-recruitment. Recruitment maneuvers may require heavy sedation to perform, and transient hypotension occasionally develops.

Inspiratory Time Manipulations

Prolonging inspiratory time may recruit more slowly recruitable alveoli (24) and improve V/Q matching (24,25). The development of intrinsic PEEP from the short expiratory times can have similar effects to that of applied PEEP. Since long inspiratory times increase the total intrathoracic pressures, cardiac output may be affected. Finally, inspiratory-to-expiratory time ratio (I/E) > 1:1—known as inverse ratio ventilation—is uncomfortable, in the absence of airway pressure release ventilation (26,27).

C. Unloading Muscles

PPMV can either partially or totally unload respiratory muscles. As mechanical loads correlate with the ventilatory muscle oxygen demands (28,29), the concept of unloading is useful in considering inspiratory muscle energy requirements during spontaneous or interactive ventilatory support (30). When referenced to muscle strength or endurance properties, load tolerance is a useful guide for setting the levels of partial ventilatory support or for predicting the spontaneous breathing capabilities (31).

Muscle loads are usually expressed as either a pressure-time product or work (W) (7,8). The pressure-time product expresses load as the integral of pressure over time (Pdt). Work expresses load as the integral of pressure over volume (PdV). Compliance, resistance, and the size of the breath all contribute to the magnitude of the load per breath. During spontaneous breaths, integrating Pes over time or volume describes the load borne by the inspiratory muscles to inflate the lungs. During a controlled breath, integrating PAO over time or volume describes the load borne by the ventilator to inflate the lungs and chest wall and integrating Pes over time or volume describes only the loads imposed by the chest wall. During interactive, partially supported breaths where load is shared between the patient and the ventilator, the sum contributions of patient and ventilator work is the same as during a controlled or spontaneous breath of the same volume and flow profile (30).

D. Patient-Ventilator Interactions

PPMV modes that permit spontaneous ventilatory activity are termed "interactive" modes, in that patients can affect various aspects of the mechanical ventilator's functions. These interactions can range from simple triggering of mechanical breaths to more complex processes affecting delivered flow patterns and breath timing. Interactive modes allow for inspiratory muscle activity which, when done at nonfatiguing or physiologic levels, may prevent muscle atrophy and facilitate recovery (31–34). Spontaneous patient ventilatory activity and comfortable interactive modes may improve ventilation and reduce the need for the sedation or neuromuscular blockers that may be required to prevent patients from "fighting" machine-controlled ventilation (27,35–37).

In synchronous interactions, the ventilator is sensitive to the initiation, modulation, and termination of a patient's effort (37). Synchrony can be assessed by noting patient "comfort" and by examining the airway pressure graphic. With synchronous gas flow, the airway pressure graphic remains convex and smooth, whereas when flow is not synchronous the airway pressure graphic is literally "sucked downward" by patient effort (Fig. 2) (38).

IV. Complications of Positive-Pressure Ventilation

A. Lung Stretch and Ventilator-Induced Lung Injury

The most recognized lung stretch injury is that of alveolar rupture presenting as extra-alveolar air, pneumo-mediastinum, pneumo-pericardium, subcutaneous emphysema, pneumothorax, and air emboli (39). The risk increases with the magnitude and duration of alveolar overdistension. Interactions between respiratory system mechanics and mechanical ventilation strategies, such as high regional VT and applied and intrinsic PEEP that increase the transpulmonary distending pressures >40 cmH_2O for prolonged periods, create alveolar units at risk for rupture (39).

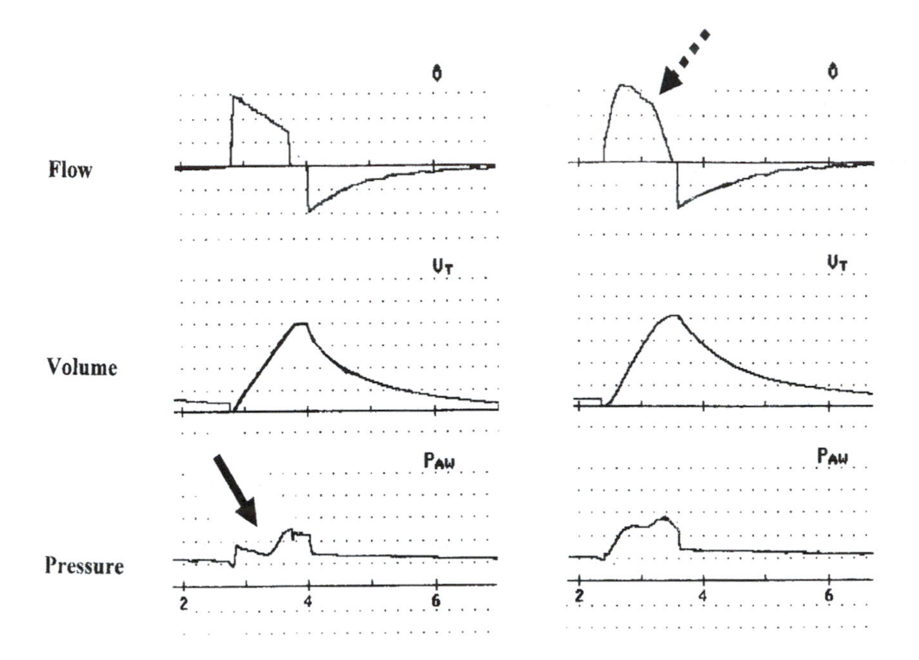

Figure 2 Flow and pressure pattern differences during dys-synchronous and synchronous breaths in a patient with a vigorous inspiratory effort. Depicted are flow (*upper panel*), volume (*middle panel*), and pressure (*lower panel*) for a dys-synchronous flow-targeted (*left panel*) and more synchronous pressure-targeted (*right panel*) breath with matched mean flow, inspiratory time, and tidal volume. Note that during the flow-targeted breaths on the left, the fixed flow does not respond to the vigorous inspiratory effort resulting in the airway pressure graphic being "sucked" downward (*solid arrow*). In contrast, with the pressure-targeted breath flow adjusts and increases to better meet the inspiratory effort (*dashed arrow*).

In animals, lung injury unassociated with extra-alveolar air can also be produced by mechanical ventilation strategies that stretch the lungs beyond the normal maximum transpulmonary distending pressures of 30 to 35 cmH_2O. This condition manifests as diffuse alveolar damage (18,40–44) and is associated with cytokine release (45,46) and bacterial translocation (47). It appears to be potentiated by a shear stress phenomenon that occurs when injured alveoli are repetitively opened and collapsed during the ventilatory cycle (44,48,49). Very rapid initial gas flow into the lung may be an additional contributing factor (50).

B. Positive-Pressure Ventilation and Cardiac Function

PPMV can also affect cardiovascular function (20,51,52) by decreasing right ventricular filling, cardiac output, and pulmonary perfusion. This complication is the rationale for using volume repletion to maintain cardiac output in the setting of high intrathoracic pressure. Reduced cardiac filling may be partially counteracted by improved left ventricular function from reduced left ventricular afterload (53).

Dyspnea, anxiety, and discomfort from inadequate ventilatory support can lead to stress-related catechol release with subsequent increases in myocardial oxygen demands and dysrhythmias (54). Coronary blood vessel oxygen delivery can also be compromised by inadequate gas exchange from the lung injury coupled with low mixed venous Po_2 due to high oxygen consumption of the ventilatory muscles.

C. Oxygen Toxicity

Oxygen concentrations approaching 100% cause oxidant injuries in airways and lung parenchyma (55). However, the safe oxygen concentration or duration of exposure is unclear, with a consensus that a fraction of inspired oxygen (F_{IO_2}) <0.4 is safe and an F_{IO_2} >0.8 should be avoided (13).

D. Inappropriate Muscle Loading

During interactive modes, insufficient unloading from either inadequate support levels or from dys-synchronous flow can produce or perpetuate muscle dysfunction, from imposed loading (35–38). Mechanical ventilation can also produce muscle dysfunction if only controlled ventilation is used for prolonged periods. This ventilator-induced diaphragmatic dysfunction is akin to muscle atrophy in other skeletal muscles (33,34).

E. Patient-Ventilator Interface Complications

The patient-ventilator interface includes the ventilator circuitry and the artificial airway. The most important complications are ventilator disconnections, reported in 8–13% of ventilated patients (56,57). Because circuit pressure and flow can still occur with the ventilator disconnected from the patient it is critical that carefully set alarms are present (3). Other complications include obstruction from secretions, circuit leaks, airway injury from inadequate heat or humidity, tracheal injury from the artificial airway, and loss of delivered VT in a compliant circuit.

F. Pulmonary Infectious Complications

Mechanically ventilated patients are at risk for pulmonary infections for several reasons (58–60). The natural glottic closure protective mechanism is compromised by an endotracheal tube. The tube itself impairs the cough reflex and serves as an additional potential portal for pathogens to enter the lungs, especially if the circuit is contaminated. The lung is more prone to infections, because of the underlying disease. And the intensive care unit environment is itself a risk for a variety of infections.

Preventing ventilator-associated pneumonias is critical, as length of stay and mortality are heavily influenced by their development (58–62). Hand washing and carefully chosen antibiotic regimens for other infections can have important beneficial effects. Management strategies that avoid breaking the integrity of the circuit, such as circuit changes only when visibly contaminated, also appear to be helpful (61–63). Finally, continuous drainage of subglottic secretions may be a simple way of reducing lung contamination with oropharyngeal material (61–63).

G. Applying Mechanical Ventilatory Support

Mechanical Ventilatory Support Involves Tradeoffs

To provide adequate support yet minimize lung injury, the need for potentially injurious pressures, volumes, and supplemental oxygen must be weighed against the benefits of gas exchange support. A rethinking of gas exchange goals has occurred over the last decade, such that pH goals as low as 7.15 to 7.20 and Po_2 goals as low as 55 mmHg are often considered acceptable if the lung can be protected from injury (13,64). However, ventilator settings must still provide enough PEEP to recruit the recruitable alveoli, and the PEEP-VT combination that overdistends the lung must be avoided. These goals represent a lung-protective strategy and guide current recommendations for the specific management of all forms of respiratory failure (13,64–67).

H. Ventilator Settings in Respiratory Failure

Parenchymal Lung Injury

Parenchymal injury produces stiff lungs and reduced lung volumes from alveolar collapse or flooding (11). Frequency–tidal volume (f-VT) settings focus on limiting end-inspiratory stretch. Large clinical trials have suggested that initial VT settings should start at 6 mL/kg ideal body weight (IBW) (65–67), less if end-inspiratory plateau pressures are >30 cmH_2O. Increasing VT might be considered if there is marked patient discomfort or suboptimal gas exchange, provided that the subsequent PAOplateau values remain <30 cmH_2O. Respiratory rate settings are then adjusted to control pH.

In the acute phases of respiratory failure, assist-control modes assure adequate support. The choice of pressure targeting versus flow-volume targeting largely depends on clinician experience with the various modes, as clinical trials showing outcome benefits to either approach do not exist. The usual I/E ratio is 1:2 to 1:4, with the flow graphics being checked to ensure adequate expiratory time, to avoid air trapping.

Inverse ratio ventilation (I/E > 1:1) can increase PEEP and improve V/Q in severe respiratory failure (24–27). This setting is applied as "airway pressure release ventilation (APRV)" (Table 1), which, although appealing, lacks good outcome studies supporting its use.

When setting the PEEP/F_{IO_2} combination to support oxygenation and minimize ventilator-induced lung injury (VILI), the PEEP/VT combination is set between the upper and lower inflection points of the static pressure-volume plot (68) or a step increase in PEEP is used to determine the PEEP level that gives the best compliance (69). F_{IO_2} adjustments are then set as low as clinically acceptable. An example of an algorithm to guide PEEP application, by providing adequate values for Pao_2 while minimizing F_{IO_2}, is shown in Table 2 (66,70). It depends on the clinician's perception of the relative "toxicities" of high thoracic pressures, high F_{IO_2}, and low Sao_2.

Obstructive Airway Disease

In respiratory failure from airflow obstruction, the increased pressures required for airflow may overload ventilatory muscles and the narrowed airways predispose to intrinsic PEEP (9). The slow expiratory phase and the increased dead space promote dynamic

Table 2 The PEEP/F_{IO_2} Table Used During the NIH ARDS Network Study (66)

F_{IO_2}	0.3	0.4	0.4	0.5	0.5	0.6	0.7	0.7	0.7	0.8	0.9	0.9	0.9	1	1	1
PEEP	5	5	8	8	10	10	12	14	14	14	16	18	18	20	22	24

Note: The clinical target is a P_{O_2} of 55–80 mmHg or an Sp_{O_2} of 88–95%. If the patient is below these target values, move up the table to the right. If the patient is above these targets, move down the table to the left.
Abbreviations: PEEP, positive end-expiratory pressure; F_{IO_2}, fraction of inspired oxygen; NIH, national institute of health; ARDS, acute respiratory distress syndrome; P_{O_2}, pressures of oxygen; Sp_{O_2}, saturation of peripheral oxygen.

hyperinflation, and overinflated regions may also compress more healthy regions of the lung-impairing V/Q matching (10,71).

VTs should be sufficiently low, for example, 6 mL/kg IBW to ensure PAOplateau <30 cmH_2O (66). As with parenchymal lung injury, VT reductions should be considered to meet PAOplateau goals. Increasing the VT for comfort or gas exchange can be considered, provided that PAOplateau does not exceed 30 cmH_2O. The elevated airway resistance and low recoil pressures of emphysema greatly increase the potential for air trapping, which limits the range breath size available (7,8). The I/E ratio is set as low as possible so as to minimize the development of air trapping.

Because alveolar recruitment is less of an issue in obstructive lung injury than in parenchymal lung injury, the need for PEEP is less. Table 2 summarizes an approach to ventilation for patients with obstructive airway disease. A role for PEEP occurs when intrinsic PEEP serves as an inspiratory threshold load for the patient attempting to trigger a breath. Under these conditions, judicious application of PEEP, up to 75–85% of measured intrinsic PEEP, can "balance" expiratory pressure throughout the ventilator circuitry to facilitate the triggering process (71,72).

Neuromuscular Respiratory Failure

The risk of VILI is less when lung mechanics are near normal and regional overdistention is less likely to occur. More "generous" VTs may be used to improve comfort, maintain recruitment, and prevent atelectasis. Maximal distending pressures should be kept as low as possible. The PAOplateau should be <30 cmH_2O. Low levels of PEEP may prevent atelectasis, as patients are often supine and incapable of secretion clearance or spontaneous sigh breaths.

V. Recent Innovations in Mechanical Ventilatory Support

In the modern microprocessor age PPMV devices are constantly being upgraded through software enhancements. This has resulted in increasingly more responsive gas delivery systems with more sophisticated monitoring. Moreover, numerous feedback enhancements have been introduced on specific machines to "automate" ventilation (Table 3) (73). While conceptually appealing, none of these feedback systems have been shown to improve outcomes. Table 3 also lists other recent innovations to improve patient-ventilator synchrony. Clinical trials with clinically relevant endpoints are important to provide justification for the adoption of these innovations.

Table 3 Recent Innovations in Mechanical Ventilation

Innovation	Clinical Applicability
New Modes	
Proportional assist ventilation	Interactive mode that adjusts pressure and flow according to spontaneous flow
Adaptive support ventilation	Feedback mode that adjusts minute ventilation to patient mechanics
Neurally adjusted ventilatory assist	Adjusts interactive support to diaphragm EMG signal
Computerized pressure support	Adjusts pressure support to the ventilatory pattern and exhaled CO_2
New Adjusters for Interactive Breaths	
Automatic tube compensation	Adjusts airway pressure to compensate for endotracheal tube resistance
Pressure slope/rise time	Adjusts rate of pressure rise for synchrony
Pressure support cycle adjust	Adjusts pressure support flow cycle criteria for synchrony
New monitors	
Esophageal pressure	Approximates pleural pressure
Trend monitors	Allows for data storage
Remote systems	Allows for central monitoring
Pressure volume plots	Allows for selection of settings that avoid overdistention and collapse/reopening
Spontaneous breathing trials	Allows for assessment of discontinuation potential

Abbreviations: EMG, electromyogram; CO_2, carbon dioxide.

VI. Conclusions

Mechanical ventilatory support is a critical component of the management of patients with respiratory failure. It must always be remembered that this technology is supportive and not therapeutic, as it cannot cure lung injury. It buys time by supporting gas exchange, without harming the lungs. Innovations must be assessed properly, especially if they are associated with significant risks or costs. Properly conducted studies with outcomes, such as mortality, ventilator-free days, barotrauma, and costs, will enable us to assess the sometimes bewildering array of new approaches to this vital life support technology.

References

1. Mushin M, Rendell-Baker W, Thompson PW, et al. Automatic Ventilation of the lungs. Oxford: Blackwell, 1980:62–160.
2. American Society for Testing and Materials. Standards specifications for ventilators intended for use in critical care. ASTM Standards. Philadelphia, PA. 1991; 36:1123–1155.
3. American Association for Respiratory Care Consensus Group. Essentials of mechanical ventilators. Respir Care 1992; 37:1000–1008.
4. Chatburn RL. Classification for mechanical ventilators. Respir Care 1992; 37:1009–1025.

5. Branson RD, MacIntyre NR. Dual control modes of mechanical ventilation. Respir Care 1996; 41:294–305.
6. MacIntyre NR, Branson RD. Feedback enhancements on ventilator breaths. In: Tobin M, ed. Principles and Practice of Mechanical Ventilation. 2nd ed. McGraw Hill, New York, NY 2006:393–400.
7. Truwit JD, Marini JJ. Evaluation of thoracic mechanics in the ventilated patient. Part I: primary measurements. J Crit Care 1988; 3:133–150.
8. Truwit JD, Marini JJ. Evaluation of thoracic mechanics in the ventilated patient. Part II: applied mechanics. J Crit Care 1988; 3:192–213.
9. Marini JJ, Crooke PS. A general mathematical model for respiratory dynamics relevant to the clinical setting. Am Rev Respir Dis 1993; 147:14–24.
10. Pepe PE, Marini JJ. Occult positive end-expiratory pressure in mechanically ventilated patients with airflow obstruction. Am Rev Respir Dis 1982; 126:166–170.
11. Pratt PC. Pathology of the adult respiratory distress syndrome. In: Thurlbeck WM, Ael MR, eds. The Lung: Structure, Function and Disease. Baltimore, MD: Williams and Wilkins Co., 1978:43–57.
12. Gattinoni L, Pesenti A, Baglioni S, et al. Inflammatory pulmonary edema and PEEP: correlation between imaging and physiologic studies. J Thorac Imaging 1988; 3:59–64.
13. Slutsky AS. ACCP consensus conference on mechanical ventilation. Chest 1993; 104:1833–1859.
14. Gattinoni L, Pelosi P, Crotti S, et al. Effects of positive end expiratory pressure on regional distribution of tidal volume and recruitment in adult respiratory distress syndrome. Am J Respir Crit Care Med 1995; 151:1807–1814.
15. Gattinoni L, Pelosi P, Suter P, et al. ARDS caused by pulmonary and extra pulmonary disease: different syndromes? Am J Respir Crit Care Med 1998; 158:3–11.
16. Gattinoni L, Caironi P, Cressoni M, et al. Lung recruitment in patients with the acute respiratory distress syndrome. N Engl J Med 2006; 354:1775–1786.
17. Kacmarek RM, Pierson DJ, eds. AARC Conference on positive end expiratory pressure. Respir Care 1988; 33:419–527.
18. Webb HJH, Tierney DF. Experimental pulmonary edema due to intermittent positive pressure ventilation with high inflation pressures: protection by positive end-expiratory pressure. Am Rev Respir Dis 1974; 110:556–526.
19. Wyszogrodski I, Kyei-Aboagye K, Taaeusch HW Jr., et al. Surfactant inactivation by hyperventilation: conservation by end-expiratory pressure. J Appl Physiol 1975; 38:461–466.
20. Pinsky MR, Guimond JG. The effects of positive end-expiratory pressure on heart-lung interactions. J Crit Care 1991; 6:1–15.
21. Crotti S, Mascheroni D, Caironi P, et al. Recruitment and derecruitment during acute respiratory failure. Am J Respir Crit Care Med 2001; 164:131–140.
22. Lim SC, Adams AB, Simonson DA, et al. Intercomparison of recruitment maneuver efficacy in three models of acute lung injury. Crit Care Med 2004; 32:2371–2377.
23. Pelosi P, Cadringher P, Bottino N, et al. Sigh in acute respiratory distress syndrome. Am J Respir Crit Care Med 1999; 159:872–880.
24. Armstrong BW, MacIntyre NR. Pressure controlled inverse ratio ventilation that avoids air trapping in ARDS. Crit Care Med 1995; 23:279–285.
25. Cole AGH, Weller SF, Sykes MD. Inverse ratio ventilation compared with PEEP in adult respiratory failure. Intensive Care Med 1984; 10:227–232.
26. Stock MC, Downs JB, Frolicher DA. Airway pressure release ventilation. Crit Care Med 1987; 15:462–466.
27. Habashi NM. Other approaches to open-lung ventilation: airway pressure release ventilation. Crit Care Med. 2005; 33(suppl 3):S228–S240.
28. MacIntyre NR, Leatherman NE. Mechanical loads on the ventilatory muscles. Am Rev Respir Dis 1989; 139(4):968–973.

29. McGregor M, Bechlake MR. The relationship of oxygen cost of breathing to mechanical work and respiratory force. J Clin Invest 1961; 40:971–980.
30. Banner MJ, Kirby RR, MacIntyre NR. Patient and ventilator work of breathing and ventilatory muscle loads at different levels of pressure support ventilation. Chest 1991; 100:531–533.
31. Bellemare F, Grassino A. Effect of pressure and timing of contraction on human diaphragm fatigue. J Appl Physiol 1982; 53:1190–1195.
32. Marini JJ. Exertion during ventilator support: how much and how important? Respir Care 1986; 31:385–387.
32a. MacIntyre NR. Weaning from mechanical ventilatory support: volume-assisting intermittent breaths versus pressure-assisting ever breath. Respir Care. 1988; 33:121–125.
33. Anzueto A, Peters JI, Tobin MJ, et al. Effects of prolonged controlled mechanical ventilation on diaphragmatic function in healthy adult baboons. Crit Care Med 1997; 25:1187–1190.
34. Vassilakopoulos D, Petrof B. Ventilator induced diaphragmatic dysfunction. Am J Respir Crit Care Med 2004; 169:336–341.
35. Sassoon CSH, Giron AE, Ely E, et al. Inspiratory work of breathing on flow-by and demand-flow continuos positive airway pressure. Crit Care Med 1989; 17:1108–1114.
36. MacIntyre NR, McConnell R, Cheng KC, et al. Pressure limited breaths improve flow dyssynchrony during assisted ventilation. Crit Care Med 1997; 25:167–171.
37. Stroetz RW, Hubmayr RD. Patient-ventilator interactions. Monaldi Arch Chest Dis. 1998; 53: 331–336.
38. Yang LY, Huang YC, MacIntyre NR. Patient-ventilator synchrony during pressure versus flow targeted small tidal volume assisted ventilation. J Crit Care 2007; 22:252–257.
39. Samuelson WN, Fulkerson WJ. Barotrauma in mechanical ventilation. Prob in Resp Care (Lippincott PA). 1991; 4:52–67.
40. Dreyfus D, Soler P, Bassett G, et al. High inflation pulmonary edema. Am Rev Respir Dis 1988; 137:1159–1164.
41. Muscedere JG, Mullen JB, Gan K, et al. Tidal ventilation at low airway pressures can augment lung injury. Am J Respir Crit Care Med 1994; 149:1327–1334.
42. Kolobow T, Morentti MP, Fumagalli R, et al. Severe impairment in lung function induced by high peak airway pressure during mechanical ventilation. Am Rev Respir Dis 1987; 135:312–315.
43. Dreyfuss D, Savmon G. Ventilator induced lung injury: lessons from experimental studies. Am J Respir Crit Care Med 1998; 157:294–323.
44. dos Santos CC, Slutsky AS. The contribution of biophysical lung injury to the development of biotrauma. Annu Rev Physiol. 2006; 68:585–618.
45. Trembly L, Valenza F, Ribiero SP, et al. Injurious ventilatory strategies increase cytokines and c-fos m-RNA expression in an isolated rat lung model. J Clin Invest 1997; 99:944–952.
46. Ranieri VM, Suter PM, Totorella C, et al. Effect of mechanical ventilation on inflammatory mediators in patients with acute respiratory distress syndrome. JAMA 1999; 282:54–61.
47. Nahum A, Hoyt J, Schmitz L, et al. Effect of mechanical ventilation strategy on dissemination of interacheally instilled E-coli in dogs. Crit Care Med 1997; 25:1733–1743.
48. Benito S, Lemaire F. Pulmonary pressure-volume relationship in acute respiratory distress syndrome in adults: role of positive and expiratory pressure. J Crit Care 1990; 5:27–34.
49. Mead J, Takishima T, Leith D. Stress distribution in lungs: a model of pulmonary elasticity. J Appl Physiol 1970; 28:596–608.
50. Rich BR, Reickert CA, Sawada S, et al. Effect of rate and inspiratory flow on ventilator induced lung injury. J Trauma 2000; 49:903–911.
51. Marini JJ, Culver BH, Butler J. Mechanical effect of lung inflation with positive pressure on cardiac function. Am Rev Respir Dis 1979; 124:382–386.
52. Scharf SM, Caldini P, Ingram RH Jr. Cardiovascular effects of increasing airway pressure in dogs. Am J Physiol 1977; 232:H35–H43.

53. Pinsky MR, Summer WR, Wise RA, et al. Augmentation of cardiac function by elevation of intrathoracic pressure. J Appl Physiol 1983; 54:950–955.
54. Lemaire F, Teboul JL, Cinotti L, et al. Acute left ventricular dysfunction during unsuccessful weaning from mechanical ventilation. Anesthesiology 1988; 69:171–179.
55. Jenkinson SG. Oxygen toxicity. New Horiz 1993; 1:504–511.
56. Betbese AJ, Perez M, Bak E, et al. A prospective study of unplanned endotracheal extubation in ICU patients. Crit Care Med 1998; 26:1180–1186.
57. Meade M, Guyatt G, Cook D, et al. Predicting success in weaning from mechanical ventilation. Chest 2001; 120(suppl 6):400S–424S.
58. Craven DE, Kunches LM, Kilinsky V, et al. Risk factors for pneumonia and fatality in patients receiving continuous mechanical ventilation. Am Rev Respir Dis 1986; 133:792–796.
59. Langer M, Mosconi P, Cigada M, et al. Long-term respiratory support and risk of pneumonia in critically ill patients. Am Rev Respir Dis 1989; 140:302–305.
60. Fagon J, Chastre J, Domart Y, et al. Nosocomial pneumonia in patients receiving continuous mechanical ventilation. Am Rev Respir Dis 1989; 139:877–884.
61. Collard HR, Saint S, Matthay M, et al. Prevention of ventilator-associated pneumonia: an evidence-based systematic review. Ann Intern Med 2003; 138:494–501.
62. Dodek P, Keenan S, Cook D, et al. Evidence-based clinical practice guideline for the prevention of ventilator-associated pneumonia. Ann Intern Med 2004; 141:305–313.
63. Kollef MH, Shapiro SD, Fraser VG, et al. Mechanical ventilation with or without seven day circuit change. Ann Intern Med 1995; 123:168–174.
64. Tremblay LN, Slutsky AS. Ventilator-induced lung injury: from the bench to the bedside. Intensive Care Med 2006; 32:24–33.
65. Amato MB, Barbas CSV, Medievos DM, et al. Effect of a protective ventilation strategy on mortality in ARDS. N Engl J Med 1998; 338:347–354.
66. NIH ARDS Network, Ventilation with lower tidal volumes as compared with traditional tidal volumes for acute lung injury and the acute respiratory distress syndrome. N Engl J Med 2000; 342:1301–1308.
67. Villar J, Kacmarek RM, Perez-Mendez L, et al. A high positive end-expiratory pressure, low tidal volume ventilatory strategy improves outcome in persistent acute respiratory distress syndrome: a randomized, controlled trial. Crit Care Med 2006; 34:1311–1318.
68. Putensen C, Bain M, Hormann C. Selecting ventilator settings according to the variables derived from the quasi static pressure volume relationship in patients with acute lung injury. Anesth Analg 1993; 77:436–447.
69. Suter PM, Fairley HB, Isenberg MD. Optimic end expiratory pressure in patients with acute pulmonary failure. N Engl J Med 1975; 292:284–289.
70. NIH ARDS Network, Higher versus lower PEEP in patients with ARDS. N Engl J Med. 2004; 351(4):327–336.
71. MacIntyre NR, McConnell R, Cheng KC. Applied PEEP reduces the inspiratory load of intrinsic PEEP during pressure support. Chest 1997; 111(1):188–193.
72. Petrof BJ, Legare M, Goldberg P, et al. Continuous positive airway pressure reduces work of breathing and dyspnea during weaning from mechanical ventilation in severe chronic obstructive pulmonary disease. Am Rev Respir Dis 1990; 141:281–289.
73. MacIntyre NR, Branson RD. Feedback enhancements on ventilator breaths. In: Tobin M, ed. Principles and Practice of Mechanical Ventilation. 2nd ed. McGraw Hill, New York, NY 2006:393–400.
74. MacIntyre NR. Mechanical ventilation. In: Murray J, Nadel J, eds. Respiratory Diseases. 4th ed. Philadelphia: WB Saunders, 2005.

3
Chronic Respiratory Failure as a Global Issue

LAURA CARROZZI
University Hospital of Pisa, Pisa, Italy

BARRY MAKE
University of Colorado School of Medicine, Denver, Colorado, U.S.A.

I. Introduction

Respiratory failure is generally considered as the inability to maintain normal arterial blood gases under resting conditions. Hypercapnic respiratory failure—also known as ventilatory failure—occurs when the arterial carbon dioxide tension ($Paco_2$) is 2 standard deviations above 40 mmHg (5.3 kPa). However, for practical purposes it is considered when the $Paco_2$ is >45 mmHg. Ventilatory failure is synonymous with alveolar hypoventilation. This may be derived from primary or secondary alterations in the central drive to breathe, neuromuscular dysfunction, chest wall restriction, or parenchymal disease resulting in increased ventilation/perfusion imbalance. Hypoxemic respiratory failure occurs when the arterial oxygen tension (Pao_2) is 2 standard deviations below the normal age adjusted level, although a value <60 mmHg (8 kPa) is most commonly used, as such values are associated with a decrease in oxygen saturation (Sao_2) and therefore a reduced arterial oxygen content. Hypercapnic and hypoxic respiratory failure can occur alone or concurrently and therefore may be difficult to separate. Noninvasive ventilation (NIV) is generally used for hypercapnic respiratory failure. Respiratory failure may present acutely, with the rapid development of dyspnea, or it may be slowly progressive, with few symptoms. It occurs in advanced stages of a variety of chronic pulmonary and nonpulmonary conditions. The management of chronic respiratory failure (CRF) is complex and has important implications for health care utilization.

CRF is increasingly recognized as an important, global, medical problem. It differs around the world, in keeping with regional differences in the incidence of the various underlying causes. Interest in the optimal management of CRF is growing, as reflected by the increasing number of publications in this area. As detailed later in this text, not only is there increasing recognition of this condition among a variety of jurisdictions, but there is also a greater understanding of the complexities associated with the medical, psychological, and social management of patients with CRF. The growing understanding of the application of NIV in the critical care environment has broadened its use in the population at risk for acute on chronic respiratory failure and led to its wider understanding, by the healthcare professionals, of the spectrum of care from the high-risk patient to the patient in the intensive care unit (ICU) and then to the rehabilitation and non-ICU management for those who remain dependent on long-term mechanical ventilation (LTMV). Similarly, patients and their families, especially those with neuromuscular conditions, have much more knowledge regarding options for the diagnosis and management of respiratory failure, as well as the need to make informed end-of-life decisions. Although estimates of the magnitude of CRF, including the numbers of patients receiving LTMV, would be useful to assist with public policy and healthcare funding, precise information remains unavailable for all but a few countries.

In this chapter we will comment on the prevalence of CRF, highlight issues in the data and its interpretation, as well as identify needs for implementing data collection to further our understanding of the management of this condition. We will also comment on the use of long-term oxygen therapy (LTOT), as many patients receiving LTMV are also receiving oxygen on a long-term basis.

II. Sources of Data on Prevalence of CRF

The healthcare impact of CRF must take into consideration the underlying condition and the prevalence of respiratory failure within the condition. Table 1 provides an overview of some of the sources of data used to gain an understanding of the magnitude of this problem around the world. When using this data for epidemiological or public health purposes, some important sources of bias should be considered. Many countries do not have such databases, and therefore some data are the property of equipment providers or home care organizations and are unavailable for general use. Moreover, data sets do not always use a common definition of CRF. One of the best proxies for diagnosed CRF is the use of LTMV as a major part of its management. The use of LTMV at home can be a good surrogate for CRF, although it includes only those diagnosed and treated with this modality, omitting patients in whom CRF has not been diagnosed and those for whom ventilatory support is either not required or is unavailable. Table 2 includes factors that can influence the reporting of home mechanical ventilation (HMV). Although indications for the use of long-term home ventilation have not been internationally standardized, two reports have included recommendations that have been well accepted and are generally followed (1,2).

In the United States, Medicare criteria for reimbursement for NIV differ slightly from the expert opinion consensus publication. Moreover, this therapy may be prescribed outside of the recommended selection criteria. Additional biases relate to the physician's or patient's preference for such treatment, biases that are likely to differ in different regions and cultures, depending on financial, medical, and political resources. Use of prescriptions for treatment also has its limitations, as patients prescribed a particular therapy may decline it, even if that treatment is available. The types of data and their sources differ in different

Table 1 Potential Sources of Data to Estimate the Burden of CRF

Estimate	Data source	Characteristics
HMV prevalence	Prescription files	Comprehensive
	Voluntary associations	Not always available
	Ventilator supply companies	Disease specific, proprietary
Mortality	Countrywide vital statistic	Always available

Abbreviations: CRF, chronic respiratory failure; HMV, home mechanical ventilation.

Table 2 Factors Influencing the Prevalence of HMV

Prevalence and incidence of underlying disorders
Recognition and diagnosis
• Of the underlying disorder leading to CRF
• Of the presence of CRF
Health care provider's understanding of treatment for CRF with NIV
• Presence, knowledge, and use of clinical guidelines and recommendations
• Health care provider's attitudes and preferences
Patient's understanding of treatment for CRF and application of NIV
• Patient's attitudes and preferences
Presence, availability, and length of experience with NIV and home care systems

Abbreviations: HMV, home mechanical ventilation; CRF, chronic respiratory failure; NIV, noninvasive ventilation.

geographic areas. These above limitations suggest why it is unlikely, in the near future, for accurate information on the global incidence and prevalence of CRF to become available.

Although there are few studies on the use of NIV as a marker for the presence of CRF, there have been some informative studies on the use of LTOT that reflect the complexity of using LTOT to estimate the prevalence of disease. LTOT is most commonly prescribed for chronic obstructive pulmonary disease (COPD), with international guidelines guiding its use. (3,4) However, criteria used to prescribe LTOT still vary by regional and national health systems (5,7). For example, LTOT may be prescribed in patients in whom the Pa_{O_2} is more than or less than the value commonly derived from clinical trials (8). In one study, patients prescribed LTOT exceeded those actually receiving LTOT by as much as 30% (9).

III. Medical and Home Care in Different Countries

The prevalence of home ventilation in different countries is based on differences in the availability of medical care as well as on the various models of home care. Contrasts between the US and French systems illustrate this point. The majority of patients receiving LTMV at home have been transitioned from the acute care or ICU environment. In France, such patients are typically offered ventilatory assistance on an elective basis, when still relatively stable, although gradually deteriorating. Elective initiation of ventilatory support among less critically ill patients is a major reason for the higher use of home ventilation in France. If the French approach was applied in the United States, there would be more than 10,000 cases of LTMV in the United States (10).

In the United States, there is no national policy, administrative structure, or organized regional clinical care system for the application of LTMV at home. In contrast, in France, a national and regional system has long been available to provide care for ventilator-assisted individuals at home, as recently reviewed by Stuart and Weinrich (11). The French national association [Association Nationale pour le Traitement à Domicile des Insuffisants Respiratoires (ANTADIR)] for care of patients with chronic respiratory insufficiency was established in 1980 for the purposes of observing the results of home care, establishing uniform services across the country, and providing cost savings. Estimates from France in 2006 indicate that more than 21,400 patients received home ventilation. Of these, two-thirds were managed by ANTADIR. This availability of a highly organized system for home care has a major influence on the high prevalence of LTMV at home, as reported in France.

IV. Prevalence of HMV

HMV is prescribed more commonly in patients with neuromuscular disorders (NMD) and thoracic restriction disorders (TRD) than in patients with COPD. Although there is a firm scientific basis for LTOT in COPD (12), the use of long-term HMV in COPD has been less well studied. A meta-analysis by Wijkstra and colleagues has evaluated the literature on randomized controlled trials of noninvasive positive-pressure ventilation (NIPPV) in patients with COPD and CRF, noting very minimal improvements in the study groups and describing some issues related to design and interpretation of the few existing studies (13). It is clear from this report that further, larger, well-designed clinical trials would be valuable. A consensus statement on the clinical indications for NIPPV in CRF attributable to various diagnostic categories was reported by National Association for Medical Directors of Respiratory Care (NAMDRC), but how extensively these criteria have been adopted is unknown (14). HMV is more demanding, more expensive, and less available and appropriate for fewer patients than is LTOT.

In 1998, Pierson summarized earlier data on HMV from Great Britain, France, and the United States (10). At that time, the U.S. government estimated there to be 4000 ventilator-assisted individuals (VAIs) for a prevalence of 1.5/100,000 population. However, this figure likely underestimates the actual number by as much as 25%. In France, LTMV at home is received by 1500 to 2000 patients. In countries such as Denmark, Spain (Catalonia), Belgium, and Switzerland, only partial information is available. Germany has prescription guidelines, but Switzerland and France have closer control of the HMV population and France has a national registry of VAIs.

The most complete European data on the use of HMV has been reported recently as the "Eurovent" study, a survey of long-term ventilator use conducted in 16 countries (15). In this survey, home ventilation was defined as ventilatory assistance for three months or more. Those receiving other forms of ventilation, such as rocking beds, negative-pressure ventilation, and phrenic nerve stimulation, were included. A total of 483 surveys were sent to the centers prescribing HMV in the 16 countries, with 329 centers (68%) responding. The numbers of patients and prevalence rates were estimated for each country. As noted in Table 3, there was a wide variation in the prevalence of HMV in Europe, ranging from 0.1/100,000 population in Poland to 17/100,000 in France. The survey identified a total of 21,526 VAIs and estimated the prevalence of HMV to be 6.6/100,000 population in Europe.

Although the Eurovent investigators reported a close relationship between the prevalence of HMV and the length of time for which HMV services had been available (15), this did not explain the variation in prevalence in countries such as France, Denmark, and Sweden, all of which have HMV registries and observation systems in place. France

Table 3 Number of Centers and Users of HMV and Prevalence of HMV

Country	Number of Centers	Users	Prevalence[a]
Austria	8	300	3.8
Belgium	23	500	5
Denmark	2	500	9.6
Finland	20	450	8.7
France	50	10,000	17
Germany	54	5,000	6.5
Greece	12	70	0.6
Ireland	15	155	3.4
Italy	70	2,200	3.9
The Netherlands	4	900	5.6
Norway	38	350	7.8
Poland	8	40	0.1
Portugal	39	933	9.3
Spain	35	2,500	6.3
Sweden	65	900	10
United Kingdom	40	2,320	4.1
All countries	483	27,118	6.6

[a]HMV/100,000 population.
Abbreviation: HMV, home mechanical ventilation.
Source: From Ref. 15.

has the highest prevalence (17/100,000), likely influenced by their unique organization of patient care and their extensive database (16). The French regional organization that provides care for HMV patients has been rated by the World Health Organization (WHO) to be the best in overall health system performance among all the 191 member states. France's chronic care by regional prevention and disease management systems is a model of cost-effective health care delivery (5,11,16,17).

V. Diagnoses of Patients Receiving LTMV at Home

Common diagnoses leading to LTMV are high cervical spinal cord injury, primary neurological disorders, and NMD. HMV users in Europe are equally distributed among patients with parenchymal lung disease (including COPD), thoracic cage restriction, and neuromuscular conditions (15). However, large variations between countries are evident, especially in relation to lung disease and NMD, as shown in Figure 1. A variety of patterns involving the use of HMV were noted in the "Eurovent" study, regarding ventilation of older patients with COPD and regarding the use of a tracheostomy for those with NMD (15).

Understandably, the diagnostic categories for CRF are different among the pediatric population. The French ANTADIR organization analyzed 287 children aged 18 years and younger who started home care for CRF (LTOT or HMV) over one year of observation (18). They represented 3.2% of the total number of patients enrolled in the association during that period. The heterogeneous causes of CRF could be divided into four groups: NMD, high cervical cord disease, nocturnal hypoventilation, and chronic lung disease.

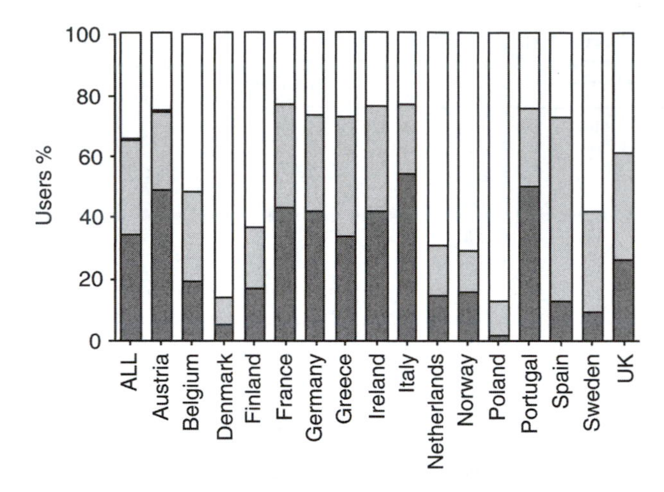

Figure 1 Percentage of HMV users in each disease category by country. Darker bars indicate lung and airway disorders; lightly shaded bars, thoracic cage disorders; open bars, neuromuscular diseases. *Abbreviation*: HMV, home mechanical ventilation. *Source*: From Ref. 15.

The specific diagnostic categories were: 30.3% NMD, 27.5% bronchopulmonary dysplasia, 8.3% cystic fibrosis (CF), 7.3% kyphoscoliosis, 4.9% cardiac disease, 3.5% stomatological disorders, 2.8% COPD, 2.1% pulmonary fibrosis, 3.1% other restrictive diseases, and 10.1% miscellaneous causes. Unlike adults, some children with CRF, such as those with bronchopulmonary dysplasia, can improve with growth to the point that ventilatory support may no longer be required. In contrast, some children have conditions associated with very limited survival (18). Other explanations for the difference in patterns of therapy between children and adults include the attitude of the pediatrician and the lifestyle requirements of the patients which vary at different ages.

VI. Mortality

Mortality records are collected worldwide and enjoy a uniformity of classification, based on the International Classification of Diseases (ICD), as to cause of death. However, coding abilities vary among health professionals and personnel from clinical records, so that not all patient groups are coded similarly. Furthermore, coding is often linked to a disease state and not specifically to the underlying diagnosis of CRF. Notwithstanding the above, mortality information does reflect health indicators and can be used to monitor and contrast specific diseases.

Table 4 illustrates the U.S. mortality (per 100 total deaths) for the different diagnoses that cause CRF. Although such data do not describe the magnitude of the population with CRF, they can be used to highlight the impact of CRF. The number of deaths related to disorders associated with CRF in the United States accounted for 5.7% of the total national mortality in 2003. Most (86%) of these deaths were attributable to COPD, with some (9.6%) attributable to interstitial disease and fewer than 1% to each of the other causes (19).

Table 4 Diagnoses of Patients Receiving LTOT

Author Year (Ref.)	Waterhouse[a,b] 1994 (9)	Miyamoto 1995 (8)	Chailleux 1996 (5)	Neri[a] 2006 (4)
Diagnosis		Number (%)		
COPD[c]	285 (60)	13,380 (41)	14,349 (54.8)	1041 (69.2)
Interstitial lung disease	55 (11.5)	5,272 (16.2)	3,417 (13.1)	169 (11.2)
Posttuberculosis	10 (2.1)	8,095 (24.8)	4,147 (15.9)	142 (9.4)
Bronchiectasis	13 (2.7)	1,217 (3.7)	1,556 (5.9)	89 (5.9)
Cancer	14 (2.8)	1,522 (4.7)	NR	50 (3.2)
Kyphoscoliosis	3 (0.6)	NR	1,574 (6)	43 (2.9)
Obesity	6 (1.3)	NR	NR	62 (4.1)
Obstructive sleep apnea	NR	NR	NR	44 (2.9)
Neuromuscular disease	5 (1.1)	119 (0.4)	1,097 (4.1)	8 (0.5)
Pulmonary hypertension/heart disease	41 (8.6)	873 (2.6)	NR	NR
Other, not classified	81 (16.9)	2,143 (6.6)		
Total number of patients	477	32,621	26,140	1,504

[a]Some patients had more than one diagnosis.
[b]Self-reported.
[c]Including asthma.
Abbreviations: COPD, chronic obstructive pulmonary disease; LTOT, long-term oxygen therapy; NR, not reported.
Source: Adapted From Refs. 4,5,8,9.

VII. Specific Disorders

A. Musculoskeletal Disorders

Musculoskeletal disorders (NMD and TRD) are relatively uncommon, but when present are often complicated by respiratory failure (20). Data on the burden of patients with CRF from musculoskeletal disorders are quite heterogeneous. Of the 79 patients who received HMV for CRF in a rehabilitation facility in California, 64% had poliomyelitis with bulbar and respiratory involvement (21), the next most common being Duchenne's muscular dystrophy. Other studies have reported CRF in scoliosis, kyphosis, and post-thoracoplasty TRD, as well as in myopathies such as Duchenne's muscular dystrophy, myotonic dystrophy, postpoliomyelitis, and amyotrophic lateral sclerosis (22).

The effects of treatments with HMV on survival have been poorly studied and the benefits of HMV over LTOT alone, or the benefits of combining both, remain unanswered (20,22). Oxygen alone is associated with poor outcomes (23). Reports on patients with muscular dystrophy in England and Wales have confirmed that even though the number of deaths per annum remains unchanged, the median survival has increased (22). Most deaths (59%) were due directly to respiratory failure, but respiratory failure may also have been a contributing factor in up to 82% of deaths. The number of new patients with muscular dystrophy who required HMV was 0.2/100,000 population per year.

B. COPD

COPD is one of the major leading causes of morbidity and mortality worldwide and is projected to move from the sixth to the third most common cause of death (24). In addition, COPD will also move from fourth to third place in the morbidity chart by 2020. Disease prevalence will continue to increase in both the developed and the developing world (24,25). It is possible that new options for management of the primary disease as well as the comorbid conditions may improve survival and quality of life.

CRF occurs in the very advanced stages of stable COPD when the degree of airflow obstruction becomes severe (26,27). In a report of hospital discharges, respiratory failure accounted for 37% of in-hospital mortality in patients with COPD, as either a primary or a secondary discharge diagnosis (28). Treatment of respiratory failure accounts for a large part of the economic burden of the disease. Admission to the hospital for COPD exacerbations, associated with respiratory failure, accounts for approximately two-thirds of the direct costs of COPD (29). The role of HMV in COPD is discussed elsewhere in this text.

C. Cystic Fibrosis

CF is one of the most common lethal genetic diseases in the Caucasian population, affecting approximately 1 in 3400 live births (31,32). Over 85% of patients with CF die from progression of their lung disease. CF has been reported as an uncommon cause of CRF in adulthood (Table 5), although the pattern of the disease is changing as patient life

Table 5 Number of Deaths and Percentage of Total Deaths in the United States for Diagnoses That May be Associated with CRF

	All		Females		Males	
Cause of death (ICD X code)	*n*	%	*n*	%	*n*	%
COPD	121,349	4.96	62,391	5.01	58,958	4.91
Pneumoconiosis/interstitial lung disease (J60, J61, J62, J63, J64, J84)	13,796	0.56	6,227	0.5	7,569	0.63
Respiratory failure (J96)	3,423	0.14	1,985	0.16	1,438	0.12
Neuromuscular disease/Myasthenia (G71.0, G70)	1,453	0.06	551	0.04	902	0.08
Sleep apnea (G47.3)	474	0.02	192	0.02	282	0.02
Cystic fibrosis (E84)	451	0.02	223	0.02	228	0.02
Scoliosis (M40; M41)	335	0.01	258	0.02	77	0.01
Sequelae of tuberculosis (B90)	80	0.003	47	0.004	33	0.002
All causes of death	2,448,288	100	1,246,324	100	1,201,964	100

Abbreviations: CRF, chronic respiratory failure; COPD, chronic obstructive pulmonary disease; ICD, international classification of disease.
Source: From Ref. 19.

expectancy is increasing. According to the Italian national registry, the proportion of adult patients more than doubled between 1998 and 2000 (41%) (33). The temporal trends in increasing median age at death have been observed in many other countries (34). This changing pattern is due both to an increase in diagnoses and improvement in survival as a result of better CF management (35). It can be expected that the importance of the management of CRF in CF will increase with time.

VIII. Clinical Comment

To monitor the prevalence and management of CRF, databases are required that will enable the prospective collection of epidemiological and clinical information. Merging data from existing national and regional registries represents a logical step toward increasing information on larger numbers of patients to allow for more specific epidemiological and clinical evaluations (36). This is occurring in amyotrophic lateral sclerosis (ALS) for which a pan-European registry has been implemented with a target population of 35.9 million people from nine countries (37). Another example is in The Netherlands, where all myopathies and polyneuropathies have been registered since 2004, with the aim of recruiting appropriate patients for population-based studies of the various NMD (31). At present, 10,313 patients with NMD have been entered in the registry. The most frequent specific diagnoses were diseases of peripheral nerves (49%), muscle diseases (29%), heritable myopathies (12%), and motor neuron disease (10%). The WHO Global Burden of Disease initiative underlines that such data are important to alert the health community and the political decision–makers to the possible underestimation of the burden of NMD. Information can be misleading if the emphasis is on mortality, rather than on prevalence and disability. A recent report has highlighted that the burden of neurological disorders has been seriously underestimated by such methods.

IX. Conclusion

Chronic conditions are the greatest cause of mortality and morbidity in the world, and chronic lung disease is one of the four leading groups of such conditions. Given the growing epidemiological and economic burden, steps to address the impact of the increase in chronic disease are needed (38,39). CRF is part of the natural history of chronic respiratory conditions and options for its management should be better recognized.

This chapter reviews the epidemiological burden of CRF and highlights several issues:

1. The sources of data on the prevalence of CRF are mostly indirect and not universally available in all countries and regions. Thus, an exact picture of CRF as a global issue remains largely incomplete, both in terms of geographical distribution and the global dimension. Multinational surveys, such as the Eurovent study, can provide insights into the use of HMV.
2. The most important cause of CRF requiring LTMV at home are neuromuscular and skeletal conditions.
3. The management of CRF varies regionally, nationally, and in different health care systems. These factors directly affect the epidemiology of CRF. The clinical and economic impact of different approaches to HMV is largely unknown.

4. The burden of CFR is apparently increasing.
5. The networks for collection of uniform data are likely to be informative. Such systems will better characterize patients, by including information on criteria for diagnosis, smoking habits, comorbidities, and socioeconomic conditions.

References

1. O'Donohue WJ Jr., Giovannoni RM, Goldberg AF, et al. Long-term mechanical ventilation: guidelines for management in the home and alternate community sites. Chest 1986; 90:1S–37S.
2. Make BJ, Hill NS, Goldberg AI, et al. Mechanical ventilation beyond the intensive care unit: report of a consensus conference of the American College of Chest Physicians. Chest 1998; 113:289S–344S.
3. Celli BR, MacNee W. Standards for the diagnosis and treatment of patients with COPD: a summary of the ATS/ERS position paper. Eur Respir J 2004; 23:932–946.
4. Neri M, Melani AS, Miorelli AM, et al. Long-term oxygen therapy in chronic respiratory failure: a multicenter Italian study on oxygen therapy adherence (MISOTA). Respir Med 2006; 100:795–806.
5. Chailleux E, Fauroux B, Binet F, et al. Predictors of survival in patients receiving domiciliary oxygen therapy or mechanical ventilation. A 10-year analysis of ANTADIR observatory. Chest 1996; 109:741–749.
6. Fauroux PH, Muir JF. Home treatment for chronic respiratory insufficiency: the situation in Europe in 1992. Eur Respir J 1994; 7:1721–1726.
7. Guyatt GH, Nonoyama M, Lacchetti C, et al. A randomized trial of strategies for assessing eligibility for long-term domiciliary oxygen therapy. Am J Respir Crit Care Med 2005; 172: 573–580.
8. Miyamoto K, Aida A, Nishimura M, et al. Gender effect on prognosis of patients receiving long-term home oxygen therapy. The Respiratory Failure Research Group in Japan. Am J Respir Crit Care Med 1995; 152:972–976.
9. Waterhouse JC, Nichol J, Howard P. Survey on domiciliary oxygen by concentrator in England and Wales. Eur Respir J 1994; 7:2021–2025.
10. Pierson DJ. Home respiratory care in different countries. Eur Respir J Suppl 1989; 7:630s–636s.
11. Stuart M, Weinrich M. Integrated health system for chronic disease management: lessons learned from France. Chest 2004; 125:695–703.
12. Medical Research Council Working Party. Long-term domicilliary oxygen therapy in chronic hypoxic cor pulmonale complicating chronic bronchitis and emphysema. Lancet 1981; 1:681–686.
13. Wijkstra P, Guyatt GH, Lacasse Y, Casanova D, Gay T, Goldstein RS. A meta analysis of nocturnal non-invasive positive pressure ventilation in patients with COPD. Chest 2003; 124 (1): 337–343.
14. Goldberg A, Leger P, Hill NS, et al. Clinical indications for noninvasive positive pressure ventilation in chronic respiratory failure due to restrictive lung disease, COPD, and nocturnal hypoventilation–a consensus conference report. Chevy Chase, MD: National Association for Medical Direction of Respiratory Care, 1999:521–534.
15. Lloyd-Owen SJ, Donaldson GC, Ambrosino N, et al. Patterns of home mechanical ventilation use in Europe: results from the Eurovent survey. Eur Respir J 2005; 25:1025–1031.
16. Stuart M and Weinrich M. Integrated health system for chronic disease management; lessons learned from France. Chest 2004; 125:695–703.
17. Veale D. Chronic respiratory care and rehabilitation in France. Chron Respir Dis 2006; 3:215–216.
18. Fauroux B, Sardet A, Foret D. Home treatment for chronic respiratory failure in children: a prospective study. Eur Respir J 1995; 8:2062–2066.

19. National Center for Health Statistics. Deaths from each cause, by month, race, and sex. Hyattsville, MD: NCHS, 2003. Available on: http://www.cdc.gov/nchs.
20. Shneerson JM, Simonds AK. Noninvasive ventilation for chest wall and neuromuscular disorders. Eur Respir J 2002; 20:480–487.
21. Baydur A, Layne E, Aral H, et al. Long term non-invasive ventilation in the community for patients with musculoskeletal disorders: 46 year experience and review. Thorax 2000; 55:4–11.
22. Buyse B, Messerman W, Demedts M. Treatment of chronic respiratory failure in kyphoscoliosis: oxygen or ventilation? Eur Respir J 2003; 22:525–528.
23. Gay PC, Edmonds LC. Severe hypercapnia after low-flow oxygen therapy in patients with neuromuscular disease and diaphragmatic dysfunction. Mayo Clin Proc 1995; 70:327–330.
24. Mannino D. Chronic obstructive pulmonary disease in 2025: where are we headed? Eur Respir J 2005; 26:189.
25. Chapman KR, Mannino DM, Soriano JB, et al. Epidemiology and costs of chronic obstructive pulmonary disease. Eur Respir J 2006; 27:188–207.
26. Gibson GJ, MacNee W. Chronic obstructive pulmonary disease: investigations and assessment of severity. In: Management of chronic obstructive pulmonary disease, Siafakas NM ed. Eur Respir Monograph 38, 2006; 11:24–40.
27. Hogg JC. Pathophysiology of airflow limitation in chronic obstructive pulmonary disease. Lancet 2004; 364:709–721.
28. Holguin F, Folch E, Redd SC, et al. Comorbidity and mortality in COPD-related hospitalizations in the United States, 1979 to 2001. Chest 2005; 128:2005–2011.
29. Croxton TL, Weinmann GG, Senior RM, et al. Clinical research in chronic obstructive pulmonary disease: needs and opportunities. Am J Respir Crit Care Med 2003; 167:1142–1149.
30. Croxton TL, Bailey WC. Long-term oxygen treatment in chronic obstructive pulmonary disease: recommendations for future research: an NHLBI workshop report. Am J Respir Crit Care Med 2006; 174:373–378.
31. Van Engelen BGM, van Veenendaal H, van Doorn PA, et al. The Dutch neuromuscular database CRAMP (computer registry of all myopathies and polyneuropathies): development and preliminary data. Neuromuscul Disord 2006; doi:10.1016/j.nmd.2006.09.017.
32. Kosorok MR, Wei WH, Farrell PM. The incidence of cystic fibrosis. Stat Med 1996; 15:449–462.
33. Viviani L, Padoan R, Giglio L, et al. Italian registry for cystic fibrosis: what has changed in the last decade. Epidemiol Prev 2003; 27:91–95.
34. Fogarty A, Hubbard R, Britton J. International comparison of median age at death from cystic fibrosis. Chest 2000; 117:1656–1660.
35. Doull IJ. Recent advances in cystic fibrosis. Arch Dis Child 2001; 85:62–66.
36. Yach D, Hawkes C, Gould CL, et al. The global burden of chronic diseases: overcoming impediments to prevention and control. JAMA 2004; 291:2616–2622.
37. Epping-Jordan JE, Galea G, Tukuitonga C, et al. Preventing chronic diseases: taking stepwise action. Lancet 2005; 366:1667–1671.
38. Calvert LD, McKeever TM, Kinnear WJ, et al. Trends in survival from muscular dystrophy in England and Wales and impact on respiratory services. Respir Med 2006; 100:1058–1063.
39. Beghi E. Workshop Report: 127th ENMC International Workshop: Implementation of a European Registry of ALS. Naarden, The Netherlands, 8–10 October 2004. Neuromuscul Disord 2006; 16:46–53.

4
Size of the Problem, What Constitutes Prolonged Mechanical Ventilation, Natural History, Epidemiology

SCOTT K. EPSTEIN
Tufts University School of Medicine, Boston, Massachusetts, U.S.A.

I. What Constitutes Prolonged Mechanical Ventilation

Approximately, 40% of patients admitted to critical care units require ventilatory support (1) and the incidence of mechanical ventilation (MV) is increasing (2,3). Most mechanically ventilated patients are easily and rapidly liberated from the ventilator after improvement or resolution of the acute precipitating illness. Five large trials conducted in the 1990s demonstrated that 65–85% of patients satisfying readiness criteria of adequate oxygenation, hemodynamic stability, and favorable respiratory physiology tolerate their first trial of spontaneous breathing and undergo extubation (4–9). Up to 20% of patients require days or weeks before they can be liberated from invasive ventilatory support and 40% of their time on MV is consumed by efforts to wean [60% for chronic obstructive pulmonary disease (COPD) patients] (10,11). In a smaller percentage of cases it is impossible to remove the patient from MV, resulting in ventilator dependence. This cohort of difficult-to-wean patients experiences prolonged ICU stays and consume a disproportionate amount of resources of up to 40% of ICU costs (12–15).

The definition of prolonged mechanical ventilation (PMV) is important and differs between regulatory agencies and clinical investigators. A standardized definition would provide a foundation for comparing studies conducted in different settings, such as long-term acute care versus the ICU, especially when comparing outcomes, such as the likelihood of weaning success, the duration of weaning, and survival. A standardized definition is also fundamental for conducting prospective epidemiological studies and for enrolling patients in randomized controlled trials.

Investigators have defined PMV as 24 hours or more to 1 month of active ventilator support (Table 1). In the United States, other investigators have used the Center for Medicare and Medicaid Services (CMS) diagnosis-related groups (DRGs), DRG 475 (respiratory disease and MV $\geq$96 hours) or DRGs 451/452 (formerly DRG 483, need for tracheostomy with MV of >96 hours with principal diagnosis, other than face, head, and neck diagnoses) to define PMV. In the past, need for tracheostomy likely identified a patient cohort requiring at least 14 to 21 days of MV, if one excluded trauma patients, but this may no longer be true as a tracheostomy is often performed earlier in the course of critical illness. Cox et al. recently found a median time to tracheostomy of just 10 days in nontrauma patients (16). In a recent randomized controlled trial, tracheostomy within 48 hours of intubation decreased the need for PMV when compared to delayed

Table 1 Definitions of Prolonged Mechanical Ventilation

Duration	Reference
>24 hr	Gillespie (104)
>2 days	Chelluri (94)
>96 hr	DRG 475(22), Douglas (35)
>7 days	Seneff (24), Esteban (23)
>10 days	Spicher (36), Martin (105)
>14 days	Carson (93), Combes (99)
>6 hr/day for 21 consecutive days	MacIntyre (22), Martin (105), Nevins (106), Scheinhorn (31), Estensorro (47)
29 days	Gracey (26)
Need for tracheostomy in the absence of face, head, and neck diagnosis	DRGs 541,542 (formerly DRG 483) (22) Nelson (52), Engoren (87), Cox (107)
Need of post-ICU mechanical ventilation	Scheinhorn (21,79)

tracheostomy of 8 to 17 days (17). Conversely, some patients with 14 or more to 21 days of MV may not undergo tracheostomy, if their prognosis is considered to be poor.

Others have characterized PMV as whenever the patient is transferred for postacute care, as the majority of patients transferred to long-term acute care have been ventilated for at least 21 days (18–21). A prospective observational study of 23 long-term hospitals found that 1419 patients were mechanically ventilated for an average of 34 days (median 25 days) before transfer to a long-term care hospital (21). Ninety-five percent of these patients had undergone tracheostomy 15 days after the initiation of invasive MV. A recent conference sponsored by the National Association of Medical Director of Respiratory Care (NAMDRC) (22) arrived at a consensus that PMV should be defined as the need for 21 or more consecutive days of MV for six or more hours a day. Most patients surviving 21 or more days of MV have likely crossed the threshold from acute to chronic critical illness. The need for more than six hours per day of MV may be too rigid as shorter periods of invasive MV still dictate continued hospitalization. On the other hand, many clinicians do not consider the need for more than six to –eight hours a day of noninvasive ventilation (NIV) as a true ventilator support. The NAMDRC Consensus Conference noted the need for a better understanding about which and how definitions of PMV are currently being employed in the United States (22).

II. Epidemiology of PMV

The prevalence of PMV depends upon the definition used. Most patients (65–85%) are easily weaned from ventilatory support after less than one week. In a multicenter observational study of >5000 medical and surgical ICU patients, 25% required greater than seven days of MV (23). In the acute physiology and chronic health evaluation III (APACHE III) database of medical and surgical ICUs, one in five patients remained ventilated for at least seven days (24). When the definition of PMV is extended to >21 days, the incidence predictably falls. In a cohort of nearly 600 medical patients admitted to a tertiary care medical intensive care unit, approximately 10% remained invasively ventilated at day 21

(25). Other single-center studies have found 3–7% of ventilated patients required more than 21 days of ventilation (20,26).

In 1985, there were 147 patients in Massachusetts, U.S.A., who required MV for more than three weeks (27), extrapolating to 6800 nationwide. A Massachusetts study performed a decade later identified a similar number of patients requiring PMV, resulting in a national estimate of 7250 patients (28). In 1990, the American Association for Respiratory Care and Gallup surveyed respiratory care directors and pulmonologists resulting in an estimate of 11,000 patients requiring MV for at least six hours a day for >30 days (29). Using DRG 483, Dewar et al. found approximately 8000 patients/yr in New York State (1992–1996) required PMV (30). Scheinhorn et al. estimated that as many as 29,000 patients with PMV are treated yearly in long-term acute care hospitals (LTACs) (31). Carson and Bach estimated there were approximately 88,000 patients coded as DRG 483 in an analysis of the 1997 National Inpatient Sample database (32). This estimation likely reflects both more patients undergoing PMV and greater use or earlier timing of tracheostomy. For example, Cox et al., analyzing patients in North Carolina, U.S.A., noted a 78% increase in patients discharged with a tracheotomy after ≥96 hours of MV when comparing data from 1993 to 2002 (16).

III. Who Becomes Difficult to Wean?

The need for PMV usually results when catastrophic acute illness occurs in a patient with chronic disease (31). Numerous factors can lead to difficulty with weaning from MV: mechanical ventilation, including systemic, e.g., severity of illness or underlying chronic lung disease; mechanical, e.g., increased work of breathing; iatrogenic- complications of mechanical ventilation or of critical illness; psychological, e.g., delirium; or process of care-the absence of weaning protocols (Table 2). Increased age appears to be a risk factor (33,34). The largest published study of patients undergoing PMV noted a mean age of 72 years (21). The presence of comorbid conditions or underlying disease also increases risk for PMV (26,35,36). In the multicenter National Association of Long-Term Hospitals (NALTH) study, Scheinhorn et al. observed 1419 patients (50% women) admitted after a median of 25 days (range, 0–1154 days) of invasive MV at the referring acute care hospital (Table 3). In this cohort, chronic conditions were common, 43% had COPD, 54% coronary artery disease or congestive heart failure, and 20% neurologic disease (21).

A. Severity of Illness

Patients requiring PMV are severely ill, as manifested by high severity of illness scores. Comparing patients transferred to Barlow Respiratory Hospital in 1996 to those transferred in 1988, Scheinhorn et al. noted lower serum albumin and higher alveolar-arterial oxygen gradients (37). The NALTH study found an APACHE III acute physiology score of 35 upon admission to long-term care, a severity of illness not markedly different from that seen for ventilated patients at the time of admission for acute care (38). In another study, trauma patients were more likely to require more than seven days of MV, if they had an injury severity score >20, PaO_2/FiO_2 <250, fluid retention of >2000 cc, or a pulmonary artery catheter placed within the first 24 hours (39). Indeed, 100% of patients with all four of these factors remained intubated for at least seven days.

Table 2 Mechanisms Associated with Prolonged Mechanical Ventilation

Systemic factors
Chronic conditions (e.g., cancer, chronic lung disease, immunocompromised host)
Severity of illness (e.g. APACHE II, SAPS)
Organ failure
Mechanical factors
Imbalance between work of breathing and respiratory muscle capacity
Critical illness polyneuropathy or myopathy
Upper airway obstruction (e.g., tracheal stenosis)
Iatrogenic factors
Acquired infection
Failure to recognize readiness for spontaneous breathing
Inappropriate ventilator settings
Imposed work of breathing from tracheostomy
Psychological factors
Excess sedation
Delirium, depression or anxiety
Sleep deprivation
Process of care factors
Absence of protocols for weaning and sedative administration
Inadequate nursing staffing
Physician experience

Abbreviations: APACHE II, acute physiology and chronic health evaluation II; SAPS, simplified acute physiology score.
Source: From Ref. 22.

Table 3 Demographics for 1419 Patients upon Admission to 23 Long-Term Care Hospitals

Variable	Value
Age, years (range)	72 (18–98)
History of smoking (% of patients)	59%
Living at home or assisted living facility (% of patients)	87%
Good premorbid functional status[a] (% of patients)	77%
Baseline comorbid conditions (per patient)	2.6
Diagnosis leading to mechanical ventilation	
Medical (% of patients)	61%
Surgical (% of patients)	39%
Hospital length of stay, days (median)	27
Duration of mechanical ventilation, days (median)	25
Time to tracheotomy, days (median)	14

[a]Assessed using the Zubrod score (108).
Source: From Ref. 21.

Another measure of severity of illness is the need for transfer back to acute care. Chan et al. found that 37% of patients transferred to a ventilator care unit required ICU readmission (40). In another study of 97 patients (71 still on MV) transferred from the ICU to long-term acute care, 23% were readmitted to ICU within 30 days (41).

B. Cause of Respiratory Failure

The cause of acute respiratory failure is among the most important determinants of whether a patient requires PMV (24). Although earlier studies found a predominance of cardiac and abdominal surgeries among such patients (26,36), medical patients now constitute the majority of those requiring PMV. For example, 61% of patients in the NALTH study were medical, while 39% were surgical. Among patients with respiratory failure secondary to medical illness, the precipitating etiology was bacterial pneumonia (34%), sepsis (21%), acute neurological disease (20%), acute exacerbation of COPD (17%), congestive heart failure (14%), and aspiration pneumonia (13%). Surgical patients were most likely to have undergone either cardiovascular (44%) or gastrointestinal (22%) procedures (21).

In a study of 183 COPD patients with acute respiratory failure, 10.4% remained mechanically ventilated 21 days after intubation (11). In the same ICU, the relative risk of remaining ventilated at day 21 was twice as high in patients intubated for acute lung injury (21 of 107) (42). One explanation for the latter observation is the presence of either critical illness polyneuropathy or ICU-acquired paresis (ICUAP). In a study of 95 patients ventilated for at least seven days, one quarter developed ICUAP, resulting in a longer duration of MV (18 vs. 8 days in patients without ICUAP) (43).

Branca et al. found that risk factors indicating preoperative medical instability, particularly cardiac or pulmonary insufficiency, predicted the highest risk of PMV (>4 days) after cardiac surgery (44). In a study of 139 cardiac surgery patients, chronic obstructive airways disease was identified as a risk factor for patients requiring seven or more days of MV postoperatively (45). In thoracic trauma patients, the presence of bilateral chest injuries, older age, and severity of concomitant head injury predicted the need for more than seven days of MV (46).

C. Renal Function

In a retrospective study of 319 patients, multivariate analysis identified shock on ICU admission day as the only independent predictor for PMV (>21 days) (47). In a preliminary study of 111 patients, increased duration of MV and need for transfer to a long-term ventilator care facility was associated with a creatinine elevation of 1.3 mg/dL anytime during the ICU stay (48). In another study, none of the 52 patients with PMV and renal failure were successfully weaned (49). Chao and colleagues reviewed >1000 patients transferred to their regional weaning center and identified 63 with renal dysfunction, with creatinine >2.5 mg/dL (40 on renal replacement therapy) (50). When compared to those with creatinine $\leq$2.5 mg/dL, patients with renal dysfunction were less likely to wean from MV (13% vs. 58%).

D. Central Nervous System Dysfunction

Central nervous system dysfunction also contributes to difficulty in weaning. Ely et al. found delirium in 82% of noncomatose ventilated ICU patients, and this finding was associated with longer hospital stay (11 vs. 21 days) and fewer ventilator-free days (51). Brain dysfunction continues to plague patients when MV becomes prolonged. Among 203 patients transferred to a respiratory care unit after tracheostomy for failure to wean, 30% were comatose throughout their stay and 32% had delirium (52). In another study of patients with PMV, a Glasgow coma score of <8 was associated with 6.5 times increased likelihood of weaning failure (53).

E. Absence of Weaning Protocols

Absence of a structured approach to weaning may increase the number of patients requiring PMV (54–56). A two-step protocol of screening combined with daily spontaneous breathing trials decreased the number of patients requiring more than 21 days of MV (54). Conversely, such protocols do not appear to shorten the duration of MV when applied to pediatric (57) and neurosurgical patients (58) or when compared to weaning conducted in an academic, well-staffed ICU (59). Two studies using historical controls suggest that protocols shorten duration of MV when applied to patients transferred to an LTAC (60,61). Duration of MV can be prolonged if managing clinicians either falsely believe weaning is not feasible or aggressive weaning efforts are not made. For example, 10% of failure to wean patients transferred to a national weaning center after 14 days of MV were successfully liberated from the ventilator within just 24 hours of arrival (62). Similarly, Vitacca et al. found that 31% of "ventilator-dependent" COPD patients (ventilated >14 days) transferred to three long-term weaning units could be immediately liberated from MV (61). Coplin et al. compared 136 brain-injured patients whose extubation was delayed compared to those who underwent timely extubation (63). The 27% of patients experiencing delayed extubation had longer duration of MV and higher mortality rates.

Approximately, 10–20% of patients who tolerate a trial of spontaneous breathing and undergo extubation require reintubation in the subsequent 48 to 72 hours (64). Reintubated patients suffer adverse outcomes when compared to patients who tolerate extubation. In a medical ICU, reintubated patients spent 12 additional days on MV (65). Reintubated patients are also more likely to undergo tracheostomy and be transferred to a long-term care facility.

F. Process of Care

Other processes of care factors contribute to PMV. Patients treated with either a sedation protocol or a strategy of daily cessation of sedation experience have a shorter duration of MV (66,67). Reductions in nursing staffing prolong time on MV. On studying COPD patients with acute respiratory failure, Thorens et al. found an increased duration of MV (seven vs. 38 days) when the effective nursing staff decreased (68). In the ICU setting, lack of daily rounds by an intensivist increases the risk for reintubation and duration of ventilation in patients after esophageal resection (69). A systematic review noted that 14 of 18 studies reported decreased ICU length of stay with high-intensity ICU physician staffing (70). One study showed a decrease in ventilator days in a closed (vs. open) ICU (71). Another investigation found that ventilator days were same despite the patients in the closed unit having a higher severity of illness (72). The role of the physician is also crucial for determining outcome in the long-term care setting. Bach et al. studied two groups of physicians at an LTAC and found faster weaning (39 vs. 59 days) and increased weaning success (46% vs. 30%) when comparing university physicians to community physicians (73). As physicians and their teams gain more experience with PMV, weaning success rate also increases (74,75).

Can the need for PMV be accurately predicted? Early identification of patients likely to require PMV is of considerable interest as allocation of ICU resources and timing of decisions to perform tracheostomy and transfer to a long-term care may be facilitated. Using clinical judgment alone at ICU day 7, the ability to predict need for MV at 21 days was no better than a chance (76). Utilizing the APACHE III database of nearly

6000 patients ventilated on ICU day 1, Seneff et al. found that duration of ventilation is principally determined by admitting diagnosis and physiological derangement (24). In a retrospective study of 319 patients, multivariate analysis identified shock on ICU admission day as the only independent predictor for PMV (47).

IV. Natural History of Patients Requiring PMV

Patients undergoing MV for acute respiratory failure are at risk for numerous complications, many of which prolong the duration of MV (77). Most complication studies focus exclusively on the acute ICU and have not examined patients undergoing PMV. Kollef and coworkers found that a witnessed aspiration event and the development of nosocomial pneumonia were risk factors for tracheostomy (78). Scheinhorn et al. examined complications in 23 long-term hospitals, combining complications present at the time of admission and those developing during hospitalization (79). Complications occurring in 10% or more of patients included urinary tract infection, lower respiratory infection, clostridium difficile colitis, sepsis without shock, line sepsis, aspiration pneumonia, and renal failure (Table 4). Duration of hospital stay and time to wean were significantly prolonged in patients with lower respiratory tract infections, urinary tract infections, and clostridium difficile colitis. Patients suffering a lower tract infection were less likely to wean successfully (48.5% vs. 56.7%) (79).

V. Weaning Outcome

The definition of "weaning" success has been variable. The process of liberation from MV can be divided into two distinct processes: freeing the patient from the mechanical ventilator (discontinuation) and endotracheal tube removal (extubation) (80). This distinction is further supported by the differences in pathophysiological causes for failure, in physiological measurements used to predict success, and in outcome for those who fail (65,81,82). Yet, in the acute ICU setting, these two processes are invariably linked with weaning success, typically defined as tolerance for a spontaneous breathing trial followed by successful extubation without need for reinstitution of ventilatory support (invasive or

Table 4 Complications in 1414 patients at 23 Long-Term Care Hospitals

Complication	Percentage of patients
Urinary tract infection	34
Lower respiratory tract infection (pneumonia, tracheobronchitis)	31
Clostridium difficile colitis	21
Sepsis without shock	14
Line associated sepsis	12
Aspiration pneumonia	10
Renal failure	10
Sepsis with shock, GI hemorrhage, thromboembolism, ileus, other infections	<10

Abbreviation: GI, gastrointestinal.
Source: from Ref. 79.

Table 5 Outcomes for Patients Requiring Prolonged Mechanical Ventilation

Author (reference)	No. of patients	Min MV (days)	Population	Hospital survival (%)	Weaned at discharge (%)
ICU Care					
Sivak (109)	15	14	60% COPD, 40% NMD	93	66
Morganroth (110)	11	30	45% postop, 18% COPD, 18% NMD, 18% other medical	73	73
Spicher (36)	245	10	56% postop, 8% CLD, 15% ALD, 12% cardiac, 9% NMD	39	NR
Gracey (26)	104	29	39% postop, 6% uncomplicated ALI, 26% MOF, 7% CLD, 7% trauma, 15% other medical	58	53
Combes (99)	347	≥14	62% cardiac surgery, ARF 19%, COPD 8%, sepsis 10%	57	NR
Cohen (85)	69	>10	31% AECOPD, 28% pneumonia	83	49
Friedrich (89)	182	42[a]	66% respiratory, 45% cardiovascular, 38% GI, 15% neurologic	68	NR
Non-ICU Care					
Indihar (75)	171	36[a]	73% CLD, 15% NMD, 12% other medical	67	34
Cordasco (111)	99	NR	50% postop, 19% CLD, 13% NMD, 12% other medical	75	25
Gracey (26)	61	21	66% surgical, 34% medical (59% CLD, 16% NMD, 8% ALI, 11% postop, 5% other medical)	90	82
Scheinhorn (112)	421	49[b]	24% postop, 24% CLD, 32% ALD, 5% cardiac 8% NMD, 7% other medical	72	53
Nava (113)	42	21	100% COPD	71	36
Gracey (114)	132	21	63% postop, 1% uncomplicated ALI, 13% CLD, 1% trauma, 23% other medical	90	78
Latriano (115)	224	23[b]	21% postop, 3% ALI, 21% MOF, 19% CLD, 9% trauma, 27% other medical	50	47
Gluck (116)	72	21	68% CLD, 8% ARDS, 8% NMD, 10% S/P CPR, 6% other medical	62	27 (at 42 days)
Gracey (117)	206	21	60% postop, 3% uncomplicated ALI, 12% CLD, 1% trauma, 24% other medical.	92	70

Scheinhorn (37)	1123	33[a]	"essentially unchanged from those reported in 1994"	71[a]	56[a]
Bagley (74)	278	NR	11% postop, 28% ALI, 31% COPD, 19% NMD, 10% other medical	52	38
Scalise (118)	47	86[b]	NR	77	62
Bach (73)	86	NR	NR	48	34
Carson (93)	133	14	5% postop, 31% ALI, 16% CLD, 16% cardiac, 20% NMD, 10% MOF	50	35
Dasgupta (119)	212	NR	33% ARDS (nonsurgical), 18% ARDS (surgical), 28% postop, 12% COPD, 4% NMD, 5% other medical	82	60
Gracey (120)	549	NR	NR (includes 206 patients from previous report)	93	60
Schonhofer (62)	403	>14	59% COPD	76	68
Iregui (121)	472	20[b]	64% medical, 23% general surgery, 7% neurologic disease/ neurosurgery, 6% thoracic surgery	82	60
Modawal (122)	145	~30[a]	42% pneumonia/neurologic, 25% postop, 15% CLD, 12% trauma	NR	50
Quinnell (84)	67	27[a]	COPD 100%	93	96
Pilcher (86)	153	26[a]	31% NMD/chest wall disease, 27% COPD, 24% surgery	73	38
Nelson (52)	203	16[a]	46% ALD, 17% CLD, 16% cardiac, 28% neurologic disease, 17% surgery, 27% sepsis/MOF	71	48
Scheinhorn (21,79)	1419	25[a]	medical 61%, surgical 39%	75	54

[a]Median.
[b]Mean.

Abbreviations: MV, mechanical ventilation; AECOPD, acute exacerbation of chronic obstructive pulmonary disease; ALD, acute lung disease; ALI, acute lung injury; ARDS, acute respiratory distress syndrome; CLD, chronic lung disease; COPD, chronic obstructive pulmonary disease; MOF, multiple organ failure; NMD, neuromuscular disease; NR, not reported.

Source: From Ref. 106.

noninvasive) within the subsequent 48 to 72 hours (83). This setting reflects the sentinel nature of removing the endotracheal tube and the probability that respiratory failure occurring >72 hours after extubation results from new or unrelated processes (81). Whether a 72-hour time threshold is appropriate for patients with PMV and tracheostomy is unclear. Tracheal tube decannulation is not a prerequisite for weaning success.

Proposed definitions of weaning success in PMV include 48 hours (61) or seven or 14 days off ventilatory support, and freedom from ventilatory support at the time of hospital discharge (20), or at six months to one year after the onset of MV (18). Standardizing the definition would allow assessment of the efficacy of weaning protocols and comparison between centers. Confounding variables include the use of NIV to facilitate liberation from invasive ventilatory support and the reinstitution of ventilatory support for factors that do not constitute a failure of the weaning process. One weaning unit reported a 68% weaning success rate but, approximately, one-third of these patients required and were discharged on NIV (62). Similarly, in a study of COPD patients requiring PMV, 40% required long-term NIV (84). Taking all these factors into account, the NAMDRC Consensus Conference defined weaning success as "complete liberation from mechanical ventilation, or a requirement for only nocturnal NIV, for 7 consecutive days"(22).

Using these various definitions, weaning success ranges from 25% to 96%, with most single-center studies reporting rates around 50% (Table 5). The multicenter NALTH study used a weaning success definition of the weaned patients at the time of discharge. Using this definition, 54% of 1414 patients successfully weaned from MV at 23 hospitals, with a range of 42–83% (79). Even after transfer, a sizeable fraction of patients, despite attaining clinical stability, cannot be weaned from the ventilator and are thus truly ventilator-dependent (85). In the NALTH study, 21% of patients were alive and ventilator-dependent at the time of hospital discharge, with a range of 0–39% in individual centers (79). In some studies, the majority of patients requiring continued ventilator support at an LTAC discharge only need MV at night (86).

VI. Survival

Short-term hospital survival for patients in the acute ICU setting ranges from 39% to 93%, depending on the patient population and the definition for PMV. (Table 5). In general, survival rates are lower for patients with PMV than for patients requiring shorter durations of MV. Hospital survival in the long-term acute care setting varies from 50% in most series to as high as 93%, depending in part on admission criteria and likelihood of transfer to a different facility when patients become acutely ill (Table 5). In the NALTH study, hospital survival was 75%, ranging from 54% to 100% among the 23 centers. Indeed, the wide variations in patient population, and admission and discharge practices, limit the importance of hospital survival as a meaningful outcome to follow across care settings. If a patient requires transfer from long-term care to acute care and then dies, he or she is considered a hospital survivor from the long-term hospital perspective.

Given these considerations, long-term outcomes, such as one-year survival, may be more meaningful and were recommended by the NAMDRC Consensus Conference (22). Reports of one-year survival from both short- and long-term care cohorts range from 29% to 58% (Table 6). Indeed, in some of these studies the majority of mortality occurred after hospital discharge (87). In the NALTH study, one-year survival was 30%, with another

Table 6 One-Year Survival for Patients with Prolonged Mechanical Ventilation

Author (reference)	Number of patients	One-year survival (%)
Spicher (36)	245	29
Gracey (26)	104	39
Scheinhorn (37)	1123	38
Carson (93)	133	23
Douglas (35)	392	34
Schonhofer (62)	403	49
Combes (99)	347	32
Engoren (87)	347	42
Pilcher (86)	153	58
Scheinhorn (21,79)	1414	30[a]

[a]One-year mortality 52%, lost or inadequate follow-up 18%.

18% lost or with incomplete follow-up (79). One-year mortality was 52% (25% inpatient and 27% after discharge). One-year survival is very relevant from a clinical perspective. PMV patients often have a high burden of underlying disease, and prolonged critical illness leaves them susceptible to recurring episodes of acute complications.

VII. Predicting Survival

Critical care physicians are well versed in predicting ICU outcome using tools, such as APACHE and simplified acute physiology score. Although such information may be insufficient to influence decision making in a given patient, it does afford general guidance and can allow for comparison of care between ICUs. Accurate estimates of survival in PMV would provide patients and families with realistic expectations for outcome, may facilitate end-of-life planning, and could help with more effective resource allocation. Regrettably, predicting outcome for patients with PMV has proved difficult (88). Intuitively, the heterogeneous nature of chronic critical illness and broad array of postacute care settings make it challenging to construct a simple, easily applied model for accurate prediction of survival. Despite this limitation, the very high morbidity, mortality, and resource utilization associated with PMV provide ample rationale for efforts to develop such a model.

Until recently, survival prediction in PMV had only been addressed in the LTAC setting. Friedrich et al. studied 182 patients with ICU stay >30 days; 181 of the patients were ventilated for a median of >40 days. Hospital survival was 58% and it decreased with increasing duration of MV. Using a multivariate model, the need for greater than 90 days of ventilation was an independent predictor of hospital mortality (89). Models, such as APACHE II, developed in acute ICU setting are insufficient discriminators of survival in the LTAC setting (90). In contrast, APACHE II can be recalibrated to help predict LTAC weaning outcome, though only for patients with duration of MV<25 days (91). A model using numbers of organ failures and presence of infection predicted LTAC survival in patients admitted to four different centers of a single hospital network (92).

A model has been developed to predict one-year survival using age, functional status prior to acute illness, and presence of diabetes (93). One-year survival was just 5% for patients older than 65 or 75 years, with poor prior functional status. In a recent report, patients requiring two or more days of MV had a 44% one-year survival. At hospital admission, survivors had fewer comorbidities, lower severity of illness, and greater functional independence than nonsurvivors. While short-term mortality was principally determined by severity of illness at ICU admission and prehospitalization, functional status had a significant association, and long-term mortality was related to age and comorbidities (94).

Further work is required to validate these models and to determine an impact on decision making. Because transfer to an LTAC involves selection based on illness severity, payer status, or rehabilitation potential, future investigations should focus on patients identified in the ICU setting.

VIII. Health-Related Quality of Life

Survival may not be the only outcome of interest for PMV patients. In one study, only 10% of PMV patients managed in a long-term care setting were functionally independent after one year (95). Despite their physical limitations, survivors usually respond that their quality of life is good and that they are living independently at home, though it appears that health-related quality of life is worse than that of the general population (35,87,96–100). When compared to a general French population, an ICU cohort ventilated for >14 days (mean 37 days) at three-year follow-up showed worse scores on the Nottingham Health Profile (99). In some cases, the disease process itself may be more important than the duration of MV. Davidson and coworkers compared acute respiratory distress syndrome survivors ventilated for less than or greater than 14 days and found no difference in the domains of either the St. George's Respiratory Questionnaire or the short-form-36 (SF-36) (101). In the NALTH study, functional status information was available in 71% (299 of 423) of one-year survivors. Functional status at long-term hospital discharge was less than that prior to admission but improved over the ensuing year in 49% of survivors (79).

These studies likely overestimate the quality of life after PMV, as many patients die within a year or are unable to respond to the interviews due to physical or cognitive limitations. Douglas et al. found that more than a quarter of patients discharged after 96 or more hours of MV had significant cognitive deficits. When symptoms for PMV patients were measured during hospitalization, the majority of patients reported significant pain, anxiety, dyspnea, and thirst (102). Identifying risk factors for severe functional limitations or nursing home admission would be of as much value for many patients as predicting hospital or long-term survival (103).

References

1. Esteban A, Anzueto A, Alia I, et al. How is mechanical ventilation employed in the intensive care unit? An international utilization review. Am J Respir Crit Care Med 2000; 161(5):1450–1458.
2. Carson SS, Cox CE, Holmes GM, et al. The changing epidemiology of mechanical ventilation: a population-based study. J Intensive Care Med 2006; 21(3):173–182.
3. Needham DM, Bronskill SE, Sibbald WJ, et al. Mechanical ventilation in Ontario, 1992–2000: incidence, survival, and hospital bed utilization of noncardiac surgery adult patients. Crit Care Med 2004; 32(7):1504–1509.
4. Brochard L, Rauss A, Benito S, et al. Comparison of three methods of gradual withdrawal from ventilatory support during weaning from mechanical ventilation. Am J Respir Crit Care Med 1994; 150(4):896–903.

5. Esteban A, Alia I, Gordo F, et al. Extubation outcome after spontaneous breathing trials with T-tube or pressure support ventilation. The Spanish Lung Failure Collaborative Group. Am J Respir Crit Care Med 1997; 156(2 pt 1):459–465.
6. Esteban A, Alia I, Tobin MJ, et al. Effect of spontaneous breathing trial duration on outcome of attempts to discontinue mechanical ventilation. Spanish Lung Failure Collaborative Group. Am J Respir Crit Care Med 1999; 159(2):512–518.
7. Esteban A, Frutos F, Tobin MJ, et al. A comparison of four methods of weaning patients from mechanical ventilation. Spanish Lung Failure Collaborative Group. N Engl J Med 1995; 332(6):345–350.
8. Vallverdu I, Calaf N, Subirana M, et al. Clinical characteristics, respiratory functional parameters, and outcome of a two-hour T-piece trial in patients weaning from mechanical ventilation. Am J Respir Crit Care Med 1998; 158(6):1855–1862.
9. Laupland KB, Kirkpatrick AW, Kortbeek JB, et al. Long-term mortality outcome associated with prolonged admission to the ICU. Chest 2006; 129(4):954–959.
10. Esteban A, Alia I, Ibanez J, et al. Modes of mechanical ventilation and weaning. A national survey of Spanish hospitals. The Spanish Lung Failure Collaborative Group. Chest 1994; 106(4): 1188–1193.
11. Nevins ML, Epstein SK. Predictors of outcome for patients with COPD requiring invasive mechanical ventilation. Chest 2001; 119(6):1840–1849.
12. Lipsett PA, Swoboda SM, Dickerson J, et al. Survival and functional outcome after prolonged intensive care unit stay. Ann Surg 2000; 231(2):262–268.
13. Stricker K, Rothen HU, Takala J. Resource use in the ICU short- vs. long-term patients. Acta Anaesthesiol Scand 2003; 47(5):508–515.
14. Wagner DP. Economics of prolonged mechanical ventilation. Am Rev Respir Dis 1989; 140 (2 pt 2):S14–S18.
15. Wong DT, Gomez M, McGuire GP, et al. Utilization of intensive care unit days in a Canadian medical-surgical intensive care unit. Crit Care Med 1999; 27(7):1319–1324.
16. Cox CE, Carson SS, Holmes GM, et al. Increase in tracheostomy for prolonged mechanical ventilation in North Carolina1, 993–2002. Crit Care Med 2004; 32(11):2219–2226.
17. Rumbak MJ, Newton M, Truncale T, et al. A prospective, randomized, study comparing early percutaneous dilational tracheotomy to prolonged translaryngeal intubation (delayed tracheotomy) in critically ill medical patients. Crit Care Med 2004; 32(8):1689–1694.
18. Scheinhorn D, Chao D, Stearn-Hassenpflug M, et al. Ventilator-dependent survivors of catastrophic illness: a multicenter outcomes study. Am J Respir Crit Care Med 2003; 167:A458.
19. Scheinhorn DJ, Chao DC, Hassenpflug MS, et al. Post-ICU weaning from mechanical ventilation: the role of long-term facilities. Chest 2001; 120(6 suppl):482S–484S.
20. Scheinhorn DJ, Chao DC, Stearn-Hassenpflug M. Post-ICU mechanical ventilation-treatment of 1575 patients over 11 years at a regional weaning center. Am J Respir Crit Care Med 2000; 161:A793.
21. Scheinhorn D, Hassenpflug M, Votto J, et al. Ventilator-dependent survivors of catastrophic illness transferred to 23 long-term care hospitals for weaning from prolonged mechanical ventilation. Chest 2007; 131(1):76–84.
22. MacIntyre NR, Epstein SK, Carson S, et al. Management of patients requiring prolonged mechanical ventilation: report of a NAMDRC consensus conference. Chest 2005; 128(6):3937–3954.
23. Esteban A, Anzueto A, Frutos F, et al. Characteristics and outcomes in adult patients receiving mechanical ventilation: a 28-day international study. JAMA 2002; 287(3):345–355.
24. Seneff MG, Zimmerman JE, Knaus WA, et al. Predicting the duration of mechanical ventilation. The importance of disease and patient characteristics. Chest 1996; 110(2):469–479.
25. Epstein SK, Vuong V. Lack of influence of gender on outcomes of mechanically ventilated medical ICU patients. Chest 1999; 116(3):732–739.

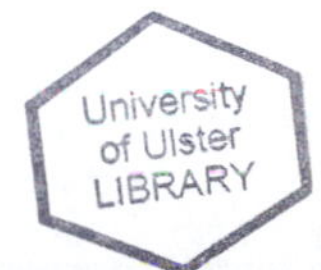

26. Gracey DR, Viggiano RW, Naessens JM, et al. Outcomes of patients admitted to a chronic ventilator-dependent unit in an acute-care hospital. Mayo Clin Proc 1992; 67(2):131–136.
27. Make B, Dayno S, Gertman P. Prevalence of chronic ventilator dependency. Am Rev Respir Dis 1986; 133:A167.
28. Harris J, Haughton J, Celli B. A survey of ventilator dependent patients in Massachusetts. Am J Respir Crit Care Med 1997; 155:A411.
29. Mulligan S. AARC and Gallup estimate numbers and costs of caring for chronic ventilator patients. AARC Times 1991; 15:30–36.
30. Dewar DM, Kurek CJ, Lambrinos J, et al. Patterns in costs and outcomes for patients with prolonged mechanical ventilation undergoing tracheostomy: an analysis of discharges under diagnosis-related group 483 in New York State from 1992 to 1996. Crit Care Med 1999; 27(12):2640–2647.
31. Scheinhorn DJ, Chao DC, Stearn-Hassenpflug M. Liberation from prolonged mechanical ventilation. Crit Care Clin 2002; 18(3):569–595.
32. Carson SS. Outcomes of prolonged mechanical ventilation. Curr Opin Crit Care 2006; 12(5):405–411.
33. Ely EW, Evans GW, Haponik EF. Mechanical ventilation in a cohort of elderly patients admitted to an intensive care unit. Ann Intern Med 1999; 131(2):96–104.
34. Esteban A, Anzueto A, Frutos-Vivar F, et al. Outcome of older patients receiving mechanical ventilation. Intensive Care Med 2004; 30(4):639–646.
35. Douglas SL, Daly BJ, Gordon N, et al. Survival and quality of life short-term versus long-term ventilator patients. Crit Care Med 2002; 30(12):2655–2662.
36. Spicher JE, White DP. Outcome and function following prolonged mechanical ventilation. Arch Intern Med 1987; 147(3):421–425.
37. Scheinhorn DJ, Chao DC, Stearn-Hassenpflug M, et al. Post-ICU mechanical ventilation: treatment of 1,123 patients at a regional weaning center. Chest 1997; 111(6):1654–1659.
38. Sirio CA, Shepardson LB, Rotondi AJ, et al. Community-wide assessment of intensive care outcomes using a physiologically based prognostic measure: implications for critical care delivery from Cleveland Health Quality Choice. Chest 1999; 115(3):793–801.
39. Velmahos GC, Belzberg H, Chan L, et al. Factors predicting prolonged mechanical ventilation in critically injured patients: introducing a simplified quantitative risk score. Am Surg 1997; 63(9):811–817.
40. Chan M, Mehta R, Vasishtha N. Ventilator care in a nursing home. Am J Respir Crit Care Med 1999; 159:A374.
41. Nasraway SA, Button GJ, Rand WM, et al. Survivors of catastrophic illness: outcome after direct transfer from intensive care to extended care facilities. Crit Care Med 2000; 28(1):19–25.
42. Zilberberg MD, Epstein SK. Acute lung injury in the medical ICU: comorbid conditions, age, etiology, and hospital outcome. Am J Respir Crit Care Med 1998; 157(4 pt 1):1159–1164.
43. De Jonghe B, Bastuji-Garin S, Sharshar T, et al. Does ICU-acquired paresis lengthen weaning from mechanical ventilation? Intensive Care Med 2004; 30(6):1117–1121.
44. Branca P, McGaw P, Light R. Factors associated with prolonged mechanical ventilation following coronary artery bypass surgery. Chest 2001; 119(2):537–546.
45. Thompson MJ, Elton RA, Mankad PA, et al. Prediction of requirement for, and outcome of, prolonged mechanical ventilation following cardiac surgery. Cardiovasc Surg 1997; 5(4):376–381.
46. Dimopoulou I, Anthi A, Lignos M, et al. Prediction of prolonged ventilatory support in blunt thoracic trauma patients. Intensive Care Med 2003; 29(7):1101–1105.
47. Estenssoro E, Gonzalez F, Laffaire E, et al. Shock on admission day is the best predictor of prolonged mechanical ventilation in the ICU. Chest 2005; 127(2):598–603.
48. Ouellette DR, Emmons EE, Gallup RA. Elevated creatinine levels are associated with failure to wean and adverse outcomes in patients receiving mechanical ventilation. Am J Resp Crit Care Med 1999; 159:A372.

49. Tafreshi M, Schneider R, Rosen M. Outcome of patients who require long-term mechanical ventilation and hemodialysis (abstract). Chest 1995; 108(suppl):134S.
50. Chao DC, Scheinhorn DJ, Stearn-Hassenpflug M. Impact of renal dysfunction on weaning from prolonged mechanical ventilation. Crit Care (Lond) 1997; 1(3):101–104.
51. Ely EW, Shintani A, Truman B, et al. Delirium as a predictor of mortality in mechanically ventilated patients in the intensive care unit. JAMA 2004; 291(14):1753–1762.
52. Nelson JE, Tandon N, Mercado AF, et al. Brain dysfunction another burden for the chronically critically ill. Arch Intern Med 2006; 166(18):1993–1999.
53. Hendra KP, Bonis PA, Joyce-Brady M. Development and prospective validation of a model for predicting weaning in chronic ventilator dependent patients. BMC Pulm Med 2003; 3(1):3.
54. Ely EW, Baker AM, Dunagan DP, et al. Effect on the duration of mechanical ventilation of identifying patients capable of breathing spontaneously. N Engl J Med 1996; 335(25):1864–1869.
55. Kollef MH, Shapiro SD, Silver P, et al. A randomized, controlled trial of protocol-directed versus physician-directed weaning from mechanical ventilation. Crit Care Med 1997; 25(4):567–574.
56. Marelich GP, Murin S, Battistella F, et al. Protocol weaning of mechanical ventilation in medical and surgical patients by respiratory care practitioners and nurses: effect on weaning time and incidence of ventilator-associated pneumonia. Chest 2000; 118(2):459–467.
57. Randolph AG, Wypij D, Venkataraman ST, et al. Effect of mechanical ventilator weaning protocols on respiratory outcomes in infants and children: a randomized controlled trial. JAMA 2002; 288(20):2561–2568.
58. Namen AM, Ely EW, Tatter SB, et al. Predictors of successful extubation in neurosurgical patients. Am J Respir Crit Care Med 2001; 163(3 pt 1):658–664.
59. Krishnan JA, Moore D, Robeson C, et al. A prospective, controlled trial of a protocol-based strategy to discontinue mechanical ventilation. Am J Respir Crit Care Med 2004; 169(6):673–678.
60. Scheinhorn DJ, Chao DC, Stearn-Hassenpflug M, et al. Outcomes in post-ICU mechanical ventilation: a therapist-implemented weaning protocol. Chest 2001; 119(1):236–242.
61. Vitacca M, Vianello A, Colombo D, et al. Comparison of two methods for weaning patients with chronic obstructive pulmonary disease requiring mechanical ventilation for more than 15 days. Am J Respir Crit Care Med 2001; 164(2):225–230.
62. Schonhofer B, Euteneuer S, Nava S, et al. Survival of mechanically ventilated patients admitted to a specialized weaning center. Intensive Care Med 2002; 28(7):908–916.
63. Coplin WM, Pierson DJ, Cooley KD, et al. Implications of extubation delay in brain-injured patients meeting standard weaning criteria. Am J Respir Crit Care Med 2000; 161(5):1530–1536.
64. Epstein SK. Decision to extubate. Intensive Care Med 2002; 28(5):535–546.
65. Epstein SK, Ciubotaru RL, Wong JB. Effect of failed extubation on the outcome of mechanical ventilation. Chest 1997; 112(1):186–192.
66. Brook AD, Ahrens TS, Schaiff R, et al. Effect of a nursing-implemented sedation protocol on the duration of mechanical ventilation. Crit Care Med 1999; 27(12):2609–2615.
67. Kress JP, Pohlman AS, O'Connor MF, et al. Daily interruption of sedative infusions in critically ill patients undergoing mechanical ventilation. N Engl J Med 2000; 342(20):1471–1477.
68. Thorens JB, Kaelin RM, Jolliet P, et al. Influence of the quality of nursing on the duration of weaning from mechanical ventilation in patients with chronic obstructive pulmonary disease. Crit Care Med 1995; 23(11):1807–1815.
69. Dimick JB, Pronovost PJ, Heitmiller RF, et al. Intensive care unit physician staffing is associated with decreased length of stay, hospital cost, and complications after esophageal resection. Crit Care Med 2001; 29(4):753–758.
70. Pronovost PJ, Angus DC, Dorman T, et al. Physician staffing patterns and clinical outcomes in critically ill patients: a systematic review. JAMA 2002; 288(17):2151–2162.
71. Multz AS, Chalfin DB, Samson IM, et al. A "closed" medical intensive care unit (MICU) improves resource utilization when compared with an "open" MICU. Am J Respir Crit Care Med 1998; 157(5 pt 1):1468–1473.

72. Carson SS, Stocking C, Podsadecki T, et al. Effects of organizational change in the medical intensive care unit of a teaching hospital: a comparison of "open" and "closed" formats. JAMA 1996; 276(4):322–328.
73. Bach PB, Carson SS, Leff A. Outcomes and resource utilization for patients with prolonged critical illness managed by university-based or community-based subspecialists. Am J Respir Crit Care Med 1998; 158(5 pt 1):1410–1415.
74. Bagley PH, Cooney E. A community-based regional ventilator weaning unit: development and outcomes. Chest 1997; 111(4):1024–1029.
75. Indihar FJ. A 10-year report of patients in a prolonged respiratory care unit. Minn Med 1991; 74(4):23–27.
76. Baudot J, Fieux F, Mokhtari M, et al. Evaluation of clinical judgment in the prediction at day 7 of the success of weaning at day 21. Am J Respir Crit Care Med 2001; 163:A889.
77. Epstein S. Complications in ventilator supported patients. In: Tobin M, ed. Principles and Practice of Mechanical Ventilation. 2nd ed. McGraw-Hill, 2006:877–902.
78. Kollef MH, Ahrens TS, Shannon W. Clinical predictors and outcomes for patients requiring tracheostomy in the intensive care unit. Crit Care Med 1999; 27(9):1714–1720.
79. Scheinhorn D, Hassenpflug M, Votto J, et al. Post-ICU mechanical ventilation at 23 long-term care hospitals: a multicenter outcomes study. Chest 2007; 131(1):85–93.
80. Epstein S. Weaning from ventilatory support. In: Crapo J, Glassroth J, Karlinsky J, King T, eds. Textbook of Pulmonary Diseases: Lippincott, Williams & Wilkins, 2003:1089–1101.
81. Epstein SK. Etiology of extubation failure and the predictive value of the rapid shallow breathing index. Am J Respir Crit Care Med 1995; 152(2):545–549.
82. Epstein SK. Predicting extubation failure: is it in (on) the cards? Chest 2001; 120(4): 1061–1063.
83. MacIntyre NR, Cook DJ, Ely EW Jr., et al, Evidence-based guidelines for weaning and discontinuing ventilatory support: a collective task force facilitated by the American College of Chest Physicians; the American Association for Respiratory Care; and the American College of Critical Care Medicine. Chest 2001; 120(6 suppl):375S–395S.
84. Quinnell TG, Pilsworth S, Shneerson JM, et al. Prolonged invasive ventilation following acute ventilatory failure in COPD: weaning results, survival and the role of noninvasive ventilation. Chest 2006; 129(1):133–139.
85. Cohen J, Starobin D, Papirov G, et al. Initial experience with a mechanical ventilation weaning unit. Isr Med Assoc J 2005; 7(3):166–168.
86. Pilcher DV, Bailey MJ, Treacher DF, et al. Outcomes, cost and long term survival of patients referred to a regional weaning centre. Thorax 2005; 60(3):187–192.
87. Engoren M, Arslanian-Engoren C, Fenn-Buderer N. Hospital and long-term outcome after tracheostomy for respiratory failure. Chest 2004; 125(1):220–227.
88. Lynn J, Teno JM, Harrell F. Accurate prognostications of death. Opportunities and challenges for clinicians. West J Med 1995; 163(3):250–257.
89. Friedrich JO, Wilson G, Chant C. Long-term outcomes and clinical predictors of hospital mortality in very long stay intensive care unit patients: a cohort study. Crit Care 2006; 10(2):R59.
90. Carson SS, Bach PB. Predicting mortality in patients suffering from prolonged critical illness: an assessment of four severity-of-illness measures. Chest 2001; 120(3):928–933.
91. Schonhofer B, Guo JJ, Suchi S, et al. The use of APACHE II prognostic system in difficult-to-wean patients after long-term mechanical ventilation. Eur J Anaesthesiol 2004; 21(7):558–565.
92. Dematte D'Amico JE, Donnelly HK, Mutlu GM, et al. Risk assessment for inpatient survival in the long-term acute care setting after prolonged critical illness. Chest 2003; 124(3): 1039–1045.
93. Carson SS, Bach PB, Brzozowski L, et al. Outcomes after long-term acute care. An analysis of 133 mechanically ventilated patients. Am J Respir Crit Care Med 1999; 159(5 pt 1): 1568–1573.

94. Chelluri L, Im KA, Belle SH, et al. Long-term mortality and quality of life after prolonged mechanical ventilation. Crit Care Med 2004; 32(1):61–69.
95. Carson SS, Bach PB. The epidemiology and costs of chronic critical illness. Crit Care Clin 2002; 18(3):461–476.
96. Teno JM, Fisher E, Hamel MB, et al. Decision-making and outcomes of prolonged ICU stays in seriously ill patients. J Am Geriatr Soc 2000; 48(5 suppl):S70–S74.
97. Heyland DK, Konopad E, Noseworthy TW, et al. Is it "worthwhile" to continue treating patients with a prolonged stay (>14 days) in the ICU? An economic evaluation. Chest 1998; 114(1):192–198.
98. Chatila W, Kreimer DT, Criner GJ. Quality of life in survivors of prolonged mechanical ventilatory support. Crit Care Med 2001; 29(4):737–742.
99. Combes A, Costa MA, Trouillet JL, et al. Morbidity, mortality and quality-of-life outcomes of patients requiring >or=14 days of mechanical ventilation. Crit Care Med 2003; 31(5):1373–1381.
100. Niskanen M, Ruokonen E, Takala J, et al. Quality of life after prolonged intensive care. Crit Care Med 1999; 27(6):1132–1139.
101. Davidson TA, Caldwell ES, Curtis JR, et al. Reduced quality of life in survivors of acute respiratory distress syndrome compared with critically ill control patients. JAMA 1999; 281(4):354–360.
102. Nelson J, Nierman D, Meier D. The symptom burden of chronic critical illness. Am J Resp Crit Care Med 2001; 163:A62.
103. Nierman DM, Schechter CB, Cannon LM, et al. Outcome prediction model for very elderly critically ill patients. Crit Care Med 2001; 29(10):1853–1859.
104. Gillespie DJ, Marsh HM, Divertie MB, et al. Clinical outcome of respiratory failure in patients requiring prolonged (greater than 24 hours) mechanical ventilation. Chest 1986; 90(3):364–369.
105. Martin CM, Hill AD, Burns K, et al. Characteristics and outcomes for critically ill patients with prolonged intensive care unit stays. Crit Care Med 2005; 33(9):1922–1927.
106. Nevins ML, Epstein SK. Weaning from prolonged mechanical ventilation. Clin Chest Med 2001; 22(1):13–33.
107. Cox C, Carson S, Howard A, et al. Tracheostomy for prolonged ventilation in North Carolina, 1993–2002. Am J Resp Crit Care Med 2004; 169:A44.
108. Zubrod C. Appraisal of methods for the study of chemotherapy of cancer in man: comparative therapeutic trial of nitrogen mustard and triethyelene fluophosphonate. J Chronic Dis 1960; 2:7–33.
109. Sivak ED. Prolonged mechanical ventilation: an approach to weaning. Cleve Clin Q 1980; 47(2):89–96.
110. Morganroth ML, Morganroth JL, Nett LM, et al. Criteria for weaning from prolonged mechanical ventilation. Arch Intern Med 1984; 144(5):1012–1016.
111. Cordasco EM, Jr., Sivak ED, Perez-Trepichio A. Demographics of long-term ventilator-dependent patients outside the intensive care unit. Cleve Clin J Med 1991; 58(6):505–509.
112. Scheinhorn DJ, Artinian BM, Catlin JL. Weaning from prolonged mechanical ventilation. The experience at a regional weaning center. Chest 1994; 105(2):534–539.
113. Nava S, Rubini F, Zanotti E, et al. Survival and prediction of successful ventilator weaning in COPD patients requiring mechanical ventilation for more than 21 days. Eur Respir J 1994; 7(9): 1645–1652.
114. Gracey DR, Naessens JM, Viggiano RW, et al. Outcome of patients cared for in a ventilator-dependent unit in a general hospital. Chest 1995; 107(2):494–499.
115. Latriano B, McCauley P, Astiz ME, et al. Non-ICU care of hemodynamically stable mechanically ventilated patients. Chest 1996; 109(6):1591–1596.
116. Gluck EH. Predicting eventual success or failure to wean in patients receiving long-term mechanical ventilation. Chest 1996; 110(4):1018–1024.

117. Gracey DR, Hardy DC, Naessens JM, et al. The Mayo ventilator-dependent rehabilitation unit: a 5-year experience. Mayo Clin Proc 1997; 72(1):13–19.
118. Scalise PJ, Gerardi DA, Wollschlager CM, et al. A regional weaning center for patients requiring mechanical ventilation: an 18-month experience. Conn Med 1997; 61(7):387–389.
119. Dasgupta A, Rice R, Mascha E, et al. Four-year experience with a unit for long-term ventilation (respiratory special care unit) at the Cleveland Clinic Foundation. Chest 1999; 116(2):447–455.
120. Gracey DR, Hardy DC, Koenig GE. The chronic ventilator-dependent unit: a lower-cost alternative to intensive care. Mayo Clin Proc 2000; 75(5):445–449.
121. Iregui M, Malen J, Tuteur P, et al. Determinants of outcome for patients admitted to a long-term ventilator unit. South Med J 2002; 95(3):310–317.
122. Modawal A, Candadai NP, Mandell KM, et al. Weaning success among ventilator-dependent patients in a rehabilitation facility. Arch Phys Med Rehabil 2002; 83(2):154–157.

5
Causes of Difficult Weaning: Which Mechanisms Are Associated with Long-Term Ventilator Dependence?

FRANCO LAGHI
Loyola University of Chicago Stritch School of Medicine and Edward Hines, Jr. Veterans Administration Hospital, Maywood, Illinois, U.S.A.

I. Introduction

Each year, over 400,000 patients in the United States receive mechanical ventilation as a result of acute or acute-on-chronic respiratory failure (1,2). About a quarter of acutely ventilated patients repeatedly fail attempts at weaning and may require prolonged mechanical ventilation (PMV) (Fig. 1) (3,4). The proportion of patients experiencing PMV ranges between 0% and 20% (5–13). Out of patients who survive PMV, 9–66% become dependent on long-term mechanical ventilation (LTMV) (4,9,14–21). Two factors account for these wide variations in the outcome. The first factor is differences in patient population. The second one is the nosology of what constitutes PMV and what constitutes LTMV is unsatisfactory.

Recovery from acute respiratory failure is determined by many factors including age of the patient (5,22), severity of precipitating disease (11), presence of preexisting or new-onset comorbidities (5,11,23–26), and organization of the intensive care unit (ICU) (27,28). Thus, designating a patient as the recipient of PMV based on a single threshold—such as the need for mechanical ventilation for more than one day (29), three days (30), four days (31), five days (32), 14 days (1), or for at least six hours per day for 21 consecutive days (6,33)—makes little sense. The situation becomes even more difficult when trying to define what LTMV is. Dependence on LTMV implies the inability (and thus dependence) of a given patient to sustain spontaneous respiration for any given period of time. To this date, however, there are no data indicating that clinicians can identify the moment at which patients transition from PMV to LTMV (6).

Due to the current limitations in nosology and the paucity of research in the field, I will discuss potential mechanisms associated with LTMV based on principles of pulmonary pathophysiology recorded in patients requiring mechanical ventilation for variable periods of time, including those in the acute care setting. Whether it is valid to extrapolate pathophysiological data recorded in the acute care setting to the chronic one is, however, unknown.

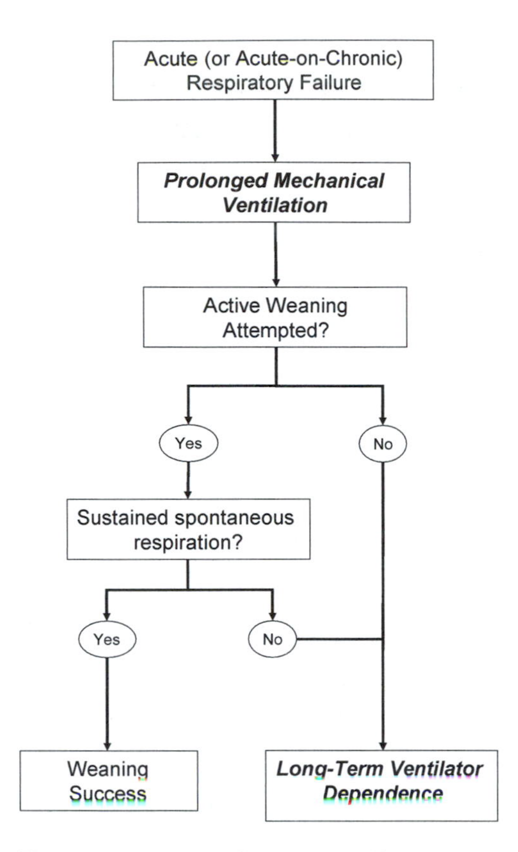

Figure 1 Conceptual framework linking acute or acute-on-chronic respiratory failure to prolonged mechanical ventilation and long-term ventilator dependence. Differences in patient population, imprecise nosology, and paucity of research make it difficult to provide solid indications for when patients may transition from one condition to the next.

II. Determinants of Long-Term Ventilator Dependence

From a pathophysiologic standpoint, it is useful to consider respiratory conditions that may result in LTMV, as those characterized by failure of the lungs as a gas-exchange unit and those characterized by a failure of the ventilatory pump (Fig. 2). In some ventilated patients, psychological factors may also contribute to their degree of impairment (34).

III. Impaired Gas Exchange

Conditions characterized by failure of the lungs as a gas-exchange unit include those associated with ventilation perfusion (V/Q) mismatching and, less often, conditions associated with increased shunt (35). The typical consequence of impaired gas exchange is hypoxemia (35). Impaired gas exchange is a common finding among patients requiring

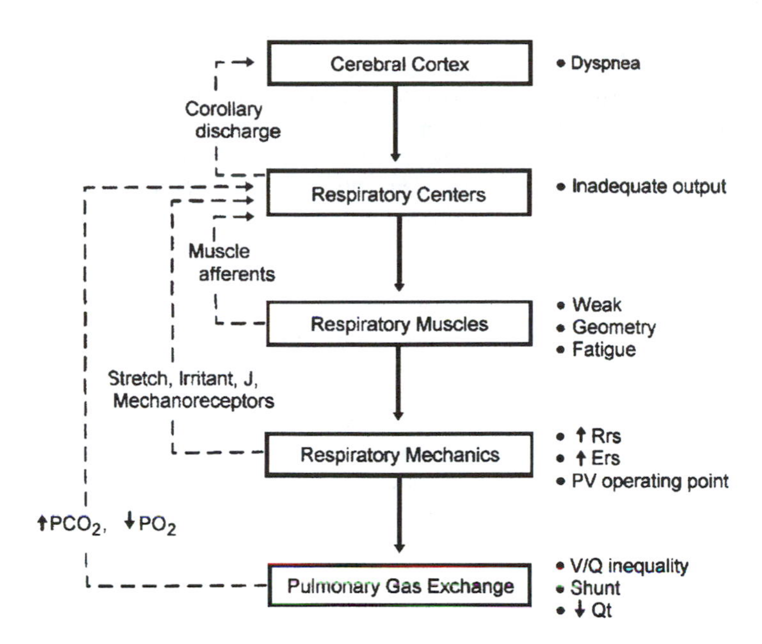

Figure 2 Model of the respiratory neuromuscular control system. Potential mechanisms of respiratory failure are listed on the right side and afferent stimuli arising at each site are shown on the left side. *Abbreviations*: Rrs, respiratory system resistance; Ers, respiratory system elastance; PV, pressure–volume; V/Q, ventilation–perfusion ratio; Qt, cardiac output; PCO_2 carbon dioxide tension; PO_2 oxygen tension. *Source*: From Ref. 127.

PMV and LTMV (18,36,37). For instance, the mean alveolar-arterial oxygen gradient in the 1419 patients enrolled in the Ventilation Outcomes Study Group was 127 mmHg (37).

The ratio of dead space to tidal volume—an approximation of impaired gas exchange due to lung units with abnormally high V/Q ratios (38)—is normally 0.3. In patients requiring PMV, the ratio can increase to above 0.74 (19). Patients can compensate for such an increase in dead space by increasing minute ventilation 2.5 times, a minor challenge when respiratory mechanics and respiratory muscles are normal. Accordingly, impaired gas exchange should not be considered the primary mechanism responsible for dependence on LTMV, unless there is a concurrent abnormality in the control of breathing, in the mechanical load of the respiratory muscles, or in their contractile performance. (35,39). Similarly, increased CO_2 production may be a contributing factor and not the sole cause of dependence on LTMV.

IV. Impaired Ventilatory Pump

Impairment of the ventilatory pump can occur in conditions characterized by decreased respiratory drive, abnormal respiratory mechanics, diminished respiratory muscle performance, and impaired cardiovascular performance.

A. Decreased Respiratory Drive

Specific conditions such as idiopathic central alveolar hypoventilation syndrome (Ondine's curse) or central alveolar hypoventilation syndrome secondary to neurological lesions (trauma, infections, infarction, Shy Drager syndrome) can cause or contribute to long-term ventilator dependence (40). In most ventilator-dependent patients, however, estimations of respiratory drive indicate that drive is increased and not decreased (18,41–43).

Purro et al. (41) measured airway occlusion pressure at 100 milliseconds ($P_{0.1}$) during trials of spontaneous respiration in patients who had been mechanically ventilated for more than three weeks. All of the weaning failures (all of whom ended up requiring LTMV) had greater $P_{0.1}$ values than the weaning successes. The high values of $P_{0.1}$ suggest an enhanced neuromuscular inspiratory drive (44). The high neuromuscular inspiratory drive, however, was poorly transformed into ventilatory output. The tidal volumes were lower in patients requiring LTMV than in weaning success patients (41). Despite these findings, in some patients, a decrease in drive relative to the ventilatory demands may still contribute to LTMV dependence. Whether hypothyroidism, metabolic alkalosis, and semistarvation may contribute to LTMV dependence by decreasing respiratory drive is unknown. Similarly, whether sleep deprivation decreases respiratory drive remains controversial (45,46).

B. Increased Mechanical Load

At the time of successful weaning, the mechanical load on the respiratory muscles of patients who had required PMV is similar to the load in stable patients with similar comorbidities (41). In contrast, patients requiring LTMV typically have 150–200% greater inspiratory resistance (41), 130–160% greater lung elastance (41,47), and up to 400% greater intrinsic positive end expiratory pressure (PEEP) (41,43) than similar patients who are not ventilator dependent. In eight ventilator-dependent patients with chronic obstructive pulmonary disease (COPD), Appendini et al. reported that 41% of the inspiratory effort was required to overcome intrinsic PEEP (42). In the same eight patients, 37% of inspiratory effort was required to overcome inspiratory resistance and 22% to overcome lung and chest wall elastic recoil (42).

Several lines of evidence support the likelihood that increased mechanical load contributes to LTMV dependence. First, mechanical load is greater in ventilator-dependent patients than in non-ventilator-dependent patients (41,43). Second, progression to successful weaning has been associated with improvement in work of breathing per liter of minute ventilation, which is a function of compliance, resistance, tidal volume, and minute ventilation (48). Third, the mean inspiratory flow produced for a given level of neuromuscular inspiratory drive is lower in LTMV-dependent patients than in patients who are successfully weaned after a period of PMV (Fig. 3) (41,43). Lastly, effective inspiratory impedance correlates with inspiratory pressure output (41). This correlation suggests worse load-capacity balance in patients who are dependent on LTMV than in patients who are successfully weaned after a period of PMV (41).

Narrowing of the tracheal lumen due to stenosis, granulation tissue, and tracheomalacia can increase the mechanical load on the respiratory muscles and contribute to prolonged ventilation (49). Reported prevalence of tracheal narrowing in prolonged ventilation ranges from 5% to 12% (49,50). As the prevalence of tracheal complications is greater in female patients, it has been speculated that the smaller tracheal lumen in female patients may make it more susceptible to damage (49–51). Whether (and how often) the

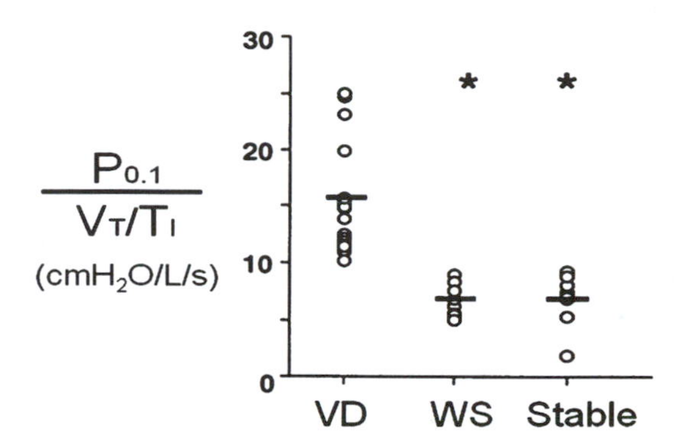

Figure 3 Effective inspiratory impedance—or drive to mean inspiratory flow ratio (P0.1/VT/TI)—during periods of unassisted breathing in ventilator-dependent patients with COPD (VD, $n = 12$), in patients with COPD who were successfully weaned after prolonged ventilation (WS, $n = 8$), and in stable patients with COPD who had not required mechanical ventilation for an average time of 18 months before data collection (stable, $n = 9$). Effective inspiratory impedance was greater in ventilator-dependent patients than in the other two groups. The higher effective inspiratory impedance in ventilator-dependent patients with COPD resulted entirely from a greater neuromuscular drive (P0.1) and not from a reduced mean inspiratory flow (VT/TI) (data not shown). Despite greater drive, the fact that the mean inspiratory flows of ventilator-dependent patients with COPD did not differ from the corresponding values in patients who were successfully weaned after prolonged ventilation indicates that for any given change in drive the flow resistance and compliance characteristics of the respiratory system in long-term ventilator-dependent patients limited the capacity of neuromuscular drive to produce the otherwise expected changes in ventilation. Horizontal bars, average values; $*p < 0.05$ for comparisons of ventilator-dependent patients versus weaning successes and stable patients. *Abbreviations*: VT, tidal volume; TI, inspiratory time; COPD, chronic obstructive pulmonary disease; VD, ventilator-dependent; WS, weaned successfully. *Source*: From Ref. 41.

work of breathing imposed by artificial airway itself contributes to PMV and its dependence on LTMV is unknown (52).

C. Inadequate Performance of the Respiratory Muscles

Respiratory muscle weakness and respiratory muscle fatigue can decrease the capacity of these muscles to generate and sustain tension. As direct quantification of respiratory muscle tension is clinically impossible, measurements of pressure elicited by respiratory muscle contractions are used to indirectly determine their contribution to ventilator dependence.

Detection of Respiratory Muscle Weakness in Mechanically Ventilated Patients

Global inspiratory muscle strength can be evaluated with measurements of airway pressure during maximal voluntary inspiratory efforts (P_{Imax}) (53). In healthy volunteers, P_{Imax} values are usually more negative than -80 cmH_2O (53). In long-term ventilator dependence, P_{Imax} values have been reported to be less negative than -30 to -60 cmH_2O (18,41–43,54).

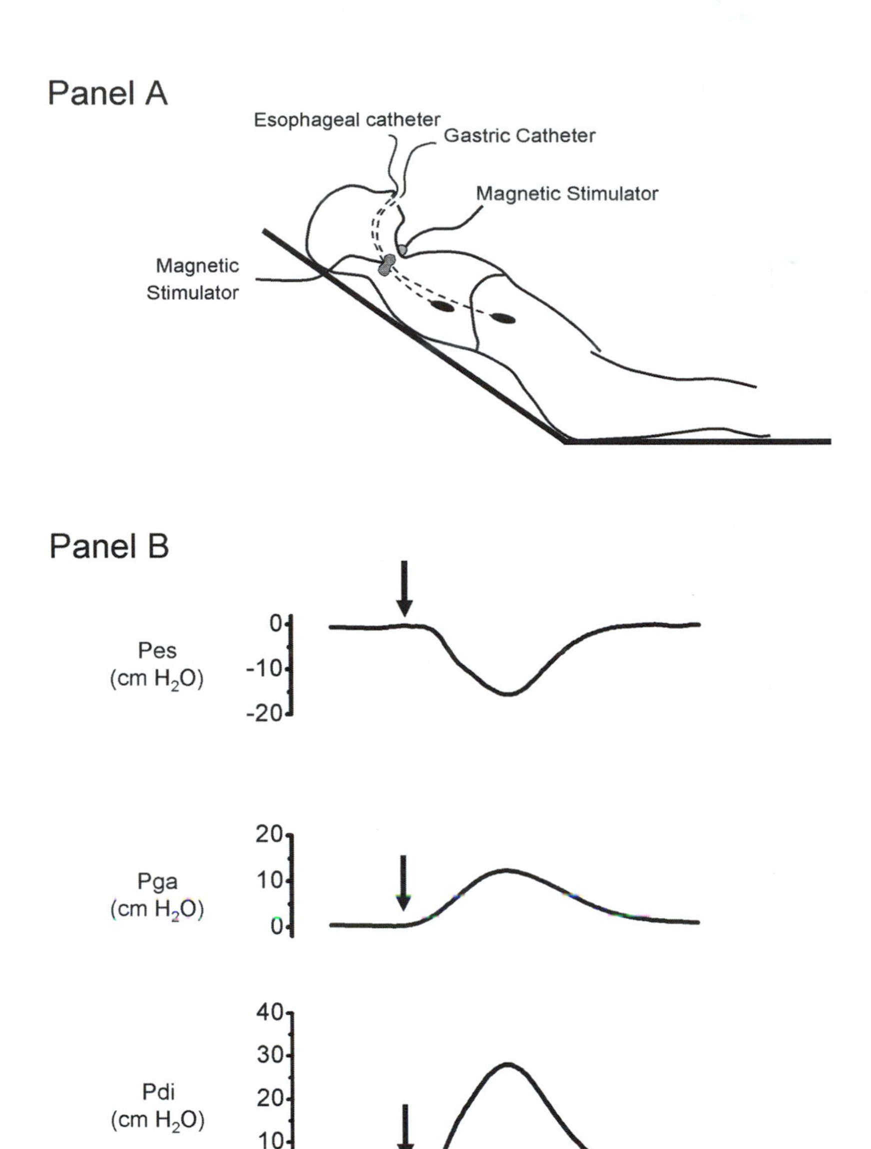

Figure 4 Technique used to record transdiaphragmatic twitch pressure (*Panel A*). An esophageal and a gastric balloon are passed through the nares. Magnetic stimulation of the phrenic nerves elicits diaphragmatic contraction. (*Panel B*) Continuous recordings of esophageal (Pes) and gastric pressures (Pga) and transdiaphragmatic pressure (Pdi)—calculated by subtracting Pes from Pga. Phrenic nerve stimulation (*arrows*) results in contraction of the diaphragm with consequent fall in intrathoracic pressure (*negative defection of Pes*) and rise in intra-abdominal pressure (*positive deflection of Pga*). These swings in pressure are responsible for the transdiaphragmatic twitch pressure. The smaller the transdiaphragmatic twitch pressure, the smaller the force-generating capacity of the diaphragm. *Abbreviations*: Pes, esophageal pressure; Pga, gastric pressure; Pdi, transdiaphragmatic pressure. *Source*: From Ref. 63.

Several lines of evidence support the likelihood that decreased inspiratory muscle strength is one of the mechanisms of dependence on LTMV (18,41,54). First, according to most (18,41,54), but not all, investigators (43) the values of P_{Imax} are less negative in LTMV-dependent patients than in patients who are successfully weaned after a period of PMV (18,41,43,54). Second, in a preliminary report of 28 patients ventilated for more than three weeks, Tulaimat et al. recorded an increase in P_{Imax} only among successfully weaned patients, with no change among those requiring LTMV (54). Three, on post-hoc analysis of 42 patients with COPD requiring PMV, P_{Imax} and $PaCO_2$ could separate patients dependent on LTMV from weaning successes with an accuracy of 84% (18). Finally, a few studies (mostly case reports) have shown that inspiratory muscle training in patients requiring PMV may decrease the need for LTMV (55–58).

P_{Imax} values depend on a level of motivation and comprehension of the maneuver that is often not obtainable in mechanically ventilated patients (59). In contrast to the voluntary nature of the P_{Imax} technique, transdiaphragmatic pressures elicited by single stimulations of the phrenic nerves—or twitch pressure—are independent of patients' motivation and eliminate the influence of the central nervous system (Fig. 4) (53).

In healthy volunteers, stimulation of the phrenic nerves elicits twitch pressures of 31 to 39 cmH_2O, whereas in patients with severe COPD, twitch pressures average 19 to 20 cmH_2O (53,60). Twitch pressures in patients recovering from an episode of acute respiratory failure are about half of those recorded in ambulatory patients with severe COPD (Fig. 5) (59,61,62). This decrease is in keeping with respiratory muscle weakness in most of these patients. Respiratory muscle weakness in mechanically ventilated patients can result from preexisting conditions or from new-onset conditions (63).

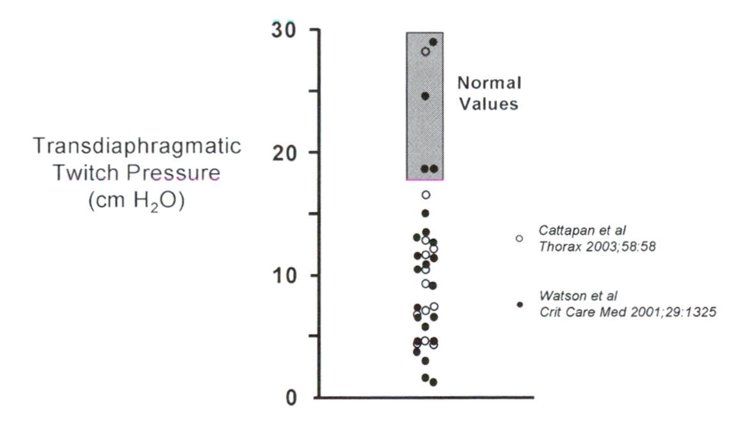

Figure 5 Transdiaphragmatic twitch pressure recorded in mechanically ventilated patients recovering from an episode of acute respiratory failure. Box represents range of transdiaphragmatic twitch pressures recorded in ambulatory patients with severe COPD. Most mechanically ventilated patients had evidence of diaphragmatic weakness [data from Ref. 62 (*open circles*), and from Ref. 61 (*closed circles*)]. *Abbreviation*: COPD, chronic obstructive pulmonary disease. *Source*: From Refs. 44.

Respiratory Muscle Weakness: Preexisting Conditions

Preexisting conditions include disorders such as neuromuscular diseases (NMD), malnutrition, endocrine disorders, and hyperinflation.

Neuromuscular Disorders

Approximately 15% of patients receiving PMV or LTMV have NMD (37,64). NMD can be grouped into disorders involving the central nervous system, such as multiple sclerosis and amyotrophic lateral sclerosis; the motor neuron, such as postpolio syndrome and amyotrophic lateral sclerosis; the peripheral nerves, such as Guillain-Barré syndrome; the neuromuscular junction, such as botulism and myasthenia gravis; and the peripheral muscles, such as inflammatory myopathies, myotonic dystrophy type 1, and Duchenne's muscular dystrophy (40).

The relationship between hypercapnia and respiratory muscle strength varies considerably among patients, with some being hypercapnic when strength falls to 39% of the predicted value (65), while others maintaining a normal partial pressure of CO_2, despite decreases in respiratory muscle strength to less than 20% of the predicted value (Fig. 6) (66). In other words, reductions in muscle strength do not consistently predict alveolar hypoventilation in this setting.

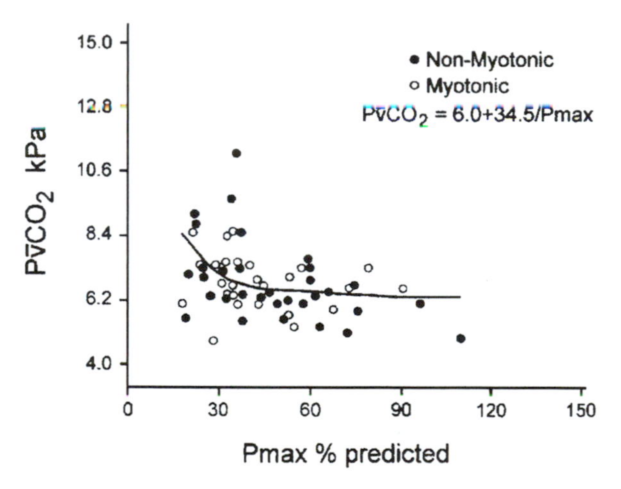

Figure 6 Relationship between muscle strength and mixed venous partial pressure of CO_2 (P_{VCO_2}) in patients with respiratory muscle weakness. Respiratory muscle strength is the arithmetic sum of maximum static inspiratory and expiratory mouth pressures ($P_{max} = P_{Imax} + P_{Emax}$). The open circles are patients with myotonic dystrophy and the closed circles are patients with a variety of nonmyotonic muscle diseases. As respiratory muscle weakness became more severe P_{VCO_2} increased, although considerable variability was observed among patients. *Abbreviations*: P_{VCO_2}, venous partial pressure of CO_2; P_{Imax}, maximum inspiratory pressure; P_{Emax}, maximum expiratory pressure. *Source*: From Ref. 66.

Hyperinflation

More than 40% of patients requiring PMV or LTMV carry a preexisting diagnosis of COPD (37). Nearly all patients with COPD requiring mechanical ventilation have expiratory flow limitation (67). Expiratory flow limitation delays lung emptying and promotes dynamic hyperinflation (40). In presence of dynamic hyperinflation, the inspiratory muscles have to offset a threshold load—termed as auto or intrinsic PEEP—before inspiratory flow can begin (40). Values of intrinsic PEEP are higher in LTMV-dependent patients with COPD than in those patients who are successfully weaned, suggesting that hyperinflation is more severe in LTMV than in weaning successes (41,43).

Hyperinflation has a number of adverse effects on inspiratory muscle function. The inspiratory muscles operate at an unfavorable position of the length–tension relationship (Fig. 7) (40). Flattening of the diaphragm decreases the zone of apposition with the result that diaphragmatic contractions cause less rib cage expansion (40). Hyperinflation adversely affects the elastic recoil of the thoracic cage with the inspiratory muscles working not only against the elastic recoil of the lungs, but also against that of the thoracic cage (40,68). Finally, hyperinflation can contribute to ineffective inspiratory efforts (Fig. 8) (41). The functional consequences of hyperinflation are probably the main cause of acute ventilatory failure and ventilator dependence in COPD (42,69).

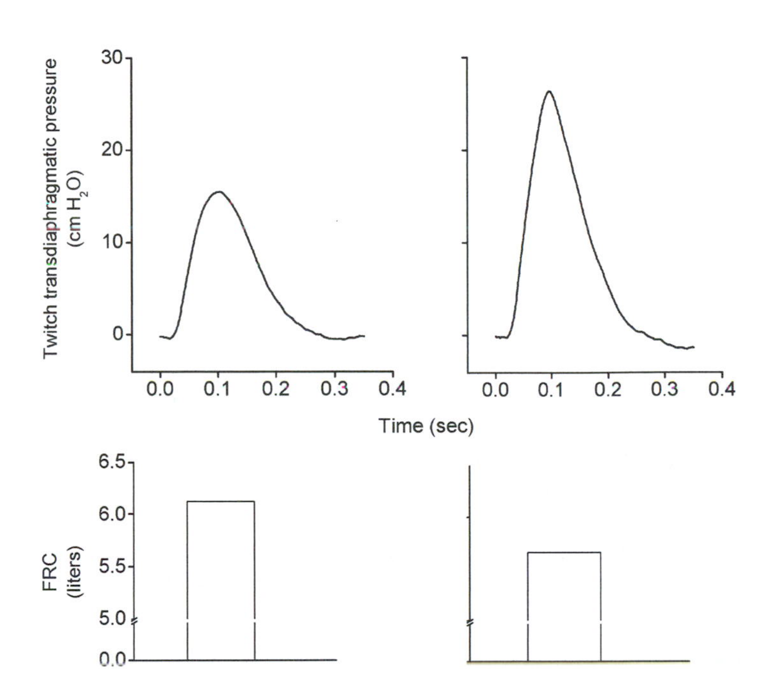

Figure 7 Twitch transdiaphragmatic pressure elicited by phrenic nerve stimulation (*upper panel*) and FRC (*lower panel*) in a patient with severe emphysema before (*left*) and after (*right*) lung volume reduction surgery. The increase in transdiaphragmatic pressure after surgery was partly due to a decrease in the operating lung volume as demonstrated by the decrease in FRC. *Abbreviation*: FRC, functional residual capacity. *Source*: Data from Ref. 128.

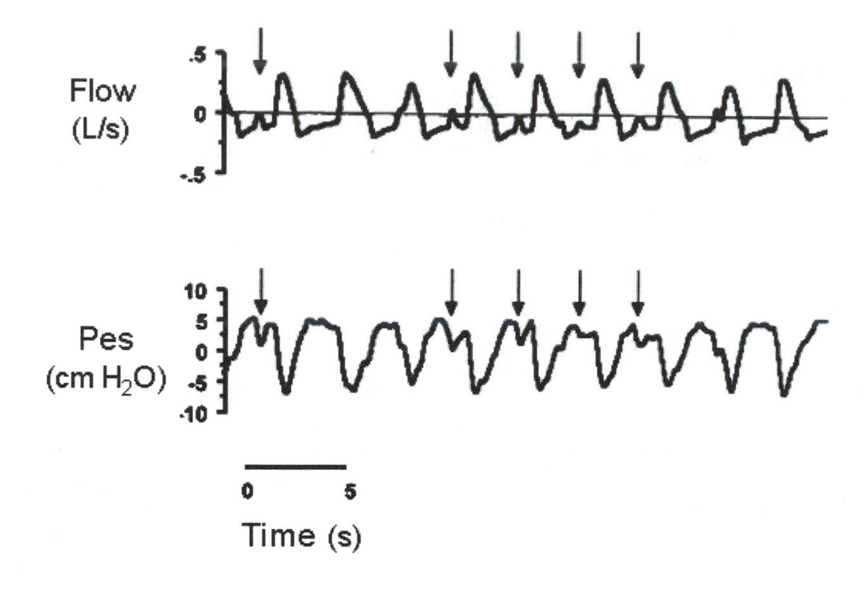

Figure 8 Continuous recordings of airflow (Flow) and esophageal pressure (Pes) in a long-term ventilator-dependent patient with COPD during a brief period of unassisted breathing. Arrows indicate ineffective inspiratory efforts—inspiratory efforts not associated with inspiratory flow. In one study (41), ineffective inspiratory efforts were recorded in 40% of long-term ventilator-dependent patients with COPD but not in patients with COPD who were successfully weaned after a period of prolonged ventilatory support. *Abbreviations*: Pes, esophageal pressure; COPD, chronic obstructive pulmonary disease. *Source*: From Ref. 41.

Malnutrition

Malnutrition is highly prevalent among patients requiring PMV (37) and LTMV (70) and is associated with poor prognosis (71). Malnutrition decreases muscle mass and respiratory muscle strength and endurance (40). These effects on the respiratory muscles are partially reversible with nutritional support. The process, however, is slow, and in laboratory animals, it can take months of refeeding for muscle mass to return to normal values (72). To date, it remains unclear whether malnutrition by itself can cause sufficient respiratory muscle weakness to produce ventilator dependence. It is more likely for malnutrition to be a contributing factor and not a sole cause of ventilator dependence.

Endocrine Disturbances

Hypothyroidism, hyperthyroidism, and acromegaly can adversely affect respiratory muscle function (40). Proteolysis of myofibrillar proteins by the ubiquitin-proteasome proteolytic system is probably responsible for respiratory muscle catabolism and weakness of hyperthyroidism (40) This mechanism is implicated in the muscle wasting associated with acidosis, renal failure, cancer, diabetes, acquired immunity deficiency syndrome, trauma, and burns (73). In contrast to other endocrine disturbances, respiratory muscle weakness is unusual in patients with Cushing's syndrome (40). Despite few case series (64,74), it is unclear whether endocrine disturbances can cause or can contribute to dependence on LTMV. In the acute setting, treatment of adrenal insufficiency is associated with increased weaning success (75).

Respiratory Muscle Weakness: New-Onset Conditions

New-onset respiratory muscle weakness may result from conditions that are unique to mechanically ventilated patients, such as ventilator-associated respiratory muscle dysfunction, sepsis-associated myopathy, and ICU-acquired paresis (63). New-onset respiratory muscle weakness may also result from conditions that are not unique to critically ill patients, such as acid–base disorders, electrolyte disturbances, decreased oxygen delivery, and medications (63).

Ventilator-Associated Respiratory Muscle Dysfunction

In laboratory animals, controlled mechanical ventilation delivered for 1 to 11 days can decrease diaphragmatic force generation by 20–50% and can cause similar decreases in diaphragmatic endurance (40). Several mechanisms, including structural injury, muscle atrophy, and oxidative stress, appear to be responsible for ventilator-associated respiratory muscle dysfunction (40). Of interest, in a study of more than 200 critically ill patients—80% of whom required acute ventilator support—duration of mechanical ventilation was nearly three days shorter in those who completed a 10-day antioxidant supplementation protocol (vitamins E and C) than in those who completed a 10-day course of placebo (76).

Whether ventilator-associated respiratory muscle dysfunction occurs in humans is unclear. In 13 infants who received uninterrupted ventilator assistance for at least 12 days before death, most diaphragmatic fibers appeared atrophic (Fig. 9) (77). These data are supported by a recent preliminary report of Levine et al. (78) who compared costal diaphragm biopsies of six brain-dead organ donors maintained on controlled mechanical ventilation for

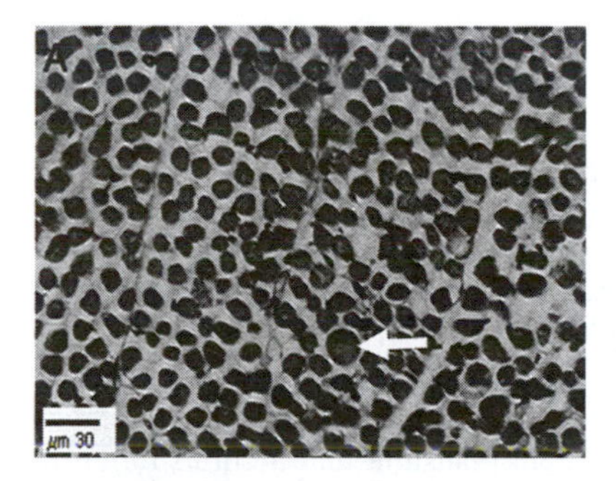

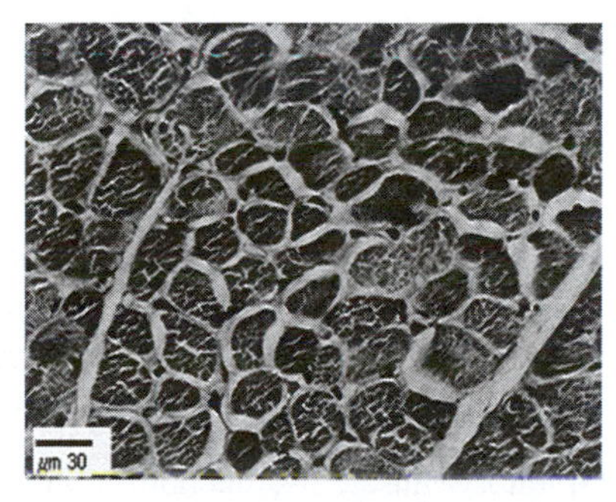

Figure 9 Photomicrographs of transverse sections of diaphragm from an infant ventilated from birth until death at day 47 (*left*) and from an infant ventilated from birth until accidental death at day 3 (*right*). Prolonged mechanical ventilation was associated with reduction in myofiber cross-sectional area. (The white arrow in the left panel indicates an early type I myofiber, also known as Wohlfart type B myofiber.) *Source*: From Ref. 77.

Table 1 Characteristics of Types of Muscle Fibers

	Type I	Type IIa	Type IIx	Type IIb
Contractile properties				
Velocity of shortening	+	++	+++	++++
Tetanic force	+	+	++	++
Endurance	++++	+++	++	+
Work efficiency[a]	+++	++	++	+
Histochemistry				
Mitochondrial volume density	+++	+++	++	+
ATP consumption rate	+	++	+++	++++
Oxidative enzymes	+++	+++	++	+
Glycolytic enzymes	+	++	+++	++++
Glycogen	+	++	++	+++
Capillary supply	+++	+++	++	+
Diameter	+	++	++	+++

A single myosin heavy chain isoform is typically expressed within an adult skeletal muscle fiber. Fibers classified as types I, IIa, IIx, and IIb express myosin heavy chain isoforms I (or slow), IIa, IIx, and IIb, respectively. Type IIx fibers have been reported in peripheral muscles of humans and animals and in the diaphragm of animals. Type IIx fibers have not been reported in the human diaphragm. More than one myosin heavy chain isoform is expressed in a few fibers (about 14% of adult rat diaphragm coexpresses myosin heavy chain isoforms IIb and IIx, and less than 1% coexpresses myosin heavy chain isoforms I and IIa). While the velocity of muscle contraction depends primarily on the myosin heavy chain isoform, the velocity of muscle relaxation is mainly determined by troponin-C calcium binding and release and by calcium reuptake by the sarco-endoplasmic reticulum calcium-adenosine triphosphatase (SERCA). Several SERCA isoenzymes have been identified: SERCA 1 is expressed in type II fibers (fast calcium reuptake); and SERCA 2a is expressed in type I (slow calcium reuptake). The density of pumping sites largely accounts for different rates of calcium uptake in fast- and slow-twitch muscle fibers. Despite this separation of tasks, velocity of contraction and velocity of relaxation tend to parallel each other; type II fibers contract and relax with a greater velocity than type I fibers. Slower velocity of relaxation allows fusion of repetitive twitches at lower frequencies of stimulation as compared with fast relaxations. Impairment of SERCA activity has been implicated in the development of fatigue and in disease states including heart failure and corticosteroid myopathy.

[a]Amount of work performed per unit of adenosine triphosphate consumed.

Abbreviation: ATP, adenosine triphosphate.

Source: From Ref. 40.

18 to 72 hours with those of nine patients ventilated for less than two hours during surgery to remove solitary pulmonary nodules. In this preliminary report, controlled PMV was associated with 40% atrophy of slow fibers and 36% atrophy of fast fibers (Table 1) (78). Atrophy was coupled with increased ubiquitin-proteasome proteolysis (79).

Given the possible relationship between decreases in protein synthesis and ventilator-associated respiratory muscle dysfunction, it would seem plausible that administration of anabolic factors, such as growth hormone, might be beneficial to ventilated patients. Unfortunately, when growth hormone was administered to patients requiring PMV, duration of mechanical ventilation was not decreased nor was muscle strength increased (80). The report that recombinant growth hormone can increase mortality of critically ill patients is a matter of concern (81).

Sepsis-Associated Myopathy

In more than 20% of patients requiring PMV or LTMV, sepsis has been identified as the likely medical diagnosis preceding respiratory failure (37). Sepsis can produce ventilatory failure by causing respiratory muscle dysfunction and by increasing metabolic demands (40). One important mechanism for respiratory muscle dysfunction in septic animals is the cytotoxic effect of nitric oxide and its metabolites (40). To determine whether the inducible nitric oxide synthase pathway contributes to impaired skeletal muscle contractility in humans as well, Lanone et al. obtained samples of the rectus abdominis in 16 septic patients and 21 control subjects (82). The muscles of the patients had lower contractile force and increase in inducible nitric oxide synthase. Immunohistochemical studies revealed the generation of peroxynitrite (a highly reactive oxidant formed by the reaction of nitric oxide with superoxide anion). Exposure of control muscles to the amount of peroxynitrite found in patients caused an irreversible decrease in force generation. These data suggest that one of the mechanisms through which sepsis decreases muscle force is the production of nitric oxide and its toxic by-products.

Intensive Care Unit–Acquired Paralysis

While cared for in the ICU, critically ill patients can develop muscle weakness and, occasionally, paralysis. Some of these patients have evidence of axonal degeneration (Table 2) and denervation atrophy (Fig. 10) (40). This constellation of findings is known as critical illness polyneuropathy. Sepsis and multiple organ failure, although common in these patients, are not essential prerequisites for the development of critical illness polyneuropathy (40). In other patients, rather than axonopathy, there is evidence of isolated myopathy (critical illness myopathy) (Fig. 11) (40). Patients developing isolated myopathy have often been treated with steroids and neuromuscular blocking agents (40).

In the last few years, it has become increasingly apparent that critical illness neuropathy and myopathy often coexist, and it has become common to refer to these patients as simply having ICU-acquired paresis (26,83). ICU-acquired paresis is an independent risk factor of prolonged weaning (26). In an investigation, tight control of hyperglycemia reduced the risk of ICU-acquired paresis and the duration of mechanical ventilation (84).

The functional outcome of ICU-acquired paresis is not uniform, with 50–60% of patients experiencing complete recovery over two weeks to six months (85–87) and 10–30% experiencing persistent disability, including tetraparesis, tetraplegia, or paraplegia (88,89). Whether ICU-acquired paresis can be prevented, and whether that would result in shorter duration of mechanical ventilation, remains unknown.

Acid–Base Disorders

Alkalosis, either metabolic or respiratory, does not affect skeletal muscle function (40). In contrast, whether acidosis, either metabolic or respiratory, impairs respiratory muscle function remains controversial.

Acid–Base Disorders: Metabolic Acidosis

Until recently, there was little doubt that metabolic acidosis could decrease muscle contractility. Purported mechanisms included inhibition of glycolytic rate, reduced Ca^{2+} release from the sarcoplasmic reticulum, and reduction of actin–myosin cross-bridge activation by H^+ competitive inhibition of Ca^{2+} binding to troponin-C (90). Despite the biological plausibility though, investigators have reported no effect or marginal effect

Table 2 Electromyographic Findings

	Axonal injury	Myelin injury	Neuromuscular conduction defect	Myopathy
Compound muscle action potential (amplitude)[a]	Reduced	Normal to slightly reduced	Normal[b]	Normal
Sensory nerve action potential (amplitude)[c]	Reduced	Normal to reduced	Normal	Normal
Conduction velocity	Normal to slightly reduced	Reduced	Normal	Normal
Spontaneous muscle depolarization[d]	Present	Absent	Absent	None to present
Amplitude of compound muscle action potential with stimulation at 3 Hz[e]	Unchanged	Unchanged	Decreased	Unchanged
Motor unit activation	Decreased	Decreased	Normal	Increased

Examples of injuries and deficits: axonal injury, critical illness myopathy; myelin injury, Guillain-Barré; neuromuscular conduction defect, myasthenia, prolonged neuromuscular blockade; myopathy, critical illness myopathy.

Although features of myopathy can be recorded by electromyographic studies, electromyography cannot always distinguish critical illness myopathy from critical illness polyneuropathy, and muscle biopsies may be needed.

[a]Elicited by motor nerve stimulation.

[b]Decreased in the Lambert–Eaton syndrome.

[c]Elicited by sensory nerve stimulation.

[d]Spontaneous muscle depolarization (caused by denervation) is detected by presence of fibrillation potentials and positive sharp waves.

[e]Repetitive nerve stimulation is performed to exclude neuromuscular transmission defects, such as prolonged neuromuscular paralysis.

Source: From Ref. 40.

(63,91) of metabolic acidosis on respiratory muscle function. These negative results are in line with some (92–95), but not all (96,97), recent investigations questioning the inhibitory role of metabolic acidosis on limb muscle contractility at physiological temperatures. Whether severe metabolic acidosis in humans might impair skeletal function by causing a reduced central nervous system drive remains to be demonstrated (63).

Acid–Base Disorders: Respiratory Acidosis

In healthy volunteers, acute increases of arterial carbon dioxide to 54 mmHg (corresponding to a pH of about 7.29) reduces the capacity of the unfatigued diaphragm to generate pressure by 10–30% (Fig. 12) (98). This direct inhibitory effect of respiratory acidosis on respiratory muscle function could provide a potential mechanism for the rapid clinical deterioration that can occur with severe asthma and during COPD exacerbations (98). Yet, the human data suggesting a direct deleterious effect of respiratory acidosis on respiratory muscle function

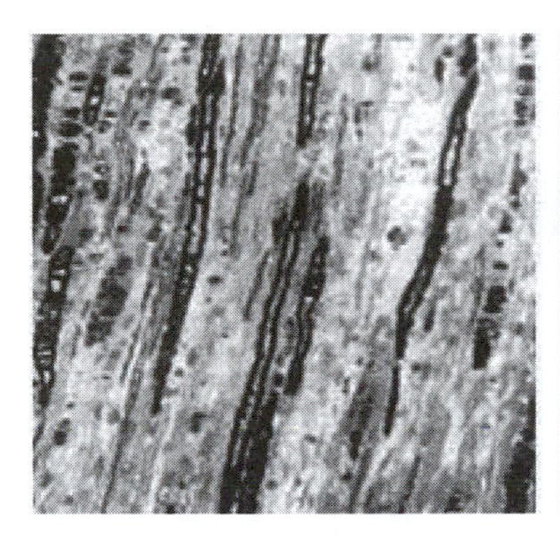
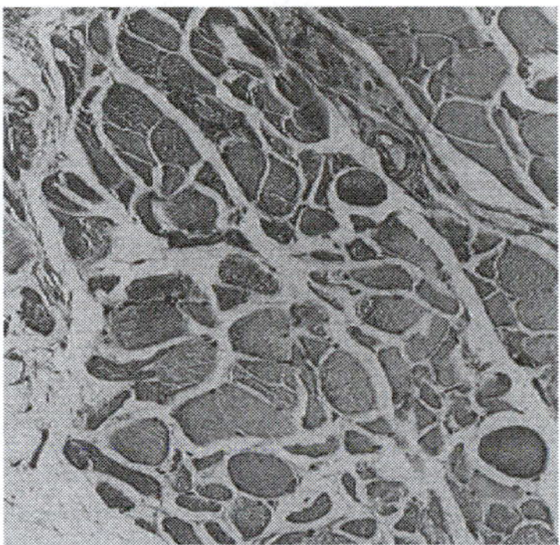

Figure 10 Critical illness polyneuropathy. Transverse section of a peripheral motor nerve (deep peroneal nerve, *left panel*) and of a skeletal muscle (intercostal, *right panel*) in patients who developed profound weakness following a prolonged hospital course characterized by sepsis, multiple organ failure syndrome, and inability to wean from mechanical ventilation. The long thin dark structures are myelin sheaths that contain axons (*left panel*). The axons are degenerating and dying. And, following death, they disintegrate. The myelin surrounding the disintegrating axons collapses around the axonal debris to form ovoids of myelin seen better on the lateral portions of the left micrograph. Amid muscle fibers that are normal in size and shape, there are atrophic ones that appear small and that have developed contours with acute angles (*right panel*). These findings are consistent with denervation atrophy secondary to axonal degeneration, so-called critical illness polyneuropathy. *Source*: From Ref. 129.

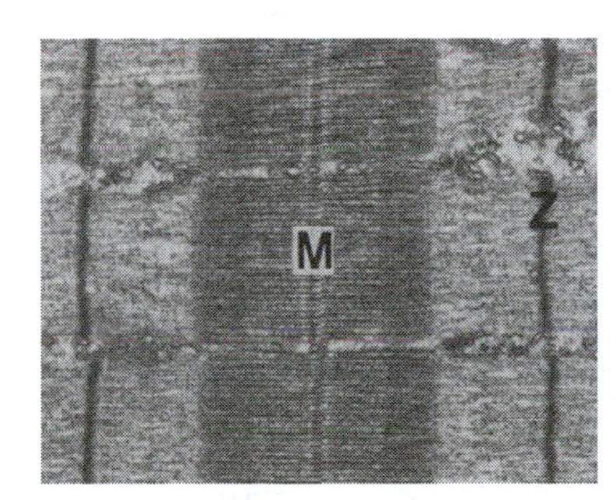

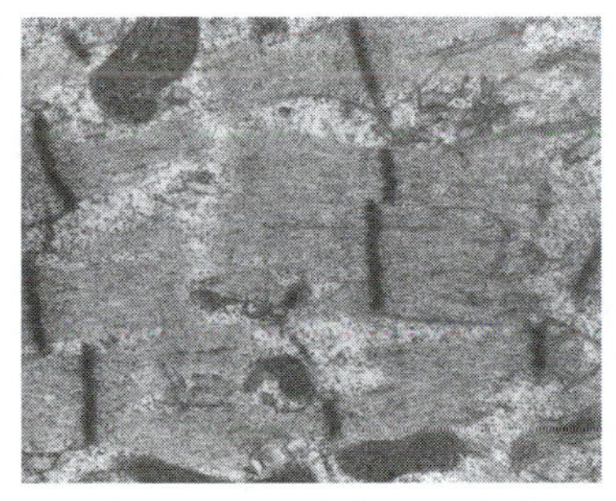

Figure 11 Critical illness myopathy. Electron micrographs of normal skeletal muscle (*right panel*) and skeletal muscle from a patient who developed critical illness myopathy and flaccid quadriplegia, as a result of administration of steroids and the neuromuscular blocking agent vecuronium during a hospitalization with status asthmaticus (*left panel*). Muscle strength returned to normal two months after discontinuation of vecuronium. Compared with the normal structure, the patient developed extensive loss of thick (myosin) myofilaments and relative preservation of thin (actin) filaments (*left panel*). Although this decrease in myosin may be important for the prolonged weakness of critical illness myopathy, impaired muscle membrane excitability is probably more critical during the acute phase (40). M = M-line formed by myosin filaments and M-line proteins; Z = Z-disk formed by a lattice of filaments that join the actin filaments of one sarcomere with the actin filaments of the adjacent sarcomere. *Source*: From Refs. 130, and 131.

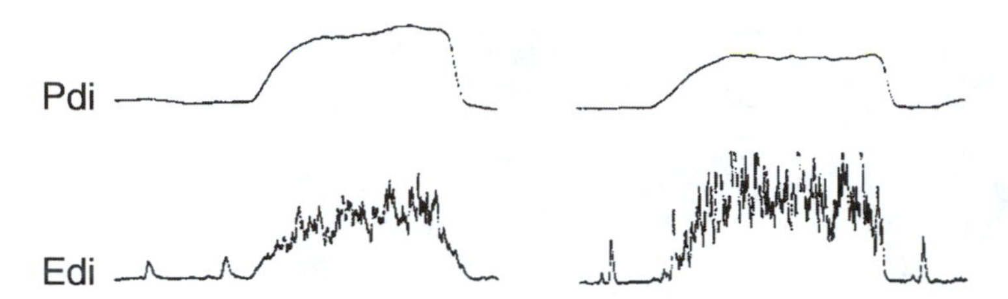

Figure 12 Transdiaphragmatic pressure (Pdi) and electrical activity of the diaphragm (Edi) during a voluntary isometric contraction in a healthy subject during normocapnia (*left panel*) and during acute hypercapnia (end-tidal CO_2, 7.5%, *right panel*). For a given Edi during hypercapnia the pressure output of the diaphragm was decreased. *Abbreviations*: Pdi, transdiaphragmatic pressure; Edi, electrical activity of the diaphragm. *Source*: From Ref. 98.

are not uniform. Some investigators report no change in diaphragmatic contractility when acute respiratory acidosis causes a decrease in pH to about 7.16 to 7.27 (99,100) and no effect on diaphragmatic fatigue 20 to 90 minutes after loading (101).

Electrolyte Disturbances

Respiratory muscle function may be impaired by decreased levels of phosphate, calcium, magnesium, and potassium (40).

Medications

Weakness can result from medications that have a direct myotoxic effect, such as blockade of myocyte glycoprotein synthesis and electron transport caused by statins (inhibitors of the hydroxy-methylglutaryl-coenzyme A reductase) used in patients with hyperlipidemia or nucleoside analogues used in patients with human immunodeficiency virus (40). Weakness can also result from neuromuscular blocking agents and aminoglycosides, which interfere with neuromuscular transmission.

In acutely ventilated patients, paralysis can persist after discontinuation of neuromuscular blocking agents (102–104). Prolonged blockade is estimated to occur in 12–44% of patients receiving pancuronium or vecuronium for one or more days (102–104). Accumulation of metabolites of the neuromuscular blocking agents is responsible for the prolonged blockade (103). In such patients, repetitive nerve stimulation demonstrates a decrement of the compound muscle action potential (Table 2). Recovery from prolonged neuromuscular blockade usually begins within two days of the last dose (102,103), and this fact contrasts with the prolonged course of critical illness like myopathy or neuropathy. It is thus unlikely, if not impossible, for prolonged neuromuscular blockade to cause long-term ventilator dependence. Monitoring of the dose of a neuromuscular blocking agent with a peripheral nerve stimulator may permit faster recovery of neuromuscular function and of spontaneous respiration (104).

Limitations in the Current Classification of Respiratory Muscle Weakness

When studying respiratory muscle weakness, it is necessary to bear in mind our current limited understanding of these disorders. One, the distinction between preexisting conditions and new-onset conditions can be arbitrary. Two, preexisting conditions, such as malnutrition and hyperinflation, can worsen during the course of an unrelated critical illness. Three, the nosology is often unsatisfactory as observed in the nebulous distinction between ICU-acquired paresis and sepsis-associated myopathy or between ICU-acquired paresis and ventilator-associated respiratory muscle dysfunction. Four, disorders in which respiratory muscle weakness is associated with muscle damage can also display some degree of muscle atrophy, as observed with diaphragmatic atrophy in cases of ventilator-associated respiratory muscle dysfunction. Five, limited laboratory specificity to differentiate the different disorders causing weakness in ventilated patients. Lastly, in any given patient more than one mechanism may be responsible for respiratory muscle weakness.

Respiratory Muscle Fatigue

Contractile fatigue occurs when a sufficiently large respiratory load is applied over a sufficiently long period (40). Contractile fatigue can be brief or prolonged. Short-lasting fatigue results from accumulation of inorganic phosphate, failure of the membrane electrical potential to propagate beyond T-tubes, and to a much lesser extent intramuscular acidosis (40). Short-lasting fatigue appears to have a protective function because it may prevent myofiber injury caused by forceful muscle contractions. Long-lasting fatigue is consistent with the development of and the recovery from muscle injury (Fig. 13) (40). Several mechanisms may contribute to muscle injury. These include activation of calpain (a calcium-dependent nonlysosomal protease) and excessive production of reactive oxygen species (40). Muscle injury can also be caused by eccentric contractions (contraction of a muscle while it is stretched by external forces) (40). Eccentric contractions can occur during ineffective

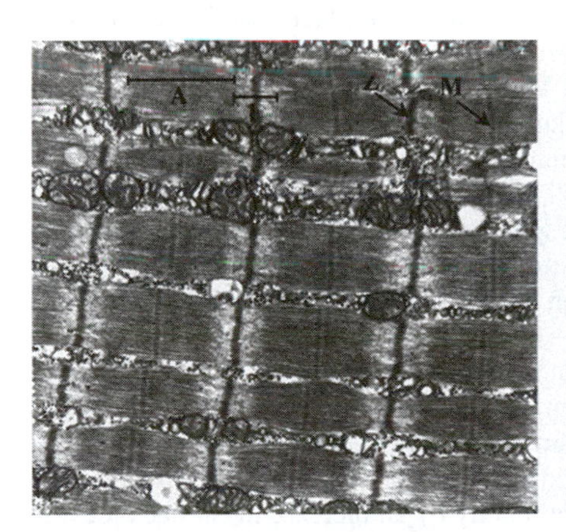

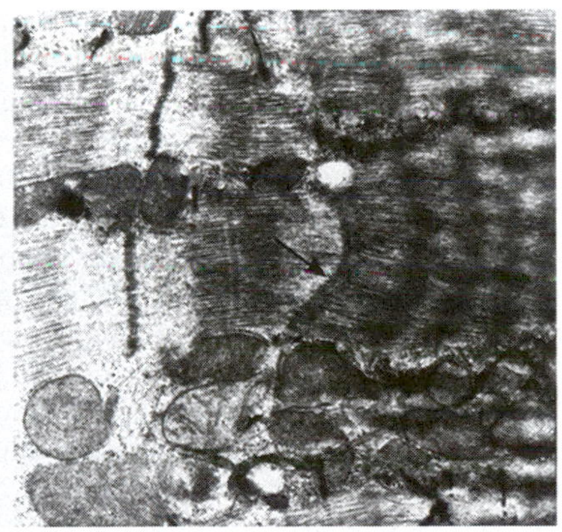

Figure 13 Electron micrographs of longitudinal sections from the costal diaphragm of a healthy control hamster (*left panel*) and a hamster exposed to six days of resistive loading (*right panel*). The left panel shows normal sarcomeres with distinct A-bands, I-bands, Z-bands, and M-lines that are aligned between adjacent myofibrils. The right panel shows load-induced damage recognizable by Z-band streaming (*arrow*) and disruption of sarcomeric structure (*right section of right panel*) with loss of distinct A-bands and I-bands. Z-band streaming is attributed to a loss of cytoskeletal protein elements, such as desmin, α-actinin, and vimentin. Magnification for both micrographs: 16,500x. *Source:* From Ref. 40.

inspiratory efforts, which have been associated with worse weaning outcome both in the acute (105) and chronic settings (106) and with ventilator dependence (41,106).

Whether or not critically ill patients develop short- or long-lasting contractile fatigue of the respiratory muscles is unclear. Patients who fail weaning are at a particular risk of developing fatigue as they experience marked increases in their respiratory load (40). Laghi et al. measured the contractile response of the diaphragm to phrenic nerve stimulation in nine patients who failed a weaning trial; seven patients who were successfully weaned served as control subjects (59). The weaning-failure patients experienced a greater respiratory load. Moreover, the tension–time index of the diaphragm, an index of diaphragm effort, was greater in the failure group than in the success group (40). Nevertheless, not a single patient developed a decrease in twitch pressure elicited by phrenic nerve stimulation (Fig. 14). The failure to develop fatigue is surprising because seven of the nine weaning-failure patients had a tension–time index above 0.15 (the putative threshold for task failure and fatigue). The increase in tension–time index over the course of the weaning trial and predicted time to task failure are shown in Figure 15 (59). At the point that the physician reinstituted mechanical ventilation, patients were predicted to be an average of 13 minutes away from task failure. In other words, patients display clinical manifestations of severe respiratory distress for a substantial time before they develop fatigue. In an ICU setting, these clinical signs will lead attendants to reinstitute mechanical ventilation before fatigue has time to develop.

D. Impaired Cardiovascular Performance

Spontaneous respiratory efforts decrease intrathoracic pressure and, thus, increase the pressure gradient for systemic venous return (107). In addition, decreases in intrathoracic pressure increase left ventricular afterload, causing additional stress on the left ventricle (107). In patients with coronary artery disease, this increased stress can alter myocardial perfusion and cause transient left ventricular dilation (108). The occurrence of myocardial ischemia during periods of spontaneous respiration has been associated with greater risks of weaning failure and ventilator dependence (109,110). Increases in transmural pulmonary artery occlusion pressure during spontaneous respiration (111) may be the central mechanism responsible for ventilator dependence in patients with myocardial ischemia (110) and in patients with impaired left ventricular function (112). Mechanisms by which increases in transmural pulmonary artery occlusion pressure can contribute to ventilator dependence include worsening pulmonary mechanics and decreased gas exchange.

In the acute setting, oxygen consumption at the completion of a weaning trial is equivalent in weaning-success and weaning-failure patients (113). The manner in which the cardiovascular system meets oxygen demands, however, differs between the two groups. In weaning successes, the increase in demand is met mainly by an increase in cardiac index. In weaning failures, the increase in demand is met by an increase in oxygen extraction, resulting in a decrease in mixed venous oxygen saturation. A decrease in mixed venous oxygen saturation is consistent with a failing cardiovascular response to an increased metabolic demand (107).

Nearly 50% of patients requiring PMV or LTMV carry a preexisting diagnosis of coronary artery disease, left ventricular failure, or right ventricular failure (37). Therefore, impaired cardiovascular performance may contribute to ventilator dependence in many patients. So far, few case reports have shown that successful diuresis and weight loss may be

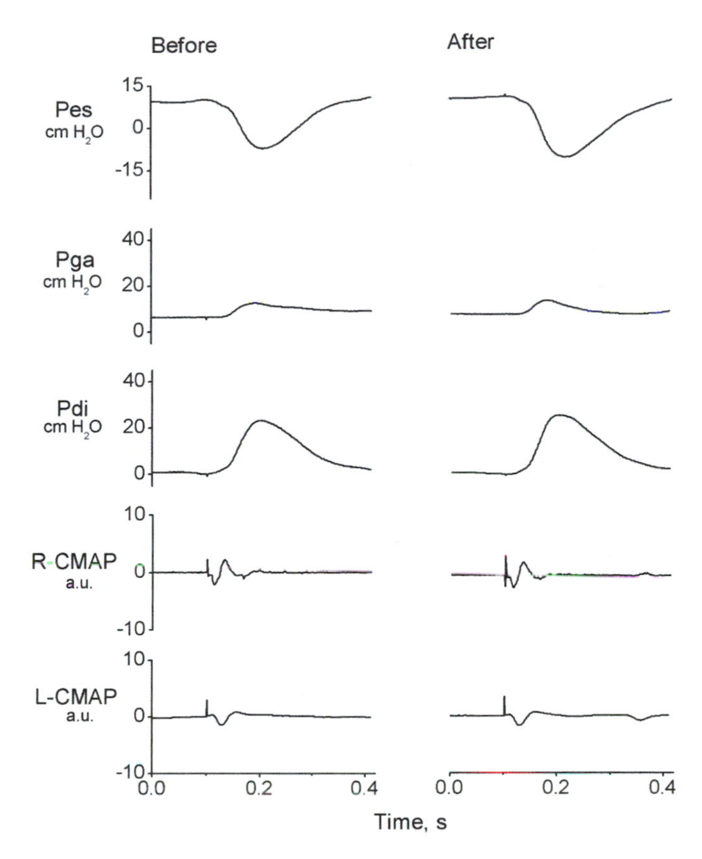

Figure 14 Esophageal pressure (Pes), gastric pressure (Pga), transdiaphragmatic pressure (Pdi), and compound motor action potentials (CAMP) of the right and left hemidiaphragms after phrenic nerve stimulation before (*left*) and after (*right*) a failed trial of weaning. The end-expiratory value of Pes and the amplitude of the right and left CAMPs were the same before and after the trial, indicating that the stimulations were delivered at the same lung volume and that the stimulations achieved the same extent of diaphragmatic recruitment. The amplitude of twitch Pdi elicited by phrenic nerve stimulation was the same before and after weaning. *Abbreviations*: Pes, esophageal pressure; Pga, gastric pressure; Pdi, transdiaphragmatic pressure; CAMP, compound motor action potentials. *Source*: From Ref. 59.

associated with weaning success (111,114). Whether intravenous inotropic agents, such as dobutamine, should be used in difficult-to-wean patients remains controversial (107,115).

V. Psychological Factors

Patients who require either PMV or LTMV are commonly affected by psychological problems, such as anxiety, agitation, delirium, depression, apathy, and posttraumatic stress disorder (21,34,116–118). In a preliminary report of 100 patients requiring prolonged

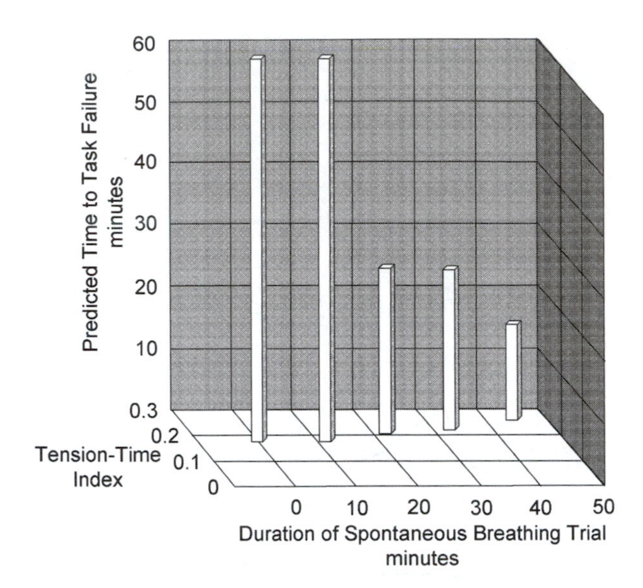

Figure 15 The interrelationship between the duration of a spontaneous breathing trial, tension–time index of the diaphragm, and predicted time to task failure in nine patients who failed a trial of weaning from mechanical ventilation. The patients breathed spontaneously for an average of 44 minutes before a physician terminated the trial. At the start of the trial, tension–time index was 0.17, and the formula of Bellemare and Grassino (132) predicted that patients could sustain spontaneous breathing for another 59 minutes before developing task failure. As the trial progressed, tension–time index increased and predicted time to the development of task failure decreased. At the end of the trial, tension–time index reached 0.26; the fact that patients were predicted to sustain spontaneous breathing for another 13 minutes before developing task failure clarifies why patients did not develop a decrease in diaphragmatic twitch pressure. In other words, physicians interrupted the trial on the basis of clinical manifestations of respiratory distress before patients had sufficient time to develop contractile fatigue. *Source*: From Ref. 40.

ventilation, Dilling et al. recorded an association between anxiety at the time of a spontaneous breathing trial and weaning failure (117).

Possible mechanisms for psychological dysfunction in ventilator-dependent patients include respiratory discomfort, severity of illness, sleep deprivation, sensory deprivation, and medication side effects (116,119,120). The delivery of mechanical ventilation itself can cause psychological dysfunction (34,116). Mechanical ventilation limits mobility, fosters isolation, impairs communication, and interferes with or blocks patient's control on the act of breathing (34).

Aggressive treatment of depression may increase the likelihood of weaning from prolonged ventilation (121,122). Biofeedback, improved patients' environment, communication and mobility, and specialized weaning centers have been used to decrease psychological problems in ventilated patients (34,123–126).

VI. Conclusion

A growing number of survivors of catastrophic diseases requires PMV and may become dependent on LTMV. Unfortunately, limited research on the pathophysiologic mechanisms for ventilator dependency has been performed. Two areas require urgent attention. First, we need a sound nosology of what constitutes prolonged ventilation. Second, once developed, such nosology should allow more meaningful investigation into the mechanisms of ventilator dependence. Identification of these mechanisms would enable a more rational approach to ventilator management of these patients.

References

1. Nava S, Vitacca M. Chronic ventilator facilities. In: Tobin MJ, ed. Principles and Practice of Mechanical Ventilation. 2nd ed. New York: McGraw-Hill Co., 2006:691–704.
2. Kahn JM, Goss CH, Heagerty PJ, et al. Hospital volume and the outcomes of mechanical ventilation. N Engl J Med 2006; 355(1):41–50.
3. Esteban A, Frutos F, Tobin MJ, et al. A comparison of four methods of weaning patients from mechanical ventilation. Spanish Lung Failure Collaborative Group. N Engl J Med 1995; 332 (6):345–350.
4. Brochard L, Rauss A, Benito S, et al. Comparison of three methods of gradual withdrawal from ventilatory support during weaning from mechanical ventilation. Am J Respir Crit Care Med 1994; 150(4):896–903.
5. Nevins ML, Epstein SK. Weaning from prolonged mechanical ventilation. Clin Chest Med 2001; 22(1):13–33.
6. MacIntyre NR, Epstein SK, Carson S, et al. Management of patients requiring prolonged mechanical ventilation: report of a NAMDRC consensus conference. Chest 2005; 128(6): 3937–3954.
7. Nevins ML, Epstein SK. Predictors of outcome for patients with COPD requiring invasive mechanical ventilation. Chest 2001; 119(6):1840–1849.
8. Herridge MS, Cheung AM, Tansey CM, et al. One-year outcomes in survivors of the acute respiratory distress syndrome. N Engl J Med 2003; 348(8):683–693.
9. Gracey DR, Viggiano RW, Naessens JM, et al. Outcomes of patients admitted to a chronic ventilator-dependent unit in an acute-care hospital. Mayo Clin Proc 1992; 67(2):131–136.
10. Kurek CJ, Cohen IL, Lambrinos J, et al. Clinical and economic outcome of patients undergoing tracheostomy for prolonged mechanical ventilation in New York state during 1993: analysis of 6,353 cases under diagnosis-related group 483. Crit Care Med 1997; 25(6):983–988.
11. Seneff MG, Zimmerman JE, Knaus WA, et al. Predicting the duration of mechanical ventilation. The importance of disease and patient characteristics. Chest 1996; 110(2):469–479.
12. HCIA Inc., Ernst & Young LLP, eds. DRG 475 1997. Respiratory system diagnosis with ventilator support. The DRG Handbook: Comparative Clinical and Financial Standards. Boston, NC: Solucient, 1997:308–313.
13. Ely EW, Wheeler AP, Thompson BT, et al. Recovery rate and prognosis in older persons who develop acute lung injury and the acute respiratory distress syndrome. Ann Intern Med 2002; 136(1):25–36.
14. Chao DC, Scheinhorn DJ, Stearn-Hassenpflug M. Impact of renal dysfunction on weaning from prolonged mechanical ventilation. Crit Care (Lond) 1997; 1(3):101–104.
15. Scheinhorn DJ, Chao DC, Stearn-Hassenpflug M, et al. Outcomes in post-ICU mechanical ventilation: a therapist-implemented weaning protocol. Chest 2001; 119(1):236–242.

16. Carson SS, Bach PB, Brzozowski L, et al. Outcomes after long-term acute care. An analysis of 133 mechanically ventilated patients. Am J Respir Crit Care Med 1999; 159(5 pt 1): 1568–1573.
17. Bach PB, Carson SS, Leff A. Outcomes and resource utilization for patients with prolonged critical illness managed by university-based or community-based subspecialists. Am J Respir Crit Care Med 1998; 158(5 pt 1):1410–1415.
18. Nava S, Rubini F, Zanotti E, et al. Survival and prediction of successful ventilator weaning in COPD patients requiring mechanical ventilation for more than 21 days. Eur Respir J 1994; 7(9):1645–1652.
19. Gluck EH. Predicting eventual success or failure to wean in patients receiving long-term mechanical ventilation. Chest 1996; 110(4):1018–1024.
20. Scheinhorn DJ, Hassenpflug MS, Votto JJ, et al. Post-ICU mechanical ventilation at 23 long-term care hospitals: a multicenter outcomes study. Chest 2007; 131(1):85–93.
21. Indihar FJ. A 10-year report of patients in a prolonged respiratory care unit. Minn Med 1991; 74(4):23–27.
22. Engoren MC, Arslanian-Engoren CM. Outcome after tracheostomy for respiratory failure in the elderly. J Intensive Care Med 2005; 20(2):104–110.
23. Garnacho-Montero J, Amaya-Villar R, Garcia-Garmendia JL, et al. Effect of critical illness polyneuropathy on the withdrawal from mechanical ventilation and the length of stay in septic patients. Crit Care Med 2005; 33(2):349–354.
24. Bagley PH, Cooney E. A community-based regional ventilator-weaning unit: development and outcomes. Chest 1997; 111(4):1024–1029.
25. Vieira JM Jr., Castro I, Curvello-Neto A, et al. Effect of acute kidney injury on weaning from mechanical ventilation in critically ill patients. Crit Care Med 2007; 35(1):184–191.
26. De Jonghe B, Bastuji-Garin S, Sharshar T, et al. Does ICU-acquired paresis lengthen weaning from mechanical ventilation. Intensive Care Med 2004; 30(6):1117–1121.
27. Topeli A, Laghi F, Tobin MJ. Effect of closed unit policy and appointing an intensivist in a developing country. Crit Care Med 2005; 33(2):299–306.
28. Thorens JB, Kaelin RM, Jolliet P, et al. Influence of the quality of nursing on the duration of weaning from mechanical ventilation in patients with chronic obstructive pulmonary disease. Crit Care Med 1995; 23(11):1807–1815.
29. Gillespie DJ, Marsh HM, Divertie MB, et al. Clinical outcome of respiratory failure in patients requiring prolonged (greater than 24 hours) mechanical ventilation. Chest 1986; 90(3): 364–369.
30. Sapijaszko MJ, Brant R, Sandham D, et al. Nonrespiratory predictor of mechanical ventilation dependency in intensive care unit patients. Crit Care Med 1996; 24(4):601–607.
31. Douglas SL, Daly BJ, Gordon N, et al. Survival and quality of life: short-term versus long-term ventilator patients. Crit Care Med 2002; 30(12):2655–2662.
32. Classification of disease and functioning and disability. ICD-9-CM National Center for Health Statistics. Available at: www.cdc.gov/nchs/icd9.htm. 2004.
33. Epstein SK. Predicting extubation failure: is it in (on) the cards? Chest 2001; 120(4): 1061–1063.
34. Martin UJ, Criner GJ. Psychological problems in the ventilated patient. In: Tobin MJ, ed. Principles and Practice of Mechanical Ventilation. 2nd ed. New York: McGraw-Hill Co., 2006:1137–1151.
35. Rossi A, Poggi R, Roca J. Physiologic factors predisposing to chronic respiratory failure. Respir Care Clin N Am 2002; 8(3):379–404.
36. Scheinhorn DJ, Hassenpflug M, Artinian BM, et al. Predictors of weaning after 6 weeks of mechanical ventilation. Chest 1995; 107(2):500–505.
37. Scheinhorn DJ, Hassenpflug MS, Votto JJ, et al. Ventilator-dependent survivors of catastrophic illness transferred to 23 long-term care hospitals for weaning from prolonged mechanical ventilation. Chest 2007; 131(1):76–84.

38. West JB. Pulmonary Pathophysiology: The Essentials. 6th ed. Philadelphia: Lippincott Williams & Wilkins, 2003:68:
39. Younes M. Mechanisms of ventilatory failure. Curr Pulmonol 1993; 14:243–292.
40. Laghi F, Tobin MJ. Disorders of the respiratory muscles. Am J Respir Crit Care Med 2003; 168 (1):10–48.
41. Purro A, Appendini L, De Gaetano A, et al. Physiologic determinants of ventilator dependence in long-term mechanically ventilated patients. Am J Respir Crit Care Med 2000; 161(4 pt 1): 1115–1123.
42. Appendini L, Purro A, Patessio A, et al. Partitioning of inspiratory muscle workload and pressure assistance in ventilator-dependent COPD patients. Am J Respir Crit Care Med 1996; 154(5):1301–1309.
43. Capdevila X, Perrigault PF, Ramonatxo M, et al. Changes in breathing pattern and respiratory muscle performance parameters during difficult weaning. Crit Care Med 1998; 26(1):79–87.
44. Laghi F. Assessment of respiratory output in mechanically ventilated patients. Respir Care Clin N Am 2005; 11(2):173–199.
45. Cooper KR, Phillips BA. Effect of short-term sleep loss on breathing. J Appl Physiol 1982; 53:4855–858.
46. Spengler CM, Shea SA. Sleep deprivation per se does not decrease the hypercapnic ventilatory response in humans. Am J Respir Crit Care Med 2000; 161(4 pt 1):1124–1128.
47. Lin MC, Huang CC, Yang CT, et al. Pulmonary mechanics in patients with prolonged mechanical ventilation requiring trachcostomy. Anaesth Intensive Care 1999; 27(6):581–585.
48. Fiastro JF, Habib MP, Shon BY, et al. Comparison of standard weaning parameters and the mechanical work of breathing in mechanically ventilated patients. Chest 1988; 94(2):232–238.
49. Rumbak MJ, Walsh FW, Anderson WM, et al. Significant tracheal obstruction causing failure to wean in patients requiring prolonged mechanical ventilation: a forgotten complication of long-term mechanical ventilation. Chest 1999; 115(4):1092–1095.
50. Law JH, Barnhart K, Rowlett W, et al. Increased frequency of obstructive airway abnormalities with long-term tracheostomy. Chest 1993; 104(1):136–138.
51. Rumbak MJ, Graves AE, Scott MP, et al. Tracheostomy tube occlusion protocol predicts significant tracheal obstruction to air flow in patients requiring prolonged mechanical ventilation. Crit Care Med 1997; 25(3):413–417.
52. Diehl JL, El Atrous S, Touchard D, et al. Changes in the work of breathing induced by tracheotomy in ventilator-dependent patients. Am J Respir Crit Care Med 1999; 159(2): 383–388.
53. Tobin MJ, Laghi F. Monitoring respiratory muscle function. In: Tobin MJ, ed. Principles and Practice of Intensive Care Monitoring. New York: McGraw-Hill Co., 1998:497–544.
54. Tulaimat A, Jubran A, Petrak RA, et al. Mortality in patients admitted to specialized facility for weaning from mechanical ventilation. Am J Respir Crit Care Med 2002; 165:A31.
55. Aldrich TK, Karpel JP, Uhrlass RM, et al. Weaning from mechanical ventilation: adjunctive use of inspiratory muscle resistive training. Crit Care Med 1989; 17(2):143–147.
56. Preusser BA, Winningham ML, Clanton TL. High- vs low-intensity inspiratory muscle interval training in patients with COPD. Chest 1994; 106(1):110–117.
57. Martin AD, Davenport PD, Franceschi AC, et al. Use of inspiratory muscle strength training to facilitate ventilator weaning: a series of 10 consecutive patients. Chest 2002; 122(1):192–196.
58. Martin AD, Davenport PW, Gonzalez-Rothi EM, et al. Inspiratory muscle strength training in failure to wean patients: interim analysis of a controlled trial. Proc Am Thorac Soc 2006, 3.A41.
59. Laghi F, Cattapan SE, Jubran A, et al. Is weaning failure caused by low-frequency fatigue of the diaphragm? Am J Respir Crit Care Med 2003; 167(2):120–127.
60. Laghi F, Jubran A, Topeli A, et al. Effect of lung volume reduction surgery on diaphragmatic neuromechanical coupling at 2 years. Chest 2004; 125(6):2188–2195.

61. Watson AC, Hughes PD, Louise HM, et al. Measurement of twitch transdiaphragmatic, esophageal, and endotracheal tube pressure with bilateral anterolateral magnetic phrenic nerve stimulation in patients in the intensive care unit. Crit Care Med 2001; 29(7):1325–1331.
62. Cattapan SE, Laghi F, Tobin MJ. Can diaphragmatic contractility be assessed by airway twitch pressure in mechanically ventilated patients? Thorax 2003; 58(1):58–62.
63. Laghi F. Hypoventilation and respiratory muscle dysfunction. In: Parrillo JE, Dellinger PR, eds. Critical Care Medicine: Principles of Diagnosis and Management in the Adult. 3rd ed. St. Louis, MO: Mosby Inc., 2007:827–851.
64. Datta D, Scalise P. Hypothyroidism and failure to wean in patients receiving prolonged mechanical ventilation at a regional weaning center. Chest 2004; 126(4):1307–1312.
65. Braun NM, Arora NS, Rochester DF. Respiratory muscle and pulmonary function in polymyositis and other proximal myopathies. Thorax 1983; 38(8):616–623.
66. Gibson GJ, Gilmartin JJ, Veale D, et al. Respiratory muscle function in neuromuscular disease. In: Jones NL, Killian KJ, eds. Breathlessness. The Campbell Symposium. Hamilton, Ontario: Boehringer-Ingelheim, 1992:66–73.
67. Calverley PM, Koulouris NG. Flow limitation and dynamic hyperinflation: key concepts in modern respiratory physiology. Eur Respir J 2005; 25(1):186–199.
68. Kimball WR, Leith DE, Robins AG. Dynamic hyperinflation and ventilator dependence in chronic obstructive pulmonary disease. Am Rev Respir Dis 1982; 126(6):991–995.
69. Coussa ML, Guerin C, Eissa NT, et al. Partitioning of work of breathing in mechanically ventilated COPD patients. J Appl Physiol 1993; 75(4):1711–1719.
70. Cano NJ, Roth H, Court-Ortune, et al. Nutritional depletion in patients on long-term oxygen therapy and/or home mechanical ventilation. Eur Respir J 2002; 20(1):30–37.
71. Cano NJ, Pichard C, Roth H, et al. C-reactive protein and body mass index predict outcome in end-stage respiratory failure. Chest 2004; 126(2):540–546.
72. Lanz JK Jr., Donahoe M, Rogers RM, et al. Effects of growth hormone on diaphragmatic recovery from malnutrition. J Appl Physiol 1992; 73(3):801–805.
73. Mitch WE, Goldberg AL. Mechanisms of muscle wasting. The role of the ubiquitin-proteasome pathway. N Engl J Med 1996; 335(25):1897–1905.
74. Pandya K, Lal C, Scheinhorn D, et al. Hypothyroidism and ventilator dependency. Arch Intern Med 1989; 149(9):2115–2116.
75. Huang CJ, Lin HC. Association between adrenal insufficiency and ventilator weaning. Am J Respir Crit Care Med 2006; 173(3):276–280.
76. Crimi E, Liguori A, Condorelli M, et al. The beneficial effects of antioxidant supplementation in enteral feeding in critically ill patients: a prospective, randomized, double-blind, placebo-controlled trial. Anesth Analg 2004; 99(3):857–863.
77. Knisely AS, Leal SM, Singer DB. Abnormalities of diaphragmatic muscle in neonates with ventilated lungs. J Pediatr 1988; 113(6):1074–1077.
78. Levine S, Nguyen T, Friscia M, et al. Ventilator-induced atrophy in human diaphragm myofibers. Proc Am Thorac Soc 2006; 3:A27.
79. Nguyen T, Friscia M, Kaiser LR, et al. Ventilator-induced proteolysis in human diaphragm myofibers. Proc Am Thorac Soc 2006; 3:A259.
80. Pichard C, Kyle U, Chevrolet JC, et al. Lack of effects of recombinant growth hormone on muscle function in patients requiring prolonged mechanical ventilation: a prospective, randomized, controlled study. Crit Care Med 1996; 24(3):403–413.
81. Takala J, Ruokonen E, Webster NR, et al. Increased mortality associated with growth hormone treatment in critically ill adults. N Engl J Med 1999; 341(11):785–792.
82. Lanone S, Mebazaa A, Heymes C, et al. Muscular contractile failure in septic patients: role of the inducible nitric oxide synthase pathway. Am J Respir Crit Care Med 2000; 162(6): 2308–2315.

83. De Jonghe B, Sharshar T, Lefaucheur JP, et al. Paresis acquired in the intensive care unit: a prospective multicenter study. JAMA 2002; 288(22):2859–2867.
84. Hermans G, Wilmer A, Meersseman W, et al. Impact of intensive insulin therapy on neuromuscular complications and ventilator dependency in the medical intensive care unit. Am J Respir Crit Care Med 2007; 175(5):480–489.
85. Leatherman JW, Fluegel WL, David WS, et al. Muscle weakness in mechanically ventilated patients with severe asthma. Am J Respir Crit Care Med 1996; 153(5):1686–1690.
86. Latronico N, Shehu I, Seghelini E. Neuromuscular sequelae of critical illness. Curr Opin Crit Care 2005; 11(4):381–390.
87. Larsson L, Li X, Edstrom L, et al. Acute quadriplegia and loss of muscle myosin in patients treated with nondepolarizing neuromuscular blocking agents and corticosteroids: mechanisms at the cellular and molecular levels. Crit Care Med 2000; 28(1):34–45.
88. de Seze M, Petit H, Wiart L, et al. Critical illness polyneuropathy. A 2-year follow-up study in 19 severe cases. Eur Neurol 2000; 43(2):61–69.
89. Fletcher SN, Kennedy DD, Ghosh IR, et al. Persistent neuromuscular and neurophysiologic abnormalities in long-term survivors of prolonged critical illness. Crit Care Med 2003; 31 (4):1012–1016.
90. Gladden LB. Lactate metabolism: a new paradigm for the third millennium. J Physiol 2004; 558(pt 1):5–30.
91. Coast JR, Shanely RA, Lawler JM, et al. Lactic acidosis and diaphragmatic function in vitro. Am J Respir Crit Care Med 1995; 152(5 pt 1):1648–1652.
92. Posterino GS, Dutka TL, Lamb GD. L(+)-Lactate does not affect twitch and tetanic responses in mechanically skinned mammalian muscle fibres. Pflugers Arch 2001; 442(2):197–203.
93. Degroot M, Massie BM, Boska M, et al. Dissociation of [H+] from fatigue in human muscle detected by high time resolution 31P-NMR. Muscle Nerve 1993; 16(1):91–98.
94. Westerblad H, Allen DG, Lannergren J. Muscle fatigue: lactic acid or inorganic phosphate the major cause? News Physiol Sci 2002; 17:17–21.
95. Nielsen OB, de Paoli F, Overgaard K. Protective effects of lactic acid on force production in rat skeletal muscle. J Physiol 2001; 536(pt 1):161–166.
96. Knuth ST, Dave H, Peters JR, et al. Low cell pH depresses peak power in rat skeletal muscle fibres at both 30 degrees C and 15 degrees C: implications for muscle fatigue. J Physiol 2006; 575(pt 3):887–899.
97. Kristensen M, Albertsen J, Rentsch M, et al. Lactate and force production in skeletal muscle. J Physiol 2005; 562(pt 2):521–526.
98. Juan G, Calverley P, Talamo C, et al. Effect of carbon dioxide on diaphragmatic function in human beings. N Engl J Med 1984; 310(14):874–879.
99. Vianna LG, Koulouris N, Moxham J. Lack of effect of acute hypoxia and hypercapnia on muscle relaxation rate in man. Rev Esp Fisiol 1993; 49(1):7–15.
100. Mador MJ, Wendel T, Kufel TJ. Effect of acute hypercapnia on diaphragmatic and limb muscle contractility. Am J Respir Crit Care Med 1997; 155(5):1590–1595.
101. Rafferty GF, Lou HM, Polkey MI, et al. Effect of hypercapnia on maximal voluntary ventilation and diaphragm fatigue in normal humans. Am J Respir Crit Care Med 1999; 160(5 pt 1): 1567–1571.
102. de Lemos JM, Carr RR, Shalansky KF, et al. Paralysis in the critically ill: intermittent bolus pancuronium compared with continuous infusion. Crit Care Med 1999; 27(12):2648–2655.
103. Segredo V, Caldwell JE, Matthay MA, et al. Persistent paralysis in critically ill patients after long-term administration of vecuronium. N Engl J Med 1992; 327(8):524–528.
104. Rudis MI, Sikora CA, Angus E, et al. A prospective, randomized, controlled evaluation of peripheral nerve stimulation versus standard clinical dosing of neuromuscular blocking agents in critically ill patients. Crit Care Med 1997; 25(4):575–583.

105. Thille AW, Rodriguez P, Cabello B, et al. Patient-ventilator asynchrony during assisted mechanical ventilation. Intensive Care Med 2006; 32(10):1515–1522.
106. Chao DC, Scheinhorn DJ, Stearn-Hassenpflug M. Patient-ventilator trigger asynchrony in prolonged mechanical ventilation. Chest 1997; 112(6):1592–1599.
107. Pinsky MR. Effect of mechanical ventilation on heart-lung interactions. In: Tobin MJ, ed. Principles and Practice of Mechanical Ventilation. New York: McGraw-Hill Co., 2006:729–757.
108. Hurford WE, Lynch KE, Strauss HW, et al. Myocardial perfusion as assessed by thallium-201 scintigraphy during the discontinuation of mechanical ventilation in ventilator-dependent patients. Anesthesiology 1991; 74(6):1007–1016.
109. Srivastava S, Chatila W, Amoateng-Adjepong Y, et al. Myocardial ischemia and weaning failure in patients with coronary artery disease: an update. Crit Care Med 1999; 27(10):2109–2112.
110. Hurford WE, Favorito F. Association of myocardial ischemia with failure to wean from mechanical ventilation. Crit Care Med 1995; 23(9):1475–1480.
111. Lemaire F, Teboul JL, Cinotti L, et al. Acute left ventricular dysfunction during unsuccessful weaning from mechanical ventilation. Anesthesiology 1988; 69(2):171–179.
112. Nozawa E, Azeka E, Ignez ZM, et al. Factors associated with failure of weaning from long-term mechanical ventilation after cardiac surgery. Int Heart J 2005; 46(5):819–831.
113. Jubran A, Mathru M, Dries D, et al. Continuous recordings of mixed venous oxygen saturation during weaning from mechanical ventilation and the ramifications thereof. Am J Respir Crit Care Med 1998; 158(6):1763–1769.
114. Scheinhorn D. Increase in serum albumin and decrease in body weight correlate with weaning from prolonged mechanical ventilation. Am Rev Respir Dis 1992; 145:A522.
115. Beach T, Millen E, Grenvik A. Hemodynamic response to discontinuance of mechanical ventilation. Crit Care Med 1973; 1(2):85–90.
116. Banzett RB, Brown R. Addressing respiratory discomfort in the ventilated patient. In: Tobin MJ, ed. Principles and Practice of Mechanical Ventilation. 2nd ed. New York: McGraw-Hill Co., 2006:1153–1162.
117. Dilling D, Duffner LA, Lawn G, et al. Anxiety levels in patients being weaned from mechanical ventilation. Proc Am Thorac Soc 2005; 2:A161.
118. Ramana RD, Lawn G, Kelly J, et al. Can anxiety be measured in patients weaning from prolonged mechanical ventilation? Proc Am Thorac Soc 2006; 3:A43.
119. Hanly PJ. Sleep in the ventilated patient. In: Tobin MJ, ed. Principles and Practice of Mechanical Ventilation. 2nd ed. New York: McGraw-Hill Co., 2006:1173–1183.
120. Dubois MJ, Bergeron N, Dumont M, et al. Delirium in an intensive care unit: a study of risk factors. Intensive Care Med 2001; 27(8):1297–1304.
121. Johnson CJ, Auger WR, Fedullo PF, et al. Methylphenidate in the 'hard to wean' patient. J Psychosom Res 1995; 39(1):63–68.
122. Rothenhausler HB, Ehrentraut S, von Degenfeld G, et al. Treatment of depression with methylphenidate in patients difficult to wean from mechanical ventilation in the intensive care unit. J Clin Psychiatry 2000; 61(10):750–755.
123. Holliday JE, Hyers TM. The reduction of weaning time from mechanical ventilation using tidal volume and relaxation biofeedback. Am Rev Respir Dis 1990; 141(5 pt 1):1214–1220.
124. Acosta F. Biofeedback and progressive relaxation in weaning the anxious patient from the ventilator: a brief report. Heart Lung 1988; 17(3):299–301.
125. Martin UJ, Hincapie L, Nimchuk M, et al. Impact of whole-body rehabilitation in patients receiving chronic mechanical ventilation. Crit Care Med 2005; 33(10):2259–2265.
126. Elpern EH, Silver MR, Rosen RL, et al. The noninvasive respiratory care unit. Patterns of use and financial implications. Chest 1991; 99(1):205–208.
127. Tobin MJ and Jubran A. Pathophysiology of failure to wean from mechanical ventilation. Schweiz Med Wochenschr 1994; 124:2139–2145.

128. Laghi F, Jubran A, Topeli A, et al. Effect of lung volume reduction surgery on neuromechanical coupling of the diaphragm. Am J Respir Crit Care Med 1998; 157:475.
129. Zochodne DW, Bolton CF, Wells GA, et al. Critical illness polyneuropathy: a complication of sepsis and multiple organ failure. Brain 1987; 110:819.
130. Eisenberg BR. In: Bradley WG, Gardner-Medwin D, Walton JN, eds. Recent Advances in Myology. Amsterdam: Excerpta Medica, 1975.
131. Danon MJ, Carpenter S. Myopathy with thick filament (myosin) loss following prolonged paralysis with vecuronium during steroid treatment. Muscle Nerve 1991; 14:1131.
132. Bellemare F and, Grassino A. Effect of pressure and timing of contraction on human diaphragm fatigue. J Appl Physiol 1982; 53:1190.

6
Weaning Protocols, Including Noninvasive Ventilation

MICHELE VITACCA
Fondazione S. Maugeri, IRCCS, Lumezzane (BS), Italy

I. Introduction

In modern clinical practice, there is considerable confusion regarding ventilator management, especially as it pertains to weaning decisions, timing of extubation, commencement of the weaning process, use of different modes of ventilation, and identification of a failed weaning trial. There is also a debate about the composition of the team involved in the weaning process, the weaning approaches for different diseases, and the definition of a failed weaning trial. During unplanned extubation, not all patients require reinstitution of mechanical ventilation (MV). It has been reported that in fully ventilated patients who experienced unplanned extubation, 23% had no further need for MV and in those already involved with the weaning process, 69% no longer required MV (1,2).

These data reinforce the idea that weaning is rarely started too early and often it may be started later than necessary. Several studies have attempted to assess the best methods for discontinuing ventilatory support at the earliest possible time. Butler et al. (3) concluded from a review of published weaning studies that they could not identify one superior weaning technique from among the three most popular modes: T-piece trial, pressure support ventilation (PSV), or synchronized intermittent mandatory ventilation (SIMV). Esteban and Brochard (4,5) performed two important multicenter trials in the mid 1990s. Both studies compared the following methods: T-piece trials, PSV, and SIMV. In Brochard's study (4) of 456 patients, the authors concluded that weaning outcome was influenced by the ventilator strategy, and that the use of PSV resulted in a significant improvement over protocols involving the other two techniques. In contrast, Esteban et al. (5), in their study of 546 patients, noted that a once-daily trial of spontaneous T-piece breathing resulted in extubation three times faster than SIMV and twice as fast as PSV, with equal success rates.

A subsequent report by Esteban et al. (6) on the same group of patients concluded that successful extubation could be achieved after a shorter period of spontaneous breathing than previously reported (30 min vs. 120 min). In both landmark studies, strict protocols were followed by experienced researchers (4,5) making it difficult to explain the different conclusions. During weaning, the method employed may be less important than the confidence and familiarity that the technique adopted and the same mode of weaning may produce different outcomes, depending on the underlying diagnostic categories.

Table 1 Tips for Implementation of Therapist-Driven Weaning Protocols

Identify the patient-care issues
Test lengths of stay and complications rates of your institution
Design evidence-based protocols that are reviewed by local experts
Change the "weaning culture"
Create a team approach to include physicians, nonphysician health professionals, managers, and ethicists
Define local goals
Promote dedicated personnel
Educate through feedback, monitoring of appropriate outcomes, and ongoing protocol review.
Avoid rigid interpretation
Preserve clinical judgment

Source: From Ref. 8.

II. Weaning Protocols

Recent papers have emphasized the value of using standardized protocols to facilitate weaning. These weaning protocols (WP) translate medical knowledge and opinion into a care plan or algorithm so that actions are directed by objective changes in patient variables (7,8). A WP team requires a physician, a nurse, and a respiratory therapist (RT) (7,8). The daily plan of a WP consists of functional activities followed by a rest period after which weaning is initiated in the optimal position, i.e., seated in bed or in a chair (7,8). Effective weaning also addresses prevention and amelioration of the deleterious effects of bed rest, ensuring good communication, and addressing emotional support to promote psychological well being (7,8). Table 1 shows recommendations and tips for implementations of these protocols and Table 2 proposes an example of a WP (9).

III. Results of Weaning Protocols

Saura et al. (10) reported that following the implementation of a WP, the initial spontaneous breathing trial was the most important factor for the success of extubation. Similar results were found by Ely (11) who demonstrated that daily screening of the respiratory function of ventilated patients, performed by nurses or RTs and followed by spontaneous breathing (SB) trials, reduced the duration of ventilation as well as the cost of intensive care and was associated with fewer complications. In this study (11) control subjects were screened daily, but did not undergo SB trials. Neither the mode of ventilation nor the weaning strategy used by the attending physicians was specified. The use of SIMV or controlled modalities could have influenced final results more than the lack of a specific therapist-driven protocol (TDP). Kollef et al. (12) also emphasized that objective "scientific" methods may improve outcomes in mechanically ventilated patients. Horst et al. (13) showed a decrease in ventilation time with a standardized WP in 515 patients admitted to a surgical intensive care unit (ICU), and both Kollef (14) and Kress (15) demonstrated that the abuse of continuous sedation prolonged weaning attempts. Despite reminders, education sessions, and team involvement, adherence to an evidence-based MV WP may be low, particularly in the larger ICUs.

Table 2 Example of a Weaning Protocol

Question 1
Is the minute ventilation $\leq$ 15 L/min; $FiO_2 \leq 60\%$; PEEP $\leq$ 10 cmH_2O; is the patient alert?
If no, re-evaluate daily.
If yes, start assisted ventilation.

Question 2
Does patient present the following parameters:
Minute ventilation < 15 L/min; $FiO_2 \leq 40\%$; PEEP $\leq$ 6 cmH_2O; HR < 140 b/min; $PaO_2/FiO_2 \geq 200$; f/VT $\leq$ 105; MIP $\geq$ 20 cmH_2O; RR < 25 a/min; pH > 7.35; systolic pressure > 100 and <150 mmHg; SaO_2 > 90%; presence of cough, good neurological status, no agitation; no sedatives; no vasopressors; no arrhythmias?
If no, reevaluate daily.
If yes, start spontaneous breathing trial with artificial nose or CPAP 5 cmH_2O or PSV 7 cmH_2O.

Question 3
Does the patient present signs of distress as RR > 35/min; SaO_2 < 90% with $FiO_2 \geq 40\%$; HR > 145 b/min or increase in HR > 20%; arrhythmias; systolic pressure > 180 or < 70 mmHg; agitation?
If no distress signs after 120 minutes, extubate patient or stop ventilation.
If yes under spontaneous breathing repeat the test during PSV 7–10 cmH_2O
If yes under spontaneous breathing and PSV 7–10 cmH_2O start the weaning process using:
Protocol A: Decrease the level of PSV by 2 cmH_2O twice a day and in case of distress, go back to previous step
Protocol B: Increase the number of times of spontaneous breathing, such as 30 minutes for 1, 2, 4, 8 hours and in case of distress, go back to previous step

Abbreviations: FiO_2, fraction of inspired O_2; PEEP, positive end-expiratory pressure; HR, heart rate; f/VT, frequency to tidal volume ratio; MIP, maximal inspiratory pressure; RR, respiratory rate; PSV, pressure support ventilation.
Source: From Ref. 9.

Implementation of a WP in the clinical setting was reported by Ely (16) who showed that implementation of a validated WP is feasible as a TDP, without daily supervision by a physician or a specific team. Scheinhorn (17) tested the variance of application of a well-constructed WP, showing that both physicians and RTs may be confident about this approach. Smyrnos (18) followed a WP over two years and noted a progressive improvement of important outcomes, such as ICU length of stay, days of MV, and costs. After implementation of a model for accelerating improvement to use WPs among a large multidisciplinary team, McLean (19) improved adherence to protocol-directed weaning, reducing the rate of unsuccessful extubations. The use of a WP has decreased the occurrence of ventilator-acquired pneumonia (VAP), especially in trauma patients (20,21). The importance of a motivated weaning team is frequently underscored (22,23), as has the importance of technology to improve the use of WPs (24), a collaborative practice program (25) and a multidisciplinary clinical pathway for long-term MV patients (26). The nurse is an essential member of the ICU weaning team because of a combination of accessibility, expertise, familiarity with the family, teaching of other staff, and fluency with protocols (26–28). Vitacca et al. (9) showed that SB trials and decreasing levels of inspiratory pressure support are equally effective in weaning chronic obstructive pulmonary disease (COPD) tracheotomized patients undergoing MV for more than 15 days. This study also showed that the application of a well-defined protocol, independent of the mode used, was associated with greater

Table 3 Summary of For and Against Opinions on Using a Weaning Protocol

For a weaning protocol
A strategy to reduce the occurrence of medical errors, omissions or delays, promotes multidisciplinary care, standardized approaches are easier to absorb, focus on weaning process, new approach with automated reminders, identification of patient's problems and assistance in overcoming barriers to weaning, a simpler approach which could be automated, easier to compare for clinical research, quality assurance and risk management.
Against a weaning protocol
Poor reliability for all conditions, differences in patient history and behavior, some not for intubated and tracheotomized patients, less useful in complex patients, omission of close attention to the patient, requirement of ongoing staff education, reduced ICU time shifts the length of stay and costs to another area, too rigid-cookbook style, not necessarily faster, nonphysician unable to modulate a therapist driven protocol, team conflicts, hard to demonstrate cost reductions

weaning success rates, shorter MV times, and shorter lengths of stay in the hospital and in the weaning unit, compared with usual clinical practice. In patients, following coronary artery bypass surgery, a standardized WP and an auto mode ventilator system able to modulate assisted and controlled assistance, further reduced the time to extubation (29).

In neurosurgical patients (30), infants or children (31), traumatic patients (32), or ICUs with physicians with a high level of interest in weaning (33), WPs have not demonstrated superiority over usual care performed by physicians. When the number of physician-hours per bed is very high (9.5 physician-hrs/bed/day) protocols may not be necessary. Some clinicians use a template to promote discussion and decisions on MV. Table 3 summarizes some for and against opinions on the use of a WP.

IV. Weaning Protocols with Noninvasive Mechanical Ventilation

In a multicenter Italian study (34), 50 patients intubated during emergency situations, were randomized to either extubation with immediate application of noninvasive ventilation (NIV) or to weaning with the endotracheal tube in place. The mean MV duration, ICU stay, and 60-day mortality were significantly reduced in the noninvasively ventilated group. None of the NIV-weaned patients developed nosocomial pneumonia whereas seven (28%) of those treated invasively did. Ferrer et al. (35) showed that the use of NIV during weaning reduced the duration of ventilation as well as infectious complications among patients unable to wean. Similarly, Squadrone et al. (36) demonstrated that continuous positive airway pressure (CPAP) decreased the incidence of endotracheal intubation in patients who developed hypoxemia after a major elective abdominal surgery. In contrast with previous experiences, a recent study by Esteban et al. (37) reported that NIV in PSV modality neither prevented the need for reintubation nor reduced mortality in unselected patients with respiratory failure after extubation. More recently, NIV was found to be more effective than standard medical therapy in preventing postextubation respiratory failure (38) and in decreasing ICU mortality (39) in a population considered at high risk for this complication. The beneficial effects of NIV in improving survival among hypercapneic patients with chronic respiratory disorders warrant new prospective clinical trials (40).

V. Final Recommendations

- Protocols and clinical guidelines have already been introduced to the ICUs and should be encouraged.
- An early SB or PSV trial should be repeated daily in difficult-to-wean patients.
- Weaning protocols are necessary to assist junior physicians, especially in ICUs where staff turnover is high.
- WPs may be especially useful when nonphysician healthcare providers play a major role in weaning or when physician availability is limited.
- A limitation of WPs is their lack of disease specificity.
- WPs should be modified to accommodate the setting, the team, the time used for the application of weaning, and the patient's underlying condition.
- Weaning is only a component of management for patients with complex multiorgan conditions.
- The potential role of NIV during weaning needs further clarification.

VI. Conclusion

In conclusion, WPs should (1) be used routinely for weaning; (2) not be too rigid but guide patient care; (3) represent an opportunity for clinical evaluation; and (4) help to safely and efficiently liberate patients from MV.

References

1. Betbesé AJ, Pérez M, Bak E, et al. A prospective study of unplanned endotracheal extubation in intensive care unit patients. Crit Care Med 1998; 26:1180–1186.
2. Epstein SK, Nevins ML, Chung J. Effect of unplanned extubation on outcome of mechanical ventilation. Am J Respir Crit Care Med 2000; 161:1912–1916.
3. Butler R, Keenan SP, Inman KJ, et al. Is there a preferred technique for weaning the difficult-to-wean patient? A systematic review of the literature. Crit Care Med, 1999; 27:2331–2336.
4. Brochard L., Rauss A, Benito S, et al. Comparison of three methods of gradual withdrawal from ventilatory support during weaning from mechanical ventilation. Am J Respir Crit Care Med 1994; 150:896–903.
5. Esteban A, Frutos F, Tobin MJ, et al. A comparison of four methods of weaning patients from mechanical ventilation. N Engl J Med 1995; 332:345–350.
6. Esteban A, Alia I, Tobin MJ, et al. Effect of spontaneous breathing trial duration on outcome of attempts to discontinue mechanical ventilation. Am J Respir Crit Care Med 1999; 159:512–518.
7. Durbin CG Jr. Therapist-driven protocols in adult intensive care unit patients. Respir Care Clin N Am 1996; 2:105–116.
8. ACCP, AARC, ACCCM task force.. Evidence based guidelines for weaning and discontinuing ventilatory support. Chest 2001; 120:75s–395s.
9. Vitacca M, Vianello A, Colombo D, et al. Comparison of two methods for weaning COPD patients requiring mechanical ventilation for more than 15 days. Am J Respir Crit Care Med 2001; 164:225–230.
10. Saura P, Blanch L, Mestre J, et al. Clinical consequences of the implementation of a weaning protocol. Intensive Care Med 1996; 22:1052–1056.
11. Ely EW, Baker AM, Dunagan DP, et al. Effect of the duration of mechanical ventilation of identifying patients capable of breathing spontaneously. N Engl J Med 1996; 335:1864–1869.

12. Kollef MH, Shapiro SD, Silver P, et al. A randomized, controlled trial of protocol-directed versus physician-directed weaning from mechanical ventilation. Crit Care Med 1997; 25:567–574.
13. Horst HM, Mouro D, Hall-Jenssens RA, et al. Decrease in ventilation time with a standardized weaning process. Arch Surg 1998; 133:483–489.
14. Kollef MH, Levy NT, Ahrens TS, et al. The use of continuous IV-sedation is associated with prolongation of mechanical ventilation. Chest 1998; 114:541–548.
15. Kress JP, Pohlman AS, O'Connor MF, et al. Daily interruption of sedative infusions in critically ill patients undergoing mechanical ventilation. N Engl J Med 2000; 342:1471–1477.
16. Ely EW, Bennett PA, Bowton DL, et al. Large scale implementation of a respiratory therapist-driven protocol for ventilator weaning. Am J Respir Crit Care Med 1999; 159:439–446.
17. Scheinhorn D, Chao DC, Stearn-Hassenpflug M, et al. Outcome in post-ICU mechanical ventilation. A therapist implemented weaning protocol. Chest 2001; 119:236–242.
18. Smyrnios NA, Connolly A, Wilson MM, et al. Effects of a multifaceted, multidisciplinary hospital-wide quality improvement program on weaning from MV. Crit Care Med 2002; 30:1224–1230.
19. McLean SE, Jensen LA, Schroeder DG, et al. Improving adherence to a mechanical ventilation weaning protocol for critically ill adults: outcomes after an implementation program. Am J Crit Care 2006; 15:299–309.
20. Marelich GP, Murin S, Battistella F, et al. Protocol weaning of mechanical ventilation in medical and surgical patients by respiratory care practitioners and nurses. Effect on weaning time and incidence of ventilator-associated pneumonia, Chest 2000; 118:459–467.
21. Dries DJ, McGonigal MD, Malian MS, et al. Protocol driven ventilator weaning reduces use of MV rate of early reintubation and VAP. J Trauma 2004; 56:943–952.
22. Henneman E, Dracup K, Ganz T, et al. Effect of a collaborative weaning plan on patient outcome in the critical care setting. Crit Care Med 2001; 29:297–303.
23. Chan PK, Fischer S, Stewart TE, et al. Practising evidence-based medicine: the design and implementation of multidisciplinary team-driven extubation protocol. Crit Care 2001; 5:349–354.
24. Iregui M, Ward S, Clinikscale D, et al. Use of handheld computer by respiratory care practitioners to improve the efficacy of weaning patients from MV. Crit Care Med 2002; 30: 2038–2043.
25. Grap MJ, Strickland D, Tormey L, et al. Collaborative practice: development, implementation, and evaluation of a weaning protocol for patients receiving mechanical ventilation. Am J Crit Care 2003; 12:454–460.
26. Burns SM, Earven S, Ficher C, et al. Implementation of an institutional program to improve clinical and financial outcomes of mechanically ventilated patients: one year outcomes and lessons learned. Crit Care Med 2003; 31:2752–2763.
27. Hoffman LA, Happ MB, Scharfenberg C, et al. Perceptions of physicians, nurses, and respiratory therapists about the role of acute care nurse practitioners. Am J Crit Care 2004; 13:480–488.
28. Tonnelier JM, Prat G, Le Gal G, et al. Impact of a nurses' protocol-directed weaning procedure on outcomes in patients undergoing mechanical ventilation for longer than 48 hours: a prospective cohort study with a matched historical control group. Crit Care 2005; 9:R83–R89.
29. Hendrix H, Kaiser ME, Yusen RD, et al. A randomized trial of automated versus conventional protocol-driven weaning from mechanical ventilation following coronary artery bypass surgery. Eur J Cardiothorac Surg 2006; 29:957–963.
30. Namen AM, Ely W, Tatter SB, et al. Predictors of successful extubation in neurological patients. Am J Respir Crit Care Med 2001; 163:658–664.
31. Randolph AG, Wypij D, Venkataraman ST, et al. Effect of mechanical ventilator weaning protocols on respiratory outcomes in infants and children. A randomized controlled trial, JAMA 2002; 288:2561–2568.

32. Duane TM, Riblet JL, Golay D, et al. Protocol driven ventilator management in a trauma Intensive care unit population. Arch Surg 2002; 137:1223–1227.
33. Krishan JA, Moore D, Robeson C, et al. A prospective controlled trial of a protocol-based strategy to discontinue mechanical ventilation. Am J Respir Crit Care Med 2004; 169:673–678.
34. Nava S, Ambrosino N, Clini E, et al. Noninvasive mechanical ventilation in the weaning of patients with respiratory failure due to chronic obstructive pulmonary disease. A randomized controlled trial. Ann Intern Med 1998; 128:721–728.
35. Ferrer M, Esquinas A, Arancibia F, et al. Non-invasive ventilation during persistent weaning failure: a randomized controlled trial. Am J Respir Crit Care Med 2003; 168:70–76.
36. Squadrone V, Coha M, Cerutti E, et al. Continuous positive airway pressure for treatment of postoperative hypoxemia. A randomized controlled trial, JAMA 2005; 293:589–595.
37. Esteban A, Frutos-Vivar F, Ferguson ND, et al. Noninvasive positive pressure ventilation for respiratory failure after extubation. N Engl J Med 2004; 350:2452–2460.
38. Nava S, Gregoretti C, Fanfulla F, et al. Noninvasive ventilation to prevent respiratory failure after extubation in high-risk patients. Crit Care Med 2005; 33:2465–2470.
39. Ferrer M, Valencia M, Nicolas JM, et al. Early noninvasive ventilation averts extubation failure in patients at risk: a randomized trial. Am J Respir Crit Care Med 2006; 173:164–170.
40. Ezingeard E, Diconne E, Guyomarch S, et al. Weaning from mechanical ventilation with pressure support in patients failing a T-tube trail of spontaneous breathing. Intensive Care Med 2006; 32:165–169.

7A
Weaning Units: The U.S. Perspective

PAUL J. SCALISE and JOHN J. VOTTO
University of Connecticut Medical School, Farmington, Connecticut, U.S.A.

I. Introduction

The care of the patient requiring prolonged mechanical ventilation (PMV) presents a logistic and financial burden to many acute care facilities. In the United States, as the cost of staying in acute care is prohibitive (1), there are multiple alternative venues. Although options include rehabilitation hospitals with ventilator weaning programs, long-term care hospitals (LTCH) is the major alternative. Most LTCHs have well-established weaning programs, with validated outcomes. Notwithstanding that LTCHs are not available in all jurisdictions, they play a vital role in the continuum of care for patients requiring PMV.

Only a small percentage of patients require ventilation for at least six hours per day for 21 days (2). These patients are often older, have more comorbid illnesses, and, frequently, have underlying obstructive lung disease (3,4). Patients who have had a shorter duration of mechanical ventilatory support during surgery are more likely to be successfully weaned (5,6).

It is estimated that 5% of all ventilated patients require PMV (7). In 1986, Make et al. reported there to be 147 patients in Massachusetts, U.S.A., who met the definition for PMV (8). In 1989, Gallup Organization estimated that in the United States 11,400 patients required PMV. Clearly, the cost to the health care system is substantial. In the Gallup survey, in 1989, the daily cost of care was $789/day, resulting in an annual cost of US $3.2 billion—a large sum for a small patient population.

The financial burden of caring for these patients has been difficult to quantify because of the lack of data on cost of (ICU) care. Recently, Dasta et al. reported on a retrospective multicenter analysis of LTCHs, noting ICU costs to be greatest on the first day, decreasing by 50% by day 2, and remaining stable after day 3 (1). Cost was greater for surgical and trauma patients than for medical patients. As ventilated patients had higher daily costs, averaging $3968 per day after day 31, it was financially prudent for patients requiring PMV to be cared for in alternative venues. Indihar noted that the prolonged respiratory care unit was cost-effective (9) and Gracey reported an institutional saving of $4.8 million over a five-year period (1988–1993) by transferring patients from ICU to a chronic ventilator-dependent unit (10).

Scheinhorn et al. recently reported on the weaning outcomes of ventilator-dependent survivors of catastrophic illness transferred to the post-ICU setting (11). The mean cost of care was approximately $63,000 and the average length of stay was 40 days. The LTCHs are less expensive in part because of the reduced overhead compared with an acute care facility. It should be noted that LTCHs offer a more limited range of services than acute care centers; for example, there are no emergency, obstetrics, or major surgery departments.

Although the clinical success of LTCH has been confirmed (3,12–14), there are no studies that compare their cost-effectiveness for PMV patients with acute care. Such studies would clearly be difficult in this small heterogeneous patient population and some would argue that it would be unethical, given the obviously large cost differences.

LTCHs benefit greatly from their committed, cost-conscious staff, dedicated to the liberation of patients from PMV. The success of units focused on the care of a well-defined group of patients is not a new concept. Indeed, an illustrative example of the results of programmatic organization of health care is the maturation of the specialty of critical care medicine. Pronovost et al. have reported on the impact of a multidisciplinary team led by an intensivist in reducing both length of stay and mortality in a closed ICU (15).

II. Etiology: The U.S. Experience

The cause of patients requiring PMV varies and there are many instances when patients with similar respiratory impairments have markedly different outcomes. Unlike patients in acute care in whom weaning is often and predictably accomplished, weaning outcome in patients requiring PMV has been correlated with the number of comorbid conditions and the duration of mechanical ventilation, with no specific predictors (3,16). Understanding why a patient does not wean is important for maximizing their chances for doing so or for counseling them on long-term ventilation. Cardiovascular and respiratory dysfunctions are the most common causes of failure to wean, with respiratory causes including abnormal gas exchange, respiratory drive, or neuromuscular function. There are many excellent reviews on the pathophysiology of failure to wean (16–18).

In our 10 years of clinical experience, patients admitted to our regional weaning center, with a left ventricular ejection fraction (LVEF) of 20% or less, were unable to be liberated from ventilation. Withdrawal of PMV increases left ventricular preload, which can increase left ventricular end-diastolic pressure and can result in acute left ventricular failure (19,20). In a study, Lemaire et al. reported on the impact of acute left ventricular dysfunction during weaning among patients with cardiopulmonary disease and noted that patients who failed to wean had increases in pulmonary artery pressure within 10 minutes of spontaneous ventilation (21). The P_{CO_2} of these patients also increased from 42 to 58 mmHg. The authors concluded that acute left ventricular dysfunction could occur in patients with chronic obstructive pulmonary disease (COPD) and preexisting arteriosclerotic heart disease (ASHD) who may not have been apparent during mechanical ventilatory support. Their findings underscore the importance of cardiopulmonary relationships being considered during weaning (21).

In addition to the cardiopulmonary dysfunction, a major factor that influences weaning is the use of sedatives and hypnotics, which depress respiratory drive and level of consciousness, leading to prolonged dependence on mechanical ventilation. Patients admitted to our regional weaning center had a mean of 12 medications prescribed prior to admission whereas on admission this could be reduced to nine medications, a reduction of 33%. Most of these medications were sedatives and hypnotics.

Nutritional status is crucial in the care of ventilated patients, as malnutrition reduces respiratory muscle mass and contributes to failure to wean from PMV (22–25). Therefore, nutritional evaluation and repletion are important to maintain and restore muscle strength. Patients admitted to regional weaning centers are often malnourished and protein depleted, which can lead to diminished respiratory and skeletal muscle strength, decreased ventilatory drive, and prolonged ventilator dependence (22,23,26).

Other metabolic factors contributing to PMV include hypophosphatemia and hypomagnesemia, both of which have been associated with diminished diaphragmatic function. Hypothyroidism is an uncommon cause of ventilator dependency (27), being associated with respiratory muscle weakness as well as altered ventilatory drive and upper airway obstruction. Hypothyroidism is a potentially treatable cause of failure to wean and it should be considered in patients with prolonged ventilator dependence.

Acute renal failure in association with respiratory failure has a mortality rate as high as 89% (28), although the influence of renal function on weaning has not been fully investigated. Scheinhorn et al. (29) included renal function in their scoring system, which is devised to predict the chance of weaning success after six weeks of ventilation. Datta and Scalise also reported that renal function correlated indirectly with weaning success (30).

III. Outcomes

The results of patients requiring PMV are difficult to generalize, given the heterogeneity of diagnostic categories regarding this population, with some studies reporting high liberation rates with low mortality rates and others reporting low liberation rates with high mortality rates (10,12,20,31,32). Studies with mainly postoperative patients report better results than studies on patients with chronic lung disease.

Scheinhorn and Gracy have reported the largest series of patients requiring PMV (10,12,13,33), with different results. In Gracy's report, 75% of patients were ventilated postoperatively, as opposed to 24% in Scheinhorn's study. The National Association of Long-Term Hospitals recently sponsored a multicenter study of patients requiring PMV. Over 1400 patients from 23 LTCHs in the United States were enrolled for a one-year period. The results, reported by Scheinhorn, revealed a 55% liberation rate and a 26% mortality rate. We believe that these findings, across a national group of diverse patient populations, are encouraging and validate the role for regional weaning centers in the care of patients requiring PMV.

Prolonged respiratory care units greatly reduce the cost of caring for PMV patients, either in regional weaning centers or in PMV units. The emergence of specialized caregivers dedicated to weaning PMV patients has been reflected in the improved care that is evident over the last 20 years. In the United States, a regional weaning center is a valuable component in the continuum of care of patients requiring PMV.

References

1. Dasta JF, McLaughlin TP, Mody SH, et al. Daily cost of an intensive care unit day: the contribution of mechanical ventilation. Crit Care Med 2005; 33(6):1266–1271.
2. Aldrich TK, Karpel JP, Uhrlass RM, et al. Weaning from mechanical ventilation: adjunctive use of inspiratory muscle resistive training. Crit Care Med 1989; 17(2):143–147.
3. Scalise PJ, Gerardi DA, Wollschlager CM, et al. A regional weaning center for patients requiring mechanical ventilation: an 18-month experience. Conn Med 1997; 61(7):387–389.

4. Nevins ML, Epstein SK. Predictors of outcome in patients with COPD requiring invasive mechanical ventilation. Chest 2001; 119(6):1840–1849.
5. Sivak ED. Prolonged mechanical ventilation: an approach to weaning. Cleve Clin Q 1980; 47:89–96.
6. Vallverdu L, Calaf N, Subirana M, et al. Clinical characteristics, respiratory function parameters, and outcomes of a two-hour T-piece trial in patients weaning from mechanical ventilation. Am J Respir Crit Care Med 1998; 158:1855–1862.
7. Pierson DJ. Long-term mechanical ventilation and weaning. Respir Care 1995; 40:289–295.
8. Make BJ, Dayno S, Gertman P. Prevalence of chronic ventilator-dependency. Am Rev Respir Dis 1986; 133:A167 (abstr).
9. Indihar FJ, Walker NE. Experience with a prolonged respiratory care unit—revisited. Chest 1984; 86:616–620.
10. Gracey DR, Hardy OC, Koenig GE. The chronic ventilator dependent unit: a lower cost alternative to intensive care. Mayo Clin Proc 2000; 75:445–449.
11. Scheinhorn DJ, Hassenpflug MS, Votto JJ, et al. Post-ICU mechanical ventilation at 23 long term care hospitals: a multicenter outcomes study. Chest 2007; 131(1):85–93.
12. Gracey DR, Naessens JM, Viggiano RW, et al. Outcome of patients cared for in a ventilator-dependent unit in a general hospital. Chest 1995; 107:494–499.
13. Gracey DR, Viggiano RW, Naessens JM, et al. Outcomes of patients admitted to a chronic ventilator-dependent unit in an acute-care hospital. Mayo Clin Proc 1992; 67(2):131–136.
14. Scheinhorn DJ, Artinian BM, Catlin JL, et al. Weaning from prolonged mechanical ventilation: the experience at a regional weaning center. Chest 1994; 105(2):534–539.
15. Pronovost PJ, Angus DC, Dorman T, et al. Physician staffing patterns and clinical outcomes in critically ill patients: a systematic review. JAMA 2002; 288(17):2151–2162.
16. Laghi F, D'Alfonso N, Tobin MJ. Pattern of recovery from diaphragmatic fatigue over 24 hours. J Appl Physiol 1995; 79:539–546.
17. Laghi F, Jubran A, Parthasarathay S, et al. Can patients who fail a fair trial of weaning develop diaphragmatic fatigue? Am J Respir Crit Care Med 2000; 161:A790 (abstr).
18. Jubran A, Tobin MJ. Pathophysiologic basis of acute respiratory distress in patients who fail a trial of weaning from mechanical ventilation. Am J Respir Crit Care Med 1997; 155:906–915.
19. Tobin MJ, Perez W, Guenther SM, et al. The pattern of breathing during successful and unsuccessful trials of weaning from mechanical ventilation. Am Rev Respir Dis 1986; 134:1111–1118.
20. Yang KL, Tobin MJ. A prospective study of indexes predicting the outcome of trials of weaning from mechanical ventilation. N Engl J Med 1991; 324:1445–1450.
21. Lemaire F, Teboul JL, Cinotti L, et al. Acute left ventricular dysfunction during unsuccessful weaning from mechanical ventilation. Anesthesiology 1988; 69:171–179.
22. Arora NS, Rochester DF. Effect of body weight and muscularity on human diaphragm muscle mass, thickness and area. J Appl Physiol 1982; 52:64–70.
23. Thurlbeck WM. Diaphragm and body weight in emphysema. Thorax 1978; 33:483–487.
24. Kelsen SG, Ference M, Kapoor S. Effects of prolonged undernutrition on structure and function of the diaphragm. J Appl Physiol 1985; 58:1354–1359.
25. Knowles JB, Fauban M, Wiggs BJ, et al. Dietary supplementation and respiratory muscle performance in patients with COPD. Chest 1988; 93:977–983.
26. Rochester DF, Esau SA. Malnutrition and the respiratory system. Chest 1984; 85:411–415.
27. Pandya K, Lal C, Scheinhorn D, et al. Hypothyroidism and ventilator dependency. Arch Intern Med 1989; 149(9):2115–2116.
28. Gillespie DJ, Marsh HMM, Divertie MB, et al. Clinical outcome of respiratory failure in patients requiring prolonged (>24 hours) mechanical ventilation. Chest 1986; 90:364–369.
29. Scheinhorn DJ, Hassenpflug M, Artinian BM, et al. Predictors of weaning after 6 weeks of mechanical ventilation. Chest 1995; 107:500–505.

30. Datta D, Scalise P. Hypothyroidism and failure to wean in patients receiving prolonged mechanical ventilation at a regional weaning center. Chest 2004; 126(4):1307–1312.
31. Cordasco EM Jr, Sivak ED, Perez-Trepichio A. Demographics of long-term ventilator-dependent patients outside the intensive care unit. Cleve Clin J Med 1991; 58:505–509.
32. Spicher JE, White DP. Outcome and function following prolonged mechanical ventilation. Arch Intern Med 1987; 147:421–425.
33. Scheinhorn DJ, Chao DC, Stern-Hassenpfllug M, et al. Post-ICU mechanical ventilation: treatment of 1123 patients at a regional weaning center. Chest 1997; 111:1654–1659.

7B
Weaning in a Specialized Facility

BERND SCHÖNHOFER
Hospital Oststadt-Heidehaus, Hannover Area Hospital, Hannover, Germany

I. Background and Rationale

A vast majority of patients can be weaned from mechanical ventilation without difficulty. Although there is no consensus on the definition of a "difficult-to-wean" patient, the period of 14 to 21 days is generally accepted as "ventilator dependent" (1). There is a small population of patients who require prolonged mechanical ventilation (PMV) because of pulmonary, cardiac, or neuromuscular disease (NMD) or because of other multisystem problems. This population consumes a large section of the overall ICU patient days and about 50% of the ICU budget (2). The number of such patients has increased in recent years (3), a trend that is likely to continue. The ICU is an inappropriate environment for patients requiring PMV, as weaning is time consuming and involves more than the choice of the best approach to ventilation for a particular patient (4,5). A recent editorial entitled "The Challenge of Prolonged Mechanical Ventilation: A Shared Global Experience" (6) stressed the need for an international consensus, based on evidence, position papers, and international conferences.

II. Weaning Facilities

Several reports have suggested that about 10% of patients in the ICU require PMV (2,7). These patients could be transferred to facilities that offer a specialized health care team with a more rehabilitative focus (Fig. 1). The main differences between ICUs and weaning facilities (WFs) are summarized in Table 1. Greater privacy and improved visitor access may accelerate the healing process and facilitate discharge, especially for patients who require long-term oxygen therapy or long-term mechanical ventilation (LTMV). WF may also be cost-effective as well as improving outcomes such as successful weaning.

III. Locations of WFs

The precise definition of WF as well as the timing and admission to them varies among different jurisdictions. Various facilities that provide PMV are summarized in Table 2.

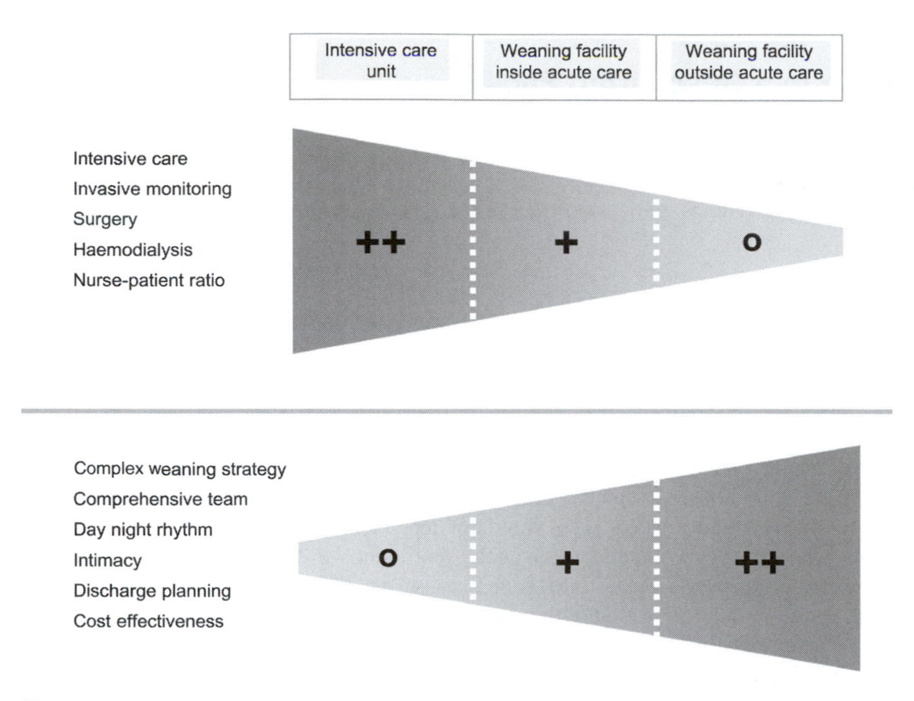

Figure 1 Strength and weaknesses, ICU, weaning units within and outside acute care hospital.

Table 1 Differences Between ICU and Weaning Facility

	ICU	WF
Noise	++	+
Day/night cycle	Disturbed	Preserved
Space in the room	+	++
Visiting time	+	++
Mobilisation-PT	+	++
Condition	+	++
Surrounding	Sterile	Intimacy encouraged
Technology	++	+
Communication	+	++
Nutrition	Tube feeding	Oral nutrition
Staff support	+	++
Psychological care	+	++
Palliative care	+	++
Discharge planning	+	++

+: Limited; ++: high level.
Abbreviation: WF, weaning facilities.

Table 2 Facilities with Different Levels of Care

Facility	Patients	Advantage	Disadvantage
ICU	Life threatened	High-tech intensive	Expensive
Step-down unit Intermediate care unit Respiratory ICU	One organ failure, clinically stable	Cost-effective for weaning success	Reduced level of care
Rehabilitation	Clinically stable	Weaning still possible Patient-centered care Lower costs Intensive PT	Reduced level of care
Nursing home	Clinically stable	Patient-centered care Lower costs	No weaning Reduced care
Home or palliative care	Clinically stable	Patient-centered care	No weaning

Abbreviations: ICU, intensive care unit; PT, physiotherapy.

IV. WF in Acute Care Hospitals

About 20 years ago, WFs started their activity within acute care hospitals aiming at an alternative therapeutic strategy and environment for ICU patients requiring PMV. A report by Smith and Shneerson in 1995 (8) described a progressive care program (PCP) for patients transferred from the ICU staffed by a dedicated multidisciplinary team of respiratory physicians and nurses. The PCP was very successful in discharging 80% of patients, of whom 76% survived for one year. WF located in acute care facilities are staffed more like an ICU than WF outside of acute care facilities, with a nurse to patient ratio of 1:2 to 1:4 (9) and a respiratory therapist permanently assigned to the unit. Medical care is provided by the medical house-staff under the direction of critical care or pneumonology specialist. The multidisciplinary team comprises a specialized nursing staff, dieticians, psychologists, physical therapists, speech therapists, social workers, and clergy, when needed. If the WF is located in an acute care hospital, diagnostic tests, such as CT and NMR, as well as therapeutic options, such as surgery, are readily available.

V. Respiratory Intermediate Care Unit

The number of respiratory intermediate care units (RICUs) in Europe is increasing. RICUs specialize in noninvasive ventilation (NIV) for acute respiratory failure (ARF) as well as PMV. Patients with chronic respiratory failure, especially those with chronic obstructive pulmonary disease (COPD), are effectively ventilated noninvasively at a lower cost, avoiding a long weaning period (59% of the total duration of invasive mechanical ventilation) (10). RICUs require fewer nursing staff (11) and enable more appropriate utilization of the ICU. Conversely, transfer from an ICU to an RICU (Fig. 2) is possible for those who become clinically stable but still require intensive nursing or physiotherapy prior to weaning (12).

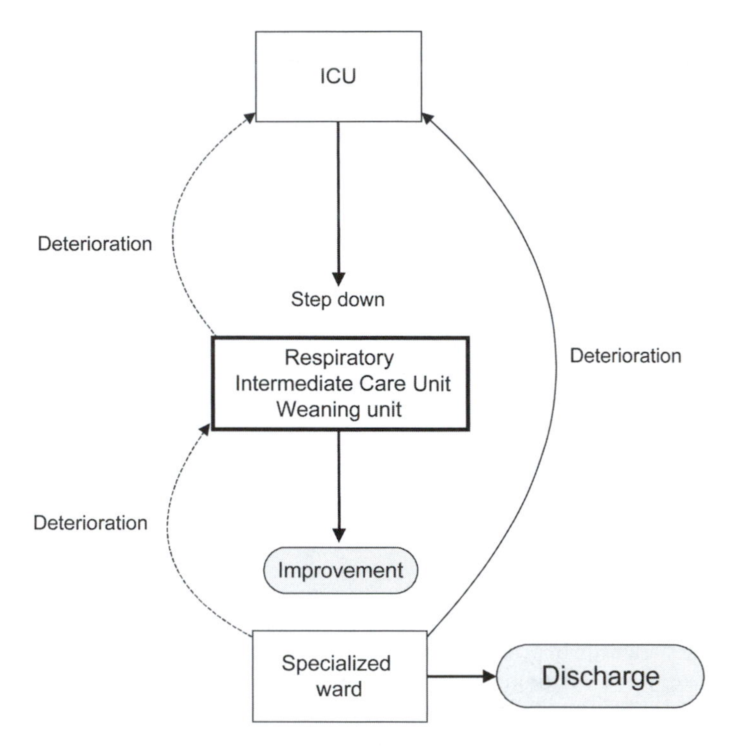

Figure 2 The central position of the respiratory intermediate care unit within the weaning process.

Reversing an earlier trend in which European respiratory specialists had only a marginal role in the management of ARF, there are now several RICUs led by experienced pneumonologists (13), utilizing a variety of organizational models.

A three-month prospective cohort study of 26 Italian RICUs reported on 756 patients (14). Of all patients receiving invasive mechanical ventilation, 61% were tracheotomized and therefore considered ventilator dependent. According to the Acute Physiology and Chronic Health Evaluation II (APACHE II) score, the predicted mortality was 22%, while the actual mortality rate was 16%. The results indicate that units with a level of care below ICU can successfully manage patients with acute-on-chronic respiratory failure.

Recently, the intensive care assembly of the European Respiratory Society published the recommendations and results of a task force that dealt with distribution, organization, and levels of service provision in RICUs (9). The task force recommended that the RICU should be located in a pneumonology unit or in an emergency department, using staffing/patient ratios or nurses/patient ratios of 1:2.5 to 1:3 (24 hours), physiotherapist/patient ratio of 1:6 (daytime), and physician/patient ratio of 1:6.5 (24 hours). Physicians, nurses, and other therapists should be experienced in emergency medicine, mechanical ventilation, and cardiopulmonary resuscitation.

The RICU was defined (Table 3) using five major and two minor criteria to identify three different levels of care (Table 4). There were no RICUs in eight of 15 countries

Table 3 Definition of Respiratory Intermediate Care Unit

Criteria for admission	Intervention equipment	Staffing
Single organ respiratory failure	Noninvasive ventilation	1:4 nursing for 24 hours
Acute respiratory failure—monitoring but not necessarily mechanical ventilation	Availability of life support—invasive ventilation followed by ICU transfer	MD available 24 hr/day
Tracheotomy patients from ICU-post acute or weaning	Minimum monitoring required—oximetry, vital signs, etc.	Unit supervised by an MD with expertise in TIPPV or NIPPV Availability of RT and PT

Abbreviations: NIPPV, noninvasive positive pressure ventilation; TIPPV, tracheotomy invasive positive pressure ventilation; RT, respiratory therapist; PT, physiotherapist; MD, medical doctor.
Source: From Ref. 9 with kind permission.

Table 4 Three Levels of Care

Major criteria	Intensive care	Intermediate care	Monitoring unit
N:P ratio	>1:3	1:3 or 1:4	<1:4
Equipment	Monitors[a] Invasive ventilators	Monitors[a] Invasive and noninvasive ventilation	Monitors[a] Noninvasive ventilation
Treatment	Single or multiorgan	Respiratory failure	Respiratory failure
Attending physician	24 hr	Available 24 hr	On call
Mechanical ventilation	IV and NIV, if needed	NIV and IV, if needed	NIV, if needed
Minor criteria			
Bronchoscopy	Inside unit	Inside unit	Inside or outside unit
ABGA	Inside unit	Inside unit	Inside or outside unit

[a]All major criteria and at least one of the minor criteria must be satisfied to include a unit at this level: oximetry, cardiogram, noninvasive blood pressure, respiratory rate.
Abbreviations: IV, invasive mechanical ventilation; NIV, noninvasive mechanical ventilation; ABGA, arterial blood gas analysis.
Source: From Ref. 9 with kind permission.

surveyed (Belgium, the Netherlands, Norway, Finland, Greece, Iceland, Portugal, and Sweden). In the remaining seven countries (Italy, Germany, France, Turkey, the United Kingdom, Spain, and Austria), 68 units were included. Their details (distribution, type, beds for each level of care) are summarized in Table 5. Of 4886 pneumonology beds, 472 were devoted to critically ill patients. Twelve units were classified as ICUs, with Italy and France sharing the highest number of units, and 42 were classified as RICUs, with Germany and

Table 5 Distribution of 68 Respiratory Units According to the Three Levels of Care

Country	Intensive care	Intermediate care	Monitoring unit	Total
Italy	4 (33.3)	13 (30.9)	7 (50)	24
Germany	1 (8.3)	15 (35.7)	2 (14.3)	18
France	4 (33.3)	5 (11.9)	0	9
Turkey	1 (8.3)	4 (9.5)	2 (14.3)	7
U.K.	1 (8.3)	3 (7.1)	3 (21.4)	7
Spain	1 (8.3)	1 (2.4)	0	2
Austria	0	1 (2.4)	0	1
Belgium	0	0	0	0
Denmark	0	0	0	0
The Netherlands	0	0	0	0
Norway	0	0	0	0
Finland	0	0	0	0
Greece	0	0	0	0
Iceland	0	0	0	0
Portugal	0	0	0	0
Sweden	0	0	0	0
Total	12	42	14	68

Source: From Ref. 9 with kind permission.

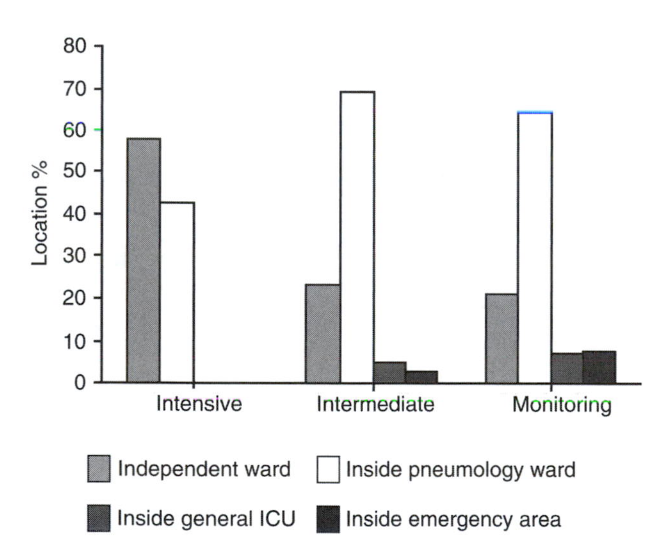

Figure 3 Location of the three different levels of care. *Source*: From Ref. 9 with kind permission.

Italy being the leading countries. As indicated in Figure 3, of the total 68 units, 17 were located in independent wards, 48 in other wards (pneumonology, 40; general ICU, 6; emergency area, 2), and three units did not provide this information.

VI. WF Outside of Acute Care Hospitals

A. Regional Weaning Centers

WFs may also be outside of acute care hospitals, as in free-standing hospitals (regional weaning centers) or in rehabilitation hospitals. The terminology used for WFs outside of acute care hospitals is given in Table 6. Such centers provide physical and pulmonary rehabilitation and offer privacy, daytime activities, longer visiting hours, and better quality sleep, all of which should improve the chances of successful weaning (15).

In Germany and Italy, about 15% of RICUs are located inside rehabilitation centers (12,16,17). Specialist physicians are responsible for medical care, with a physician/patient ratio of about 1:8 (9,13,14).

B. Nursing Homes

In the United States, nursing homes, either within larger facilities or as stand-alone facilities, have reported success in weaning (18). In Europe, such facilities are uncommon (19). There is no standardization of criteria for admission or staffing, other than for those requiring 24-hour nursing care owing to cognitive or a physical impairment. Nurses are trained to perform specific procedures, such as suctioning, tracheotomy care, and basic monitoring of ventilation parameters.

VII. Staffing Issues in WF

Although there is heterogeneity in training and expertise, WF staff are trained in life-saving procedures as well as protocols, such as airway care, secretion management etc., for PMV. In a WF, the staff may help the clinicians to decide on care issues such as decannulation (20,21). Vitacca et al. noted that in the first two days after admission, the time consumed by a ventilator-dependent patient was approximately 45% of a nurse's shift (22). Respiratory therapists and nurses are trained in weaning protocols, clinical tests, such as bronchoscopy and other respiratory approaches that assist clinicians, as well as the secondary psychological issues that accompany prolonged ventilation (23).

Table 6 Terminology of Weaning Facilities Outside Acute Care Hospitals

Outside Acute Care Hospitals
• Regional weaning center
• VD rehabilitation center
• Extended care facilities
• Prolonged respiratory care unit
• Long-term acute care unit
• Chronic VD unit
• Respiratory intermediate care unit

Abbreviation: VD, ventilator dependent.

VIII. Admission Criteria

Some WFs accept all ventilator-dependent patients, but most have admission criteria. The American College of Critical Care Medicine has recommended that "medically stable ventilator patients for weaning and chronic care" are the ideal candidates (24). Some centers accept exclusively tracheotomized patients, assuming that the tracheotomy itself indicates ventilator dependency. Frequently used criteria for admission include clinically stable patients with single organ failure (respiratory), dependency >14 to 21 days on invasive ventilation, two failed weaning trials, potential for weaning, adequate oxygenation, and no other issues that might impair weaning, such as hemodynamic instability, sepsis, renal failure, altered level of consciousness, surgical problems, or need for sedation.

IX. Outcome and Effectiveness

Table 7 shows characteristics and outcome data of patients admitted to nonacute settings for weaning attempts taken from both American and European studies. WFs have clinical and financial advantages over ICU care, although comparison studies are few (7,25,26). Gracey reported a marked reduction in mortality after a dedicated ventilator unit was opened inside an acute care hospital (27). A randomized, controlled trial of ventilator-dependent patients managed in the ICU ($n = 75$ patients) or in a special care unit ($n = 145$), managed mainly by specialized nurses, noted similar mortality rates but fewer re-admissions and shorter stays in the special care unit (28). Observational studies have shown that about 50% of so-called "unweanable" patients can be weaned in a WF (12,27,29–35). Most reports are from single centers and may lack generalizeability despite a consensus that they are valuable for weaning or for preparation for home mechanical ventilation (HMV). The outcome of PMV depends on their underlying disease, with outcomes being best for postoperative patients and those with acute lung injury and lowest in COPD or NMD (36). In our patient population, survival rate was worse in patients with severe COPD than in non-COPD patients (16).

Nava et al. showed a successful weaning rate of 55% in 42 patients with COPD in whom rehabilitation was continued after the ICU (12), and Scheinhorn reported improvements in survival, after discharge, with time probably due to the improved expertise of the personnel (30). In survivors of PMV, physical function is often limited after discharge (8,16,37). Quality of life has been defined not only as good, quite good, reasonable, or normal, but also as severely reduced, in a minority of studies (8,37); often it had improved by 6 to 12 months after discharge (38,39).

X. Financial Issues

In Europe, treatment is reimbursed through a diagnosis-related group (DRG)-based system including beds for chronically ill patients, if they are located in rehabilitation wards of acute care hospitals. If they are independently structured in rehabilitation hospitals, reimbursement is on a per diem basis, with adjustments based on the DRG classification. Most studies estimate care costs in a WF as less than in an ICU (17,40,41) mainly due to staff salaries, NIV, and fewer diagnostic tests. Seneff et al. evaluated mortality and costs over six months

Table 7 Studies of Weaning Outcomes

	First author and reference					
	Nava (12)	Pilcher (17)	Schönhofer (45)	Gracey (46)	Scheinhorn (47)	Bagley (36)
Patients (*n*)	42	153	232	132	421	278
Mean age (yr)	67	62	65	67	70	67
Diagnosis						
COPD	100%	27%	54%	13%	24%	30%
Surgery	—	24%	7%	63%	24%	11%
ALS	—	—	5%	1%	32%	28%
Neuromuscular	—	31%	16%	—	8%	19%
Miscellaneous	0%	18%	18%	23%	12%	12%
Weaning						
Ventilation days	13	26	44	14	49	—
Days to wean	30	19	7.5	16	39	—
Weaning success (%)	54%	38%	65%	70%	53%	38%
Survival						
At discharge (%)	71%	73%	72%	90%	71%	53%
Long-term (%)	55%-(1 yr)	73%	64% (3 mo)	—	28%-(1 yr)	—

Abbreviations: COPD, chronic obstructive pulmonary disease; ALS, amyotrophic lateral sclerosis.

in 54 acute care hospitals and 26 long-term acute care institutions and noted that transfer to a WF reduced costs without adversely affecting mortality (42).

XI. Organized Discharge

Discharge management from a WF gives the patient and caregivers confidence and skills, helps to soothe emotional issues in those at home, and is a valuable use of staff time.

XII. Home Mechanical Ventilation (HMV)

Stoller described ICU-discharge survival rate as 32% at two years, with a slower decline up to five years for ventilator-independent patients (43). We found the use of NIV at home in 31.5% of patients following PMV (16). Survival rates were poor (49% at one year and worse) in patients with COPD. In a research series by Pilcher, 38% of patients were fully weaned and 35% required HMV, most of the latter needing only nocturnal noninvasive support. Patients with NMD and transfusion-related diseases (TRD) were less likely to be weaned but had a reduced mortality, compared with those with COPD in whom survival rate was 58% at one year and 47% at three years (17).

According to recent reports, 71% and 80% of patients, respectively, were directly discharged after weaning (8,17). Although HMV requires more careful discharge planning, its increased use may significantly improve prognosis in patients who require PMV. There are few controlled studies in this area, especially among patients with COPD.

HMV is not without technical issues, and a recent European survey noted that quality control procedures showed considerable inter- and intra-country variability, there was poor communication between the prescribing centers and equipment suppliers, equipment quality control was limited, and only a few centers were associated with HMV-patient associations (44).

XIII. Conclusions

Clinical experience supported by observational studies would suggest that weaning success is higher in dedicated WFs, with improved outcomes at reduced costs, provided patients are selected carefully. An international consensus on the management of difficult and prolonged weaning was recently published (48). Prospective randomized controlled trials that evaluate the influence of WF on weaning success are yet to be established.

References

1. Scheinhorn DJ, Stearn-Hassenpflug M. Provision of long-term mechanical ventilation. Crit Care Clin 1998; 14:819–832.
2. Cohen IL, Booth FV. Cost containment and mechanical ventilation in the United States. New Horiz 1994; 2:283–290.
3. Cox CE, Carson SS, Holmes GM, et al. Increase in tracheostomy for prolonged mechanical ventilation in North Carolina, 1993–2002. Crit Care Med 2004; 32:2219–2226.
4. Brochard L, Rauss A, Benito S, et al. Comparison of three methods of gradual withdrawal from ventilatory support during weaning from mechanical ventilation. Am J Respir Crit Care Med 1994; 150:896–903.
5. Esteban A, Frutos F, Tobin MJ, et al. A comparison of four methods of weaning patients from mechanical ventilation. Spanish Lung Failure Collaborative Group. N Engl J Med 1995; 332:345–350.
6. Chao DC, Stearn-Hassenpflug M, Scheinhorn DJ. The challenge of prolonged mechanical ventilation: a shared global experience. Respir Care 2003; 48:668–669.
7. Robson V, Poynter J, Lawler PG, et al. The need for a regional weaning centre, a one-year survey of intensive care weaning delay in the Northern Region of England. Anaesthesia 2003; 58:161–165.
8. Smith IE, Shneerson JM. A progressive care programme for prolonged ventilatory failure: analysis of outcome. Br J Anaesth 1995; 75:399–404.
9. Corrado A, Roussos C, Ambrosino N, et al. Respiratory intermediate care units: a European survey. Eur Respir J 2002; 20:1343–1350.
10. Esteban A, Alia I, Ibanez J, et al. Modes of mechanical ventilation and weaning. A national survey of Spanish hospitals. The Spanish Lung Failure Collaborative Group. Chest 1994; 106:1188–1193.
11. Elpern EH, Silver MR, Rosen RL, et al. The noninvasive respiratory care unit. Patterns of use and financial implications. Chest 1991; 99:205–208.
12. Nava S, Rubini F, Zanotti E, et al. Survival and prediction of successful ventilator weaning in COPD patients requiring mechanical ventilation for more than 21 days. Eur Respir J 1994; 7:1645–1652.
13. Nava S, Confalonieri M, Rampulla C. Intermediate respiratory intensive care units in Europe: a European perspective. Thorax 1998; 53:798–802.

14. Confalonieri M, Gorini M, Ambrosino N, et al. Respiratory intensive care units in Italy: a national census and prospective cohort study. Thorax 2001; 56:373–378.
15. Nava S. Rehabilitation of patients admitted to a respiratory intensive care unit. Arch Phys Med Rehabil 1998; 79:849–854.
16. Schönhofer B, Euteneuer S, Nava S, et al. Survival of mechanically ventilated patients admitted to a specialised weaning centre. Intensive Care Med 2002; 28:908–916.
17. Pilcher DV, Bailey MJ, Treacher DF, et al. Outcomes, cost and long term survival of patients referred to a regional weaning centre. Thorax 2005; 60:187–192.
18. Lindsay ME, Bijwadia JS, Schauer WW, et al. Shifting care of chronic ventilator-dependent patients from the intensive care unit to the nursing home. Jt Comm J Qual Saf 2004; 30:257–265.
19. Schmidt-Ohlemann M. Ventilation in nursing homes. Management of ventilator-dependent patients in inpatient facilities for handicapped—a report of experiences. Med Klin (Munich) 1996; 91(suppl 2):56–58.
20. Brook AD, Ahrens TS, Schaiff R, et al. Effect of a nursing-implemented sedation protocol on the duration of mechanical ventilation. Crit Care Med 1999; 27:2609–2615.
21. Ely EW. The utility of weaning protocols to expedite liberation from mechanical ventilation. Respir Care Clin N Am 2000; 6:303–319.
22. Vitacca M, Clini E, Porta R, et al. Preliminary results on nursing workload in a dedicated weaning center [in process citation]. Intensive Care Med 2000; 26:796–799.
23. Ceriana P, Carlucci A, Navalesi P, et al. Weaning from tracheotomy in long-term mechanically ventilated patients: feasibility of a decisional flowchart and clinical outcome. Intensive Care Med 2003; 29:845–848.
24. Nasraway SA, Cohen IL, Dennis RC, et al. Guidelines on admission and discharge for adult intermediate care units. American College of Critical Care Medicine of the Society of Critical Care Medicine. Crit Care Med 1998; 26:607–610.
25. Fox AJ, Owen-Smith O, Spiers P. The immediate impact of opening an adult high dependency unit on intensive care unit occupancy. Anaesthesia 1999; 54:280–283.
26. Heyland DK, Konopad E, Noseworthy TW, et al. Is it 'worthwhile' to continue treating patients with a prolonged stay (>14 days) in the ICU? An economic evaluation. Chest 1998; 114:192–198.
27. Gracey DR, Hardy DC, Naessens JM, et al. The Mayo ventilator-dependent rehabilitation unit: a 5-year experience. Mayo Clin Proc 1997; 72:13–19.
28. Rudy EB, Daly BJ, Douglas S, et al. Patient outcomes for the chronically critically ill: special care unit versus intensive care unit. Nurs Res 1995; 44:324–331.
29. Carson SS, Bach PB, Brzozowski L, et al. Outcomes after long-term acute care. An analysis of 133 mechanically ventilated patients. Am J Respir Crit Care Med 1999; 159:1568–1573.
30. Scheinhorn DJ, Chao DC, Stearn-Hassenpflug M, et al. Post-ICU mechanical ventilation: treatment of 1,123 patients at a regional weaning center. Chest 1997; 111:1654–1659.
31. Menzies R, Gibbons W, Goldberg P. Determinants of weaning and survival among patients with COPD who require mechanical ventilation for acute respiratory failure. Chest 1989; 95:398–405.
32. Spicher JE, White DP. Outcome and function following prolonged mechanical ventilation. Arch Intern Med 1987; 147:421–425.
33. Elpern EH, Larson R, Douglass P, et al. Long-term outcomes for elderly survivors of prolonged ventilator assistance. Chest 1989; 96:1120–1124.
34. Indihar FJ. A 10-year report of patients in a prolonged respiratory care unit. Minn Med 1991; 74:23–27.
35. Vitacca M, Vianello A, Colombo D, et al. Comparison of two methods for weaning patients with chronic obstructive pulmonary disease requiring mechanical ventilation for more than 15 days. Am J Respir Crit Care Med 2001; 164:225–230.
36. Bagley PH, Cooney E. A community-based regional ventilator weaning unit: development and outcomes. Chest 1997; 111:1024–1029.

37. Ambrosino N, Bruletti G, Scala V, et al. Cognitive and perceived health status in patient with chronic obstructive pulmonary disease surviving acute on chronic respiratory failure: a controlled study. Intensive Care Med 2002; 28:170–177.
38. Chatila W, Kreimer DT, Criner GJ. Quality of life in survivors of prolonged mechanical ventilatory support. Crit Care Med 2001; 29:737–742.
39. Euteneuer S, Windisch W, Suchi S, et al. Health-related quality of life in patients with chronic respiratory failure after long-term mechanical ventilation. Respir Med 2006; 100:477–486.
40. Dasgupta A, Rice R, Mascha E, et al. Four-year experience with a unit for long-term ventilation (respiratory special care unit) at the Cleveland Clinic Foundation. Chest 1999; 116:447–455.
41. Gracey DR, Hardy DC, Koenig GE. The chronic ventilator-dependent unit: a lower-cost alternative to intensive care. Mayo Clin Proc 2000; 75:445–449.
42. Seneff MG, Wagner D, Thompson D, et al. The impact of long-term acute-care facilities on the outcome and cost of care for patients undergoing prolonged mechanical ventilation. Crit Care Med 2000; 28:342–350.
43. Stoller JK, Xu M, Mascha E, et al. Long-term outcomes for patients discharged from a long-term hospital-based weaning unit. Chest 2003; 124:1892–1899.
44. Farre R, Lloyd-Owen SJ, Ambrosino N, et al. Quality control of equipment in home mechanical ventilation: a European survey. Eur Respir J 2005; 26:86–94.
45. Schönhofer B, Haidl P, Kemper P, et al. Entwöhnung vom Respirator ("Weaning") bei Langzeitbeatmung. Dtsch Med Wochenschr 1999; 124:1022–1028.
46. Gracey DR, Naessens JM, Viggiano RW, et al. Outcome of patients cared for in a ventilator-dependent unit in a general hospital. Chest 1995; 107:494–499.
47. Scheinhorn DJ, Artinian BM, Catlin JL. Weaning from prolonged mechanical ventilation. The experience at a regional weaning center. Chest 1994; 105:534–539.
48. Boles JM, Bion J, Connors A, et al. Weaning from mechanical ventilation. Eur Respir J 2007; 29:1033–1056.

8
Organization of Rehabilitation in the ICU

DEBBIE FIELD
Lane Fox Respiratory Intensive Care Unit, St. Thomas' Hospital, London, U.K.

I. Introduction

The lack of a clear definition for the term "rehabilitation" has resulted in a lack of understanding among practitioners of what rehabilitation has to offer to patients. What is clear from current literature, however, is that rehabilitation has evolved from its original concept described by Howard Rusk (1) of being the "third phase of medicine" to a new paradigm of early rehabilitation. It is now accepted that the earlier the rehabilitation strategies are begun, the greater are their effects (2). Although the benefits of rehabilitation for individuals with COPD, heart failure, spinal injury, and neurological conditions have been well described, in terms of symptom control, reduced admission to an acute facility and increase in quality of life and life satisfaction; there is limited information regarding the impact of rehabilitation on ICU patients receiving mechanical ventilation (MV). The question remains as to whether early and continuous rehabilitation in the ICU can influence patient outcome by enhancing functional capacity physiologically and psychologically as well as by reducing the risks associated with the ICU.

This chapter addresses the importance of integrating the process of rehabilitation within the milieu of critical care. A conceptual model will be presented to show how rehabilitation can be organized within the ICU, incorporating the whole of the patient's journey irrespective of their length of stay (LOS) within the ICU. The chapter will focus on those patients who require prolonged mechanical ventilation (PMV), i.e., >21 days and will be presented from a U.K. perspective. Case examples from my own critical care practice will be used to demonstrate how a rehabilitation framework of care impacts upon patient mortality, quality of care, and ICU costs. Finally, recommendations will be made for future practice.

II. Why Should Rehabilitation Be Integrated into ICU?

Thomas et al. (3) state that the aim of rehabilitation is to achieve the greatest return of physical, psychological, social, vocational, recreational, and economic functions within the limits imposed by the illness and physical or mental impairment. This aim can best be achieved if rehabilitation is established early in a patient's illness. Patients experience physiological and psychological complications that impair their recovery, particularly if their stay in the ICU is prolonged (4,5). Table 1 lists some of the major issues associated with patients requiring ICU admission. They are important, as ICU patients have high mortality (6) and morbidity and their care involves considerable costs (7).

Table 1 Signs and Symptoms Commonly Manifested or Reported by ICU Patients

- Respiratory and skeletal muscle weakness
- Sleep deprivation
- Cognitive dysfunction
- Loss of control
- Delirium
- Dyspnea
- Lack of energy
- Pain
- Anxiety and fear
- Thirst
- Difficult communication
- Boredom
- Sensory deprivation

Health care providers often see rehabilitation as something that takes place post-ICU after an acute episode of illness and is organized by a specialized rehabilitation facility. However, there is often little opportunity to send post-ICU patients to a specialized rehabilitation facility at the time they require such an intervention. Figure 1 shows data from two general ICUs in the south of England from 2004 to 2005, noting the time that 13 patients spent waiting for placement in a rehabilitation facility. These patients had already spent more than 21 days in the ICU!

In the past 20 years, in the United Kingdom, ICUs have developed the concept of ICU follow-up clinics to try and meet the needs of patients who find it difficult to adjust once they have gone home (8). Although these clinics have been important for a small group of patients, it is the author's opinion that there would be a better chance of improving quality of life, and reducing morbidity, and mortality, if there was a rehabilitative focus during the patients' ICU stay.

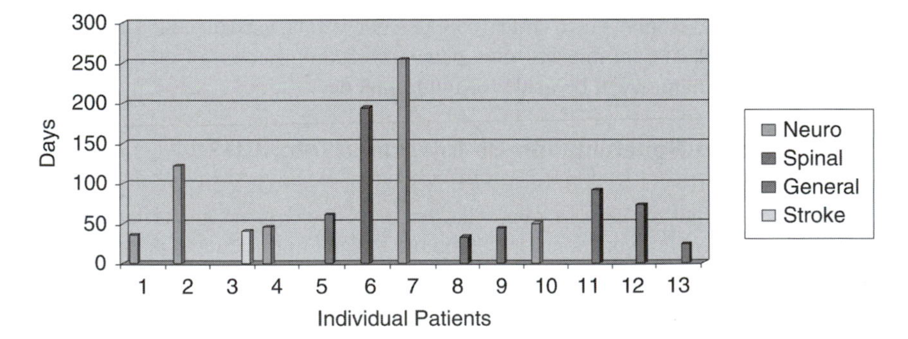

Figure 1 LOS for patients, from two ICUs in south England, waiting for placement in a rehabilitation unit after >21 days in the ICU (2004–2005). *Abbreviations*: LOS, length of stay; ICU, intensive care unit.

III. Organization of Rehabilitation in the ICU

Comparisons between countries are difficult because of differences in health care systems—especially funding, training, and education of health care professionals. In the United Kingdom, rehabilitation is not seen as an essential component of ICU care, as it is less exciting, time consuming, and slower than the acute, fast-responsive philosophy of critical care. Although there is not a generally accepted model for early rehabilitation in the ICU, a national consensus conference on rehabilitation management of the traumatic brain injured (TBI) patient considered the following as essential interventions during the acute ICU phase (9):

- Repeated postural changes during the day as well as passive mobilization
- Structured ongoing monitoring of patients' responsiveness
- Respiratory rehabilitation including facilitation of bronchial drainage, progressive weaning from controlled ventilation, and switching to assisted or spontaneous ventilation
- Uniformity and consistency of information given by the medical team to patients' families as well as psychological and practical support.

These interventions could easily be adapted and applied to a rehabilitative model of care for all ICU patients. Outcomes of early rehabilitation in patients with TBI were reported by Mammi et al. (10) to reduce care costs and LOS without affecting outcome.

Rehabilitation in the acute phase of ICU should be an integral part of nursing care, as it is designed to prevent complications and to maintain and restore functioning. Interventions, such as frequent repositioning, titrating drugs to maintain hemodynamic stability, adjusting ventilation to reduce dyspnea, touching the patient, and talking to the patients and their relatives, are implicit in nursing care, and the staff may not realize that they are part of the process of rehabilitation. Although physical therapists (PTs) provide other rehabilitation interventions, such as secretion clearance, there is often little interdisciplinary communication that the overall rehabilitation process remains uncoordinated. The concept of "care bundles" originated in North America as a simple method of ensuring the delivery of evidence-based care in a systematic way while also providing the means to audit the care and outcomes (11). Care bundles, especially the ventilator care bundle (Table 2), have been well integrated into the United Kingdom critical care health care system (12). Although originally not described as a rehabilitation intervention, this systematic approach does reduce complications, especially in the acute phase of ICU.

Many of the rehabilitation strategies for critically ill patients are organized in facilities for long-term mechanical ventilation (LTMV) or within specialized respiratory ICUs. Patients are transferred to these facilities when their LOS in ICU exceeds a set criterion (often 21 days) or when the patient is perceived as difficult to wean. Several investigators have

Table 2 Ventilator Care Bundle Example

- Head of bed elevation >30°
- Deep vein thrombosis prophylaxis
- Gastric ulcer prophylaxis
- Daily sedation hold
- Screen for readiness to wean from mechanical ventilation

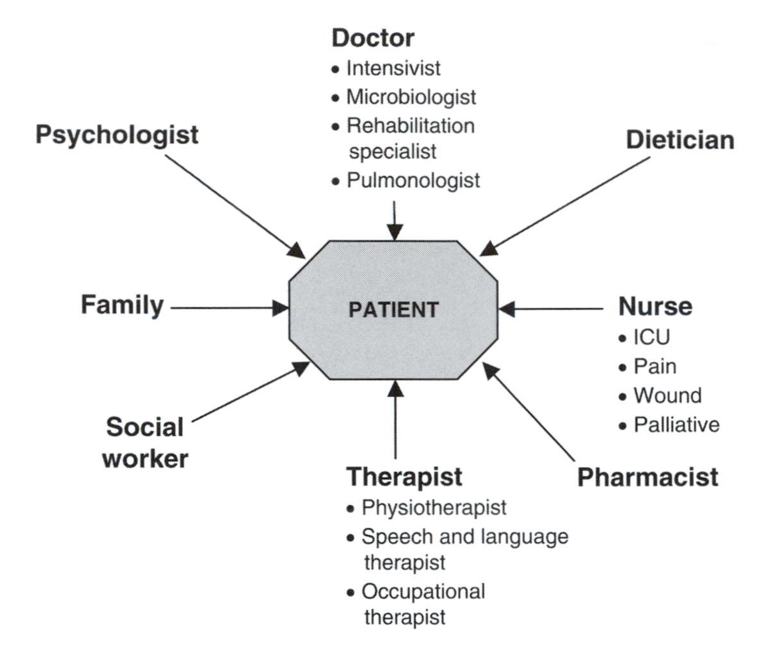

Figure 2 Comprehensive interdisciplinary rehabilitation team-skill sets are listed under the name of the discipline. *Abbreviation*: ICU, intensive care unit.

noted the benefits for patients on LTMV in which a multidisciplinary rehabilitation team (Fig. 2) provides comprehensive rehabilitation, even though some patients will only make a limited recovery and others may not recover at all (13–18). Although not all the skills sets can be represented in separate individuals, they can be made available, either from additional training and experience within a discipline or on a part-time consulting basis.

In the United Kingdom, there are few specialized facilities for LTMV, as a result, patients may need to be managed for protracted periods within the ICU. The core team usually consists of the intensivist, nurse, and PT, with dieticians, pharmacists, and microbiologists making up the peripheral ICU team on a part-time basis (Fig. 3). The rehabilitation process should exist within a practical framework, coordinated by enthusiastic, knowledgeable, experienced, and motivated professionals.

Stucki et al. (2) has suggested that the principles of early rehabilitation can be classified into (1) nonspecialized rehabilitation and (2) specialized rehabilitation.

This classification is a useful distinction that can be applied to the conceptual rehabilitation model and framework (Figs. 4 and 5). The core ICU team undertakes the acute and intermediate phase of nonspecialized rehabilitation. The long-term phase is specialized rehabilitation and again undertaken by the core ICU team but in collaboration with other relevant specialist practitioners, such as speech and language and occupational therapy, to optimize the patients' rehabilitation potential.

Within the ICU, a team of motivated people who coordinate the different phases to ensure continuity and consistency are needed. Thorens and Engoren have emphasized the importance of sufficient experienced practitioners for optimal weaning (19,20).

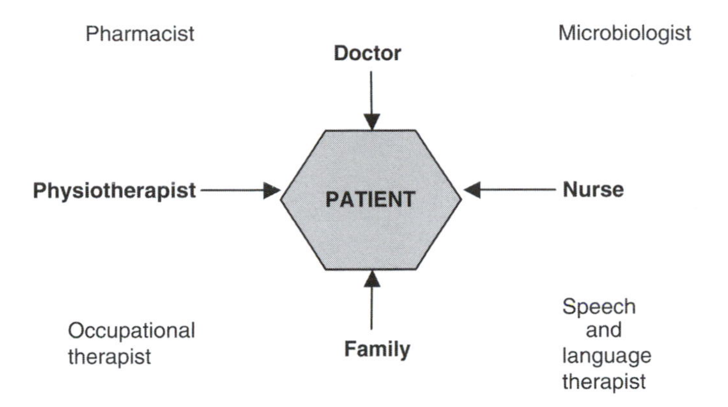

Figure 3 Core U.K. ICU rehabilitation team. *Abbreviation*: ICU, intensive care unit.

A. A Model of Organization

Figure 4 shows a conceptual model that encompasses the phases of the patient's potential journey through ICU. Inevitably, these phases overlap. As the LOS increases there are greater risks of secondary infections and acute events that require management. Therefore, the intermediate or long-term phases pause, although rehabilitation should never be stopped, but

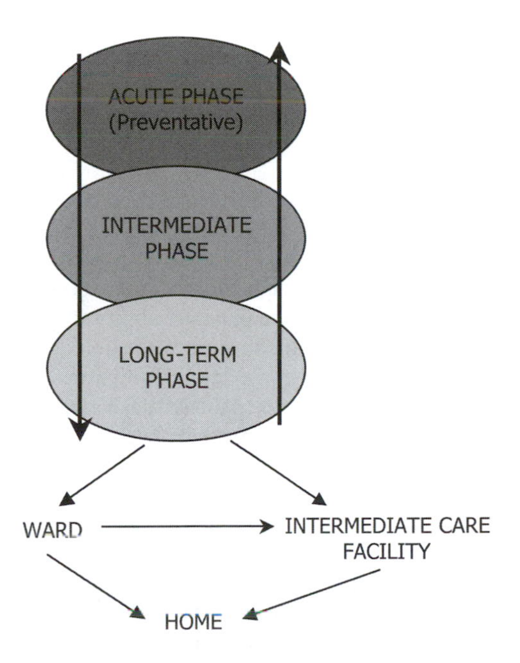

Figure 4 Conceptual model of rehabilitation for each phase of a patient's potential journey through ICU. *Abbreviation*: ICU, intensive care unit.

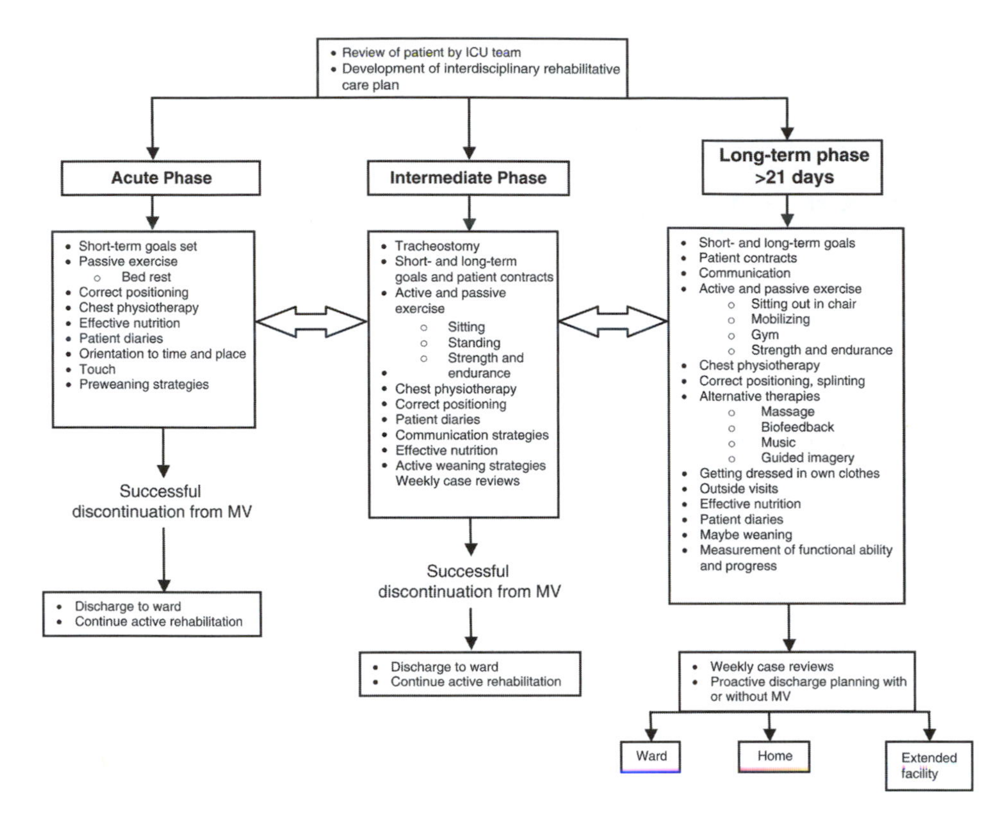

Figure 5 Template for a rehabilitation framework.

should continue even postdischarge from hospital. Short- and long-term goals should be set as the patient is transferred to the ward from ICU and eventually discharged home.

Figure 5 outlines a template of management, recognizing that the acute and the intermediate phases of rehabilitation will be limited by the patient's medical condition, surgical procedure, monitoring, intravenous lines, availability of staff, and the patient's ability to participate. During the acute phase, exercise is mainly passive, focusing on correct positioning of the patient and the patient's limbs to reduce contracture, joint damage, compression neuropathies, and tissue destruction. Patient diaries are introduced to help the patients make sense of their stay (21). Nutritional intake and requirements are calculated. As patients become intermediate (post tracheostomy and when sedation is reduced), exercise becomes more active, but positioning continues to be paramount. Diaries continue all through these phases. During the long-term phase, emphasis is on strength and endurance as well as enabling patients to have a sense of control. Discharge is carefully planned, especially for those requiring PMV.

This framework embraces the concept of whole-body rehabilitation, as described by Martin et al. (17), including physical and psychological aspects of care during the ICU stay. An essential component is the appointment of a coordinator, particularly in the intermediate and long-term phases, to ensure continuity and consistency. In the United Kingdom, the PT and nurse in the ICU are in a prime position to take on such a role.

B. Demonstration of the Framework: A Personal Experience

During my time as nurse consultant (NC) to the Surrey Wide Critical Care Network (SWCCN) in southeast England, I was responsible for developing and implementing the rehabilitation framework (Fig. 5) for patients with an ICU LOS >21 days. To demonstrate the framework's efficacy and to encourage all ICUs within the SWCCN to integrate it into their own unit's philosophy of care, I implemented the long-term phase of the rehabilitation framework for difficult-to-wean patients who had been in the ICU for more than 21 days (2,4). The patients were in two separate ICUs, both of which had an established weaning protocol and were using the ventilator care bundle. One senior PT in each unit volunteered to help coordinate the framework.

Case Study 1: Sarah

Sarah, a 32-year-old woman with severe kyphoscoliosis, was admitted to ICU when she contracted a community-acquired pneumonia. Her respiratory failure required intubation and ventilation on admission. After 24 hours, she developed adult respiratory distress syndrome. She was acutely ill for four weeks and had paralysis. During this time, she required hemodynamic support, hemofiltration, controlled ventilation, prone positioning, high positive end-expiratory pressure (PEEP), and full sedation. A tracheostomy was carried out on day 21 of admission, as prior to this time she had been too unstable for surgery. Five weeks following admission, she met the weaning criteria, using the unit ventilator care bundle, and was placed on a weaning protocol that consisted of gradual reduction of pressure support (PS) and tracheostomy mask trials.

I was asked to pilot the long-term phase of the rehabilitation framework on Sarah after several failed attempts at weaning. She had been ventilated in the ICU for 85 days. She had had a total of four weaning episodes (Table 3) lasting for on average 11.75 days. The PS during weaning was erratic and inconsistent with the PS levels set for initiation of the long-term phase of the rehabilitation framework (Figs. 6 and 7). Reasons for her failure to wean are summarized in Table 4.

Following implementation of the long-term phase of the rehabilitation framework, she was weaned and decannulated within 21 days. Her total LOS in the ICU was 106 days at a cost of £159,000 ($301,221). She was transferred to the ward and went home 14 days later on an individual pulmonary rehabilitation program. At six months Sarah was back at work full time and has had no further physiological or psychological problems. Appendix 1 shows Sarah's specific rehabilitation and weaning plan.

Table 3 Sarah's Weaning Episodes Prior to Commencing the Long-Term Phase of the Rehabilitation Framework

Weaning episodes	Days
Episode 1	13
Episode 2	13
Episode 3	9
Episode 4	12

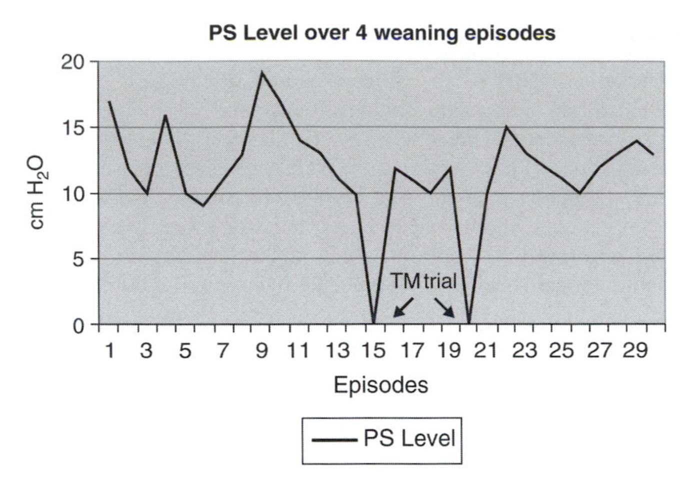

Figure 6 PS level during four episodes of weaning prerehabilitation framework. *Abbreviations*: PS, pressure support; TM, trache mask.

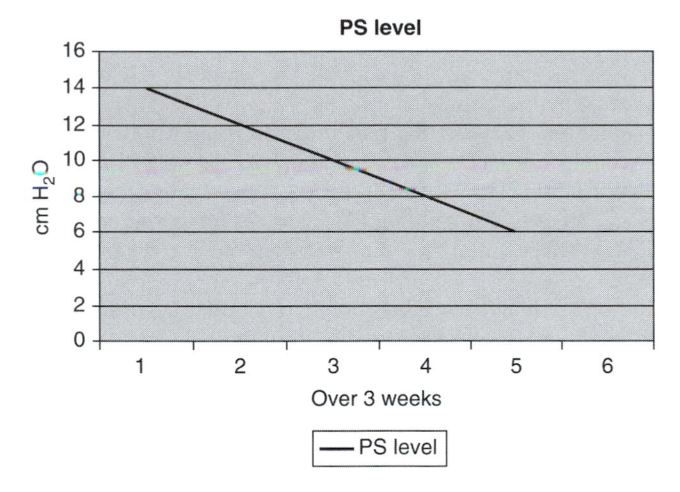

Figure 7 PS level following implementation of the long-term phase of the rehabilitation framework. *Abbreviation*: PS, pressure support.

Case Study 2: May

May, a 75-year-old lady with diverticular disease and hypertension, was admitted to ICU following a colectomy. On day 2 of her ICU stay, she suffered a cardiac event and ventilated for further three days, followed by a failed wean. She was transferred to another

Table 4 Reasons for Sarah's Failure to Wean

- Two episodes of sepsis—during weaning episodes 1 and 2
- Respiratory load and capacity imbalance complicated by thoracic restriction
- Critical care polyneuropathy
- Nonpulmonary factors
  - Sleep deprivation
  - Delirium
  - Anxiety and panic attacks
  - Pain
  - Thirst
  - Communication
- Acute critical care philosophy

hospital where five days later a tracheostomy was performed. She returned to her previous ICU where weaning continued for a further 41 days (six episodes lasting an average of seven days). Her total LOS in ICU was 51 days before she entered the long-term phase of the rehabilitation framework.

Figure 8 shows May's PS level on MV during her six weaning episodes, which again was erratic and lacked consistency compared with the PS level set once the long-term phase of the rehabilitation framework had been implemented (Fig. 9). Her night-time PS was increased to overcome her nocturnal hypoventilation. Her reasons for failing to wean can be seen in Table 5.

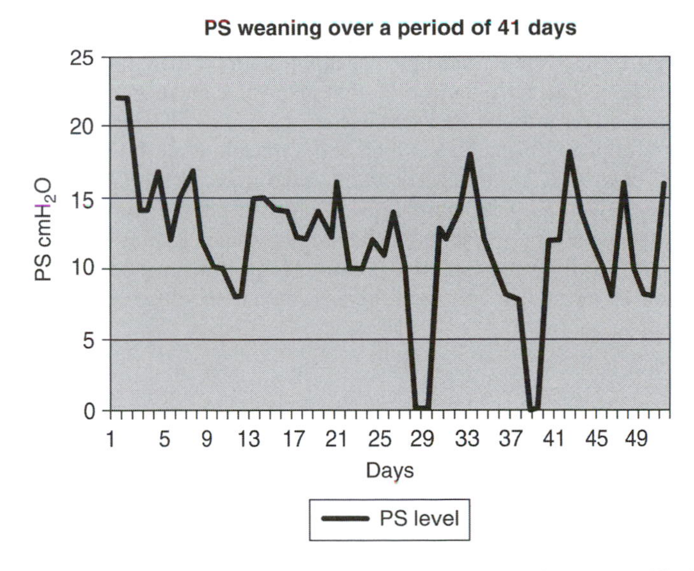

Figure 8 PS level during six episodes of weaning prior to rehabilitation framework. *Abbreviation*: PS, pressure support.

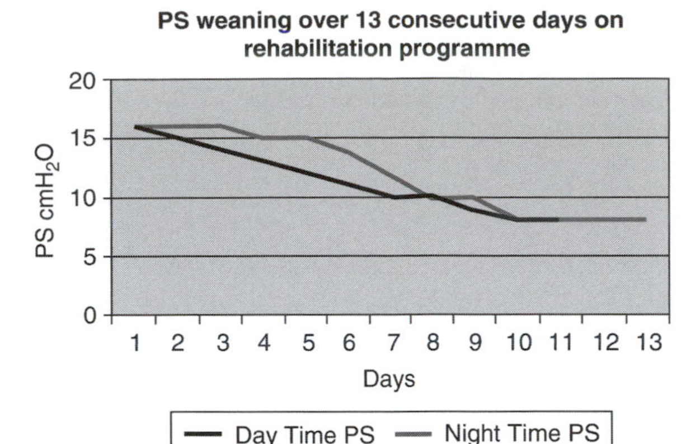

Figure 9 PS level following implementation of rehabilitation framework. *Abbreviation*: PS, pressure support.

Following implementation of the rehabilitation framework, May was weaned from MV and decannulated within 21 days. Her total LOS was 72 days at a cost of £108,000 ($204,588). She was transferred to the ward but waited for another 33 days before being transferred to a rehabilitation facility, where she stayed for 21 days. Now, one year later, May lives at home, cares for herself, socializes, and is making good progress.

Case Conclusion

The above two cases illustrate the importance of implementing a coordinated long-term rehabilitative plan in the ICU. In each case, multiple weaning attempts had failed for reasons outlined in Tables 4 and 5. The introduction of this plan by a nurse intensivist, together with a PT and a physician, streamlined care and hastened weaning. The economic cost of caring for the long-term critically ill patient is high and a rehabilitation framework implemented at the beginning of their ICU admission would have reduced the LOS and therefore the care costs in these two cases. In case 1, beginning an active whole-body rehabilitation program during the acute care phase, after the second weaning failure, might have saved 26 days of PMV in the ICU. Moreover, there is a need for follow-up studies that embrace quality of life as well as morbidity and mortality. However, these two patients

Table 5 Reasons for May's Failure to Wean

- Respiratory and skeletal muscle weakness
- Cardiac failure
- Nocturnal hypoventilation
- Pain
- Feelings of dyspnea
- Fear and anxiety
- Sleep deprivation
- Communication
- Cognitive impairment

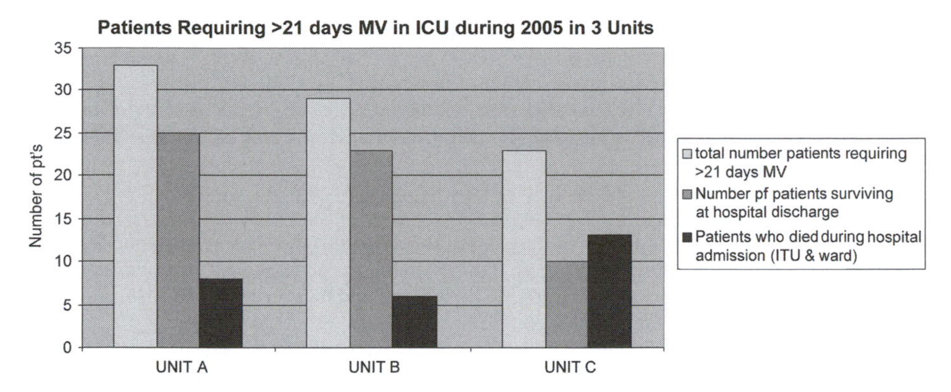

Figure 10 Patients requiring >21 days MV in 3 separate ICUs across the SWCCN during 2005. *Abbreviation*: MV = mechanical ventilation.

have encouraged both the ICUs to fully implement a rehabilitation framework by developing a core team of staff and formally appointing a coordinator. In these instances, the coordinators were the two senior PTs.

The rehabilitation framework implemented in these two ICUs has positively influenced patient outcomes. Figure 10 shows survival, in 2005, of patients who required MV more than 21 days in 3 separate ICUs within SWCCN. Although the patients had similar demographics and clinical characteristics, mortality in ICU C was 57% compared to ICU A and ICU B, where mortality were 24% and 20%, respectively. There are great opportunities for a more formal evaluation of the influence of this rehabilitation framework.

IV. Recommendations for Future Practice

- Introduction of a general rehabilitation framework across all general ICUs to promote rehabilitation as an integral part of intensive care management.
- Development of generic education and training courses in critical care rehabilitation.
- Development of research strategies to measure patient outcomes.
- Development of specialized respiratory support units for the LTMV.
- Addressing the prolonged LOS in ward before transferring to a specialized rehabilitation facility or home.
- Introduction of rehabilitation programs for post-ICU patients after they are discharged.

References

1. Rusk HA. Rehabilitation: the third phase of medicine. R I Med J 1960; 43:385–387.
2. Stucki G, Stier-Jarmer M, Grill E, et al. Rationale and principles of early rehabilitation care after an acute injury or illness. Disabil Rehabil 2005; 27:353–359.
3. Thomas DC, Kreizman IJ, Mekhiarre P, et al. Rehabilitation of the patient with chronic critical illness. Crit Care Clin 2002; 18:695–715.

4. Nelson JE, Meier DE, Litke A, et al. The symptom burden of chronic critical illness. Crit Care Med 2004; 32:1527–1534.
5. Nierman DM, Nelson JE, eds. Chronic critical illness. Crit Care Clin 2002; 18:461–715.
6. Knaus WA. Prognosis with mechanical ventilation: the influence of disease, severity of disease, age and chronic health status on survival from an acute illness. Am Rev Respir Dis 1989; 140: S8–S13.
7. Criner GJ. Care of the patient requiring invasive mechanical ventilation. Respir Care Clin N Am 2002; 8:575–592.
8. Griffiths RD, Jones CJ, eds. Intensive Care Aftercare. Oxford:Butterworth Heinmann, 2002.
9. Taricco M, De Tanti A, Boldrini P, et al. The rehabilitation management of traumatic brain injury patients during the acute phase: criteria for referral and transfer from intensive care units to rehabilitative facilities. Eura Medicophys 2006; 42:73–84.
10. Mammi P, Zaccaria B, Franceschini M. Early rehabilitative treatment in patients with traumatic brain injuries: outcome at one year follow up. Eura Medicophys 2006; 42:17–22.
11. Pronovost P, Berenholtz S, Ngo K, et al. Developing and pilot testing quality indicators in the intensive care unit. J Crit Care 2003; 18:145–155.
12. Crunden E, Boyce C, Woodman H, et al. An evaluation of the impact of the ventilator care bundle. Nurs Crit Care 2005; 10:242–246.
13. Dasgupta A, Rice R, Mascha E, et al. Four year experience with a unit for long-term ventilation (respiratory special care unit) at the Cleveland Clinical Foundation. Chest 1999; 116:447–455.
14. Pilcher DV, Bailey MJ, Treacher DF, et al. Outcomes, cost and long term survival of patients referred to a regional weaning centre. Thorax 2005; 60:187–192.
15. Scheinhorn DJ, Chao DC, Stearn-Hassenpflug M, et al. Post ICU mechanical ventilation: treatment of 1,123 patients at a regional weaning centre. Chest 1997; 111:1654–1659.
16. Gracy DR, Hardi DC, James MN, et al. The Mayo ventilator-dependent rehabilitation unit: a 5 year experience. Mayo Clin Proc 1997; 72:13–19.
17. Martin UJ, Hincapie L, Nimchuck M, et al. Impact of whole body rehabilitation in patients receiving chronic mechanical ventilation. Crit Care Med 2005; 3:2259–2265.
18. Schonhofer B, Euteneyer S, Nava S, et al. Survival of mechanically ventilated patients admitted to a specialized weaning centre. Intensive Care Med 2002; 28:908–916.
19. Thorens JB, Kaelin RM, Jolliet P, et al. Influence of the quality of nursing on the duration of weaning from mechanical ventilation in patients with chronic obstructive pulmonary disease. Crit Care Med 1995 23:1807–1815.
20. Engoren M. Marginal cost of liberating ventilator dependent patients after cardiac surgery in a step down unit. Ann Thorac Surg 2000; 70:182–185.
21. Storli SL, Lind R, Viotti I-L. Using diaries in intensive care: a method for following up patients. The World of Critical Care Nursing 2003; 2:103–108.

Appendix 1. Rehabilitation and Weaning Plan for the Case Report

Once Sarah was placed into the long-term phase of the rehabilitation framework, all active weaning from MV was stopped and the nurse consultant, the lead doctor, and the PT made a comprehensive and holistic assessment. Further advice was sought from the dietician, the speech and language therapist, and the pharmacist. An overall plan was then developed, which included the following:

1. Providing full support for respiratory muscles during and between exercise sessions.
2. Increasing PS, PEEP, and Fio_2 during exercises.
3. Decreasing ventilatory support only after Sarah demonstrated significant improvement in exercise tolerance, as measured by maximum inspiratory measure (P_{imax}), modified Borg scale, and functional independence measure.
4. Setting daily goals with Sarah, team, and family.
5. Sarah, dressing in her normal clothes during the day.
6. Not stopping therapy, but adapting it to meet Sarah's ability and medical condition.
7. Establishing communication strategies through leak speech.
8. Increasing calories when exercise tolerance increased.
9. Establishing following alternative therapies:
   - Pet therapy once per week
   - Music
   - Art
   - Guided imagery
   - Biofeedback
   - Reflexology
10. Monitoring reduced to a minimum.

Specific exercise program:

1. To sit out twice daily, progressing to all day
2. Standing transfers, bed to chair
3. Hourly breathing exercises
4. Resisted upper limb exercises using weights
5. Resisted trunk exercises
6. Treadmill work in the gym, while on portable ventilator.
   - Progression in time or speed as per tolerance—defined as ↓ $Spo_2 < 85\%$ or patient fatigue using a dyspnea visual analogue scale.
   - Use of Heliox during treadmill exercise entrained through the ventilator
7. Step ups.

Within three weeks of starting rehabilitation Sarah was weaned and decannulated.

Table A1 shows Sarah's exercise tolerance over the three-week period.

Table A1 Sarah's Rehabilitation Exercise Progress

Day 1, week 1	4 m (on pressure support ventilation)
Day 5, week 1	120 m (on pressure support ventilation)
Week 2	288 m (on pressure support ventilation)
Day 18, week 3	108 m (using entrained heliox via ventilator on reduced pressure support)
Day 20, week 3	67 m on a tracheostomy mask using heliox
Day 21, week 3	80 m following decannulation
Day 25	120 m prior to discharge on oxygen only

9
Indications and Physiological Basis of Rehabilitation in the ICU

ENRICO M. CLINI
University of Modena, Modena, and Ospedale Villa Pineta, Pavullo (MO), Italy

NICOLINO AMBROSINO
Pulmonary and Respiratory Intensive Care Unit-University Hospital Pisa, Italy and Pulmonary Rehabilitation and Weaning Center, Auxilium Vitae, Volterra (PI), Italy

I. Introduction

In developed countries, rehabilitation is considered an integral part of the management of patients in the intensive care unit (ICU), especially those who have overcome the acute stage of their condition. The intent is to apply advanced, cost-effective therapeutic modalities that maximize the patient's autonomy by improving function and preventing complications that might lead to rehospitalization and a poor prognosis (1,2). In other words, the two major end points of rehabilitation are restoring both respiratory and physical autonomy and decreasing the risks associated with prolonged bed rest. Both weaning from mechanical ventilation (MV) and physiotherapy will speed up the patient's recovery. By increasing patient mobility as well as secretion clearance, the early initiation of physiotherapy might well expedite weaning (3).

Table 1 summarizes the spectrum of rehabilitation for patients in the ICU. Given the costs associated with ICU management, health care specialists, including physiotherapists, must provide evidence-based practice. The precise role of the physiotherapist and the choice of techniques used vary among different ICUs, according to local practice, staff availability, and expertise (1,4,5). In some units, physiotherapists assess all patients and in others, patients are seen only by referral from the medical staff (1). In this chapter, we review the indications and the rationale for referring ICU patients for rehabilitation as well as the pathophysiological basis of the major interventions.

II. Weaning

A. Rationale and Outcome

Acute respiratory failure is the most common reason for admission to an ICU and 80% of mechanically ventilated patients resume spontaneous breathing after a few days (6). Of the remaining patients who cannot be weaned, those with chronic obstructive pulmonary disease (COPD) are often the most difficult to separate from the ventilator (7). Common obstacles to weaning include immobility and deconditioning prior to

Table 1 Components of Rehabilitation in Critical Care

Activity	Technique
Difficult weaning	
Team intervention	TDPs
Physiotherapy	
Mobilization	Postures
	Passive and active limb exercises
	CRT
Chest physiotherapy	MH
	Percusssion/vibration
	Manually or mechanically assisted cough suctioning
Muscle retraining	Respiratory muscle training
	Peripheral muscle training
	NMES

Abbreviations: TDP, therapist-driven protocols; CRT, continuous rotational therapy; MH, manual hyperinflation; NMES, neuromuscular electrical stimulation.

respiratory failure, systemic corticosteroids, neuromuscular blocking agents that promote immobility, disuse atrophy, malnutrition, and severe gas exchange abnormalities (6). Weaning can be considered as a specific rehabilitative intervention, aiming at restoring respiratory autonomy (8).

B. Therapist-Driven Protocols

Standardized weaning protocols are useful approaches for the difficult-to-wean patients (9–13). Therapist-driven protocols (TDPs) are daily care plans, which are drawn up by experienced staff and designed to be responsive to changes in the patient's condition, the latter being measured objectively by tracking physiological and clinical variables.

The plan requires a daily assessment of the ventilated patient, with a special emphasis on patient-to-ventilator synchrony (Fig. 1). On the basis of this assessment, the staff makes decisions, such as decreasing the level of assistance or changing a ventilation strategy, to follow a patient's need. The use of TDPs for weaning in the ICU reduces days of MV (11,13), costs, and complications (11).

When using a protocol-based strategy, the weaning success rate for difficult-to wean-patients is about 60% (6,8,14). Interestingly, the precise technique involved may be less important than the confidence and familiarity of the staff with the adopted protocol, or the underlying diagnosis (15).

III. Physiotherapy

A. Rationale and Outcome

The goals of physiotherapy (PT) are to prevent and treat pulmonary complications, such as infections, as well as minimizing the consequences of immobility (Fig. 2). The approaches involve secretion clearance techniques and exercises to restore mobility. Muscle mass and aerobic exercise performance decline during inactivity (16), with muscle strength declining

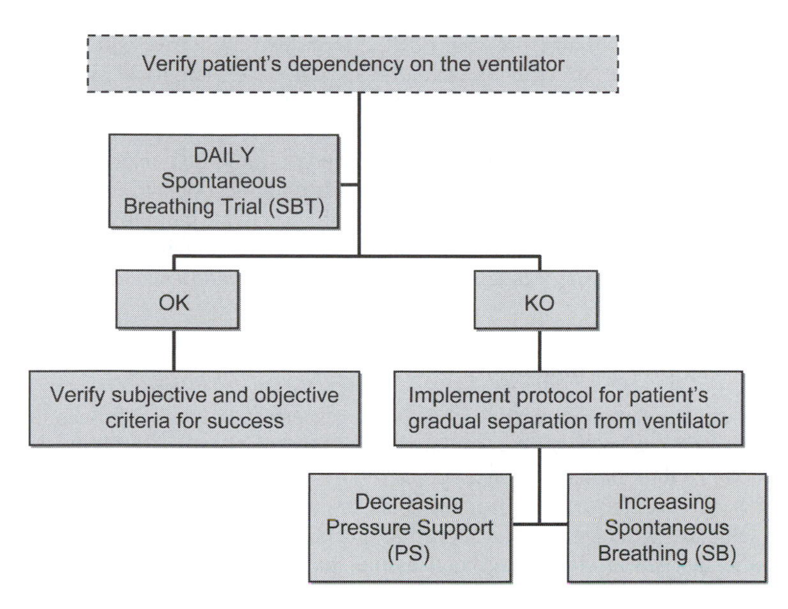

Figure 1 Therapist-driven protocol. Algorithm for daily assessment during weaning attempt.

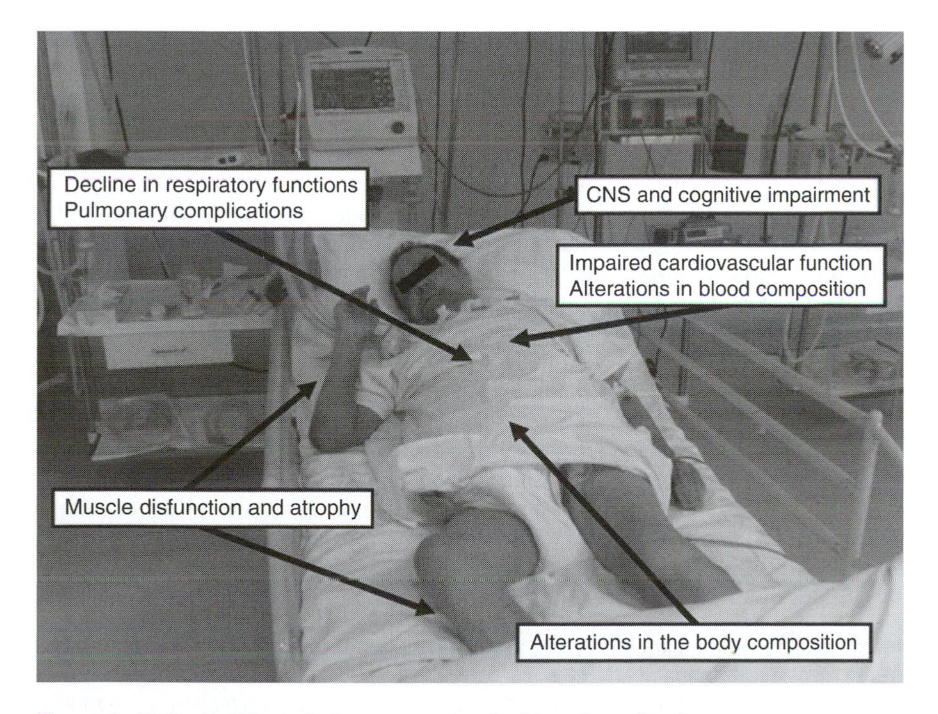

Figure 2 Pathophysiological changes associated with prolonged bed rest.

by 40% during the first week (17). Therefore, one of the simplest rehabilitative end points in the ICU is a return of muscle strength to enable basic daily life activities, such as washing, dressing and cooking, as well as the ability to walk independently.

Although clinically appealing, it should be noted that there is only limited evidence to support the notion that any specific PT intervention will improve morbidity or mortality, facilitate weaning, shorten the length of stay in ICU, or decrease complications. In one study (18), the addition of PT-postural drainage and manual hyperinflation twice daily to standard nursing care significantly reduced the incidence of nosocomial pneumonia. Such studies are difficult to standardize in the ICU, where diagnostic categories, comorbidities, and clinical interventions, vary considerably.

B. Effect on Respiratory Function

Several observational studies have reported on the short-term effect of chest PT on pulmonary function among ICU patients receiving invasive MV (19,20–24). Postural drainage and manual percussion or vibration have been associated with significant improvements in lung compliance (20), gas exchange, and intrapulmonary shunt (19,23), lasting for two hours (23) in some subjects, with other studies reporting no change (21,22,24). These trials were hampered by the absence of controls as well as the spontaneous variability in outcomes such as arterial blood gases (25).

C. Effect on Hemodynamics and Metabolism

Manual percussion in alternate side–lying positions, followed by suction in the supine position, in MV patients increases heart rate, systolic and mean arterial blood pressure, cardiac output, oxygen consumption, and carbon dioxide production for the duration of treatment (26). This increased metabolic demand resembles an exercise response, resulting from increased muscular activity (27). Indeed, oxygen consumption could be significantly reduced by pretreating patients with the paralytic agent vecuronium, but not by the hypnotic agent midazolam. Several other studies in ICUs documented both detrimental hemodynamic effects (28) and increased metabolic responses (29,30) associated with chest PT. These effects were present only during the application of treatment and lasted no more than half an hour after stopping it (31).

In a study of 72 critically ill patients, cardiac arrhythmias were noted in some following postural drainage and percussion (32). Minor (<6 premature atrial or ventricular contractions) and major (>6 premature ventricular contractions) arrythmias were recorded in 25% and 11% of patients, respectively, with none being life-threatening and all stopping on cessation of treatment. Suction and manual hyperinflation also increased intracranial pressure (32,33), although cerebral perfusion pressure was maintained at adequate levels. Although it is unlikely that chest PT would be dangerous or life-threatening in ICU patients, these possible side effects should be noted, especially when treating neurosurgical patients.

D. Effect of PT on Incidence and Course of Pulmonary Complications

Although reduction in pulmonary infections is one of the reasons for PT in the ICU, a combined intervention of postural drainage and manual hyperinflation resulted in only a slightly lower incidence of nosocomial pneumonia among MV patients, compared with a control group who received standard nursing care (13% vs. 16%, respectively) (18).

In two randomized controlled trials among postoperative and neurological ICU patients with acute lobar atelectasis, PT treatment, consisting of postural drainage, percussion, vibration, manual hyperinflation, and deep breathing with suction or coughing, resulted in conflicting outcomes (34,35) when compared with bronchoscopy secretion clearance techniques. Nonetheless, observational (19,36) and controlled studies (37) using combined PT techniques have underlined the favorable effect of PT on the resolution of acute lobar atelectasis. In clinical practice, pulmonary complications in intubated patients are usually managed by means of chest PT.

E. Effect on Muscles

Another important aspect of PT in the ICU is the prevention or treatment of immobility to reduce the complications associated with prolonged bed rest (38). An end point of rehabilitation would be a return of a muscle function sufficient to allow self-grooming activities and the ability to walk independently. There are several good reasons to increase mobility. First, ICU-associated bed rest influences skeletal muscle function and promotes disuse atrophy, which may be further aggravated by paralytic or corticosteroid medications. Prolonged bed rest and deconditioning causes a selective transformation, known as "slow to fast" transformation, of type IIa fibers to type IIb fibers, the former having a higher aerobic capacity (39). Immobility is also associated with a reduction in the number and density of mitochondria. The extent of the muscle atrophy depends on the location and the function of a specific muscle group. The antigravity muscles, such as the calf or back muscles, lose strength faster than the muscle groups associated with grip strength in the upper body (40,41). Passive training with neuromuscular electrical stimulation has been shown to improve lower limb muscle strength and to decrease the number of days needed for bed-bound ventilated COPD patients to transfer from a bed to a chair (42).

Second, the cardiovascular response to submaximal exercise is altered after a period of bed rest. The cardiac output and the stroke volume decrease and the heart rate increases (43,44). The cardiovascular adjustment to changing posture from supine to sitting is impaired in bed-ridden patients (45).

Third, immobility contributes to bone demineralization as well as protein and mineral wasting (46), which accounts, at least in part, for the loss of body weight and the relative increase in the fat mass.

Finally, immobility influences both the central and the peripheral nervous systems, reducing cognitive performance (47) and peripheral muscle function (48). These disorders, which develop during an ICU stay, can be classified as diseases of both peripheral nerves, neuromuscular synapses, and muscle fibers. The clinical appearance resembles a polyneuropathy whose severity correlates with the length of stay (48), sometimes leading to quadriplegia (49). In recent years, this new ICU-associated syndrome has been defined as the "critical illness myopathy and neuropathy" (50,51). It is distinct from the specific changes associated with bed rest and its occurrence has a negative correlation with the success of weaning (52).

Abnormal gas exchange, malnutrition, and prolonged use of controlled ventilation, leading to selective diaphragmatic muscle atrophy, add to peripheral and respiratory muscle weakness (38). Many of the above reasons make it likely that patients will benefit from PT that targets respiratory and skeletal muscle function, although clearer evidence of positive outcomes is still required (53). Inspiratory muscle training has been shown to facilitate weaning in an unselected ICU population (54). In one retrospective study of 49 difficult-to-wean patients (55), whole-body rehabilitation improved peripheral and respiratory muscle strength, thus allowing all the patients to become independent in both ambulation and ventilation. Two randomized ICU trials have reported on the effects of peripheral muscle retraining in COPD patients recovering from an acute episode of hypercapnic respiratory failure (56,57). In the first trial by Nava (56), a step-by-step retraining program was associated with a more significant improvement in the patient's exercise capacity and symptom scores, compared with controls. In the second trial by Porta (57), arm-ergometer training improved strength and endurance of the upper limbs in patients recently weaned from MV.

IV. Conclusions

There is some evidence to support PT rehabilitation in the ICU (2) as an aid to earlier discharge and improved recovery (58), although the evidence that it results in long-term gains remains to be established. Since ICU care is associated with reduced survival in the following year (59,60), any treatment that might enhance the patient's functional capacity and independence is of great interest (61). It is likely that the earlier the rehabilitation can begin, the greater the potential for it to address the effects of immobility and prolonged bed rest.

Although TDPs for difficult-to-wean patients are well established (62), evidence supporting other PT treatments is limited by the paucity of well-designed long-term controlled trials. The details of the various airway clearance techniques are addressed elsewhere in this text. The effect of mobilization on weaning from MV and the influence of PT on improving muscle strength and function provide stimulating clinical research topics for the rehabilitation community. Assessment of the patient's perspective may also help in understanding the optimum time for introducing rehabilitation in the ICU (63).

References

1. Stiller K. Physiotherapy in intensive care. Towards an evidence-based practice. Chest 2000; 118:1801–1813.
2. Clini E, Ambrosino N. Early physiotherapy in the respiratory intensive care unit. Respir Med 2005; 99:1096–1104.
3. Topp R, Ditmyer M, King K, et al. The effect of bed rest and potential of prehabilitation on patients in the intensive care unit. AACN Clin Issues 2002; 13:263–276.
4. Casaburi R. Deconditioning. In: Fishman AP ed. Pulmonary Rehabilitation. New York: Marcel Dekker, 1996:213–230.
5. Norrenberg M, Vincent JL. A profile of European intensive care unit physiotherapists. Intensive Care Med 2000; 26:988–994.
6. ACCP, AARC, ACCCM task force. Evidence based guidelines for weaning and discontinuing ventilatory support. Chest 2001; 120:375s–395s.
7. Brochard L, Rauss A, Benito S, et al. Comparison of three methods of gradual withdrawal from ventilatory support during weaning from mechanical ventilation. Am J Respir Crit Care Med 1994; 150:896–903.
8. Scheinhorn DJ, Chao DC, Stearn-Hassenpflug M, et al. Post-ICU mechanical ventilation treatment of 1123 patients at a regional weaning center. Chest 1997; 111:1654–1659.

9. Butler R, Keenan SP, Inman KJ, et al. Is there a preferred technique for weaning the difficult-to-wean patient? A systematic review of the literature. Crit Care Med 1999; 27:2331–2336.
10. Vitacca M, Vianello A, Colombo D, et al. Comparison of two methods for weaning COPD patients requiring mechanical ventilation for more than 15 days. Am J Respir Crit Care Med 2001; 164:225–230.
11. Ely EW, Baker AM, Dunagan DP, et al. Effect of the duration of mechanical ventilation of identifying patients capable of breathing spontaneously. N Engl J Med 1996; 335:1864–1869.
12. Kollef MH, Shapiro SD, Silver P, et al. A randomized controlled trial of protocol-directed versus physician directed weaning from mechanical ventilation. Crit Care Med 1997; 25:567–574.
13. Saura P, Blanch L, Mestre L, et al. Clinical consequences of the implementation of a weaning protocol. Intensive Care Med 1996; 22:1052–1056.
14. Schonhofer B, Euteneuer S, Nava S, et al. Survival of mechanically ventilated patients admitted to a specialized weaning center. Intensive Care Med 2002; 28:908–916.
15. Vitacca M. Therapist driven protocols. Monaldi Arch Chest Dis 2003; 59:342–324 (review).
16. Bloomfield SA. Changes in musculoskeletal structure and function with prolonged bed rest. Med Sci Sports Exerc 1997; 29:197–206.
17. Fowles JR, Sale DG, MacDougal JD. Reduce strength after passive stretch of the human plantar flexors. J Appl Physiol 2000; 89:1179–1188.
18. Ntoumenopoulos G, Presneill JJ, Mc Elholum M, et al. Chest physiotherapy for the prevention of ventilator associated pneumonia. Intensive Care Med 2002; 28:850–856.
19. Stiller K, Jenkins S, Grant R. Acute lobar atelectasis: a comparison of five physiotherapy regimens. Physiother Theory Pract 1996; 12:197–209.
20. Mackenzie CF, Shin B. Cardiorespiratory function before and after chest physiotherapy in mechanically ventilated patients with post-traumatic respiratory failure. Crit Care Med 1985; 13:483–486.
21. Novak RA, Shumaker L, Snyder JV, et al. Do periodic hyperinflations improve gas exchange in patients with hypoxemic respiratory failure? Crit Care Med 1987; 15:1081–1085.
22. Poelaert J, Lannoy B, Vogelaers D, et al. Influence of chest physiotherapy on arterial oxygen saturation. Acta Anaesthesiol Belg 1991; 42:165–170.
23. Jones AYM, Hutchinson RC, Oh TE. Effects of bagging and percussion on total static compliance of the respiratory system. Physiotherapy 1992; 78:661–666.
24. Eales CJ, Barker M, Cubberley NJ. Evaluation of a single chest physiotherapy treatment to post-operative, mechanically ventilated cardiac surgery patients. Physiother Theory Pract 1995; 11:23–28.
25. Sasse SA, Chen PA, Mahutte CK. Variability of arterial blood gas values over time in stable medical ICU patients. Chest 1994; 106:187–193.
26. Cohen D, Horiuchi K, Kemper M, et al. Modulating effects of propofol on metabolic and cardiopulmonary responses to stressful intensive care unit procedures. Crit Care Med 1996; 24:612–617.
27. Horiuchi K, Jordan D, Cohen D, et al. Insights into the increased oxygen demand during chest physiotherapy. Crit Care Med 1997; 25:1347–1351.
28. Paratz J. Haemodynamic stability of the ventilated intensive care patient: a review. Aust J Physiother 1992; 38:167–172.
29. Weissman C, Kemper M, Harding J. Response of critically ill patients to increased oxygen demand: hemodynamic subsets. Crit Care Med 1994; 22:1809–1816.
30. Harding J, Kemper M, Weissman C. Pressure support ventilation attenuates the cardiopulmonary response to an acute increase in oxygen demand. Chest 1995; 107:1665–1672.
31. Harding J, Kemper M, Weissman C. Midazolam attenuates the metabolic and cardiopulmonary responses to an acute increase in oxygen demand. Chest 1994; 106:194–200.
32. Hammon WE, Connors AF, McCaffree DR. Cardiac arrhythmias during postural drainage and chest percussion of critically ill patients. Chest 1992; 102:1836–1841.

33. Ersson U, Carlson H, Mellstrom A, et al. Observations on intracranial dynamics during respiratory physiotherapy in unconscious neurosurgical patients. Acta Anaesthesiol Scand 1990; 34:99–103.
34. Stiller K, Geake T, Taylor J, et al. Acute lobar atelectasis: a comparison of two chest physiotherapy regimens. Chest 1990; 98:1336–1340.
35. Fourrier F, Fourrier L, Lestavel P, et al. Acute lobar atelectasis in ICU patients: comparative randomized study of fiberoptic bronchoscopy versus respiratory therapy. Intensive Care Med 1994; 20:S40.
36. Hammon WE, Martin RJ. Chest physical therapy for acute atelectasis. Phys Ther 1981; 61:217–220.
37. Raoof S, Chowdhrey N, Raoof S, et al. Effect of combined kinetic therapy and percussion therapy on the resolution of atelectasis in critically ill patients. Chest 1999; 115:1658–1666.
38. Cirio S, Piaggi GC, De Mattia E, et al. Muscle retraining in ICU patients. Monaldi Arch Chest Dis 2003; 59:300–303.
39. Bloomfield SA. Changes in musculoskeletal structure and function with prolonged bed rest. Med Sci Sports Exerc 1997; 29:197–206.
40. Coyle EF, Martin WH, Bloomfield SA, et al. Effects of detraining on response to submaximal exercise. J Appl Physiol 1985; 59:853–859.
41. Geboers JF, Van Tuijl JH, Seelen HA, et al. Effect of immobilization on ankle dorsiflexion strength. Scand J Rehabil Med 2000; 32:66–71.
42. Zanotti E, Felicetti G, Maini M, et al. Peripheral muscle strength training in bed-bound patients with COPD receiving mechanical ventilation. Effect of electrical stimulation. Chest 2003; 124:2992–2996.
43. Hung J, Goldwater D, Convertino VA, et al. Mechanism for decreased exercise capacity after bed rest in normal middle-aged men. Am J Cardiol 1983; 51:344–348.
44. Martin WH, Coyle EF, Bloomfield SA, et al. Effects of physical deconditioning after intense endurance training on left ventricular dimension and stroke volume. J Am Coll Cardiol 1986; 7:982–989.
45. Fareeduddin K, Abelmann WH. Impaired orthostatic tolerance after bed rest in patients with myocardial infarction. N Engl J Med 1969; 280:345–350.
46. Bortz WM. Disuse and aging. JAMA 1982; 248:1203–1208.
47. Downs F. Bed rest and sensory disturbances. Am J Nurs 1974; 74:434–438.
48. Witt NJ, Zochodne DW, Bolton CF, et al. Peripheral nerve function in sepsis and multiple organ failure. Chest 1991; 99:176–184.
49. Berek K, Margreiter J, Willeit J, et al. Polyneuropathies in critically ill patients: a prospective evaluation. Intensive Care Med 1996; 22:849–855.
50. Latronico N, Fenzi F, Recupero D, et al. Critical illness neuropathy and myopathy. Lancet 1996; 347:1579–1582.
51. De Jonghe B, Cook D, Sharshar T, et al. Acquired neuromuscular disorders in critically ill patients: a systematic review. Intensive Care Med 1998; 24:1242–1250.
52. De Jonghe B, Bastuji-Garin S, Sharshaar T, et al. Does ICU-acquired paresis lengthen weaning from mechanical ventilation? Intensive Care Med 2004; 30:1117–1121.
53. Lötters F, Van Tol B, Kwakkel G, et al. Effects of controlled inspiratory muscle training in patients with COPD: a meta-analysis. Eur Resp J 2002; 20:570–577.
54. Martin DA, Davenport PD, Franceschi AC, et al. Use of inspiratory muscle strength training to facilitate ventilator weaning. Chest 2002; 122:192–196.
55. Martin UJ, Hincapie L, Nimchuk M, et al. Impact of whole-body rehabilitation in patients receiving chronic mechanical ventilation. Crit Care Med 2005; 33:2259–2265.
56. Nava S. Rehabilitation of patients admitted to a respiratory intensive care unit. Arch Phys Med Rehabil 1998; 79:849–854.

57. Porta R, Vitacca M, Gilè S, et al. Supported arm training in patients recently weaned from mechanical ventilation. Chest 2005; 128:2511–2520.
58. Jones C, Skirrow P, Griffiths RD, et al. Rehabilitation after critical illness: a randomized, controlled trial. Crit Care Med 2003; 31:2456–2461.
59. Stoller JK, Xu M, Mascha E, et al. Long-term outcomes for patients discharged from a long-term hospital-based weaning unit. Chest 2003; 124:1892–1899.
60. Niskanen M, Kari A, Halonen P. Five-year survival after intensive care. Comparison of 12,180 patients with the general population. Finnish ICU Study Group. Crit Care Med 1996; 24:1962–1667.
61. Ambrosino N, Porta R. Rehabilitation and acute exacerbations of chronic obstructive pulmonary disease. In: Siafakas NM, Anthonisen NR, Georgopoulos D, eds. Acute Exacerbations of Chronic Obstructive Pulmonary Disease. New York: Marcel Dekker, 2004:507–530.
62. Kollef MH, Shapiro SD, Clinkscale D, et al. The effect of respiratory therapist-initiated treatment protocols on patient outcomes and resource utilization. Chest 2000; 117:467–475.
63. Zibrak JD, Rosseti P, Wood E. Effect of reductions in respiratory therapy on patient outcome. N Engl J Med 1986; 315:292–295.

10
Peripheral and Respiratory Muscle Training

RIK GOSSELINK, THIERRY TROOSTERS*, and MARC DECRAMER
University Hospitals Leuven and Katholieke Universiteit Leuven, Leuven, Belgium

I. Introduction

The progress of intensive care medicine has dramatically improved the survival of critically ill patients, especially in patients with acute respiratory distress syndrome (ARDS) (1,2). This improved survival rate is, however, associated with general deconditioning, muscle weakness, dyspnea, depression and anxiety, and reduced health-related quality of life after intensive care unit (ICU) discharge (3–5). Deconditioning and, specifically, muscle weakness are suggested to have a key role in impaired functional status after ICU stay (3). Indeed, optimal physiological functioning depends on the upright position (6–9), so bed rest and limited mobility during critical illness result in profound physical deconditioning and dysfunction of the respiratory, cardiovascular, musculoskeletal, neurological, renal, and endocrine systems. These effects can be exacerbated by inflammation and pharmacological agents, such as corticosteroids, muscle relaxants, neuromuscular blockers and antibiotics. Denervation atrophy may also complicate critical illness and sepsis has been shown to be one of the most important determinants of critical illness polyneuropathy (10). Ginz et al. reported 20–40% reductions in involuntary muscle force of the ankle dorsiflexors upon peroneal nerve stimulation in critically ill patients who were immobilized for a week (11). These data are in line with findings in which stimulation of the ulnar nerve was used (–40% in patients, compared to controls) (12). Consecutive muscle biopsies of the tibialis anterior in critically ill patients showed 3–4% reduction per day in fiber cross-sectional area in both type I and type II fibers (13). The prevalence of skeletal muscle weakness in the ICU is poorly investigated. In a prospective study, De Jonghe et al. investigated 95 of 206 patients ventilated for more than seven days. Twenty-five percent of the patients developed clinically significant muscle weakness (14). In another study, prospectively investigating patients with multiple organ failure, half of the patients developed some focal or diffuse weakness and 26% developed severe muscle weakness (15). In addition, a patient with underlying chronic disease may already have muscle weakness before being admitted to the ICU. In animal experiments, it was shown that as few as 24 hours of mechanical ventilation does induce changes in muscle regulatory factors (MyoD, myogenin), in the diaphragm, and gastrocnemius muscle (16). It is clear that these changes were induced long before the "critical illness myopathy." Hence, it is important to realize that even in patients not formally diagnosed with critical illness myopathy, muscle dysfunction may be present.

*Post-doctoral Fellow of FWO-Vlaanderen.

Development of neuropathy or myopathy also contributes to weaning failure (17). Although most patients under mechanical ventilation are extubated in less than three days, still approximately 20% require prolonged support (18). Chronic ventilator dependence is not only a major medical problem, but is also an extremely uncomfortable state for a patient, carrying important social implications. There is accumulating evidence that weaning problems are associated with failure of the respiratory muscles to resume ventilation and inspiratory muscle training might therefore be beneficial in patients with weaning failure.

The above mentioned changes in peripheral and respiratory functions not only indicate the need for rehabilitation after ICU stay (5,19), but also underscores the need for measures to prevent muscle deconditioning during ICU stay.

II. Peripheral Muscle Training

Although bed rest is required to support recovery, the risks associated with rest have been well documented (20) and it needs to be used judiciously (20–23). To avoid or minimize physical deconditioning and other complications, short duration of mechanical ventilation with early extubation are prime goals of the critical care team. Early mobilization was shown to reduce the time to wean from mechanical ventilation and is the basis for long-term functional recovery (21,23). Evidence for the benefits of body positioning, mobilization, exercise, and muscle training, on the prevention and treatment of deconditioning in other patient groups (24), as well as in healthy subjects, lends support for the use of these interventions in the management of critically ill patients.

Mobilization has been part of the physiotherapy management of acutely ill patients for several decades (25,26). Mobilization in this context differs from nursing care and refers to physical activity sufficient to elicit acute physiological effects that enhance ventilation, central and peripheral perfusions, circulation, muscle metabolism, and alertness. Strategies, in order of intensity, include active and passive turning and moving in bed, active-assisted and active exercises, use of cycling pedals in bed or at the bedside, sitting at the edge of the bed, standing, stepping in place, transferring to bed and from the bed to chair, chair exercises, and walking. Exercise and walking are countermeasures for venous stasis and deep vein thrombosis. Patients with identifiable risk factors, such as advancing age, history of smoking, obesity, general anesthesia, malignancy, or circulatory disease, particularly warrant prophylactic treatment of deep vein thrombosis. Standing and walking frames (Fig. 1) enable the patient to mobilize safely with attachments for bags, lines, and leads that cannot be disconnected. The arm support on a frame or rollator has been shown to increase ventilatory capacity in patients with severe chronic obstructive pulmonary disease (COPD) (27). The frame needs to be able to accommodate either a portable oxygen tank or a portable mechanical ventilator and seat, or a suitable trolley for equipment can be used. Walking and standing aids and tilt tables enhance physiological responses (28,29) and promote early mobilization of critically ill patients (30,31). The tilt table may be used to effect gravitational stress; however, the patient is unable to move the legs to counter dependent fluid displacement and may be at risk of orthostatic intolerance. Abdominal belts need to be carefully positioned to support, not restrict, respiration during mobilization. In patients with spinal cord injury, this improves vital capacity (32). Transfer belts facilitate heavy lifts and protect both the patient and the physiotherapist. Noninvasive ventilation (NIV) during mobilization may improve exercise tolerance for nonintubated patients,

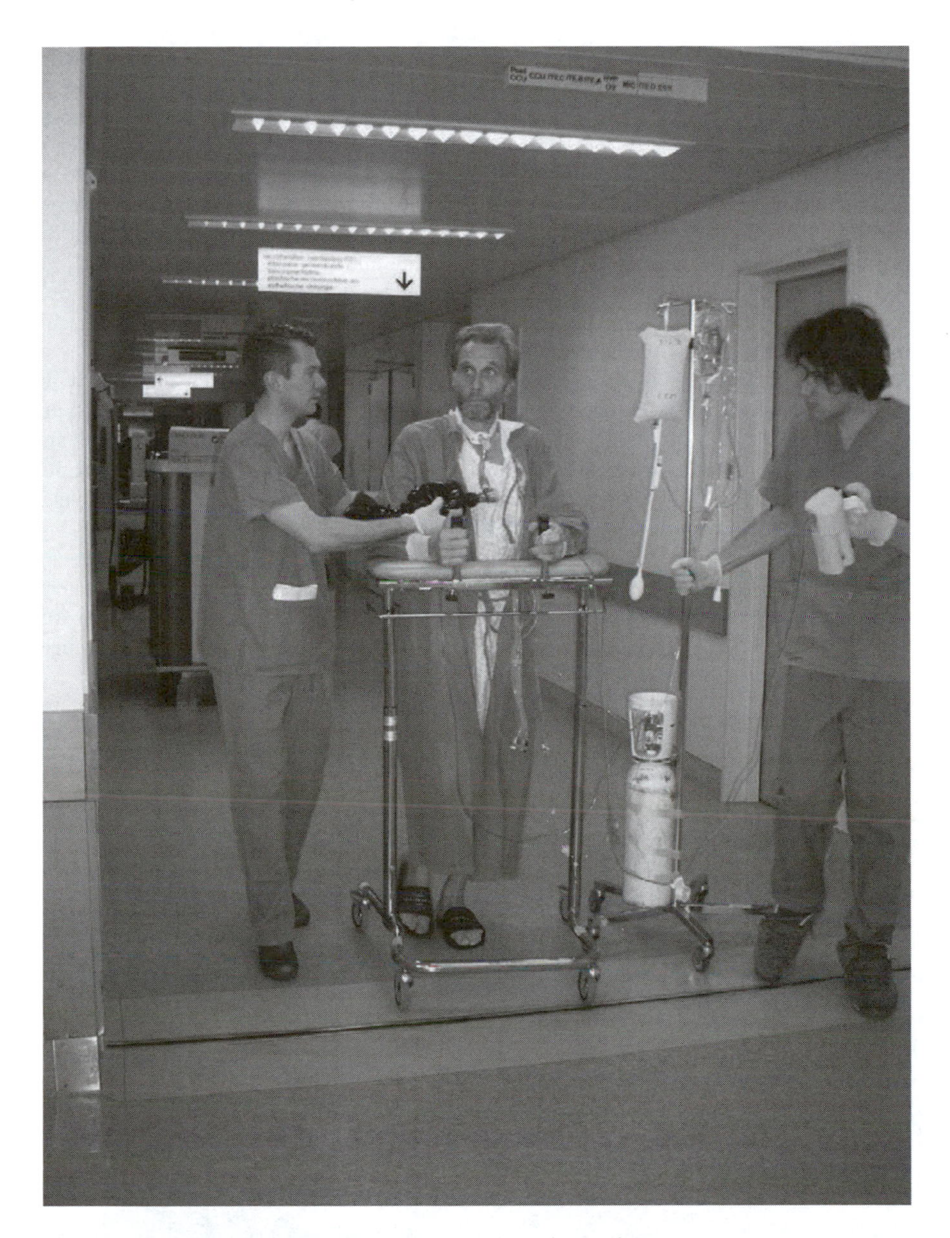

Figure 1 Walking frame to assist a ventilator-dependent patient.

similar to that demonstrated in patients with stable COPD (33). However, no randomized trials have been performed in this setting. In ventilated patients, the ventilator settings may require adjustment to the patient's needs (i.e., increased minute ventilation).

Aerobic training and muscle strengthening, in addition to routine mobilization, improved walking distance more than mobilization alone in patients on long-term mechanical ventilation and chronic critical illness (34). A recent randomized controlled trial showed that a six-week upper and lower limb training program improved limb muscle strength, ventilator-free time, and functional outcomes in patients requiring long-term mechanical ventilation compared to a control group (35). These results are in line with a retrospective analysis of patients on long-term mechanical ventilation who participated in whole-body training and respiratory muscle training (36). In patients recently weaned from mechanical ventilation (37), the addition of upper-limb exercise enhanced the effects of chest physiotherapy on exercise endurance performance and dyspnea.

The application of exercise training in the early phase of ICU admission is often more complicated because of cooperation and clinical status of the patient. Recent technological development resulted in equipment for (active or passive) leg cycling during bed rest (Fig. 2). The application of active cycling on this device in hospitalized patients with exacerbations of severe COPD has been reported to double oxygen consumption (38), while passive cycling also significantly increased oxygen consumption (38). An interim analysis of a randomized controlled trial of early application of leg cycling in critically ill patients showed improved functional status at hospital discharge compared to patients receiving standard physiotherapy without leg cycling (39).

Low-resistance multiple repetitions of resistive muscle training can augment muscle mass, force generation, and activate oxidative enzymes. This increase, in turn, can improve O_2 extraction and efficiency of muscle O_2 kinetics (40). Sets of repetitions [3 sets of 8–10 repetitions at 50–70% of 1 repetition maximum (RM)] (41) within the patient's tolerance

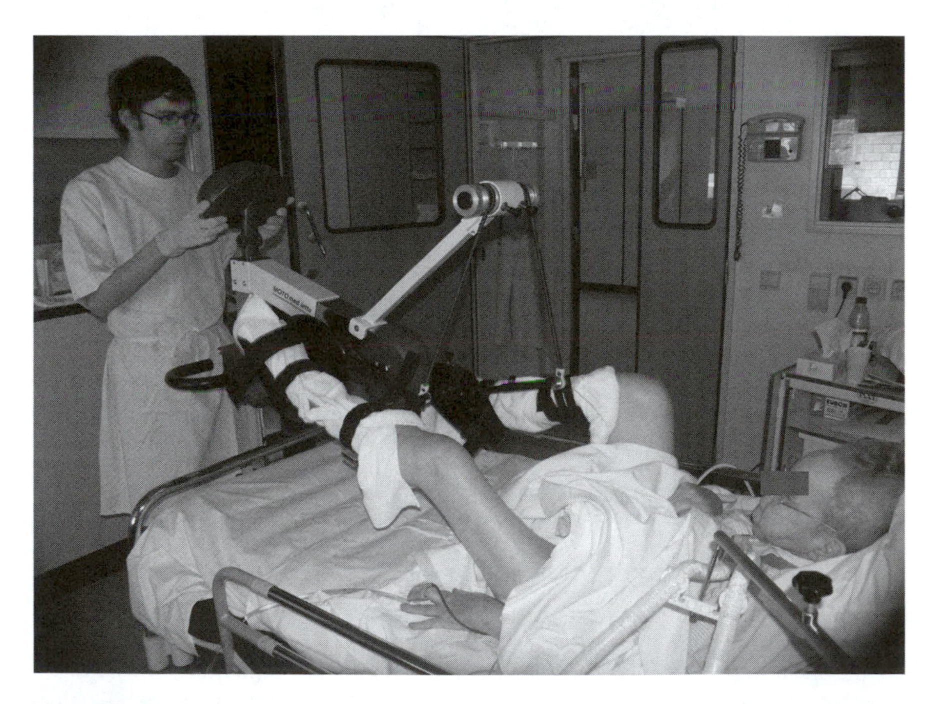

Figure 2 Device for active and passive cycling in a bedridden patient in the intensive care unit.

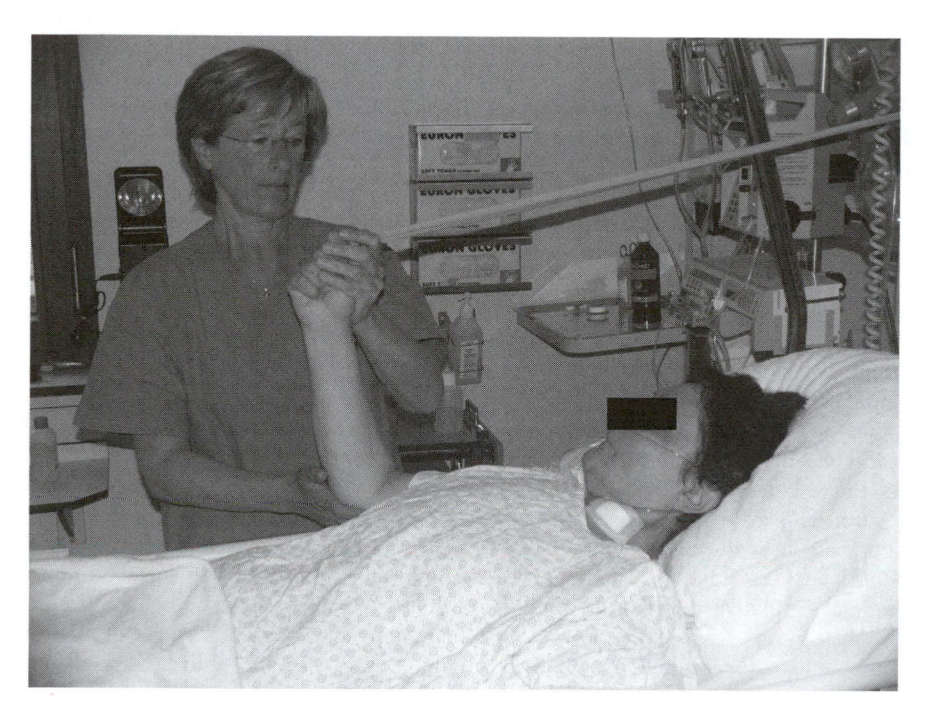

Figure 3 Resistance muscle training for lower limbs in a patient with critical illness with elastic straps.

can be scheduled daily, commensurate with their goals. Resistive muscle training can include the use of pulleys, elastic bands, and weight belts (Fig. 3). Patients with cardiovascular dysfunction may benefit from resistance training, although high resistance of large muscle masses may have detrimental cardiovascular effects in elderly subjects with cardiovascular disease.

In patients unable to perform voluntary muscle contractions, electrical muscle stimulation (EMS) (Fig. 4) has been used to prevent disuse muscle atrophy. In patients with

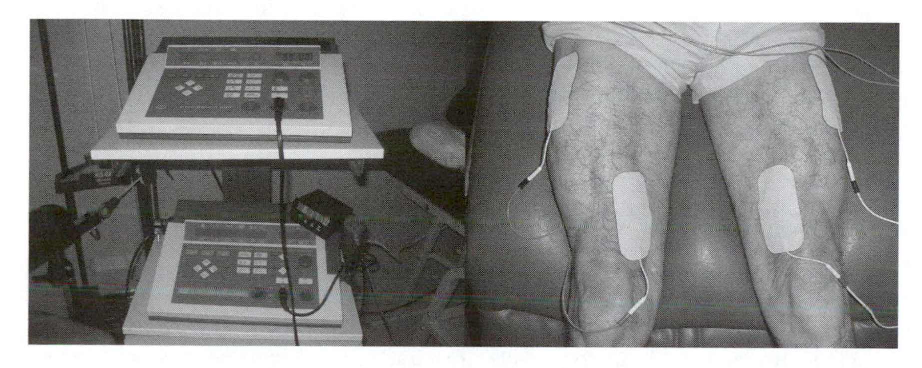

Figure 4 Neuromusclar stimulation of the quadriceps femoris muscles.

lower limb fractures and cast immobilization for six weeks, daily EMS for at least one hour reduced the decrease in cross-sectional area of the quadriceps and enhanced normal muscle protein synthesis (42). In patients with COPD in the ICU, EMS of the quadriceps, in addition to active limb mobilization, enhanced muscle strength and hastened independent transfer from bed to chair (43).

Alternatively, passive stretching or range of motion exercise may have a particularly important role in the management of patients who are unable to move spontaneously. Studies in healthy subjects have shown that passive stretching decreases stiffness and increases extensibility of the muscle (44,45). Passive stretching for at least 30 minutes a day prevented loss of joint mobility and muscle mass in an animal model (46). Passive movement has been shown to enhance ventilation in neurological patients in high-dependency units (47). In other patient groups, evidence for using continuous dynamic stretching is based on the observation that continuous passive motion (CPM) prevents contractures and promotes muscle function. It appears particularly effective in patients with intra-articular fractures (48,49). CPM has been assessed in patients with critical illness subjected to prolonged inactivity (50). In critically ill patients, three hours of CPM per day reduced fiber atrophy and protein loss, compared with passive stretching for five minutes, twice daily (50).

For patients who cannot be actively mobilized and have high risk of soft tissue contracture, such as following severe burns, trauma, and some neurological conditions, splinting may be indicated. Splinting of the periarticular structures in the stretched position for more than 11 hours a day was shown to have a beneficial effect on the range of motion in an animal model (51). In burns patients, fixing the position of joints reduced muscle and skin contractions (52). In patients with neurological dysfunction, splinting may reduce muscle tone (53).

The prescription of exercise intensity, duration, and frequency is response dependent rather than time dependent and is based on clinical challenge tests, such as the response to a nursing or investigative procedure or to a specific mobilization challenge. Exercise should be safely tolerated in any treatment session and, if the patient responds positively, greater intensity and duration can be applied. For acutely ill patients, frequent short sessions (analogous to interval training) allow for greater recovery than the less frequent, longer sessions prescribed for patients with chronic stable conditions (54). Patients with hemodyamic instability, or with little to no O_2 transport reserve capacity (e.g., those on high concentrations of O_2 and high levels of ventilatory support, or those with anemia or cardiovascular instability), are not candidates for aggressive mobilization. The risk of moving a critically ill patient is weighed against the risk of immobility and recumbency and, when employed, requires stringent monitoring to ensure that the mobilization is instituted appropriately and safely (55). Stiller and Philips have outlined the steps involved in safe mobilization of critically ill patients (55).

III. Weaning and Respiratory Muscle Training

Only a small proportion of patients fail to wean from mechanical ventilation, but they require a disproportionate amount of resources. Weaning failure has been extensively studied in the clinical literature and several factors are likely to contribute to it. These factors include inadequate ventilatory drive, respiratory muscle weakness, respiratory muscle fatigue, increased work of breathing, or cardiac failure. There is accumulating evidence that weaning problems are associated with failure of the respiratory muscles to resume ventilation (56–58). Respiratory muscle weakness is often observed in patients with weaning failure. Patients who had received mechanical ventilation for more than 48 hours had reduced inspiratory muscle endurance that worsens with the duration of mechanical ventilation and is present following successful weaning. These data suggest that patients needing prolonged mechanical ventilation are at risk of respiratory muscle fatigue (58). Indeed, a high ratio of respiratory muscle workload and muscle capacity [inspiratory pressure/maximal inspiratory pressure (P_I/P_{Imax})] is a major cause of ventilator dependency and predicts the outcome of successful weaning (56).

Since inactivity ("ventilator induced diaphragm dysfunction") is suggested to be an important cause of respiratory muscle failure and intermittent loading of the respiratory muscles have been shown to attenuate respiratory muscle deconditioning (59), inspiratory muscle training might be beneficial to patients with weaning failure. Some investigators might argue against the application of loaded breathing in the treatment of weaning failure on the basis of studies showing subcellular diaphragm muscle damage after loaded breathing (60,61). However, these changes were observed after continuous loading instead of intermittent loading as applied during inspiratory muscle training (eight contractions repeated in three series). An improvement in inspiratory muscle function and a reduction in duration of mechanical ventilation and weaning time was observed in more recent uncontrolled trials of inspiratory muscle training (threshold loading) (Fig. 5) (62,63).

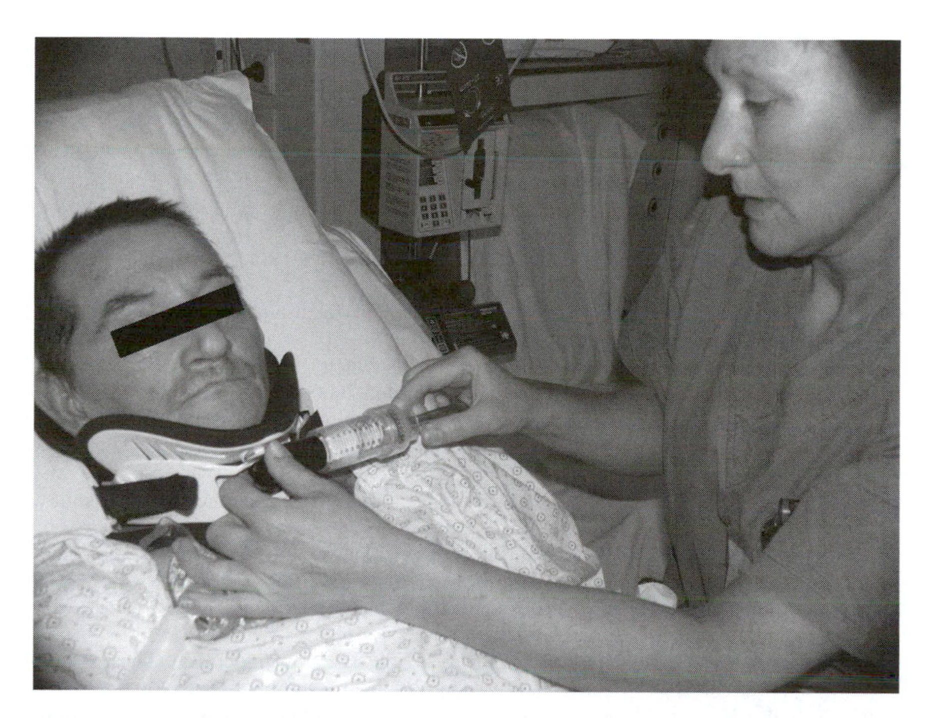

Figure 5 Respiratory muscle resistive training with threshold loading in a patient weaning from mechanical ventilation.

Interim analysis of a randomized controlled trial comparing inspiratory muscle training at moderate intensity (~50% P_{Imax}) versus sham training in patients with weaning failure showed that a statistically significant larger proportion of the training group (76%) could be weaned compared to the sham group (35%) (64). Alternatively, in patients unable to cooperate with respiratory muscle training, intermittent electrical stimulation of the diaphragm through phrenic nerve pacing might be applied (65). So far, only studies in patients with spinal cord injury were reported to support this concept.

References

1. Milberg JA, Davis DR, Steinberg KP, et al. Improved survival of patients with acute respiratory distress syndrome (ARDS): 1983–1993. JAMA 1995; 273:306–309.
2. Eisner MD, Thompson T, Hudson LD, et al. Efficacy of low tidal volume ventilation in patients with different clinical risk factors for acute lung injury and the acute respiratory distress syndrome. Am J Respir Crit Care Med 2001; 164:231–236.
3. Herridge MS, Cheung AM, Tansey CM, et al. One-year outcomes in survivors of the acute respiratory distress syndrome. N Engl J Med 2003; 348:683–693.
4. Montuclard L, Garrouste-Org, Timsit JF, et al. Outcome, functional autonomy, and quality of life of elderly patients with a long-term intensive care unit stay. Crit Care Med 2000; 28:3389–3395.
5. Fletcher SN, Kennedy DD, Ghosh IR, et al. Persistent neuromuscular and neurophysiologic abnormalities in long-term survivors of prolonged critical illness. Crit Care Med 2003; 31:1012–1016.
6. Convertino VA G-factor as a tool in basic research: mechanisms of orthostatic tolerance. J Gravit Physiol 1999; 6:73–76.
7. Dittmer DK, Teasell R. Complications of immobilization and bed rest. Part 1: Musculoskeletal and cardiovascular complications. Can Fam Physician 1993; 39:1428–1427.
8. Morishima K, Sekiya N, Miyashita S, et al. Effects of 20 days horizontal bed rest on maintaining upright standing posture in young persons. J Gravit Physiol 1997; 4:S41–S45.
9. Teasell R, Dittmer DK. Complications of immobilization and bed rest. Part 2: other complications. Can Fam Physician 1993; 39:1440–1446.
10. Eikermann M, Koch G, Gerwig M, et al. Muscle force and fatigue in patients with sepsis and multiorgan failure. Intensive Care Med 2006; 32:251–259.
11. Ginz HF, Iaizzo PA, Girard T, et al. Decreased isometric skeletal muscle force in critically ill patients. Swiss Med Wkly 2005; 135:555–561.
12. Harris ML, Luo YM, Watson AC, et al. Adductor pollicis twitch tension assessed with magnetic stimulation of the ulnar nerve. Am J Respir Crit Care Med 2000; 162:240–245.
13. Helliwell T, Wilkinson A, Griffiths RD, et al. Muscle fibre atrophy in critically ill patients is associated with the loss of myosin filaments and the presence of lysomal enzymes and ubiquitin. Neuropath Appl Neurobiol 1998; 24:507–517.
14. De Jonghe B, Sharshar T, Lefaucheur JP, et al. Paresis acquired in the intensive care unit: a prospective multicenter study. JAMA 2002; 288:2859–2867.
15. Bednarik J, Lukas Z, Vondracek P. Critical illness polyneuromyopathy: the electrophysiological components of a complex entity. Intensive Care Med 2003; 29:1505–1514.
16. Racz GZ, Gayan-Ramirez G, Testelmans D, et al. Early changes in rat diaphragm biology with mechanical ventilation. Am J Respir Crit Care Med 2003; 168:297–304.
17. Hund EF. Neuromuscular complications in the ICU: the spectrum of critical illness-related conditions causing muscular weakness and weaning failure. J Neurol Sci 1996; 136:10–16.
18. Esteban A, Frutos F, Tobin MJ, et al. A comparison of four methods of weaning patients from mechanical ventilation. N Engl J Med 1995; 332:345–350.

19. Jones C, Skirrow P, Griffiths RD, et al. Rehabilitation after critical illness: a randomized, controlled trial. Crit Care Med 2003; 31:2456–2461.
20. Allen C, Glasziou P, Del Mar C. Bed rest: a potentially harmful treatment needing more careful evaluation. Lancet 1999; 354:1229–1233.
21. Topp R, Ditmyer M, King K et al. The effect of bed rest and potential of prehabilitation on patients in the intensive care unit. AACN Clin Issues 2002; 13:263–276.
22. Dock W. The evil sequelae of complete bed rest. JAMA 1944; 125:1083–1085.
23. Thomas DC, Kreizman IJ, Melchiorre P, et al. Rehabilitation of the patient with chronic critical illness. Crit Care Clin 2002; 18:695–715.
24. Smidt N, de Vet HC, Bouter LM, et al. Effectiveness of exercise therapy: a best-evidence summary of systematic reviews. Aust J Physiother 2005; 51:71–85.
25. Dripps RD, Waters RM. Nursing care of surgical patients. Am J Nurs 1941; 41:530–534.
26. Dean E, Ross J. Discordance between cardiopulmonary physiology and physical therapy. Toward a rational basis for practice. Chest 1992; 101:1694–1698.
27. Probst VS, Troosters T, Coosemans I, et al. Mechanisms of improvement in exercise capacity using a rollator in patients with COPD. Chest 2004; 126:1102–1107.
28. Chang AT, Boots RJ, Hodges PW, et al. Standing with the assistance of a tilt table improves minute ventilation in chronic critically ill patients. Arch Phys Med Rehabil 2004; 85:1972–1976.
29. Zafiropoulos B, Alison JA, McCarren B. Physiological responses to the early mobilization of the intubated, ventilated abdominal surgery patient. Aust J Physiother 2004; 50:95–100.
30. Chang AT, Boots R, Hodges PW, et al. Standing with assistance of a tilt table in intensive care: a survey of Australian physiotherapy practice. Aust J Physiother 2004; 50:51–54.
31. Yohannes AM, Connolly MJ. Early mobilization with walking aids following hospital admission with acute exacerbation of chronic obstructive pulmonary disease. Clin Rehabil 2003; 17:465–471.
32. Goldman JM, Rose LS, Williams SJ, et al. Effect of abdominal binders on breathing in tetraplegic patients. Thorax 1986; 41:940–945.
33. Van't Hul A, Kwakkel G, Gosselink R. The acute effects of noninvasive ventilatory support during exercise on exercise endurance and dyspnea in patients with chronic obstructive pulmonary disease: a systematic review. J Cardiopulm Rehabil 2002; 22:290–297.
34. Nava S. Rehabilitation of patients admitted to a respiratory intensive care unit. Arch Phys Med Rehabil 1998; 79:849–854.
35. Chiang LL, Wang LY, Wu CP, et al. Effects of physical training on functional status in patients with prolonged mechanical ventilation. Phys Ther 2006; 86:1271–1281.
36. Martin UJ, Hincapie L, Nimchuk M, et al. Impact of whole-body rehabilitation in patients receiving chronic mechanical ventilation. Crit Care Med 2005; 33:2259–2265.
37. Porta R, Vitacca M, Gile LS, et al. Supported arm training in patients recently weaned from mechanical ventilation. Chest 2005; 128:2511–2520.
38. Galetke W, Randerath W, Pfeiffer M, et al. [Spiroergometry in patients with severe chronic obstructive pulmonary disease confined to bed]. Pneumologie 2002; 56:98–102.
39. Burtin C, Clerckx B, Robbeets C, et al. Effectiveness of early exercise in critically ill patients: preliminary results. Intensive Care Med 2006; 32:109.
40. Green HJ, Jones S, Ball-Burnett ME, et al. Early muscular and metabolic adaptations to prolonged exercise training in humans. J Appl Physiol 1991; 70:2032–2038.
41. Kraemer WJ, Adams K, Cafarelli E, et al. American college of sports medicine position stand. Progression models in resistance training for healthy adults. Med Sci Sports Exerc 2002; 34:364–380.
42. Gibson JNA, Smith K, Rennie MJ. Prevention of disuse muscle atrophy by means of electrical stimulation: maintenance of protein synthesis. Lancet 1988; 2:767–769.
43. Zanotti E, Felicetti G, Maini M, et al. Peripheral muscle strength training in bed-bound patients with COPD receiving mechanical ventilation. Effect of electrical stimulation. Chest 2003; 124:292–296.

44. McNair PJ, Dombroski EW, Hewson DJ, et al. Stretching at the ankle joint: viscoelastic responses to holds and continuous passive motion. Med Sci Sports Exerc 2001; 33:354–358.
45. Reid DA, McNair PJ. Passive force, angle, and stiffness changes after stretching of hamstring muscles. Med Sci Sports Exerc 2004; 36:1944–1948.
46. Williams PE. Use of intermittent stretch in the prevention of serial sarcomere loss in immobilised muscle. Ann Rheum Dis 1990; 49:316–317.
47. Chang A., Paratz J, Rollston J. Ventilatory effects of neurophysiological facilitation and passive movement in patients with neurological injury. Aust J Physiother 2002; 48:305–310.
48. Salter RB. The physiologic basis of continuous passive motion for articular cartilage healing and regeneration. Hand Clin 1994; 10:211–219.
49. Namba RS, Kabo JM, Dorey FJ, et al. Continuous passive motion versus immobilization. The effect on posttraumatic joint stiffness. Clin Orthop 1991; 267:218–223.
50. Griffiths RD, Palmer A, Helliwell T, et al. Effect of passive stretching on the wasting of muscle in the critically ill. Nutrition 1995; 11:428–432.
51. Cummings GS, Tillman LJ. Remodeling of dense connective tissue in normal adult tissue. In Currier DP, Nelson RM, eds. Dynamics of Human Biologic Tissues. Philadelphia FA Davis Co, 1992:45–68.
52. Kwan MW, Ha KW. Splinting programme for patients with burnt hand. Hand Surg 2002; 7:231–241.
53. Hinderer SR, Dixon K. Physiologic and clinical monitoring of spastic hypertonia. Phys Med Rehabil Clin N Am 2001; 12:733–746.
54. Vogiatzis I, Nanas S, Roussos C. Interval training as an alternative modality to continuous exercise in patients with COPD. Eur Respir J 2002; 20:12–19.
55. Stiller K, Philips A. Safety aspects of mobilising acutely ill patients. Physiother Theory Pract 2003; 19:239–257.
56. Vassilakopoulos T, Zakynthinos S, Roussos C. The tension-time index and the frequency/tidal volume ratio are the major pathophysiologic determinants of weaning failure and success. Am J Respir Crit Care Med 1998; 158:378–385.
57. Zakynthinos SG, Vassilakopoulos T, Roussos C. The load of inspiratory muscles in patients needing mechanical ventilation. Am J Respir Crit Care Med 1995; 152:1248–1255.
58. Chang AT, Boots RJ, Brown MG, et al. Reduced inspiratory muscle endurance following successful weaning from prolonged mechanical ventilation. Chest 2005; 128:553–559.
59. Gayan-Ramirez G, Testelmans D, Maes K, et al. Intermittent spontaneous breathing protects the rat diaphragm from mechanical ventilation effects. Crit Care Med 2005; 33:2804–2809.
60. Orozco-Levi M, Gea J, Lloreta JL, et al. Subcellular adaptation of the human diaphragm in chronic obstructive pulmonary disease. Eur Respir J 1999; 13:371–378.
61. Orozco-Levi M, Lloreta J, Minguella J, et al. Injury of the human diaphragm associated with exertion and chronic obstructive pulmonary disease. Am J Respir Crit Care Med 2001; 164:1734–1739.
62. Aldrich TK, Karpel JP, Uhrlass RM, et al. Weaning from mechanical ventilation: adjunctive use of inspiratory muscle resistive training. Crit Care Med 1989; 17:143–147.
63. Martin, AD, Davenport PD, Franceschi AC, et al. Use of inspiratory muscle strength training to facilitate ventilator weaning: a series of 10 consecutive patients. Chest 2002; 122:192–196.
64. Martin D, Davenport PW, Gonzalez-Rothi J, et al. Inspiratory muscle strength training improves outcome in failure to wean patients. Eur Respir J 2006; 28:369s.
65. Pavlovic D, Wendt M. Diaphragm pacing during prolonged mechanical ventilation of the lungs could prevent from respiratory muscle fatigue. Med Hypotheses 2003; 60:398–403.

11
Transcutaneous Electrical Muscle Stimulation

CAROLYN L. ROCHESTER
Yale University School of Medicine, New Haven and VA Connecticut Healthcare System, West Haven, Connecticut, U.S.A.

I. Introduction

Intolerance to physical exertion is one of the most disturbing symptoms of chronic obstructive pulmonary disease (COPD). Dyspnea, leg fatigue, weakness, and discomfort are crucial factors contributing to exercise limitation (1), and are major causes of disability, even among medically stable ambulatory outpatients with moderate-to- severe disease. Significant worsening of muscle function and decline in functional status are common during periods of immobility, such as those resulting from acute disease exacerbations or hospitalizations for acute illness (2). Persons who are significantly immobilized during episodes of respiratory failure require mechanical ventilatory assistance, prolonged weaning from the ventilator, or long-term ventilatory support, and are especially at risk. The decline in functional status associated with acute illness or prolonged immobilization may persist for weeks or months following hospital discharge (3). Increased disability over prior baseline, with associated impairment in quality of life, lasts indefinitely in some persons. As such, implementations of rehabilitative strategies that prevent functional status decline are crucial for both stable outpatients and persons with acute and/or chronic ventilatory failure. This chapter will focus on the use of transcutaneous electrical muscle stimulation (TCEMS), a newly emerging approach in the rehabilitation of patients with chronic respiratory disease.

II. The Basis of Exercise Limitation in COPD

Exercise limitation and functional disability in COPD have a complex, multifactorial basis. Ventilatory limitation is caused by increased airways resistance, static and dynamic hyperinflation, increased elastic load to breathing, gas exchange disturbances, and mechanical disadvantage and/or weakness of the respiratory muscles (4–6). Cardiocirculatory disturbances (7,8), nutritional factors (9), and psychological factors, such as anxiety and fear, also contribute commonly to exercise intolerance. Skeletal muscle dysfunction is characterized by reductions in muscle mass (10,11), atrophy of type I (slow twitch, oxidative, endurance) (12,13) and type IIa (fast twitch) muscle fibers (14), altered myosin heavy chain expression (15), as well as reductions in fiber capillarization (16) and oxidative enzyme capacity (17,18). Such a dysfunction is another key factor that contributes to exercise limitation in COPD (19,20). Muscle metabolism and bioenergetics are impaired both at rest and during exercise because of these structural and functional changes (18,19,21,22), and resultant lowering of lactate threshold can further increase ventilatory demand (23). COPD patients with skeletal muscle dysfunction experience reduced muscle strength (10,11), reduced endurance (19,24,25), and impaired exercise capacity (10,26,27). They also demonstrate increased utilization of health care resources (28) and have reductions in quality of life and survival (9). Deconditioning and muscle disuse, nutritional impairments with loss of fat-free mass, oxidative stress, systemic inflammation, and muscle apoptosis all likely contribute to the structural and functional changes in skeletal muscle among patients with COPD (19,23,29–34). Hypoxemia, electrolyte disturbances, and corticosteroid-induced myopathy may also play a role in some persons (19). Each of the conditions thought likely to contribute to skeletal muscle dysfunction is likely to develop or worsen during periods of acute illness, particularly those associated with exacerbations of airflow obstruction, infection, ventilatory failure, or prolonged hospitalization. Immobilization associated with acute illness is well known to increase skeletal muscle catabolism (35) and atrophy, with associated reductions in muscle strength, endurance, and coordination (2,36). Loss of muscle mass may occur during periods of immobility despite adequate nutritional supplementation (37) and may be further exaggerated in patients who have conditions wherein adequate nutritional supplementation may be temporarily unfeasible.

In individual patients with COPD, both ventilatory limitation and skeletal muscle dysfunction lead to exercise intolerance and functional impairment, to differing degrees. Whereas disabling dyspnea associated with severe ventilatory limitation is the principal contributing factor for some persons (38), skeletal muscle dysfunction and associated leg weakness or discomfort are the major causes of limitation for others. Many patients are limited by both types of symptoms (1). Optimal management of these processes must include efforts to correct nutritional impairments and electrolyte disturbances and/or hypoxemia, to optimize pharmacologic therapy, to minimize ventilatory limitation, and to address the skeletal muscle dysfunction by incorporating rehabilitation that includes exercise and muscle training.

III. The Rationale for TCEMS as a Strategy for Rehabilitation

Exercise training and pulmonary rehabilitation (PR) have been shown convincingly to improve muscle dysfunction and exercise capacity for patients with COPD (5,19,23,39–41). Although the benefits of traditional aerobic/endurance and strength training are well established, individual patient responses are variable, and, indeed, some patients fail to achieve gains in exercise tolerance despite full participation in an exercise training program. The percentage of "nonresponders" to PR varies across studies, depending on the patient population and exercise training regimen undertaken, but ranges from 10% to 50% (38,42–44). Although the factors that determine which COPD patients are most likely to benefit from rehabilitation are not completely understood, existing studies suggest that patients with a predominance of severe ventilatory limitation (42–44) or dyspnea (38) are less likely to improve than those whose exercise tolerance is limited predominantly by peripheral muscle dysfunction and/or other nonventilatory factors.

Moreover, some patients experience such disabling dyspnea, gas exchange disturbances, or fear that they are unwilling or unable to undertake exercise, or they may be too disabled to leave their home. Logistic difficulties, such as lack of transportation and travel distance to a rehabilitation facility and financial considerations, can lead to lack of patient access to rehabilitation. Importantly, conventional exercise training is often unfeasible during periods of acute illness, hospitalization, and/or ventilatory failure. As such, novel approaches to maintaining and/or restoring muscle function are needed.

IV. TCEMS as an Alternate Rehabilitation Strategy

TCEMS is an alternate, simple, safe, and well-tolerated rehabilitation technique wherein muscle contraction is elicited; muscle can thereby be trained without the requirement for conventional exercise. Electrical impulses are delivered to the muscle via self-adhering surface electrodes placed on the skin, in a manner that leads to contraction of the muscles targeted for activation (Fig. 1). Both console-based, and small, portable, battery-powered TCEMS systems are currently available (45). TCEMS can be applied to train muscles throughout the body, including those of the lower and upper extremities, torso, and face. Some systems are designed to enable delivery of the combination of TCEMS and other forms of conventional exercise, such as cycling or rowing (46,47). Electrical stimulation of the muscle must be delivered according to a specific protocol in which the intensity, frequency, duration, and waveform of the stimulus are chosen to achieve the desired muscle response (48). The electrical stimulus amplitude (intensity) determines the strength of muscle contraction. The stimulus amplitude is generally chosen according to individual patient tolerance or is delivered as a percentage of amplitude that elicits a maximal voluntary contraction.

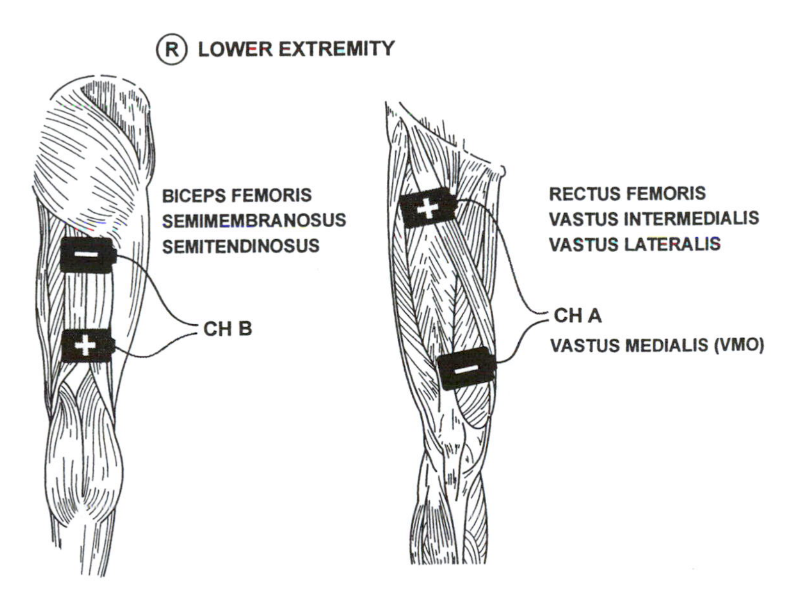

Figure 1 Example of electrode placement for electrical stimulation of the quadriceps and hamstring muscles. *Source*: From accelerated clinical practice, chronic obstructive pulmonary disease, www.acplus.com (45).

Stimulus amplitudes of up to 100 mA typically lead to muscle contraction and are well tolerated (49–51). The stimulus duration is the total time of each electrical impulse, and the pulse frequency is the time between the start of one impulse and that of the next impulse. The duration of groups (trains) of pulses and the interval between trains of pulses are also chosen (48). Additionally, as for any form of muscle training, the total duration of each TCEMS session, number of training sessions per week, and total training duration must also be specified. Clinical benefits of TCEMS have been demonstrated in varying patient populations following a broad range of TCEMS training regimens, including pulse frequencies from 10 to 2500 Hz and session durations ranging from as few as 10 to 15 muscle contractions per day up to 8 to 12 hours of continuous stimulation per day, three to seven sessions per week, for periods ranging from 10 days to 6 weeks (49,52–54).

TCEMS has potential advantages over (or may be useful in conjunction with) conventional exercise in several situations. First, selected muscles that may be particularly impaired can be chosen for stimulation therapy so that particular aspects of impaired function can be addressed. Small, portable TCEMS machines can be used alone or in combination with voluntary exercise, such as resistance exercise, walking [even among persons who require adaptive equipment, such as walkers (Fig. 2)], or cycling. Muscle contraction induced by electrical stimulation bypasses the cognitive, motivational, and psychological aspects involved in conventional exercise that may hinder or prevent effective exercise training (54). Importantly, unlike conventional exercise training, TCEMS-induced muscle contraction does not lead to dyspnea and, as such, can improve skeletal muscle function for persons with severe ventilatory or cardiac limitation (including hospitalized patients) without posing additional ventilatory or cardiocirculatory demand

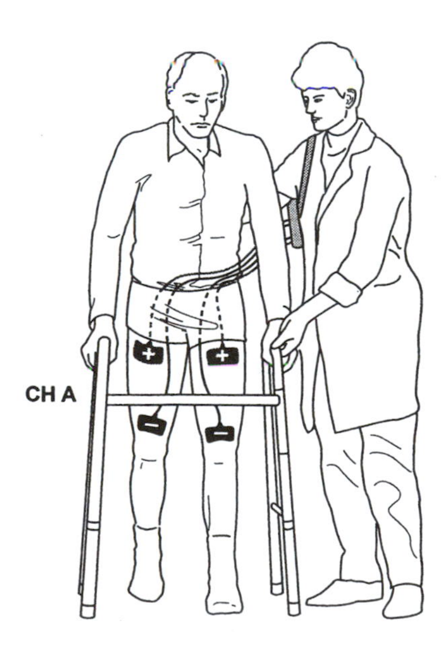

Figure 2 Use of TCEMS combined with walking exercise. *Abbreviation*: TCEMS, transcutaneous electrical muscle stimulation. *Source*: From accelerated clinical practice, chronic obstructive pulmonary disease, www.acplus.com (45).

(55–57). Therefore, it is potentially an excellent strategy for providing effective muscle rehabilitation to either improve or prevent decline in function among patients who do not achieve gains in exercise tolerance during conventional exercise training in PR, or who are unable to participate in conventional exercise training methods during periods of acute illness, immobilization, and/or respiratory failure. Small, relatively inexpensive, portable electrical stimulators are also suitable for home use and, therefore, may benefit persons who are too disabled to leave their homes, require home mechanical ventilation, or lack access to traditional PR programs. Home use of TCEMS may also reduce costs associated with outpatient PR and/or enhance benefits achieved in such programs.

V. Clinical Benefits of TCEMS in Non-COPD Patient Populations

TCEMS was initially used to enhance exercise performance among healthy athletes. It improves muscle strength of healthy persons to a comparable extent, as conventional exercise training (49,58). TCEMS has also been used widely to improve and restore (or prevent decline in) muscle function and to reduce disability among persons with orthopedic injury (51,59), major abdominal surgery (60), and immobility caused by acute illness (61), stroke (62,63), or spinal cord injury (46,64). Noted benefits in these patient populations include increased muscle strength (47,54,62,63,65–70), girth or mass (37,71), prevention of atrophy (36,60,72), increased endurance (47,73), as well as improvements in walking and mobility (51,59,62,63,67–69) and decreased length of hospital stay (74).

Particularly relevant to patients with advanced chronic respiratory disease, many of whom also have concurrent cardiac disease, is the recent demonstration that TCEMS is a beneficial method of exercise training even among patients with severe exercise limitation due to advanced refractory congestive heart failure (CHF), many of whom have evidence of skeletal muscle dysfunction with morphological and functional features similar to those found in COPD (75,76). For example, TCEMS delivered to the quadriceps and calf muscles for one hour per session, for five days per week, and for five weeks at a frequency of 10 Hz and maximal tolerated amplitude, in the absence of additional exercise training, led to significant improvements in muscle volume, walking endurance (assessed by the six-minute walk distance test), maximal oxygen consumption (V_{O_2}max), and delay in anaerobic threshold among 14 patients with severe stable chronic CHF (mean left ventricular ejection fraction, 22.3%) (56). The magnitude of gains in these parameters was comparable to those seen historically following conventional exercise training among comparable patient groups. Similarly, the randomized controlled trial conducted by Quittan and colleagues demonstrated that TCEMS delivered at a frequency of 50 Hz at an amplitude chosen to induce muscle contractions at 25% to 30% of the magnitude of a maximal voluntary contraction induced significant increases in strength and cross-sectional area of the thigh muscles among a cohort of 42 patients with severe, stable CHF awaiting heart transplantation (57). These changes were associated with reduction in muscle fatigue and improvement in quality of life. Importantly, in both of these studies, TCEMS led to improvements in the New York Heart Association (NYHA) functional class (56,57) and was well tolerated, yet did not induce any significant changes in heart rate, systemic blood pressure, or cardiac output. Since then, additional studies have confirmed that TCEMS leads to gains in exercise endurance (measured by six-minute walk test and treadmill

Table 1 Comparison of Electrical Stimulus Regimens Among Studies of TCEMS in Patients with CHF and COPD

Author and reference	Amplitude	Frequency	Wave form	Training duration	Benefits noted
CHF					
Maillefert (56)	Maximum tolerated up to 60 mA	10 Hz (200 msec), duty cycle 20 sec on, 20 sec off	Biphasic	1 hr each limb 5 days/wk for 5 wk	Increased muscle volume Increased walk distance Increased VO_2max Increased anaerobic threshold Improved NYHA functional class
Quittan (57)	25–35% of maximal voluntary contraction	50 Hz (0.7 msec), duty cycle 2 sec on, 6 sec off	Symmetric biphasic	Up to 60 min/day each limb 5 days/wk for 8 wk	Increased muscle strength Increased muscle CSA
Harris (77)	Set to create visible contraction as tolerated	25 Hz, 5 sec on, 5 sec off	Not specified	30 min each limb 5 days/wk for 6 wk	Increased walking endurance Increased muscle strength Reduced muscle fatigue
Deley (78)	Maximum tolerated	10 Hz (200 msec), duty cycle 12 sec on, 8 sec off	Biphasic	1 hr each limb 5 days/wk for 5 wk	Increased muscle strength Increased 6-min walk distance Increased VO_2max Increased Wmax
COPD					
Bourjeily-Habr (55)	Set to create visible muscle contraction, increase by 5 mA/wk, up to mean 95 ± 4.2 mA	Bursts of impulses, 50 Hz (200 msec) every 1500 msec	Symmetric square wave	20 min each limb 3 days/wk for 6 wk	Increased muscle strength Increased shuttle walk distance Reduced dyspnea

Neder (79)	As tolerated, up to final 100 mA	50 Hz (300–400 msec), variable duty cycle	Symmetric biphasic square wave	15 min each limb during week 1, then 30 min each limb 5 days/wk for 6 wk	Increased muscle strength Increased Vo_2max Increased endurance Improved dyspnea scores (CRQ)
Vivodtzev (80)	Maximum tolerated, increase by 1–5 mA/day, final 46 ± 24 mA	35 Hz (400 msec) lasting 7 sec, alternate with 5 Hz (400 msec) lasting 8 sec	Symmetric biphasic square wave	30 min each limb 4 days/wk for 4 wk	Increased muscle strength Increased walking distance Reduced dyspnea with daily activities
Zanotti (61)	Not specified	5 min at 8 Hz (250 msec), alternating with 25 min at 35 Hz (350 msec)	Bipolar, biphasic, asymmetric, rectangular wave	Up to 30 min each limb 5 days/wk for 4 wk	Increased muscle strength Decreased respiratory rate Shorter time to transfer bed to chair
Dal Corso (81)	Set to create visible contraction, increase by 5 mA/wk, as tolerated	50 Hz (400 msec), variable duty cycle	Not specified	15 min each limb during week 1, then 30 min each limb 5 days/wk for 6 wk	No clear effect on muscle strength, mass, or walking capacity Increased type II fiber CSA

Abbreviations: TCEMS, transcutaneous electrical muscle stimulation; CHF, congestive heart failure; COPD, chronic obstructive pulmonary disease; Vo_2max, peak oxygen consumption; NYHA, New York heart association; CSA, cross-sectional area; Wmax, maximal workload; CRQ, chronic respiratory disease questionnaire.

endurance time), maximal leg strength, and reduced muscle fatigue at a degree comparable to that achieved following conventional bicycle or multimodality exercise training among patients with chronic heart failure (77,78). In the study by Harris (77), the TCEMS was conducted successfully in the patients' home setting, but increases in V_{O_2}max were not achieved. In the study by Deley and colleagues (78), patients with NYHA class II and III chronic heart failure due to dilated or ischemic cardiomyopathy whose activity was limited by fatigue and exertional dyspnea were randomized to receive either low frequency (10 Hz) TCEMS of the quadriceps and calf muscles at an amplitude set to patient tolerance or conventional treadmill, cycling, and arm ergometer exercise training for one hour per session, for five days per week, for five weeks. Patients in both training groups achieved comparable gains in V_{O_2}max, peak workload and increased workload at ventilatory threshold, as well as shorter time to recover half of peak V_{O_2}, increased knee extensor muscle strength, six-minute walk test distance, and reduced time to cover a 200-m walk distance. Collectively, these studies demonstrate that TCEMS is an effective muscle training regimen that can result in significant gains in muscle strength, endurance, and in some cases, maximal exercise capacity (peak workload) and V_{O_2}max, even among patients with severe impairment in cardiac function, without directly imposing an increased demand on cardiac performance. Differences in the precise electrical stimulus regimen chosen (Table 1), with resultant differential effects at the level of the skeletal muscle, may account for variability in findings with regard to whether patients achieved gains in V_{O_2}max in these studies.

VI. Effects of TCEMS on Muscle Function and Exercise Tolerance Among Patients with COPD

Five studies have thus far evaluated TCEMS as a mode of rehabilitation for patients with COPD. Four of these studies have investigated the effects of TCEMS among persons with severe airflow obstruction and/or significant baseline exercise impairment and debility. The electrical stimulus regimens used in these studies are shown in Table 1. In our randomized, controlled, double-blind trial of TCEMS of the quadriceps and calf muscles in 18 medically stable outpatients with severe COPD [forced expiratory volume in one second (FEV_1), 18% predicted], poor baseline exercise tolerance, and low ventilatory reserve, TCEMS led to a significant (30–40%) improvement in maximum quadriceps and hamstring strength, a 36% increase in incremental shuttle walk distance (an index of both exercise endurance and maximal exercise capacity) (Fig. 3) and reductions in dyspnea (assessed by the Borg scale of perceived exertion), compared to the sham-treated group (55). Similarly, Neder and colleagues (79) randomized 15 patients with severe stable COPD (FEV_1, 38–39% predicted) and severe breathlessness to receive either six weeks of TCEMS of the leg muscles or a six-week control (no TCEMS) period before undergoing TCEMS. TCEMS led to significant improvements in maximal isokinetic strength (peak torque) and reduction in muscle fatigue. An 84% increase in endurance capacity and a 16% increase in V_{O_2}max were also noted. These benefits were associated with improved dyspnea and reduced sense of leg fatigue during exercise. Importantly, the four patients who experienced COPD exacerbations during the study period were able to continue the TCEMS training program despite the exacerbations. Recently, a group of malnourished patients with low body mass index, severe airflow limitation, and severe deconditioning following hospitalizations for acute exacerbations of COPD were shown to achieve greater improvements in leg muscle strength and dyspnea

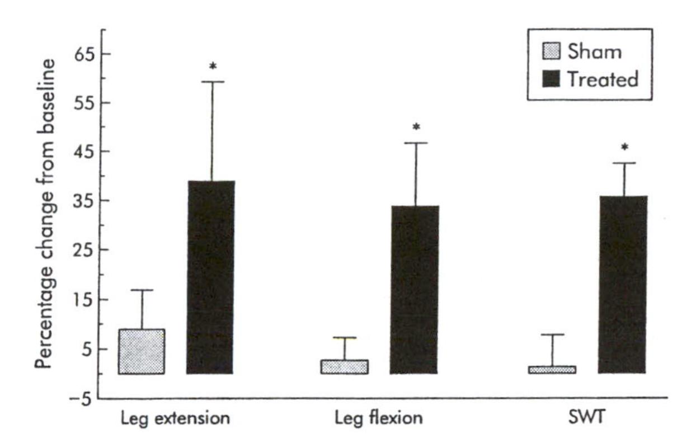

Figure 3 Improvements in leg muscle strength and incremental shuttle walk distance following TCEMS among patients with severe, stable COPD. *Abbreviation*: TCEMS, transcutaneous electrical muscle stimulation. *Source*: From Ref. 55.

during daily activities following treatment for four weeks with TCEMS and "usual rehabilitation" (UR) as compared with UR alone (80) (Fig. 4). Gains in strength correlated with changes in muscle mass. Notably, patients in this study were severely debilitated, as the UR was limited to a regimen of active limb mobilization performed with the patient lying supine, and the strongest patients had a regimen of slow treadmill walking and 5 to 10 minutes of low-intensity arm-lifting exercise. Although patients who received TCEMS and UR also achieved gains in walking distance, the difference between gains in walking distance made following TCEMS and UR did not reach statistical significance as compared to those made following UR alone. In the study by Zanotti and colleagues, the effects of TCEMS were evaluated in a group of 24 bed-bound patients with chronic hypercapnic respiratory failure due to COPD who were receiving mechanical ventilation (61). TCEMS combined with active limb mobilization significantly improved muscle strength, respiratory rate, and time needed to perform transfer from bed to chair compared with active limb mobilization alone among these patients (61). Taken together, these studies demonstrate that as for other disorders TCEMS is a safe and effective intervention for improving muscle function and exercise capacity of patients with COPD. Importantly, to date, it has been shown to be most effective among persons with severe baseline exercise tolerance, low ventilatory reserve, and severe breathlessness. Notably, the limited data currently available suggests it can be used during acute exacerbations and is also effective for those with advanced respiratory failure who are severely immobilized and limited in their ability to undertake conventional exercise training due to requirement for mechanical ventilation.

However, it is unclear whether TCEMS is as effective for COPD patients with a higher degree of baseline exercise tolerance. In the only study to examine this issue, to date, six weeks of high frequency (50 Hz) electrical stimulation of the quadriceps femoris did not lead to significant changes in muscle strength (peak torque), leg muscle mass, or six-minute walking distance as compared to sham stimulation among 17 patients with moderate-to-severe airflow obstruction (mean FEV_1, 49.6 ± 13.4% predicted) with well-preserved baseline functional capacity, muscle strength, and mass (81). Moreover, although TCEMS did induce a slight degree of type II (fast twitch) muscle fiber hypertrophy, no correlation was identified between

A

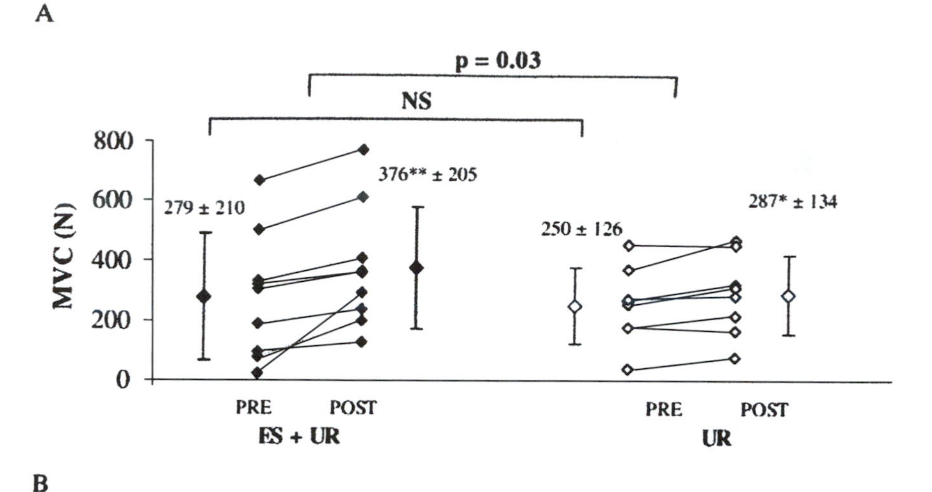

B

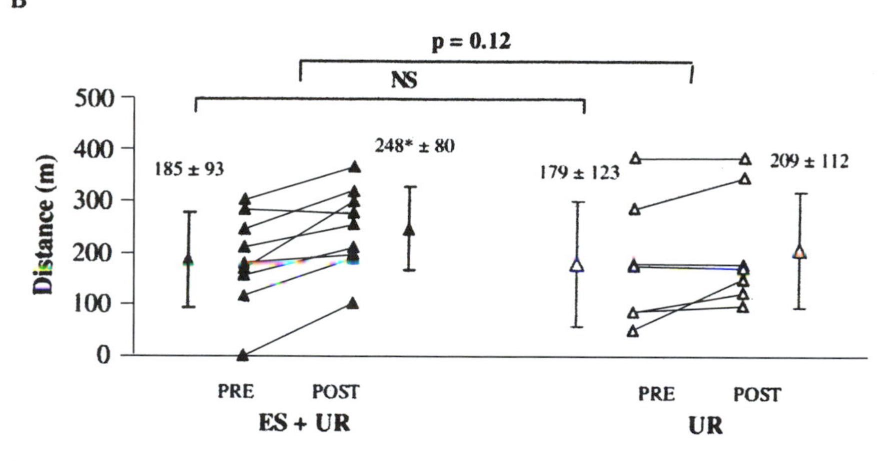

Figure 4 Improvements in muscle strength (maximal voluntary contraction) and walking distance following TCEMS plus usual rehabilitation as compared with usual rehabilitation alone among severely debilitated patients with COPD. *Abbreviations*: TCEMS, transcutaneous electrical muscle stimulation; COPD, chronic obstructive pulmonary disease. *Source*: From Ref. 80.

changes in type II fiber cross-sectional area and changes in muscle strength. Further work is needed to confirm whether the benefits of TCEMS are limited to patients with more advanced degrees of disability and skeletal muscle dysfunction as well as to address whether there may be subpopulations of patients with preserved functional capacity and muscle strength who may also benefit from TCEMS, applied either alone or in combination with other muscle training interventions. The precise electrical stimulation protocol chosen may also impact the outcomes of TCEMS among COPD patients with a lesser degree of baseline disability.

VII. Mechanisms and Duration of Improvement in Muscle Function

The mechanisms by which TCEMS improves muscle function and exercise capacity or performance are incompletely understood. Animal studies have demonstrated structural and biochemical changes in muscle following electrical stimulation (82–89). Similarly, in investigations done to date in non-COPD populations, TCEMS can increase oxidative enzyme capacity (90,91), muscle capillarity (91), and the proportion of type I muscle fibers (90,92) in humans. These findings are intriguing, since disturbances in each of these parameters contribute to the skeletal muscle dysfunction in COPD (see above). TCEMS-induced improvements in these processes could account for some of the gains in exercise tolerance, particularly the improvements in muscle endurance. Improved tissue blood flow (93), increased protein synthesis (60), muscle hypertrophy (53,94), enhanced neural recruitment (62), altered muscle expression of growth factors (95), and/or reduction in protein breakdown (96) are additional mechanisms by which TCEMS may lead to improvements in muscle strength, mass, and function.

The pattern of activation of muscle fibers and physiologic results of the contraction during TCEMS may differ from activation of muscle fibers that takes place during voluntary muscle contraction. First, with TCEMS the firing frequency is preset and, as such, specific fiber types may be selected for activation. This differs from voluntary contraction wherein one can activate additional motor units after those initially recruited became fatigued (97). Second, during voluntary contraction, slow-twitch (type I, high oxidative capacity, fatigue resistant) fibers are recruited first, followed by fast-twitch (lower oxidative capacity, more fatigue-prone fibers) type IIa and IIx fibers (designed to perform bursts of activity) (98). In contrast, the order of TCEMS-induced motor unit recruitment may depend on several factors, including the distance between the stimulating electrode and axon, the tendency for largest diameter motor units (predominantly, fast-twitch fibers) to be superficially located, the potential for activation of axon collaterals, a lower excitability threshold of nerves supplying fast-motor units, as well as the potential for TCEMS to activate sensory afferent nerve endings in muscle that might affect sensorimotor control (99). Indeed, some investigators believe TCEMS leads to preferential recruitment of fast-twitch fibers, i.e., a reversal of the order of motor unit recruitment as compared with voluntary contraction (97,100). Such preferential recruitment of fast-twitch fibers might render the muscle more prone to fatigue. Other investigators believe, however, that TCEMS leads to a nonselective, synchronous pattern of muscle-fiber activation (97). Indeed, it has been suggested that the ability of TCEMS to activate both fast-twitch and slow-twitch fibers may enable TCEMS to induce changes in muscle strength, cross-sectional area, and endurance that may not be likely to occur otherwise in a severely disabled population of patients performing low-intensity rehabilitative muscle exercise (97).

Importantly, the precise electrical stimulus protocol chosen also impacts the training effect on the muscle. In particular, the frequency of stimulus delivered likely determines the types of muscle fibers activated. Slow-twitch fibers normally have a firing frequency of ~10 Hz, whereas fast-twitch fibers have a firing frequency of ~30 Hz (97). A TCEMS stimulus frequency up to 10 Hz would, therefore, preferentially activate slow-twitch fibers and may selectively improve resistance to fatigue (101), whereas frequency greater than 30 Hz may activate both types of fibers or may selectively recruit fast-twitch fibers and enhance power (58). In this light, studies conducted to date have demonstrated clinical benefits of TCEMS among patients with COPD, wherein gains in both muscle strength and endurance have been noted, and have utilized stimulus frequencies ranging from 5 to 50 Hz (55,61,79,80). Many electrical stimulators enable ramping and modulation of the pulse amplitude, duration, and frequency. In rodents, such modulation allows progressive recruitment and derecruitment of motor units, with resultant augmentation of fiber-type changes and delay in muscle fatigue (99). Some investigators, therefore, advocate delivery of a combination of stimulus frequencies during TCEMS training to most closely mimic normal motor neuron firing patterns and have maximal impact on muscle function (102–104).

It is intriguing to note that in some, but not all, studies, including those among patients with COPD (79) and advanced CHF (78), TCEMS has not only been able to induce gains in muscle strength and walking endurance, but has also been able to induce physiologic gains in aerobic fitness, such as increased $V_{O_2}max$, even in the absence of demonstrable increases in cardiac output (56) and resting or peak heart rate (78). The metabolic basis for inducing these training effects at the level of the skeletal muscle, i.e., whether these benefits are based on increases in oxidative enzyme capacity that can be seen following high-intensity conventional exercise training among patients with COPD (105), remains unknown.

Finally, the duration of benefits in muscle function following a limited (e.g., several weeks) period of TCEMS muscle training has not, to date, been studied in patients with lung disease. In one study, six weeks training of the rectus femoris and flexor digitorum brevis muscles (30 min/day, 5 days/wk) among seven untrained healthy young male subjects led to gains in maximum voluntary contraction and muscle endurance that persisted six weeks after completion of training (99). Further work is needed to assess the duration of benefits of TCEMS among patients with COPD and other forms of respiratory disease.

VIII. Patient Candidacy and Safety

There are no formal patient candidacy guidelines for TCEMS or precise recommendations regarding persons in whom TCEMS should be avoided. TCEMS is generally safe and well tolerated. The adverse effect reported most commonly is mild muscle soreness that usually resolves after the first few TCEMS sessions (55–57), and is comparable to that expected for any person who may undertake any form of exercise training after a period of relative inactivity. The development of muscle soreness, in part, relates to the stimulus amplitude and frequency chosen. Pulse amplitudes greater than 100 mA or pulse frequencies greater than 5000 Hz may lead to intolerable muscle discomfort (45). At the start of TCEMS training, stimulus amplitudes that lead to nonpainful muscle contraction are applied and incremental gains in the stimulus amplitude are made over the course of the training program, according to patient tolerance.

Concerns regarding other potential adverse effects of TCEMS largely relate to situations in which the delivery of an electrical stimulus applied externally could possibly cause harm to the patient. Current recommendations regarding which patients should not receive TCEMS are primarily based on expert opinion and common sense, rather than evidence-based data. To this end, most care providers and clinical researchers do not perform TCEMS on patients with any implanted electrical devices, such as pacemakers or implanted defibrillators and persons with seizure disorder, uncontrolled cardiac arrythmias (particularly ventricular), unstable angina, recent myocardial infarction, or intracranial clips (56,57,78,106). Inappropriate shock from an implanted defibrillator has been reported following use of transcutaneous electrical nerve stimulation (107,108). Patients with severe osteoarthritis of the joints to be mobilized by the muscles to be stimulated or those with severe peripheral edema or other skin problems wherein desired placement of electrodes would be limited may also be poor candidates for TCEMS. A case of ischemic colitis has also been reported following the application of TCEMS to the lower abdominal muscles (109).

IX. Questions for the Future

Several important questions remain regarding the use of TCEMS as a rehabilitative strategy for patients with chronic respiratory disease. Overall, to date, the evidence base regarding use of TCEMS for patients with respiratory disease remains small, and existing studies have included relatively small numbers of patients with selected characteristics. As such, the role of TCEMS as a routine component of PR remains undefined. It will be important to learn more about which groups of patients with COPD can benefit most—in particular, to compare outcomes of TCEMS among medically stable outpatients with or without severe debility due to skeletal muscle dysfunction (including reductions in muscle mass, strength, endurance) as well as persons with or without severe ventilatory limitation. Additional studies are needed to determine the duration of benefits from TCEMS-based training compared with that of conventional PR, whether TCEMS can add to gains made in conventional PR, and whether those persons who fail to make gains in conventional PR can achieve gains following TCEMS. Moreover, although it is known that TCEMS can be tolerated during COPD exacerbations, further studies are needed to determine whether delivery of TCEMS during exacerbations can truly prevent decline in muscle function and overall disability that typically results from these episodes. Likewise, more work is needed to evaluate whether TCEMS can prevent decline in functional status, minimize dsypnea, and preserve quality of life among patients with and without respiratory failure who are immobilized due to hospitalization and/or due to short- or long-term mechanical ventilation.

Importantly, also, much more information is needed regarding how to optimize TCEMS training regimens. Currently, little is known about how the choice of particular stimulus protocols affects patient outcomes and induces structural and functional changes in the skeletal muscle. More knowledge is needed in this area to enable individualization of the treatment plan to achieve the desired muscle training effect according to patient needs. The optimal duration and frequency of electrical stimulation sessions, best means of maintaining the benefits of TCEMS on muscle performance, and optimal ways to combine TCEMS with other forms of exercise remain unknown at this time. Finally, since patients with chronic respiratory diseases other than COPD have similar symptoms, and likely to have at least some features of skeletal muscle dysfunction in common with COPD, it will be important to learn whether TCEMS can be beneficial among persons with other forms of chronic lung disease and persons with combined respiratory and cardiac disease. It may be of particular interest in the treatment of disorders, such as interstitial lung disease or pulmonary hypertension, in which the patients' ability to tolerate conventional exercise training may be limited. Many additional studies are needed to answer these questions. In conclusion, TCEMS is an exciting, novel rehabilitative strategy with great potential for preventing decline or restoring muscle function and preventing disability, and in turn, preserving quality of life for patients with chronic respiratory disease.

References

1. Killian KJ, LeBlanc P, Martin DH, et al. Exercise capacity and ventilatory, circulatory and symptom limitation in patients with chronic airflow obstruction. Am Rev Respir Dis 1992; 146:935–940.
2. Vallbona C. Bodily responses to immobilization. In: Kottke FJ, Stillwell GK, Lehmann JF, eds. Krusen's Handbook of Physical Medicine and Rehabilitation. Philadelphia: WB Saunders Co, 1982:963–976.
3. Herridge MS, Cheung AM, Tansey CM, et al. One-year outcomes in survivors of the acute respiratory distress syndrome. N Engl J Med 2003; 348(8):683–693.
4. Gallagher CG. Exercise limitation and clinical exercise testing in chronic obstructive pulmonary disease. Clin Chest Med 1994; 15:305–326.
5. Rochester CL. Exercise training in chronic obstructive pulmonary disease. J Rehabil Res Dev 2003; 40(5 suppl 2):59–80.
6. O'Donnell DE. Ventilatory limitations in chronic obstructive pulmonary disease. Med Sci Sports Exerc 2001; 33(suppl 7):S 647–655.
7. O'Donnell DE, Revill SM, Webb KA. Dynamic hyperinflation and exercise intolerance in chronic obstructive pulmonary disease. Am J Respir Crit Care Med 2001; 164:770–777.
8. Sietsema K. Cardiovascular limitations in chronic obstructive pulmonary disease. Med Sci Sports Exerc 2001; 33 (suppl 7):S656–S661.
9. Schols AMWJ, Wouters EFM. Nutritional abnormalities and supplementation in chronic obstructive pulmonary disease. Clin Chest Med 2000; 21(4):753–762.
10. Baarends EM, Schols AMWJ, Mostert R, et al. Peak exercise response in relation to tissue depletion in patients with chronic obstructive pulmonary disease. Eur Respir J 1997; 10:2807–2813.
11. Bernard S, Le Blanc P, Whittom F, et al. Peripheral muscle weakness in patients with chronic obstructive pulmonary disease. Am J Respir Crit Care Med 1998; 158:629–634.
12. Hilderbrand IL, Sylven C, Esbjonrsson M, et al. Does chronic hypoxemia induce transformation of fiber types? Acta Physiol Scand 1991; 141(3):435–439.
13. Jakobsson P, Jordfelt I, Brundin A. Skeletal muscle metabolites and fiber types in patients with advanced COPD with and without chronic respiratory failure. Eur Respir J 1990; 3:192–196.
14. Hughes RL, Katz H, Sahgal JA, et al. Fiber size and energy metabolites in five separate muscles from patients with chronic obstructive pulmonary disease. Respiration 1983; 44:321–328.
15. Maltais F, Sullivan MJ, LeBlanc P, et al. Altered expression of myosin heavy chain in the vastus lateralis muscle in patients with COPD. Eur Respir J 1999; 13:850–854.
16. Simard C, Maltais F, Le Blanc P, et al. Mitochondrial and capillarity changes in vastus lateralis muscle of COPD patients: electron microscopy study. Med Sci Sports Exerc 1996; 28:S95.
17. Jakobsson P, Jordfelt I, Henriksson J. Metabolic enzyme activity in the quadriceps femoris muscle in patients with severe COPD. Am J Respir Crit Care Med 1995; 151:374–377.
18. Maltais F, Simard AA, Simard C, et al. Oxidative capacity of the muscle and lactic acid kinetics during exercise in normal subjects and in patients with COPD. Am J Respir Crit Care Med 1996; 153:288–293.
19. American Thoracic Society/European Respiratory Society. Skeletal muscle dysfunction in chronic obstructive pulmonary disease. Am J Respir Crit Care Med 1999; 159:S1–S40.
20. Casaburi R. Skeletal muscle dysfunction in chronic obstructive pulmonary disease, Med Sci Sports Exerc 2001; 33(suppl 7):S662–S670.
21. Maltais F, Jobin J, Sullivan MJ, et al. Metabolic and hemodynamic responses of lower limb during exercise in patients with COPD. J Appl Physiol 1998; 84:1573–1580.
22. Kutsuzawa T, Shioya S, Kurita D, et al. Muscle energy metabolism and nutritional status in patients with chronic obstructive pulmonary disease: a 31P magnetic resonance study. Am J Respir Crit Care Med 1995; 152:647–652.

23. Troosters T, Casaburi R, Gosselink R, et al. Pulmonary rehabilitation in chronic obstructive pulmonary disease: state of the art. Am J Respir Crit Care Med 2005; 172:19–38.
24. Mador MJ, Kufel TJ, Pineda L. Quadriceps fatigue after cycle exercise in patients with chronic obstructive pulmonary disease. Am J Respir Crit Care Med 2000; 161:447–453.
25. Allair J, Maltais F, Doyon JF, et al. Peripheral muscle endurance and the oxidative profile of the quadriceps in patients with COPD. Thorax 2004; 59:673–678.
26. Gosselink R, Troosters T, Decramer M. Peripheral muscle weakness contributes to exercise limitation in COPD. Am J Respir Crit Care Med 1996; 153:976–980.
27. Hamilton AL, Killian KJ, Summers E, et al. Muscle strength, symptom intensity, and exercise capacity in patients with cardiorespiratory disorders. Am J Respir Crit Care Med 1995; 152:2021–2031.
28. Decramer M, Gosselink R, Troosters T, et al. Muscle weakness is related to utilization of health care resources in COPD patients. Eur Respir J 1997; 10:417–423.
29. Debigare R, Cote CH, Maltais F. Peripheral muscle wasting in chronic obstructive pulmonary disease: clinical relevance and mechanisms. Am J Respir Crit Care Med 2001; 164:1712–1717.
30. Jagoe RT, Engelen MPKJ. Muscle wasting and changes in muscle protein metabolism in chronic obstructive pulmonary disease. Eur Respir J 2003; 22(suppl 46):52S–63S.
31. Couillard A, Maltais F, Saey D, et al. Exercise-induced quadriceps oxidative stress and peripheral muscle dysfunction in patients with chronic obstructive pulmonary disease. Am J Respir Crit Care Med 2003; 167:1664–1669.
32. Couillard A, Prefaut C. From muscle disuse to myopathy in COPD: potential contribution of oxidative stress. Eur Respir J 2005; 26(4):703–719.
33. Agusti AG. Systemic effects of chronic obstructive pulmonary disease. Proc Am Thorac Soc 2005; 2(4):367–370.
34. Agusti AGN, Sauleda J, Miralles C, et al. Skeletal Muscle Apoptosis and weight loss in chronic obstructive pulmonary disease. Am Respir Crit Care Med 2002; 166:485–489.
35. Moore FD, Brennan MF. Surgical injury: body composition, protein metabolism, and neuro-endocrinology. In: American College of Surgeons: Pre- and Post-operative care. Philadelphia: WB Saunders Co, 1975.
36. Eriksson E, Haggemark T. Comparison of isometric muscle training and electrical stimulation supplementing isometric muscle training in the recovery after major knee ligament surgery. Am J Sports Med 1979; 7:169–176.
37. Buckley DC, Kudsk KA, Rose B, et al. Transcutaneous muscle stimulation promotes muscle growth in immobilized patients. J Parenter Enteral Nutr 1987; 11:547–551.
38. Wedzicha JA, Bestall JC, Garrod R, et al. Randomized controlled trial of pulmonary rehabilitation in severe COPD patients, stratified with the Medical Research Council Dyspnoea scale. Eur Respir J 1998; 12:363–369.
39. Nici L, Donner C, Wouters E, et al. American Thoracic Society/European Respiratory Society statement on pulmonary rehabilitation. Am J Respir Crit Care Med 2006; 173(12):1390–1413.
40. ACCP and AACVPR. Pulmonary Rehabilitation: joint ACCP and AACVPR evidence-based guidelines. Chest 1997; 112(5):1363–1396.
41. American Thoracic Society Statement. Pulmonary Rehabilitation. Am J Respir Crit Care Med 1999; 159:1666-–1682.
42. Troosters T, Gosselink R, Decramer M. Exercise training in COPD: how to distinguish responders from non-responders. J Cardiopulm Rehabil 2001; 21:10–17.
43. ZuWallack RL, Patel K, Reardon JZ, et al. Predictors of improvement in the 12-minute walk distance following a 6-week outpatient pulmonary rehabilitation program. Chest 1991; 99: 805–808.
44. Plankeel JF, McMullen B, MacIntyre NR. Exercise outcomes after pulmonary rehabilitation depend on the initial mechanism of exercise limitation among non-oxygen-dependent COPD patients. Chest 2005; 127:110–116.

45. Nyland J, Nolan MF. Therapeutic modality: rehabilitation of the injured athlete. Clin Sports Med 2004; 23:299–313.
46. Wheeler GD, Psych C, Andrews B, et al. Functional electrical stimulation-assisted rowing: increasing cardiovascular fitness through functional electrical stimulation rowing training in persons with spinal cord injury. Arch Phys Med Rehabil 2002; 83:1093–1099.
47. Hooker SP, Figoni SF, Rodgers MM, et al. Physiologic effects of electrical stimulation leg cycle exercise training in spinal cord injured persons. Arch Phys Med Rehabil 1992; 73:470–476.
48. Eberstein A, Eberstein S. Electrical stimulation of denervated muscle: is it worthwhile? Med Sci Sports Exerc 1996; 28(12):1463–1469.
49. Currier DP, Mann R. Muscular strength development by electrical stimulation in healthy individuals. Phys Ther 1983; 63(6):915–921.
50. Morrissey MC, Brewster CE, Shields CL. The effects of electrical stimulation on quadriceps during postoperative knee immobilization. Am J Sports Med 1985; 13(1):40–45.
51. Lamb SE, Oldham JA, Morse RE. Neuromuscular stimulation of the quadriceps muscle after hip fracture: a randomized controlled trial. Arch Phys Med Rehabil 2002; 83:1087–1092.
52. Paternostro-Sluga T, Fialka C, Alacamliogliu Y, et al. Neuromuscular electrical stimulation after anterior cruciate ligament surgery. Clin Orthop Relat Res 1999; 368:166–175.
53. Cabric M, Appell HJ, Resic A. Fine structural changes in electrostimulated human skeletal muscle. Eur J Appl Physiol 1988; 57:1–5.
54. Delitto A, Rose SJ, McKowen JM, et al. Electrical stimulation versus voluntary exercise in strengthening thigh musculature after anterior cruciate ligament surgery. Phys Ther 1988; 68 (5):660–663.
55. Bourjeily-Habr G, Rochester CL, Palermo F, et al. Randomized controlled trial of transcutaneous electrical muscle stimulation of the lower extremities in patients with chronic obstructive pulmonary disease. Thorax 2002; 57:1045–1049.
56. Maillefert JF, Eicher JC, Walker P, et al. Effects of low-frequency electrical stimulation of quadriceps and calf muscles in patients with chronic heart failure. J Cardiopulm Rehabil 1998; 18:277–282.
57. Quittan M, Wiesinger GF, Sturm B. et al. Improvement of thigh muscles by neuromuscular electrical stimulation in patients with refractory heart failure: a single-blind, randomized, controlled trial. Am J Phys Med Rehabil 2001; 80:206–214.
58. Selkowitz DM. Improvement in isometric strength of the quadriceps femoris muscle after training with electrical stimulation. Phys Ther 1985; 65:186–196.
59. Avramidis K, Strike PW, Taylor PN. Effectiveness of electric stimulation of the vastus medialis muscle in the rehabilitation of patients after total knee arthroplasty. Arch Phys Med Rehabil 2003; 84:1850–1853.
60. Vinge O, Edvardsen L, Jensen F, et al. Effect of transcutaneous electrical muscle stimulation on post-operative mass and protein synthesis. Br J Surg 1996; 83:360–363.
61. Zanotti E, Felicetti G, Maini M, et al. Peripheral muscle strength training in bed-bound patients with COPD receiving mechanical ventilation: effect of electrical stimulation. Chest 2003; 124:292–296.
62. Newsam CJ, Baker LL. Effect of electric stimulation facilitation program on quadriceps motor unit recruitment after stroke. Arch Phys Med Rehabil 2004; 85:2040–2045.
63. Glanz M, Klawansky S, Stason W, et al. Functional electrostimulation in post-stroke rehabilitation: a meta-analysis of the randomized controlled trials. Arch Phys Med Rehabil 1996; 77:549–553.
64. Scremin AME, Kurta L, Gentili A, et al. Increasing muscle mass in spinal cord injured persons with a functional electrical stimulation exercise program. Arch Phys Med Rehabil 1999; 80:1531–1536.

65. Snyder-Mackler L, Ladin Z, Schepsis AA, et al. Electrical stimulation of thigh muscles after reconstruction of the anterior cruciate ligament. J Bone Joint Surg 1991; 73A:1025–1036.
66. Lewek M, Stevens J, Snyder-Mackler L. The use of electrical stimulation to increase quadriceps femoris muscle force in an elderly patient following a total knee arthroplasty. Phys Ther 2001; 81(9):1565–1571.
67. Munsat T, McNeal D. Effects of nerve stimulation on human muscle. Arch Neurol 1976; 33:608–616.
68. Takebe K, Kukulka C, Naraya MG, et al. Peroneal nerve stimulator in rehabilitation of hemiplegic patients. Arch Phys Med Rehabil 1975; 56:237–240.
69. Cozean CD, Pease WS, Hubbell SL. Biofeedback and functional electrical stimulation in stroke rehabilitation. Arch Phys Med Rehabil 1988; 69:401–405.
70. Belanger M, Stein RB, Wheeler GD, et al. Electrical stimulation: can it increase muscle strength and reverse osteopenia in spinal cord injured individual? Arch Phys Med Rehabil 2000; 81:1090–1098.
71. Currier DP, Ray JM, Nyland J, et al. Effects of electrical and electromagnetic stimulation after anterior cruciate ligament reconstruction. J Orthop Sports Phys Ther 1993; 17:177–184.
72. Baldi JC, Jackson RD, Moraille R, et al. Muscle atrophy is prevented in patients with acute spinal cord injury using functional electrical stimulation. Spinal Cord 1998; 36:463–469.
73. Petrofsky JS, Laymon M. The effect of previous weight training and concurrent weight training on endurance for functional electrical stimulation cycle ergometry. Eur J Appl Physiol 2004; 91:392–398.
74. Gotlin RS, Hershkowitz S, Juris PM, et al. Electrical stimulation effect on extensor lag and length of hospital stay after total knee arthroplasty. Arch Phys Med Rehabil 1994; 75:957–959.
75. Gosker, HR, Lencer NHMK, Franssen FME, et al. Striking similarities in systemic factors contributing to decreased exercise capacity in patients with severe chronic heart failure or COPD. Chest 2003; 123:1416–424.
76. Troosters T, Gosselink R, Decramer M. Chronic obstructive pulmonary disease and chronic heart failure: two muscle diseases? J Cardiopulm Rehabil 2004; 24:137–145.
77. Harris S, LeMaitre JP, Mackenzie G, et al. A randomized study of home-based electrical stimulation of the legs and conventional bicycle exercise training for patients with chronic heart failure. Eur Heart J 2003; 24(9):871–878.
78. Deley G, Kervio G, Verges B, et al. Comparison of low-frequency electrical myostimulation and conventional aerobic exercise training in patients with chronic heart failure. Eur J Cardiovasc Prev Rehabil 2005; 12:226–233.
79. Neder JA, Sword D, Ward SA, et al. Home based neuromuscular electrical stimulation as a new rehabilitative strategy for severely disabled patients with chronic obstructive pulmonary disease (COPD). Thorax 2002; 57:333–337.
80. Vivodtzev I, Pepin J-L, Vottero G, et al. Improvement in quadriceps strength and dyspnea in daily tasks after 1 month of electrical stimulation in severely deconditioned and malnourished COPD. Chest 2006; 129:1540–1548.
81. Dal Corso S, Napolis L, Malaguti C, et al. Skeletal muscle structure and function in response to electrical stimulation in moderately impaired COPD patients. Respir Med 2007; 101:1236–1243.
82. Bigard AX, Lienhard DM, Serrurier B, et al. Effects of surface electrostimulation on the structure and metabolic properties in monkey skeletal muscle. Med Sci Sports Exerc 1993; 25 (3):355–362.
83. Kirschbaum BJ, Helig A, Hartner KT, et al. Electrostimulation-induced fast-to-slow transitions of myosin light and heavy chains in rabbit fast-twitch muscle at the mRNA level. FEBS Lett 1989; 243:123–126.
84. Hudlicka O, Dodd L, Renkin M, et al. Early changes in fiber profile and capillary density in long-term stimulated muscles. Am J Physiol 1982; 243:H528–H535.

85. Heilmann C, Muller W, Pette D. Correlation between ultrastructural and functional changes in sarcoplasmic reticulum during chronic stimulation of fast muscle. J Membr Biol 1981; 59:143–149.
86. Brown MD, Cotter MA, Hudlicka O, et al. The effects of different patterns of muscle activity on capillary density, mechanical properties and structure of slow and fast rabbit muscles. Pflugers Arch 1976; 361:241–250.
87. Brownson C, Isenberg H, Brown W, et al. Changes in skeletal muscle gene transcription induced by chronic stimulation. Muscle Nerve 1988; 11:1183–1189.
88. Salmons S, Gale DR, Sreter FA. Ultrastructural aspects of the transformation of skeletal muscle fibre type by long-term stimulation: changes in Z discs and mitochondria. J Anat 1978; 127:17–31.
89. Brunotte F, Thompson CH, Adamopoulos S, et al. Rat skeletal muscle metabolism in experimental heart failure: effects of physical training. Acta Physiol Scand 1995; 154:439–447.
90. Grimby G, Nordwall A, Hulten B, et al. Changes in histochemical profile of muscle after long-term electrical stimulation in patients with idiopathic scoliosis. Scand J Rehabil Med 1985; 17:191–196.
91. Cabric M, Appell HJ, Resic A. Stereological analysis of capillaries in electrostimulated human skeletal muscles. Int J Sports Med 1987; 8:327–330.
92. Wright J, Hebert MA, Velasquez R, et al. Morphologic and histochemical characteristics of skeletal muscle after long-term intramuscular electrical stimulation. Spine 1992; 17:767–770.
93. Vanderthommen M, Depresseux JC, Dauchat L, et al. Blood flow variation in human muscle during electrically stimulated exercise bouts. Arch Phys Med Rehabil 2002; 83:936–941.
94. Neumayer C, Happack W, Kern H, et al. Hypertrophy and transformation of muscle fibers in paraplegic patients. Artif Organs 1997; 21:188–190.
95. Aaron RK, Boyan BD, Ciombor D, et al. Stimulation of growth factor synthesis by electric and electromagnetic fields. Clin Orthop 2004; 419:30–37.
96. Bouletreau P, Patricot MC, Saudin F, et al. Effects of intermittent electrical stimulations on muscle catabolism in intensive care patients. J Parenter Enteral Nutr 1987; 11(6):552–555.
97. Gregory CM, Bickel CS. Recruitment patterns in human skeletal muscle during electrical stimulation. Phys Ther 2005; 85(4):358–364.
98. Henneman E, Somjen G, Carpenter DO. Functional significance of cell size in spinal motoneurons. J Neurophysiol 1965; 28:560–580.
99. Marqueste T, Hug F, Decherchi P, et al. Changes in neuromuscular function after training by functional electrical stimulation. Muscle Nerve 2003; 28(2):181–188.
100. Requena Sanchez B, Padial Puche P, Gonzalez-Badillo JJ. Percutaneous electrical stimulation in strength training: an update. J Strength Cond Res 2005; 19(2):438–448.
101. Kwende MM, Jarvis JC, Salmons S. The input output relations of skeletal muscle. Proc Biol Sci 1995; 261:193–201.
102. Callaghan MJ, Oldham JA. Electric muscle stimulation of the quadriceps in the treatment of patellofemoral pain. Arch Phys Med Rehabil 2004; 85:956–962.
103. Burke RE, Rudomin P, Zajac FE. Catch property in single mammalian motor units. Science 1970; 168:122–124.
104. Burke RE, Rudomin P, Zajac FE. The effect of activation history in tension production by individual muscle units. Brain Res 1976; 109:515–529.
105. Maltais F, LeBlanc P, Jobin J, et al. Intensity of training and physiologic adaptation in patients with COPD. Am J Respir Crit Care Med 1997; 155(2):555–561.
106. Nuhr MJ, Pette D, Berger R, et al. Beneficial effects of chronic low-frequency stimulation of thigh muscles in patients with advanced chronic heart failure. Eur Heart J 2004; 25:136–143.
107. Siu CW, Tse HF, Lau CP. Inappropriate implantable cardioverter defibrillator shock from a transcutaneous muscle stimulation device therapy. J Interv Card Electrophysiol 2005; 13(1): 73–75.

108. Glotzer TV, Gordon M, Sparta M, et al. Electromagnetic interference from a muscle stimulation device causing discharge of an implantable cardioverter defibrillator: epicardial bipolar and endocardial bipolar circuits are compared. Pacing Clin Electrophysiol 1998; 21 (10):1996–1998.
109. Tsujimoto T, Takano M, Ishikawa M, et al. Onset of ischemic colitis following use of electrical muscle stimulation (EMS) exercise equipment. Intern Med 2004; 43(8):693–695.

12
Psychological Aspects in Patients with Chronic Respiratory Failure

SHARON JANKEY
West Park Healthcare Centre, Toronto, Ontario, Canada

CLAUDIO F. DONNER
Mondo Medico, Multidisciplinary and Rehabilitation Outpatient Clinic, Borgomanero, Novara, Italy

I. Introduction

Advances in medical science have enabled persons with ventilatory failure from a variety of diagnoses to prolong their lives by opting for long-term mechanical ventilation (LTMV). In addition to their various medical issues, such patients also have psychological responses to both their physical status and their need for prolonged mechanical ventilation (PMV). The impact of living with an unremitting, life-threatening condition can overwhelm a person's coping resources and result in reactive psychological disorders, which must be addressed for their medical treatment to be maximally effective. The effects of LTMV are also experienced by the family, who may be profoundly impacted by their relative's change in physical and emotional function. Such changes influence marital and family roles and relationships.

Caring for a patient group with a myriad of physical and psychosocial needs poses challenges for the clinical staff and caregivers who are required to manage the needs of both patients and families. In this chapter, we comment on some key psychological issues that arise when working with patients in ventilatory failure receiving LTMV.

II. Psychological and Psychosocial Factors

The impact of LTMV varies with the underlying disease and its management. However, as in many medical illnesses, the impact of the condition is mediated by psychological factors. For those working with LTMV patients, an understanding of the basic assumption of the biopsychosocial model, proposed by Engel in 1977, is useful (1). In this model, both psychological and social factors influence and are influenced by the underlying pathology. This model asserts that the medical team must be sensitive to the patient's psychological issues whereas the mental health professionals must develop an understanding of the patient's health status and the potential impact of medical treatments on the patient's function and prognosis.

Being dependent on life support poses unique demands and stressors on LTMV patients, which result in psychological difficulties. These may include loss of autonomy and control, disruption of plans for the future, uncertainty about the future, permanent changes in physical appearance and bodily function, inability to communicate effectively, and diminished roles and responsibilities in the family and the society.

Symptoms of anxiety and panic are commonly associated with a dependency on life support, communication difficulties, and uncertainty regarding health status (2). Many patients meet the Diagnostic and Statistical Manual of Mental Disorders-IV (DSM-IV) criteria for diagnosis of an anxiety disorder or a panic disorder. Posttraumatic stress disorder is sometimes the result of being close to death as well as the subsequent ICU experiences (3). If unmanaged, such psychiatric conditions will have important clinical consequences on adherence to recommended care and participation in rehabilitation. They will undoubtedly also influence health-related quality of life.

Depression relates to the loss of autonomy, control and physical function, as well as altered family roles and relationships. Many patients meet DSM-IV criteria for the diagnosis of a major depressive episode or disorder. Feelings of helplessness, frustration, guilt, fear, and despair have also been reported among the LTMV population (4–6). Substance abuse also may increase among those with LTMV, requiring that the staff be sensitive to this issue (7).

III. Factors Associated with Adjustment and Coping

Although the literature in this field includes primarily qualitative studies, with small sample sizes that limit generalization, evidence has been presented to suggest that the following factors are important to the psychological response of persons with LTMV.

1. *Communication*. A number of studies have highlighted the stress associated with communication difficulties in the LTMV population (6,8). One of the most widely reported stressors is when patients cannot speak or make themselves understood, or understand what their caregivers are trying to communicate. Therefore, health care professionals need to facilitate communication to reduce the frustration and stress of the patient. When speech is severely impaired, communication board or computer-based communication is associated with much less frustration (6).
2. *Social support*. Social support is very helpful in fostering good coping for LTMV patients (9–11). A study of adult amyotrophic lateral sclerosis (ALS) patients on LTMV highlighted the importance of human interaction, verbal or electronic conversation, and discussion groups in increasing social support (9). A similar finding was found in a study of children with Duchenne's muscular dystrophy on LTMV (11).
3. *Family*. Family adjustment has a positive impact on patient adjustment. Family caregivers who are able to spend time away from home and do not feel guilty about ensuring that their own needs are met are able to provide more positive support to their family member on LTMV. Studies of family caregiver burden have documented that lack of funding assistance, equipment issues, social isolation, and financial difficulties result in emotional strain (12). Psychological problems, such as fatigue and depression, have been reported in studies of the impact on caregivers of persons with LTMV (13).
4. *Finding meaning*. Spirituality is of assistance to those on LTMV coping with adversity (9,10). It appears that spiritual beliefs foster hope in these individuals, enhancing their coping ability.

5. *Managing physical symptoms*. Physical and emotional symptoms were noted to correlate in patients on LTMV (14,15), with persons experiencing more severe physical symptoms having greater emotional and social difficulties (14). Unalleviated pain and ventilator difficulties were also associated with greater emotional distress (15). Comfort enhances coping and self-care activities, such as bathing and dressing. Massage has also been associated with greater patient satisfaction (9).
6. *Managing emotions*. Individual and group interventions can assist patients in managing their emotions. Management includes techniques, such as relaxation, training, music therapy, education, and information sharing (15).
7. *Meaningful activities*. Participation in individually relevant activities, such as hobbies, religious activities, and recreational activities, are reported to be sources of happiness among persons with ALS (9). Similar findings have been reported among children. Getting out of the house and engaging in social activities increases satisfaction (10).

IV. Assessing and Diagnosing Psychological Disorders

Unfortunately, mental health professionals, such as psychologists and psychiatrists, are often not part of the multidisciplinary team responsible for LTMV patients. Therefore, an efficient referral system to access mental health professionals must be in place, so that psychological issues can be addressed before they become major comorbidities. Optimal care should include simple screening for psychological symptoms at the same time as the physical assessment, and on an annual basis thereafter (16). The screening can be conducted by any health care professional able to administer the screening tool. Suitable tools are brief, easy to administer, and have known psychometric properties.

The following are examples of useful screening tools for identifying the presence of psychological symptoms.

Symptom Checklist-90-Revised (SCL-90-R). The SCL-90-R is a 90-item, self-administered, inventory developed by Derogatis in 1977 and is derived from the Hopkins Symptom Checklist (17). The inventory was developed to screen for psychopathology and assesses symptomatic distress in nine primary dimensions and three global indices of distress. The dimensions include somatization, obsessive-compulsive features, interpersonal sensitivity, depression, anxiety, hostility, phobic anxiety, paranoid ideation, and psychoticism. The measure takes 15 to 20 minutes to complete. It has been used widely with community adolescents and adults, inpatients, and outpatients. It has been shown to have good reliability and validity (18).

Brief Symptom Inventory (BSI). The BSI, developed by Derogatis in 1983, is the shorter form of the SCL-90-R (19). It is also self-administered and assesses the same nine symptom dimensions as the SCL-90-R and three global indices using 53 items. Dimension scores correlate highly with comparable SCL-90-R scores and it shares most psychometric characteristics. It takes 10 to 15 minutes to complete and is used widely with community adolescents and adults, inpatients, and outpatients. The BSI demonstrates good reliability and validity (18).

The Hospital Anxiety and Depression Scale (HADS). The HADS was developed by Zigmond and Snaith in 1983 (20) as a self-administered questionnaire with subscales for anxiety and depression. It takes five to seven minutes to complete. Although originally designed for hospital patients, it is used extensively in the community. It has 14 items, each on a four-point verbal rating scale and it can be used to provide measures of anxiety (7 items), depression (7 items), or emotional distress (all 14 items). The HADS has been shown to demonstrate good reliability and validity (21).

The following is a useful screening tool for cognitive dysfunction:

The Mini-Mental Status Examination, developed by Folstein et al. in 1973 (22), is widely used across a variety of populations. It includes 11 questions and requires 5 to 10 minutes to administer. It is divided into two sections, the first of which requires oral responses only and covers orientation, memory, and attention. The second part assesses the ability to name, follow verbal and written commands, write sentences spontaneously, and copy a complex figure. The measure has demonstrated good reliability and validity (22).

V. Comprehensive Assessments

Referral to a mental health professional for a diagnostic assessment may be made for any of the following reasons: if a patient demonstrates significant psychopathology or if they score above the cutoff on the screening questionnaires; if evidence exists of an underlying personality disorder; if a patient's personality traits are impacting on the ability of the staff to provide them with optimal medical care; and if educational or cultural issues preclude the use of screening tools.

Behavioral assessments may be undertaken when it is essential for the patient's clinical team to develop a better understanding of the triggers of a particular behavior that is impacting on their ability to care for the patient, such as repeated call bell pressing (23). Such assessments, although often time intensive, provide valuable information and allow for a more organized and consistent approach to addressing a target behavior.

Comprehensive cognitive assessments should be undertaken if a LTMV patient shows evidence of low cognitive functioning, such as disinhibition, poor judgment, or memory impairment, or if simple screening scores are below the cutoffs. Disordered cognition may influence the patient's ability for self-care or for making decisions about financial or medical management. Mental health professionals may be required to assess a patient's mental capacity for making end-of-life-related decision, such as discontinuation of ventilatory support.

VI. Treatment Approaches

A. Psychological Interventions

A treatment that allows patients to communicate their difficulties and to develop strategies to address them is the most helpful approach. Assisting patients to better understand the connection between their thoughts and feelings can provide an important tool to allow them to better manage their difficult emotions. Enhancing self-efficacy, which may have been diminished with the loss of physical functioning, is a key component to assisting the patient to improve their feelings of control over themselves and their environment. Training patients to communicate their symptoms and to direct their care are important vehicles for their gaining greater control over their environment. Assisting persons on LTMV to answer the question "How do I go on from here?" is critical in assisting them to reframe their situation. Meaningful activities help reduce the sense of loss, especially if these are activities that the patient has previously enjoyed. Assisting with helping patients find meaning in adversity is also a useful technique.

Specific interventions that counter anxiety arousing include relaxation training (15). The mindfulness approach, as popularized by Jon Katat-Zinn (24), assists patients to focus on the here and now. Music therapy has also been shown to have positive results in reducing anxiety for patients on LTMV (25). Professional support is valuable when addressing sensitive issues, such as end-of-life decisions and advanced directives for medical care. For terminally ill patients, family members can be assisted in expressing their loss, grief, and guilt.

B. Pharmacological Intervention

Medications may enhance psychological interventions although there are no published guidelines for psychotherapeutic medications in the LTMV population. Commonly used selective serotonin reuptake inhibitors, with antidepressant and anxiolytic properties, can be useful in treating this population. Benzodiazepines can also be used to treat anxiety and to manage sleep difficulties although caution must be exercised to avoid their addictive properties. Antipsychotics may be helpful, if agitation is high.

VII. Assistance for Family and Caregivers

A. Support for Families

Whether the LTMV patient is living at home or in an institution, family support is critical for coping with the demands of a ventilated patient. Provision of professional support to help address specific issues of concern is recommended to ease the burden for families (12,26). Interventions to enhance a family's advocacy skills, for patients, can also be helpful in increasing a family member's sense of control and self-efficacy. For palliative patients, providing family members with the opportunity to discuss their own feelings related to guilt and grief can be beneficial.

B. Support for Caregivers

Caregiver support to assist staff caregivers in addressing the psychosocial needs of their patients is prudent, given that the staff report greater difficulty while attempting to meet these psychological needs than the patients' physical needs (27). Given the stress associated with working with a patient group with such complex needs, support to assist caregivers to manage the unique stressors of caring for LTMV patients is important.

VIII. Conclusion

Treating persons requiring LTMV is a challenging but rewarding experience. The clinical staff and caregivers will observe not only some of the most severe forms of emotional distress but also some of the most heroic adjustments of any patient group. Becoming sensitive to these patients' psychological difficulties as well as their many stressors is essential, if their comprehensive medical care is to include their psychological as well as their medical needs. With appropriate support, patients on LTMV have been shown to attain a good quality of life (28,29). Substantial demands are placed on the caregivers, both the family and the health care professionals. Therefore, support for the caregivers is essential for optimizing patient care, managing the various psychological responses and assisting those requiring LTMV to achieve a satisfying and meaningful life.

References

1. Engel GL. The need for a new medical model. A challenge to biomedicine. Science 1977; 196:129–136.
2. Nelson JE, Meier DE, Litke A, et al. The symptom burden of chronic critical illness. Crit Care Med 2004; 32(7):1527–1534.
3. Granberg A, Engberg JB, Lundberg D. Patients experience of being critically ill or severely injured and care for in an intensive care unit in relation to the ICU syndrome. Part 1. Intensive Crit Care Nurs 1998; 14:294–307.
4. Gipson WT, Sivak ED, Gutledge AD. Psychological aspects of ventilator dependency. Psychol Med 1987; 5(3):245–255.
5. Cobb AK. Illness experience in a chronic disease: ALS. Soc Sci Med 1986; 23:641–650.
6. Wojnicki-Johnson G. Communication between nurse and patient during ventilator treatment: patient report and RN evaluators. Intensive Crit Care Nurs 2000; 17:29–39.
7. Heinmann AW, Doll MD, Armstrong RJ, et al. Substance use and receipt of treatment by persons with long-term spinal cord injuries. Arch Phys Med Rehabil 1991; 72:482–487.
8. Bergom-Engberg I, Hadjumac R. Assessment of patients' experience of discomfort during respirator therapy. Crit Care Med 1989; 19(10):1068–1092.
9. Hirano YM, Yamazaki Y, Shimizu J, et al. Ventilator dependence and expressions of need: a study of patients with amyotrophic lateral sclerosis in Japan. Soc Sci Med 2005; 62:1403–1413.
10. Miller JR, Colbert AP, Osbery JS. Ventilator dependency: decision making, daily functioning and quality of life for patients with Duchenne Muscular Dystrophy. Dev Med Child Neurol 1990; 32:1078–1096.
11. Gelinas DFO'Connor P, Miller RG. Quality of life for ventilator dependent ALS patients and their caregiver. J Neurol Sci 1998; 160(1):S1234–S1236.
12. van Resteren RG, Velthius B, von Leyden LW. Psychosocial problems arising from home ventilation. Am J Phys Med Rehabil 2001; 80(6):439–446.
13. Douglas, SL. Caregivers of long-term ventilator patients: physical and psychological outcomes. Chest 2003; 123(4):1073–1081.
14. Nelson JE, Meier DE, Litke A, et al. The symptom burden of chronic illness. Crit Care Med 2004; 32(7):1527–1534.
15. Thomas LA. Clinical management of stressors perceived by patient on mechanical ventilation. AACN Clin Issues 2003; 14(1):73–81.
16. Derogatis LR, Fleming MP, Sudler NC, et al. Psychological assessment. In: Nicasso PM, Smith TW, eds. Managing Chronic Illness: A Biopsychological Perspective. Vol 59. Washington, D.C.: American Psychological Association, 1995:115.
17. Derogatis LR, Liman RS, Rickels K, et al. The Hopkins Symptom Checklist (HSCL). In: Pinchot P, ed. Psychological Measurement in Psychopharmacology. Basel, Switzerland: Karger Press 1974:79–111.
18. Derogatis LR, Lazarus L. The SCL 90-R. Brief symptom inventory and matching clinical rating scales. In: Maruish M, ed. The Use of Treatment Planning and Outcome Assessment. L. Erlbaum Associates, Hillsdale, New Jersey 1994:217–248.

19. Derogatis LR, Melisaratos N. The brief symptom inventory: an introductory report. Psychol Med 1983; 13:595–605.
20. Zigmond AS, Snaith R. The hospital anxiety and depression scale. Acta Psychiatr Scand 1983; 67:361–370.
21. Snaith RP. The hospital anxiety and depression scale. Health Qual Life Outcomes 2003; 1:29.
22. Folstein M, Folstein S, McHugh P. Mini mental state. J Psychiatr Res 1975; 12:189–198.
23. Matthies BK, Kreutzer JS, West DD. The Behavioral Handbook. San Antonio, Texas: Therapy Skill Builders, 1997.
24. Katbat-Zinn J. Full Catastrophe Living: Using the Wisdom of Your Body and Mind to Face Stress, Pain, and Illness. New York: Delta, 1991.
25. Wong HLC, Lopez-Nahas V, Molassiotis A. Effects of music therapy on anxiety in ventilator dependent patients. Heart Lung 2001; 30(5):376–387.
26. Findeis A, Larson JL, GalloA, et al. Caring for individuals using home ventilators: an appraisal of family caregivers. Rehabil Nurs 1994; 19(1):6–11.
27. Hewitt-Taylor J. Children who require long-term ventilation: staff education and training. Intensive Crit Care Nurs 2004; 20:93–102.
28. Bach JR, Campagnolo D. Psychosocial adjustment of post poliomyelitis ventilator assisted individuals. Arch Phys Med Rehabil 1992; 173(10):934–939.
29. Bach JR, Barnett V. Ethical considerations in the management of individuals with severe neuromuscular disorders. Am J Phys Med Rehabil 1994; 73(2):134–140.

13
Definition and Indications for Prolonged Mechanical Ventilation (PMV)

GERARD J. CRINER and VICTOR KIM
Temple University School of Medicine, Philadelphia, Pennsylvania, U.S.A.

I. Introduction

Recent advances in intensive care have resulted in an increased salvage of critically ill patients; a number of patients have become dependent upon mechanical ventilation as a chronic form of life support (1). The increased use of prolonged mechanical ventilation (PMV) has led to greater intensive care unit (ICU) bed use, resource consumption, and costs (2,3). It is important to characterize such patients to define treatment goals and expectations, to establish ventilatory care units for their specialized care, and to provide prognostic information for overall survival, morbidities, and health-related quality of life. The goals of this chapter are to provide definitions of PMV, to characterize the patient population requiring this modality of treatment, and to briefly describe a multidisciplinary approach to treatment.

II. Definition

Until recently there was no consensus on what constitutes PMV, the definition having varied from >24 hours (4,5) to >29 days (6). Alternatively, PMV has been defined as the need for mechanical ventilation after discharge from the ICU (7). The literature on chronic ventilation has been difficult to summarize because of these varied definitions, heterogeneous patient groups, and measured outcomes.

In 2004, the National Association for Medical Direction of Respiratory Care (NAMDRC) sponsored a conference on the care and management of patients requiring PMV (8). The members of this panel consisted of representatives from multiple organizations, including the American College of Chest Physicians, the American Thoracic Society, the American College of Physicians, the American Academy of Home Care Physicians, the American Association for Respiratory Care, and the Society of Critical Care Medicine, and sponsors from industry. They defined PMV to standardize interpretation of the literature, analyze outcomes of data, and guide treatment decisions. In the United States, the definition also has implications for service reimbursement and the placement of patients in long-term ventilator facilities or weaning facilities. PMV was defined as ≥21 consecutive days of mechanical ventilation for ≥6 hr/day. This definition was based on stipulations of the Center for Medicare and Medicaid Services (CMS) Diagnosis Related Groups (DRGs) for mechanical ventilatory support as well as on observational studies that demonstrated that the majority of patients transferred to a long-term acute care hospital had been ventilator dependent for at least 21 days (9,10). The NAMDRC did recognize that the criteria of ≥6 hours per day might be too strict. The requirement of mechanical ventilation for any period of time has important implications for patient disposition, such as a weaning facility or a long-term care ventilator facility as well as equipment and staffing needs. The threshold of six hours per day may exclude some patients who require chronic ventilation.

The introduction of noninvasive positive pressure ventilation (NPPV) has led to a substantial increase in the utilization of chronic ventilation. Although there is no consensus on what defines the chronic use of NPPV, earlier literature has considered chronic NPPV to be from 4.3 hours nocturnally for 2 weeks to 10 hours nocturnally for 6 months (11,12). This lack of consensus is compounded by the different outcomes reported. As opposed to PMV, where the goal of therapy is ventilatory support for chronic respiratory failure, the goals of NPPV can vary from prevention of acute bouts of respiratory failure (13) to improvement in sleep quality (14), respiratory muscle rest (15), decreased dyspnea (16), and improved gas exchange (13). The decision to use NPPV and the goals of treatment should be determined for each individual according to their disease category and achievable goals. Agreement on a definition for NPPV is important to summarize the current literature.

III. Epidemiology

The incidence of PMV varies on the basis of the setting studied and the definitions used. Prospective cohort studies have estimated that 5–20% of ICU patients will require mechanical ventilation for ≥4 days (17–19). An international prospective cohort study of intubated patients in 361 ICUs in Europe estimated that 25% of patients required ventilation for ≥7 days (20). Studies using the definition of >21days have shown a more conservative estimate of 3–7% of patients (21,22). However, these single center studies may have underestimated the incidence of PMV.

Data over the last two decades suggest that the prevalence of PMV is on the rise. A statewide survey of acute care hospitals in Massachusetts, U.S.A., estimated that there were 6800 ventilator-dependent patients in the United States in 1983 (23). Fifteen years later, this estimate has risen more than 10-fold. In 1997, an analysis of the National Inpatient Sample, a database containing information on all discharges from multiple hospitals in 22 states, estimated that 88,000 patients were discharged with DRG 483 (tracheostomy with mechanical ventilation >96 hours with principal diagnosis except for face, head, and neck diagnoses) (24). Analyses of two statewide databases revealed 66% and 78% increases in the number of adult discharges with DRG 483 in the mid 1990s (25,26). In parallel with this rise, the average age of patients requiring PMV has decreased from 65 years, in 1993, to 62 years, in 2002, and the number of comorbid illnesses has increased.

The expanding use of NPPV, especially for averting or weaning from invasive ventilation, should reduce the population of patients requiring PMV. Despite the

Table 1 General Characteristics of Patients Requiring Prolonged Mechanical Ventilation

Absent or severely impaired spontaneous breathing efforts
Central disorders (i.e., major strokes, central hypoventilation)
Major insults to the respiratory system, secondary to catastrophic medical or surgical illnesses
s/p ARDS
Cardiomyopathy
Chronic disorder that precipitates recurrent bouts of respiratory failure
Severe COPD
Severe kyphoscoliosis

Abbreviations: ARDS, acute respiratory distress syndrome; COPD, chronic obstructive pulmonary disease.
Source: From Travaline JM, Criner GJ. Management and monitoring of long-term invasive mechanical ventilation. In: Hill NS, ed. Long-Term Mechanical Ventilation. New York: Marcel Dekker, Inc., 2000:216.

increased utilization of NPPV, the literature has not indicated any decline in this population as yet.

IV. Indications for Chronic Ventilatory Assistance

The indications for PMV are summarized in Table 1; indications for the chronic use of NPPV are addressed elsewhere in this textbook. The most obvious group of patients have absent or severely impaired spontaneous breathing, as in hypoventilation secondary to depressed central ventilatory drive, for example, intracranial disorders or central hypoventilation. Patients who fail repeated attempts at weaning from ventilation represent another group of patients who may require PMV. They have often experienced acute respiratory failure and, despite reversal of the acute problem, they are unable to sustain adequate unassisted ventilation. This failure may have occurred as a result of a severe medical illness or a postoperative catastrophe, or as an acute illness superimposed on a chronic disorder that further impairs an already compromised respiratory pump, such as, malnutrition, advanced age, cardiac disease, or a systemic infection. The third and potentially the largest group of patients who may require PMV are those with chronic disorders associated with recurrent episodes of respiratory failure. Examples of this group include neuromuscular conditions, thoracic restriction, and parenchymal lung disease.

V. Outcome

Unselected patients receiving PMV, if not screened by the severity or nature of their underlying disease, extent of multiple organ dysfunction, rehabilitative potential, and functional preadmission status, have a greatly reduced chance of survival. Those who do survive have limited improvements in functional status and health-related quality of life. However, patients receiving PMV have a much better prognosis if they are appropriately selected and if they receive aggressive rehabilitation. Data from two of the U.S. Health Care Financing Administration (HCFA) chronic ventilator demonstration sites suggested that the survival of some patients requiring invasive long-term ventilation has improved.

Gracey et al. reported the outcomes in 206 consecutive patients admitted to the Mayo Clinic Ventilator-Dependent Unit during a five-year study period (27). Two hundred and six patients who met the current definition of PMV were admitted; 92% (190) were discharged of which 77% returned to their homes, and 153 of the patients were weaned totally from mechanical ventilation, whereas 37 remained completely or partially ventilator dependent. Of the patients receiving mechanical ventilation at the time of discharge, 73% received it only nocturnally. The four-year survival rate of the patients was 53%. However, a significant number (60%) of patients received prolonged ventilation as a result of postoperative conditions, which may have skewed the results to a more optimistic report.

In a report by Criner et al. (28) from another HCFA Chronic Ventilator Demonstration Project Clinical Unit of 77 patients, in which 74% had medical causes, the findings were similar to Gracey's. Ninety-three percent of patients were discharged, 82% were alive at 6 months, and 61% at 12 months. Eighty-six percent of the patients were completely weaned from mechanical ventilation, 11% required continuous ventilation, and 10% had nocturnal ventilation at the time of discharge. In those discharged, there was a significant increase in functional status at 5 and 12 months.

Overall, both these studies suggest that when patients receiving PMV were properly selected, they had an acceptable clinical outcome with a return to preadmission functional status and successful home discharge.

VI. Location of Care

Patients requiring PMV account for a disproportionate amount of health care costs and resources, with those who are ventilator dependent in the ICU for >21 days accounting for 37% of all ICU costs (29). Therefore, there has been a significant drive to improve outcomes and to increase non-ICU facilities, where such patients can receive appropriate care. The decision to transfer a patient who requires PMV may be difficult. Clinical stability and a determination that the patient's staffing needs will be met are necessary before transfer to a step-down unit. A noninvasive respiratory care unit is less expensive than an ICU, allows for more effective transition home or to a nonacute care location, fosters patient independence, and improves quality of life (Fig. 1).

At our facility, the Temple University Hospital, which is one of four HCFA Chronic Ventilator-Demonstration sites, the complex and diverse problems of PMV patients are treated by a diverse team comprises pulmonologists, respiratory nurses, nutritionists, psychologists, physical therapists, speech therapists, and a social worker (Fig. 2). This unit emphasizes rehabilitation and restoration of functional status despite requirements for prolonged ventilation. Special needs of patients that require PMV addressed in this unit include evaluation of the optimum form of ventilator support, special attention to swallowing dysfunction, impaired communication skills, psychological dysfunction, nutritional repletion, respiratory muscle and whole body reconditioning, as well as close attention to new or changing medical conditions.

Criteria for admission are summarized in Table 2. Patients must have been ventilator dependent for at least 21 consecutive days for >6 hr/day and be willing to participate in rehabilitation. They must have a stable airway in place as afforded by a tracheostomy and

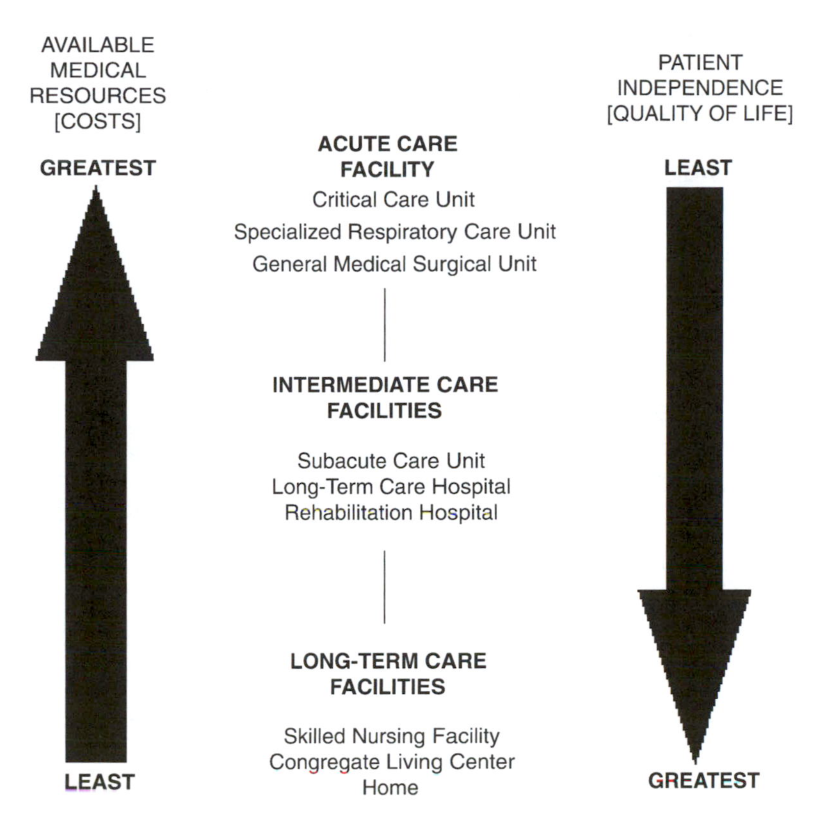

Figure 1 Potential sites of care for patients requiring PMV. Sites toward the bottom of the figure have fewer medical resources and lower costs but allow greater patient independence and a higher quality of life. *Abbreviation*: PMV, prolonged mechanical ventilation. *Source*: From Make BJ, Hill NS, Goldberg AI, et al. Mechanical ventilation beyond the intensive care unit: report of a consensus conference of the American college of chest physicians. Chest 1998; 113:295S.

they must have manageable secretions. They should not be on sophisticated modes of mechanical ventilation and their requirements for supplemental oxygen or positive end-expiratory pressure should be modest. In addition, comorbid conditions, such as cardiac, hematological, or fluid and electrolyte imbalances, must be stable and the patients should have secure routes for medication access and alimentation.

Multidisciplinary rehabilitation is vital to the care of the patient requiring PMV, not only to maximize functional capacity and independence, but also to increase the chances of a weaning success. Martin et al. found that aggressive whole body and inspiratory muscle training improved strength, functional status, and weaning in debilitated chronically ventilated patients (30). This finding supports recent literature demonstrating that patients recently weaned from PMV had reduced respiratory muscle strength (31) and that inspiratory muscle and upper extremity training improved general physical conditioning and weaning outcome (32,33).

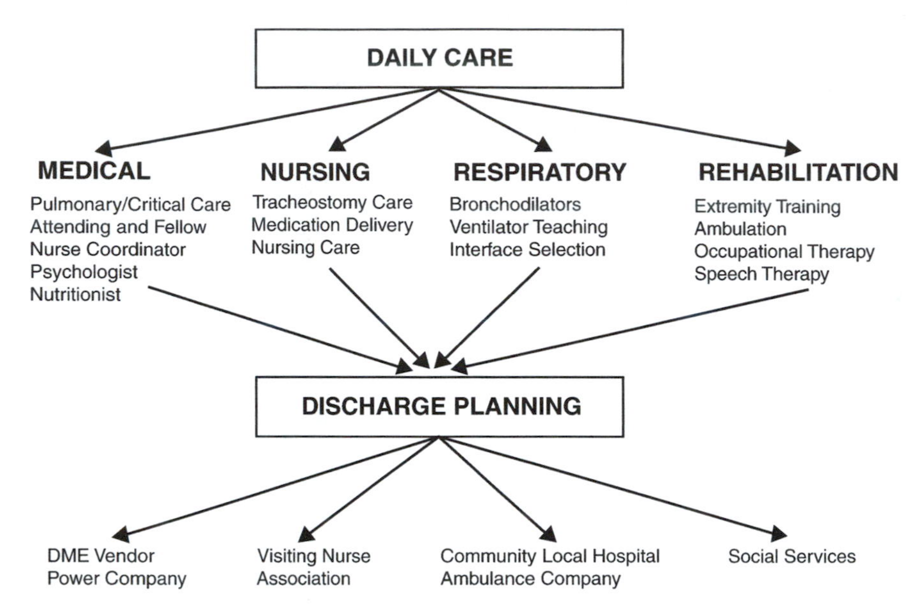

Figure 2 Multidisciplinary plan of patient care in the ventilator rehabilitation unit at Temple University Hospital. Patients' daily care is divided into four components: medical, nursing, respiratory, and rehabilitative. All four groups deliver the care as indicated daily. Team members meet for discharge planning once a week and communicate with outpatient resources and the outpatient clinic staff. *Source*: From Criner GJ. Respir Care Clin N Am 2002; 8:580.

Table 2 Criteria for Transfer from the ICU to the VRU

Respiratory criteria	Nonrespiratory criteria
Ventilator dependent for >6 hr/day for >21 days	Willingness to participate in rehabilitation
Failed >2 weaning attempts	Controlled sepsis
Secure airway: tracheostomy	No uncontrolled hemorrhage
Manageable secretions with infrequent suctioning	No uncontrolled arrhythmias, CHF, or unstable angina
Adequate oxygenation: $Fio_2 \leq 50\%$, PEEP $\leq 5 cmH_2O$, $Sao_2 > 92\%$	No coma
Stable ventilator settings, no sophisticated modes	Secure parenteral line
Able to tolerate >30 min SBT via tracheostomy	Secure alimentation route

Abbreviations: VRU, ventilator rehabilitation unit; PEEP, positive end-expiratory pressure; Sao_2, oxygen saturation; SBT, spontaneous breathing trial; Fio_2, fraction of inspired oxygen; CHF, congestive heart failure.

Source: From Make BJ, Hill NS, Goldberg AI, et al. Mechanical ventilation beyond the intensive care unit: report of a consensus conference of the American college of chest physicians. Chest 1998; 113:299S.

VII. Summary and Recommendations

In summary, individuals requiring PMV-ventilator dependence for >6 hr/day for >21 days comprise a growing population of patients that account for increased health care utilization and costs. Because this group continues to grow, physicians must know when and how to transition care from the ICU setting to another. Ultimate disposition depends on clinical stability, the ability to provide ventilator and tracheostomy care, and the functional status of the patient. Transition from the ICU to one that can provide these special needs, while focusing on rehabilitation, will restore functional status and improve health related quality of life, while decreasing the costs of hospital care. Contrary to earlier beliefs, chronic ventilation is associated with an acceptable long-term outcome in carefully selected patients.

References

1. Mulligan S. AARC and Gallup estimate numbers and costs for chronic ventilator patients. Am Assoc Respir Care Times 1991; 150:30–36.
2. Cohen IL, Booth FVM. Cost containment and mechanical ventilation in the United States. New Horiz 1994; 2:283–290.
3. Scheinhorn DJ, Char DC, Hassenpflug MS, et al. Post-ICU weaning from mechanical ventilation: the role of long-term facilities. Chest 2001; 120:482S–484S.
4. Gillespie DJ, Marsh HM, Divertie MB, et al. Clinical outcome of respiratory failure in patients requiring prolonged (greater than 24 hours) mechanical ventilation. Chest 1986; 90:364–369.
5. Spicher JE, White DP. Outcome and function following prolonged mechanical ventilation. Arch Intern Med 1987; 147:421–425.
6. Gracey DR, Viggiano RW, Naessens JM, et al. Outcomes of patients admitted to a chronic ventilator-dependent unit in an acute-care hospital. Mayo Clin Proc 1992; 67:131–136.
7. Scheinhorn D, Chao D, Stearn-Hassenpflug M, et al. Ventilator-dependent survivors of catastrophic illness: a multicenter outcomes study. Am J Respir Crit Care Med 2003; 167:A458 (abstr).
8. MacIntyre NR, Epstein SK, Carson S, et al. Management of patients requiring prolonged mechanical ventilation: report of a NAMDRC consensus conference. Chest 2005; 128: 3937–3954.
9. Scheinhorn DJ, Chao DC, Hassenpflug MS, et al. Post-ICU weaning from mechanical ventilation: the role of long-term facilities. Chest 2001; 120(suppl):482S–484S.
10. Scheinhorn DJ, Chao DC, Stearn-Hassenpflug M. Post-ICU mechanical ventilation-treatment of 1,575 patients over 11 years at a regional weaning center. Am J Respir Crit Care Med 2000; 161: A793 (abstr).
11. Lin CC. Comparison between nocturnal nasal positive pressure ventilation combined with oxygen therapy and oxygen monotherapy in patients with severe COPD. Am J Respir Crit Care Med 1996; 154:353–358.
12. Elliott MW, Steven MH, Phillips GD, et al. Non-invasive mechanical ventilation for acute respiratory failure. BMJ 1990; 300:358–360.
13. Clinical indications for noninvasive positive pressure ventilation in chronic respiratory failure due to restrictive lung disease, COPD, and nocturnal hypoventilation—a consensus conference report. Chest 1999; 116:521–534.
14. Krachman SL, Quaranta AJ, Berger TJ, et al. Effects of noninvasive positive pressure ventilation on gas exchange and sleep in COPD patients. Chest 1997; 112:623–628.
15. Braun NM, Marino WD. Effect of daily intermittent rest of respiratory muscles in patients with severe chronic airflow limitation (CAL). Chest 1984; 85:59S–60S.

16. Clini E, Sturani C, Rossi A, et al. The Italian multicentre study on noninvasive ventilation in chronic obstructive pulmonary disease patients. Eur Respir J 2002; 20:529–538.
17. Epstein SK, Voung V. Lack of influence of gender on outcomes of mechanically ventilated medical ICU patients. Chest 1999; 116:732–739.
18. Rady MY, Ryan T. Perioperative predictors of extubation failure and the effect on clinical outcome after cardiac surgery. Crit Care Med 1999; 27:246–247.
19. Conner B, Branca P, Butka B, et al. Ventilator dependence after cardiac surgery. Chest 2000; 118(suppl):162S (abstr).
20. Esteban A, Anzueto A, Frutos F, et al. Characteristics and outcomes in adult patients receiving mechanical ventilation: a 28-day international study. JAMA 2002; 287:345–355.
21. Gracey DR, Viggiano RW, Naessens JM, et al. Outcomes of patients admitted to a chronic ventilator-dependent unit in an acute-care hospital. Mayo Clin Proc 1992; 67:131–136.
22. Bureau of Data Management and Strategy. 100% MEDPAR inpatient hospital fiscal year 1998, 6/99 update. United States Health Care Finance Administration. Washington, DC:US Government Printing Office, 1999.
23. Make B, Dayno S, Gertman P. Prevalence of chronic ventilator-dependency. Am Rev Respir Dis 1986; 133:A167 (abstr).
24. Carson SS, Bach PB. The epidemiology and costs of chronic critical illness. Crit Care Clin 2002; 18:461–476.
25. Dewar DM, Kurek CJ, Lambrinos J, et al. Patterns in costs and outcomes for patients with prolonged mechanical ventilation undergoing tracheostomy: an analysis of discharges under diagnosis-related group 483 in New York State from 1992 to 1996. Crit Care Med 1999; 27:2640–2647.
26. Cox C, Carson S, Howard A, et al. Tracheostomy for prolonged ventilation in North Carolina, 1993–2002. Am J Respir Crit Care Med 2004; 169:A44 (abstr).
27. Gracey DR, Hardy DC, Naessens JM, et al. The Mayo ventilator-dependent rehabilitation unit: a 5-year experience. Mayo Clin Proc 1997; 72:13–19.
28. Criner GJ, Kreimer DT, Pidloan L. Patient outcome following prolonged mechanical ventilation (MV) via tracheostomy. Am Rev Respir Dis 1993; 147:A874 (abstr).
29. Wagner DP. Economics of prolonged mechanical ventilation. Am Rev Respir Dis 1989; 140 (suppl):S14–S18.
30. Martin UJ, Hincapie L, Nimchuk M, et al. Impact of whole-body rehabilitation in patients receiving chronic mechanical ventilation. Crit Care Med 2005; 33:2259–2265.
31. Chang AT, Boots RJ, Brown MG, et al. Reduced inspiratory muscle endurance following successful weaning from prolonged mechanical ventilation. Chest 2005; 128:553–559.
32. Aldrich TK, Karpel JP, Uhrlass RM, et al. Weaning from mechanical ventilation: adjunctive use of inspiratory muscle resistive training. Crit Care Med 1989; 17:143–147.
33. Porta R, Vitacca M, Gile LS, et al. Supported arm training in patients recently weaned from mechanical ventilation. Chest 2005; 128:2511–2520.

14
Clinical Settings for Ventilator-Assisted Individuals—When and Why—LTAC-SNF-CAVC

ANDREA VIANELLO
Respiratory Pathophysiology Unit, University Hospital, Padova, Italy

NICOLINO AMBROSINO
Pulmonary and Respiratory Intensive Care Unit-University Hospital Pisa, Italy and Pulmonary Rehabilitation and Weaning Center, Auxilium Vitae, Volterra (PI), Italy

I. Introduction

Long-term mechanical ventilation (LTMV) has existed for over 50 years, with polio survivors of the mid-20th century representing the first generation of ventilator-assisted individuals (VAIs) (1). LTMV was initially conceived as a hospital-centered treatment, and intensive care units (ICU) remained the primary sites for treatment of most of the long-term VAIs until the end of the 1980s (2,3).

However, in the early 1990s, the management of VAIs in ICU became complicated by three new critical elements, i.e., the increasing number of VAIs, increasing costs of their treatment, and greater emphasis on their quality of life.

A. Increasing Number of VAIs and Increasing Costs

The number of VAIs has fluctuated from decade to decade. As the need for LTMV for polio patients declined, the number of patients with spinal cord injuries or progressive neuromuscular disease (NMD) increased due to better acute care. Therefore, the number of patients administered LTMV has progressively increased, due both to advances in medical care and to the more widespread application of invasive mechanical ventilation in the acute setting. The increasing number of VAIs can be documented by comparing surveys performed in the last two decades. Regional surveys carried out in Minnesota, United States, in 1986 and 1992, documented that the prevalence of ventilatory assistance rose from 2.4/100,000 in 1986 to 4.9/100,000 in 1992 (2). Extrapolation of these data would suggest that in the United States, the potential number of VAIs rose from 5777 in 1986 to 12,279 in 1992 (4).

As a consequence of their growing numbers, prolonged care of a VAI (>30 days) in the ICU has rapidly increased the costs to the health care system: in the United States, it has been estimated that patients requiring prolonged mechanical ventilation (PMV) account for as much as 40% of the ICU budget (5). Nevertheless, in 1995, a U.S. survey of 300 randomly selected acute care units reported that over 11,000 patients had received PMV at a cost of $9 million per day. Of these patients, 17% were awaiting placement outside the ICU, and 12% remained in ICU as they could not be reimbursed for care elsewhere (6). Although in Europe, the exact number of VAIs awaiting placement outside the ICU is not known, the pressure to relieve ICU beds is quite similar (4).

B. Increased Emphasis on Quality of Life

Several reports have commented on the optimal site for LTMV. The ICU often involves activities with regard to the patients, such as physical restraint, sedation, and depersonalization. It also lacks a rehabilitative focus, fosters dependence, and disrupts family life (7) and is therefore inappropriate for stable ventilator-dependent patients. As a consequence, several alternative locations for LTMV have been proposed.

Although a great deal of effort has been expended to transform LTMV from a hospital-centered to a home-centered treatment, many VAIs cannot return home due to medical, psychosocial, environmental, technical, and financial reasons. Alternative options vary in complexity and intensity of care provided. They may exist within acute care hospitals, rehabilitation hospitals, skilled nursing facilities, or be freestanding institutions (8,9). Patients may transition through these sites according to their changing medical and social circumstances.

In this chapter, we describe possible alternate settings for a VAI unsuitable for the ICU or the home environment. We discuss outcomes of care and provide indications for making decisions regarding the most appropriate site for long-term ventilation.

II. Transfer from ICU to Alternative Sites of Care

There is evidence that VAIs may derive significant advantages in transferring from the ICU to specialized facilities that provide appropriate care (Table 1) (10). However, careful evaluation is required before transfer to an extended care facility. Accelerated discharge practices may result in readmission to a tertiary care hospital within 30 days and a diminishing one-year survival (11).

Clinical stability, defined in Table 2, is a key factor for determining the chances for successful LTMV at a non-ICU care facility. In 1996, an evidence-based test [Kindred Admission Screening Tool (KAST)] was developed to assess which ICU patients may be candidates for a long-term facility (12). This decision supporting tool provides three concise reports that may help physicians in identifying patients at high risk of requiring PMV and facilitates a more timely selection and transfer of VAIs to an appropriate long-term facility, before their reentering the community. It should also result in cost reductions at the acute care hospital (Fig. 1).

III. Clinical Settings for VAIs

In the United States, the growing influence of capitated care has driven the development of alternative care sites for a VAI. By 1997, there were 200 long-term acute care (LTAC) hospitals nationwide, with a capacity for 15,000 patients (13). The presence of intermediate and long-term facilities in Europe for the management of a VAI varies in different jurisdictions. In France, a well-developed system of care includes extended care facilities, which provide long-term care for VAIs or respite care for patients whose families need relief from

Table 1 Potential Advantages for VAIs in Transferring from ICU to a VAI-Focused Environment

ICU	VAI-focused intermediate or long-term care
Noise	Relative quiet
Light	Day/night cycles
Limited view of world	Outdoors easily visible
Crowded/cramped	Relatively roomy
Supportive visitors restricted	Supportive visitors encouraged
Immobilized	Mobility increased
Sterile surroundings	Personal objects permitted
Communication limited	Time and devices increase communication
Tube feeding	Transition to oral feeding
Continued deconditioning with little opportunity for physical or occupational therapy	More time, space, personnel for reconditioning
High reliance on technology	More reliance on patient interaction
Limited staff nurturing time	Emphasis on staff nurturing
Limited psychological, social, religious counseling	More time and opportunity for counseling
Limited application of palliative care	Time and space for patient/family palliative care
Ward-geared discharge planning	Home-geared discharge planning

Abbreviations: VAI, ventilator-assisted individuals; ICU, intensive care units.
Source: From Ref. 9

Table 2 Criteria for Discharging VAI from ICU to an Alternative Clinical Setting

1. Absence of sustained dyspnea or severe dyspneic episodes or tachypnea
2. Acceptable arterial blood gas levels, with $FiO_2 < 0.40$
3. Absence of life-threatening cardiac dysfunction or arrythmias
4. Ability to clear secretions or presence of a tracheostomy
5. Evidence of gag-cough reflex or protected airway
6. Adequate nutrition
7. Ability to communicate with caregivers and to self-direct care
8. Motivation to be moved outside the ICU

home care (14). Few other European countries have an equivalent integrated health system for the management of VAI.

Facilities vary in admission criteria, care levels, nursing skills, and diagnostic and therapeutic capabilities (15). Sites may be divided into intermediate care facilities and long-term care facilities (Table 3).

A. Intermediate Care Facilities

LTAC Hospital

Long-term acute care (LTAC) hospitals are for patients who need less intensive monitoring and intervention than ICU patients, but require treatment that is too complex for

Consultation Report

- Patient Background
- Severity of Illness (APACHE III, Acute Physiology Score)
- Expected Mortality
- Expected ICU LOS
- Estimated Cost of ICU Care
- Expected Hospital Reimbursement
- Clinical Variables (eg. VS, laboratory values, GCS, DNR and dialysis status)
- Case Notes

Financial Summary Report

- Patient Background
- Estimated Cost of ICU Care
- Expected Hospital Reimbursement
- Remaining Hospital Days Before Costs > Reimbursement
- Remaining Hospital Days Before Costs > Reimbursement
- Cost-Reimbursement Trend (graph)
- Summary

Clinical Summary Report

- Patient Background
- Severity of Illness (APACHE III, Acute Physiology Score
- Expected Mortality
- Expected ICU LOS
- Clinical Variables (e.g., VS, laboratory values, GCS, DNR, and dialysis status)
- Case Notes

APACHE, acute physiologic and chronic health evaluation; ICU, Intensive Care Unit; LOS, length of stay; VS, vital signs; GCS, Glasgow Coma Score; DNR, do not resuscitate.

Figure 1 Kindred Admission Screening Tool (KAST) client reports. *Source*: From Ref. 35.

Table 3 Characteristics of Alternative Site of Care for Long-Term Mechanical Ventilation

Site	Patient type	Advantages	Disadvantages
LTAC unit	All except very acute	Individualized comprehensive treatment	High cost
CAVC unit	Stable	Intensive nursing and respiratory care, patient focused, lower cost	Unable to provide intensive care, limited weaning
Rehabilitation hospital	Stable; able to participate in rehabilitation program	Round-the-clock rehabilitation nursing, patient focused, lower cost	Unable to provide intensive care
SNF	Stable	Patient focused, lowest cost	Unable to provide intensive and/or acute care, no weaning
Group-living environment	Stable	Respiratory care, nursing care	Unable to provide acute care

Abbreviations: LTAC, long-term acute care; CAVC, chronic assisted ventilatory care; SNF, skilled nursing facility.

conventional skilled nursing facilities. Patients requiring continuous inotropic or vasopressor support, hemodialysis, or total parenteral nutrition are not uncommon. LTAC units provide care to patients with subacute or chronic respiratory failure, with the goal of providing a comprehensive treatment plan intended to restore VAIs to their fullest respiratory autonomy. These facilities may be inside acute hospitals or separate free-standing facilities. They have their own fully equipped ICU and may perform low-level surgical procedures. Some have a designated step-down unit.

In the United States, LTAC hospitals were expected to maintain a mean length of stay of >25 days. The number of LTAC hospitals has increased substantially to become one of the fastest-growing cost components of the U.S. Medicare program (10,16,17). As a consequence, there is now a capped payment system based on the assessment of the needs for patient care.

LTAC outcomes report survival until discharge from 48% to 93% and long-term survival from 23% to 53% at one and four years, respectively (18). Scheinhorn et al. (19) surveyed 1123 consecutive patients at an LTAC unit for attempted weaning over an eight-year period. Patients had chronic lung disease (28%), acute lung disease (29%), and postoperative ventilatory failure (22.5%). More than 50% of the patients were successfully weaned, with 29 days of median time to wean, and 38% of them had a one-year survival postdischarge. Carson reported on 133 VAIs who were ventilated >14 days in an ICU and then transferred to a single LTAC hospital (20). Sixty-six (50%) patients died during hospitalization at the LTAC hospital, 47 (70%) discharged patients were weaned, but only 30 (23%) were still alive at one year. These authors concluded that patients who require prolonged LTMV after an acute illness, admitted to an LTAC unit, had a low one-year survival rate and after one year, few managed independent living. In contrast, other studies have suggested that 34–60% of ventilator-dependent patients discharged from ICU can be weaned effectively in an LTAC hospital (21) and that survival after hospital discharge was reasonable depending on the underlying disease (22). Adopting a fixed weaning protocol increases the weaning success rate in the LTAC setting and may decrease weaning time (23,24). The LTAC units with more restrictive admission criteria have reported higher success rates in weaning as well as the best survival (25,26).

Several reports have suggested that age >75 years, lack of functional independence before the acute care hospital admission, duration of stay in the ICU, renal failure, and diabetes herald a greater chance of weaning failure and decreased one-year survival (20,22). Based on these criteria, VAIs with extremely poor prognoses may be offered other options that are more focused on palliation or hospice care.

LTAC hospitals have higher patient-to-nurse ratios, standardized services, and standard protocols for weaning. Nevertheless, a study of 7440 patients transferred from 155 acute care hospitals to LTAC units reported that costs remain high for PMV patients (usually reimbursed under DRG 483), even in an LTAC hospital, and concluded that this subgroup of patients is still a source of uncompensated care (27).

CAVC Unit

Chronic assisted ventilatory care (CAVC) units are often not-for-profit or government-supported facilities, designed to provide extended medical and rehabilitative care for VAIs who remain ventilator dependent and require care by a multidisciplinary team with the goal of optimizing their level of function. Causes of chronic respiratory failure include both obstructive and nonobstructive conditions. General guidelines for admission include (1) a tracheostomy, (2) failure of all attempts at weaning, (3) ventilation for >two months, (4) medical complexity, and (5) inadequate social support precluding community-based care.

CAVC units include multidisciplinary teams and are led by a physician, preferably a respiratory or rehabilitation specialist with experience in LTMV. Nurses provide medications, airway care hygiene, and skin care. Respiratory therapists supervise all aspects of ventilation, in collaboration with the physician. Other team members, such as occupational and physical therapists, supervise exercise, mobility, and communication issues. Detailed descriptions of the multidisciplinary team are found elsewhere in this text.

Votto (28) and Wijkstra (29) have both reported their experience with CAVC units. Chronic obstructive pulmonary disease (COPD) patients had the worst outcomes and many NMD patients were discharged to a more independent community-based environment. The approach to the management of VAIs must be individualized, with the goal of addressing their specific needs.

Rehabilitation Hospital

Rehabilitation hospitals admit VAIs who require therapy before reentering the community. They must be able to participate in three hours or more of physical therapy per day. Most admissions are from acute care hospitals (85%), and the mean length of stay is approximately 30 days. Many patients (20%) are discharged to a skilled nursing facility (SNF) (30). Patients participate actively, with minimum restrictions and maximum therapy by the multidisciplinary team that often includes physical, occupational, and respiratory therapist, prosthetist-orthotist, rehabilitation nurse, speech pathologist, psychologist, social worker, and vocational counselor (31).

B. Long-Term Care Facilities

Skilled Nursing Facility

Nursing homes have created units to care for noncritically ill VAIs who are free from acute medical problems. A rehabilitation nurse is often the principal provider of care, including education on self-management. The nurse, social worker, recreation therapist, and dietician work together to coordinate a program that best fits the patient. Ongoing access to an inpatient medical service is usually provided.

Ankrom reported a five-year experience in a 19-bed chronic ventilator unit located in a SNF, for which there were no predetermined requirements for VAI admission except that the patients do not require intensive monitoring, nursing, or technology (32). Patients had failed weaning trials over several weeks, had a tracheostomy and required LTMV. Of the 95 VAIs, 26 lived more than 12 months; 15 patients were weaned, 13 elected to discontinue ventilator support, and 13 were still alive in the nursing home but required LTMV. The one-year survival in a SNF was similar to that of an ICU. Care of VAI in a SNF is less costly than at home (33).

Group-Living Environment

These facilities usually consist of private residences or apartments housing six to 10 patients, with therapeutic services contracted by the facility and caregiver support. Not much available in the United States, these facilities are frequently used in many other countries (34).

IV. Conclusion

The management of clinically stable, ventilator-dependant individuals is a challenge both in terms of achieving the best quality of care and in reducing healthcare resources. Given that VAIs are best managed away from the ICU, those who cannot return home require safe locations that maximize their quality of life. Careful selection of patients, close attention to their required level of care, and ongoing collection of valid outcome data will facilitate the optimum management at the lowest cost, for these patients.

References

1. Hodes HL. Treatment of respiratory difficulties in poliomyelitis. In: Poliomyelitis: papers and discussion presented at the Third International Poliomyelitis Conference. Philadelphia: Lippincott; 1955:91–113.
2. Make B, Dayno S, Gertman P. Prevalence of chronic ventilator-dependency. Am Rev Respir Dis 1986; 132(suppl):A167.
3. Milligan S. AARC and Gallup estimate numbers and costs of caring for chronic ventilator patients. AARC Times 1991; 15(1):30–36.
4. Simonds AK. From intensive care unit to home discharge in the 24 h ventilator dependent patient. In: C. Roussos, ed. Mechanical Ventilation from Intensive Care to Home Care. Sheffield: European Respiratory Society Journal Ltd, 1998:364–379.
5. Halpern NA, Bettes L, Greenstein R. Federal and nationwide intensive care units and healthcare costs: 1986-1992. Crit Care Med 1994; 22(12):2001–2007.
6. Make BJ. Indications for home ventilation in critical care unit patients. In: Robert D, Make BJ, Leger P, et al., eds. Home Mechanical Ventilation. Paris: Arnette Blackwell, 1995:229–240.
7. Goldstein RS. Home mechanical ventilation: demographics and user perspectives. Monaldi Arch Chest Dis 1998; 53(5):560–563.
8. Prentice WS. Placement alternatives for long-term ventilator care. Respir Care 1986; 31 (4):199–204.
9. Ambrosino N, Vianello A. Where to perform long-term ventilation. Respir Care Clin N Am 2002; 8(3):463–478.
10. MacIntyre NR, Epstein SK, Carson S, et al. Management of patients requiring prolonged mechanical ventilation. Report of a NAMDRC Consensus Conference. Chest 2005; 128 (6):3937–3954.
11. Naseaway SA, Button GJ, Rand WM, et al. Survivors of catastrophic illness: outcome after direct transfer from intensive care to extended care facilities. Crit Care Med 2000; 28(1):19–28.
12. Seneff MG, Zimmerman JE, Knaus WA, et al. Predicting the duration of mechanical ventilation: the importance of disease and patient characteristics. Chest 1996; 110:469–479.
13. Campbell S. HCFA clamping down on long term acute care "hospitals within hospitals". Health Care Strateg Manage 1997; 15(8):12–13.
14. Kurz C. National survey by ANTADIR of patients treated at home for chronic respiratory insufficiency in corresponding sector. Soins 1984; 423(1):33–36.
15. Reinhardt UE. Spending more through "cost control": our obsessive quest to gut the hospital. Health Aff (Millwood) 1996; 15(8):145 154.
16. Hotes LS, Kalman E. The evolution of care for the chronically critically ill patients. Clin Chest Med 2001; 22(1):1–11.
17. Scheinhorn DJ, Chao DC, Stearn-Hassenpflug M, et al. Post-ICU weaning from mechanical ventilation. The role of long-term facilities. Chest 2001; 120(6):482S–484S.

18. Dematte D'Amico JE, Donnelly HK, Mutlu GM, et al. Risk assessment for inpatient survival in the long-term acute care setting after prolonged critical illness. Chest 2003; 124(3):1039–1045.
19. Scheinhorn DJ, Chao DC, Stearn-Hassenpflug M, et al. Post-ICU mechanical ventilation. Treatment of 1,123 patients at a regional weaning centre. Chest 1997; 111(6):1654–1659.
20. Carson SS, Bach PB, Brzozowski L, et al. Outcomes after long-term acute care. An analysis of 133 mechanically ventilated patients. Am J Respir Crit Care Med 1999; 159(5):1568–1573.
21. Chan L, Koepsell TD, Deyo RA et al. The effect on Medicare's payment system for rehabilitation hospitals on length of stay, charges, and total payments. N Engl J Med 1997; 337 (14):978–985.
22. Pilcher DV, Bailey MJ, Treacher DF, et al. Outcomes, cost and long-term survival of patients referred to a regional weaning centre. Thorax 2005; 60(3):175–182.
23. Vitacca M, Vianello A, Colombo D, et al. Comparison of two methods for weaning patients with chronic obstructive pulmonary disease requiring mechanical ventilation for more than 15 days. Am J Respir Crit Care Med 2001; 164(2):225–236.
24. Scheinhorn DJ, Chao DC, Stearn-Hassenpflug M, et al. Outcomes in post-ICU mechanical ventilation: a therapist-implemented weaning protocol. Chest 2001; 119(1):236–242.
25. Gracey DR, Hardy DC, Naessens JM, et al. The Mayo Ventilator-Dependent Rehabilitation Unit: a 5 year experience. Mayo Clin Proc 1997; 72(1):13–19.
26. Smith IE, Shneerson JM. A progressive care program for prolonged ventilatory failure: analysis of outcome. Br J Anaesth 1995; 75(4):399–404.
27. Seneff MG, Wagner D, Thompson D, et al. The impact of long-term acute-care facilities on the outcome and cost of care for patients undergoing prolonged mechanical ventilation. Crit Care Med 2000; 28(2):342–350.
28. Votto J, Brancifort JM, Scalise PJ, et al. COPD and other diseases in chronically ventilated patients in a prolonged respiratory care unit: a retrospective 20-year survival study. Chest 1998; 113(1):86–90.
29. Wijkstra PJ, Avendano MA, Goldstein RS. Inpatient chronic assisted ventilatory care. A 15-year experience. Chest 2003; 124(3):850–856.
30. Liu K, Baseggio C, Wissoker D, Maxwell S, et al. Long-term care hospitals under Medicare: facility-level characteristics. Health Care Financ Rev 2001; 23(2):1–18.
31. DeLisa J, Bach JR. Overview of rehabilitation, general evaluation, principles and the rehabilitation team. In: JR Bach, ed. Pulmonary Rehabilitation. The Obstructive and Paralytic Conditions. Philadelphia: Hanley & Belfus, 1996:1–25.
32. Ankrom MA, Barofsky I, Georas SN, et al. What happens to patients in a nursing home-based, chronic ventilator unit: a five-year retrospective review of patients and outcomes. Ann Long-Term Care 1998; 6(10):309–314.
33. American College of Chest Physician. Mechanical ventilation beyond the intensive care unit. Chest 1998; 113(5 suppl):289s–344s.
34. Goldberg AI. Home care for life-supported persons: is a national approach the answer? Chest 1986; 90(5):744–749.
35. Lusk R, O'Bryan L. Evaluation of critically ill patients for transfer to long-term acute-care facilities. Lippincott Case Manag 2002; 7(1):24–26.

15

The Multidisciplinary Team Training and Experience

MIGUEL DIVO

Caritas St. Elizabeth's Medical Center, Tufts University School of Medicine, Boston, Massachusetts, U.S.A.

I. Introduction

Multidisciplinary team work has been widely recognized as an important approach in health care (1) and few will dispute the critical role of this approach for patients receiving prolonged mechanical ventilation (PMV). Teams make fewer mistakes than individuals, especially when each team member knows his or her responsibilities as well as those of other team members (2,3). The effectiveness of a team resides in having each member perform predetermined tasks simultaneously, thus reducing complex processes into concise manageable components (4,5). However, teamwork is not an automatic consequence of colocating people together. Regardless of each member's individual skills, it depends more on the member's willingness to cooperate, communicate, and share a common goal. For decades, commercial aviation has shifted from individual pilot skill training to an interdisciplinary team training program that incorporates proven methods for team management (2,3,6). The essence of these methods consists of training the crew in a cluster of specific knowledge, skills, and attitudes that facilitate coordination and adaptation as well as providing support to the objectives and mission of the other teammates (7,8).

In medicine, not only are members of multidisciplinary teams rarely trained together, but they come from separate disciplines and diverse educational programs (1). Achieving safe patient care that results from the interaction of multidisciplinary teams is difficult to accomplish without adequate understanding of the contributions of each member and the mechanisms that enhance interaction among each other.

In this chapter, we will review the importance of the multidisciplinary team approach and the role of the team members in the care of PMV patients. We will also suggest a structure to enhance effective teamwork.

II. The Role of Multidisciplinary Team Caring for Ventilator-dependent Patient Through Continuum of Care

Advances in critical care and mechanical ventilation (MV) have greatly improved the long-term survival of critically ill patients. Up to 25% may require PMV (9,10). These survivors leave the ICU with ongoing morbidity, neurocognitive impairment, and decreased quality of life. They create stressful situations for families and caregivers as well as an economic impact to the patient, family, and society (11). Managing patients with PMV involves a more comprehensive patient-centered approach to care, rather than the life-support model found in the ICU (12). This patient-centered, rehabilitative model of care (13–15) is a complex multilayered process that requires expertise in different disciplines (Table 1).

Table 1 Components of Rehabilitative Model of Post-ICU Weaning

Component
Physician services
Physician experienced in PMV and weaning leads multidisciplinary team, assesses patients daily, plans treatment, and approves nonphysician care protocols
Clinical case manager
Experienced nurse in PMV leads weekly multidisciplinary conferences, ensures communication between team members, execution of care plan, uniformity of policy and procedure, monitors protocol adherence
Nutrition support
Registered dietitian performs initial and follow-up clinical assessments and laboratory tests, sets goals for nutritional mode and content modified for comorbidities
Bedside nursing
Registered nurses, licensed practical nurse, assistants with experience in PMV, cross-trained in airway and secretion management provide patient and family education. Nursing care by protocols, e.g., tracheostomy care, indwelling lines, feeding tubes, bowel routines, bladder catheters, skin care, and communication with other team members
Respiratory therapist
Certified, registered therapist, competent in all equipment procedures associated with ventilation and airway care, assesses patients for dyspnea, gas exchange, comfort and anxiety, manages weaning protocols, and communicates with patient and team
Pharmacy support
Registered pharmacist reviews medication profiles to minimize overuse and minimize sedatives, educates patient, family, and staff
Physical therapist
Peripheral and respiratory muscle training, ambulation, assists with secretion clearance
Occupational therapist
Activities of daily living, environmental aids, seating and mobility, modified for PMV
Speech therapist
Swallowing evaluation and management, speech and alternative communication tools
Psychological services
Psychologist with psychiatry support, patient and family evaluation, formulation of comorbidities—anxiety, depression, delirium, counsels patients, family and team, knowledgeable in palliative care and end-of-life decision making
Social services
Experienced social workers with access to pastoral care. Patient and family education and counseling, palliative care and discharge planning. Liaison with equipment vendors, home care nurses, home team, local community hospital, local family physician, ambulance and power companies
Recreational Therapy
Leisure, social, and recreational needs within and outside (gardens, shows) the facility

Abbreviation: PMV, prolonged mechanical ventilation.
Source: From Ref. 15 (Table 5, p. 3946) Consensus Statement (www.chestjournal.org)

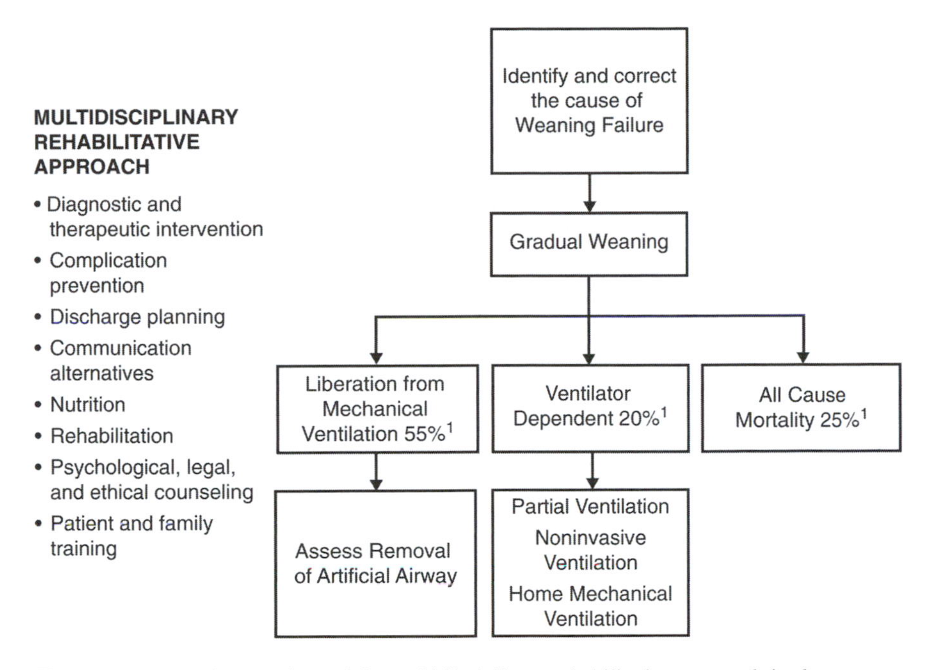

Figure 1 Schematic overview of the multidisciplinary rehabilitative approach in the care process of prolonged mechanically ventilated patients.

While not all of these modalities contribute equally, they share interdependent tasks and contribute to the common goal of inspiring patients to reach their maximal functional independence.

Figure 1 represents a schematic view of the care process and outcomes for PMV patients. The care goal can shift from aggressive weaning intervention to alternative ventilation modes, including facilitating home mechanical ventilation (HMV) or providing palliative care for patients approaching the end of their lives.

The multidisciplinary team is better suited to approach the physical and emotional stresses associated with continued weaning efforts as well as the provision of spiritual and emotional support during the healing or dying process (12).

The team can also assess the impact of repeated weaning failures; specifically when to consider noninvasive ventilation, nocturnal ventilation, or HMV as well as how to best address issues that impact health-related quality of life, such as speech, swallowing, and mobility.

When there are outstanding issues with the patient and family on goal setting and discharge planning, the team can offer counseling, palliative care services, pastoral care, and social services.

III. The Multidisciplinary Team Members

As PMV patients move through the care continuum (Fig. 2), team structure (Table 1) and expertise can be modified according to intensity (y-axis), acuity (x-axis), and available resources.

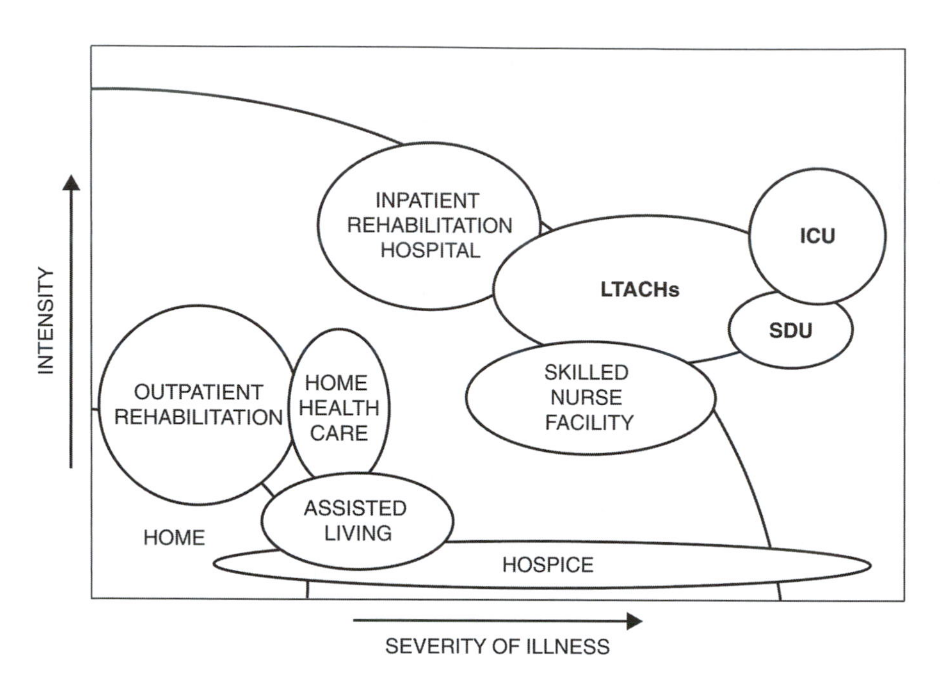

Figure 2 Overview of the continuum of care for prolonged mechanically ventilated patients according to severity of illness (x-axis) and intensity of care (y-axis). *Abbreviations*: SDU, step-down unit; LTACH, long-term acute care hospital. *Source*: Illustration courtesy of Dr. Sean Muldoon, Kindred Healthcare.

IV. Multidisciplinary Team Training

Maintaining team competencies such as skill, knowledge, and attitudes is a dynamic process that requires a structured approach as opposed to a short course, if lifelong teamwork habits are expected to occur. One approach is based on a framework that seeks opportunities to entrench those competencies during the routine care of PMV patients. Key items include:

1. Multidisciplinary team rounds that emphasize communication, coordination, and collective orientation
2. Simulation training in "hyper-acute" scenarios, such as mock arrests and rapid response teams that promote skills, collaboration, supportive behavior, and adaptability
3. Revision and update of evidence-based best practices (EBBP), using formal and informal formats, to answer high prevalence, high impact clinical questions that update knowledge and collaboration
4. Development of protocols that standardize routine tasks and promote the effective implementation of EBBP

V. Multidisciplinary Rounds

The multidisciplinary rounds provide the unique opportunity to collectively communicate, discuss, and coordinate all aspects of a patient's care plan. This powerful tool can overcome cultural barriers and politics by finding a common interest among caregivers, namely that of focusing efforts exclusively on patient care.

Table 2 provides a template for the rounds structure, which the reader can modify to meet the needs of specific patients, locations, and resources. Points to consider include:

Table 2 Proposed Multidisciplinary Round Structure and Objectives

Presenter	Topic	Category/application of EBBP
Physician	Brief history Active medical problems Medication list review DVT prophylaxis appropriate?	Medications error prevention, drug-drug interaction, side effects, cost reduction
Respiratory therapy	Mechanical ventilation mode/type Airway/interface size/type O_2 requirements (taper?) Actively weaning Y/N stage Home ventilation training VAP prevention orders	VAP prevention bundle
Rehabilitation services	Cognitive level	Delirium prevention
Physical therapist Occupational therapist	Physical activity level Activities of daily living Safety awareness Self-care	 Fall prevention
Speech language pathologist	Swallowing retraining Communication and alternatives	Quality of life Quality of life
Nursing	Current nursing issues Lines and catheters Skin integrity Fall risk assessment	 Catheter-related infection prevention Pressure ulcer prevention Fall prevention
Dietician	Current weight/ideal weight Diet: according to medical condition Route Laboratory monitoring: albumin, prealbumin, etc.	
Patient/family	Perspective and concerns	Quality of life
Social worker	Summation of barriers to discharge Estimated length of stay	
Case manager	Care coordination	

Abbreviations: EBBP, evidence-based best practices; DVT, deep vein thrombosis; VAP, ventilatory-associated pneumonia.

Frequency: determined by the intensity of patient care. As patients move through the care continuum (Fig. 2), multidisciplinary rounds decrease in frequency from daily (or twice daily) in the ICU and step-down units to weekly in the long-term acute care hospital (LTACH) (although physician visit is required daily) and skilled nursing facility and to a frequency that resembles outpatient follow-up after discharge with HMV.

Patient-centered care emphasizes the need to empower patients or the health care proxy: to participate in medical decision making. Integrating the patient in the multidisciplinary team promotes patient participation in a therapeutic alliance, identifying stresses and maladaptive assimilation of their chronic condition. It is also a more compassionate format for communicating bad news.

Implementation of EBBP and preventive care: by incorporating the best available evidence together with the patients' values and providers' preferences that impact clinical and financial outcomes (16).

There is no single approach that will impact behavioral changes and the universal application of EBBP (17). However, a combination of strategies (12,17–22) can be integrated into the meeting format. These strategies are:

Limiting reliance on memory and using reminders and checklists. Several team members can ensure that a particular therapy or process occurs. Examples: ventilator-associated pneumonia (VAP), catheter-related blood stream infection, and reminder of whether catheter could be removed.

The use of a goal sheet for each patient, which clearly states the short-, medium-, and long-term plans, which can be reassessed at each multidisciplinary team meeting (20,21).

Orders sets and protocols, which reduce practice variations among caregivers.

VI. Conclusion

Managing patients with PMV involves a more comprehensive patient-centered, rehabilitative model of care that requires expertise in different disciplines. Although not all of these disciplines contribute equally, they share interdependent tasks and contribute to the common goal of inspiring patients to reach their maximal functional independence. However, teamwork is not an automatic consequence of colocating people together but requires an interdisciplinary team-training program that incorporates a cluster of specific knowledge, skills, and attitudes that facilitate coordination and support to the objectives and mission of the other teammates. One approach is based on a framework that entrench those competencies during the routine care of PMV patients, which include multidisciplinary team rounds, simulation training in "hyper-acute" scenarios, revision and update of EBBP, and development of protocols that standardize routine tasks and promote the effective implementation of EBBP. Multidisciplinary teamwork should be widely supported as an important approach for patients receiving PMV.

References

1. Baker DP, Salas E, King H, et al. The role of teamwork in the professional education of physicians: current status and assessment recommendations. Jt Comm J Qual Patient Saf 2005; 31(4):185–202.
2. Salas E, Cannon-Bowers J. The science of training: a decade of progress. Annu Rev Psychol 2001; 52:471–499.

3. Salas E, Wilson KA, Burke CS, et al. Using simulation-based training to improve patient safety: what does it take? Jt Comm J Qual Patient Saf 2005; 31:363–371.
4. Smith-Jentsch K, Salas E, Baker D. Training team performance-related assertiveness. Pers Psychol 1996; 49:909.
5. Lanzetta JT, Roby TB. Effects of work-group structure and certain task variables on group performance. J Abnorm Psychol 1956; 53(3):307–314.
6. Stammers RB, Hallam J. Task allocation and the balancing of task demands in the multi-man-machine system—some case studies. Appl Ergon 1985; 16(4):251–257.
7. Baker DP, Gustafson S, Beaubien J, Salas E, Barach P. *Medical Teamwork and Patient Safety: The Evidence-based Relation.* Literature Review. AHRQ Publication No. 05-0053, April 2005. Agency for Healthcare Research and Quality, Rockville, MD. http://www.ahrq.gov/qual/medteam/
8. Parry S. Just what is a competency (and why should we care)? Training 1998; 35:58.
9. Brochard L, Rauss A, Benito S, et al. Comparison of three methods of gradual withdrawal from ventilatory support during weaning from mechanical ventilation. Am J Respir Crit Care Med 1994; 150(4):896–903.
10. Esteban A, Frutos F, Tobin MJ, et al. A comparison of four methods of weaning patients from mechanical ventilation. Spanish Lung Failure Collaborative Group. N Engl J Med 1995; 332(6): 345–350.
11. Angus DC, Carlet J. Surviving intensive care: a report from the 2002 Brussels Roundtable. Intensive Care Med 2003; 29(3):368–377.
12. Burns SM, Marshall M, Burns JE, et al. Design, testing, and results of an outcomes-managed approach to patients requiring prolonged mechanical ventilation. Am J Crit Care 1998; 7(1): 45–57.
13. Bagley PH, Cooney E. A community-based regional ventilator weaning unit: development and outcomes. Chest 1997; 111(4):1024–1029.
14. Criner GJ. Long-term ventilation introduction and perspectives. Respir Care Clin N Am 2002; 8(3):345–353.
15. MacIntyre NR, Epstein SK, Carson S, et al. Management of patients requiring prolonged mechanical ventilation: report of a NAMDRC consensus conference. Chest 2005; 128(6): 3937–3954.
16. Sackett DL, Rosenberg WM, Gray JA, et al. Evidence based medicine: what it is and what it isn't. BMJ 1996; 312(7023):71–72.
17. Berenholtz S, Pronovost PJ. Barriers to translating evidence into practice. Curr Opin Crit Care 2003; 9(4):321–325.
18. Cook DJ, Montori VM, McMullin JP, et al. Improving patients' safety locally: changing clinician behaviour. Lancet 2004; 363(9416):1224–1230.
19. Davis DA, Taylor-Vaisey A. Translating guidelines into practice. A systematic review of theoretic concepts, practical experience and research evidence in the adoption of clinical practice guidelines. CMAJ 1997; 157(4):408–416.
20. Narasimhan M, Eisen LA, Mahoney CD, et al. Improving nurse-physician communication and satisfaction in the intensive care unit with a daily goals worksheet. Am J Crit Care 2006; 15(2):217–222.
21. Pronovost P, Berenholtz S, Dorman T, et al. Improving communication in the ICU using daily goals. J Crit Care 2003; 18(2):71–75.
22. Pronovost P, Weast B, Schwarz M, et al. Medication reconciliation: a practical tool to reduce the risk of medication errors. J Crit Care 2003; 18(4):201–205.

16
Clinical Experience in a CAVC Unit

MONICA AVENDANO and CHRISTINA HURTADO
West Park Healthcare Centre, Toronto, Ontario, Canada

ROGER S. GOLDSTEIN
West Park Healthcare Centre, University of Toronto, Toronto, Ontario, Canada

I. Introduction

Prolonged mechanical ventilation (PMV) has been defined as the need for ventilatory support for >21 consecutive days for >6 hr/day (1). Patients who require PMV could be classified as chronically critically ill, as they depend on life support for survival. PMV is part of the continuum of critical care medicine.

Most patients requiring PMV do not need the sophisticated monitoring available in the intensive care unit (ICU). However, they are often obliged to remain in the ICU due to their need for PMV. This results in a disproportionately high number of ICU beds occupied by patients requiring PMV, beds that are therefore unavailable for acutely ill patients, requiring intensive care. It also results in patients who are clinically stable and alert, but ventilator dependent, being housed in an environment with at best a minimal rehabilitative focus.

Patients requiring PMV are increasingly related both to improved ICU management and the increasing number of patients with chronic respiratory failure resulting from a variety of pathologies such as thoracic restriction (TR) or neuromuscular disease (NMD), for whom long-term ventilation prolongs survival.

A recent Canadian report, conducted on behalf of the Ontario Ministry of Health and Long-Term Care (MOHLTC), noted that in Ontario, over a nine-year period, there had been a steady increase in the use of mechanical ventilation (MV) and therefore a concomitant increase in inpatient bed days attributed to PMV (2). The increase in the use of MV has been attributed to the aging of the population as well as the increase in complex chronic diseases and their comorbidities, rather than to the increased availability of technology. This report also highlighted the increasingly important impact of PMV on health care resource utilization, both in the ICU and the broader medical system.

In the ICU, a small number of patients become clinically stable but remain ventilator dependent. Some patients are successfully weaned from the ventilator in units dedicated to that activity (3). However, failure to wean leaves these patients on PMV for the rest of their lives. The ICU environment is not geared to the care of patients who are not acutely critically ill, and therefore these ventilator-dependent individuals might actually be neglected in favor of the more immediate needs of those who are acutely critically ill.

Long-term mechanical ventilation (LTMV) in the home setting is a "very rewarding challenge for the clinically stable patient, the health care team and the caregivers" (4).

Unfortunately, it is not always possible—often because of the lack of family support and the unavailability of home care. One of the most viable alternatives is the chronic assisted ventilatory care unit (CAVC). In this chapter, we will discuss CAVC, based on our experience in such a unit, located in a center that specializes in rehabilitation and complex continuing care center.

II. The Chronic Assisted Ventilatory Care Unit

Long-term care has evolved from being essentially custodial to offering more comprehensive management for complex patients with multiple comorbidities. The CAVC unit is an example of this direction.

The unit has demonstrated that ongoing ventilatory support can be safely provided outside of the acute care setting. Its main achievements include providing a safe environment with a rehabilitative focus that will promote functional ability and autonomy among ventilator-assisted individuals (VAI).

Since its inception in 1986 in response to the growing need for a more appropriate environment for LTMV patients, our unit has expanded from 5 to 22 beds. For the CAVC unit to be successful, it is important to carefully select patients who meet written admission criteria, to have an interdisciplinary clinical team with technical knowledge and experience, and to have the capability for the ongoing monitoring of ventilation and gas exchange.

An example of admission criteria is found in Table 1. All patients have a preadmission assessment by the multidisciplinary team to ensure that they are appropriate to the CAVC environment and can safely be cared for outside of the acute care environment. A smooth transition from acute care is very important, especially for individuals who have been in such a sheltered ICU environment for a long time. Patients and families are usually apprehensive about leaving the intensive nursing and monitoring environment of the ICU. Therefore, patients able to be transported to the CAVC unit are assessed there to provide them and their families the opportunity to visit the unit, thus making the subsequent transfer a little less stressful.

The multidisciplinary team is experienced in addressing the physical and neuropsychological complications, both of the underlying disease and the prolonged ICU stay (5,6). Communication among disciplines is facilitated by weekly care conferences in which the patient's status is documented and management plans updated. Families and caregivers

Table 1 Admission Criteria

- Aged ≥18 years and require invasive ventilation for all or part of the day
- Stable-free of continuous cardio-respiratory monitoring or monitoring lines
- Motivation to function at their optimum level with the possibility of community reintegration
- Must be able to direct their own care
- Must be able to access a call bell system and be able to exercise appropriate judgment as to when to request assistance
- Nonsmokers
- Motivated to interact in a wider hospital environment
- Able to communicate their needs (we sometimes modify this admission criterion, provided full time attendant care is available for patients who cannot operate a call bell)

are involved whenever possible. It is important for them to be trained in suctioning techniques as well as manual ventilation as such training will enable the patients to enjoy more freedom for family visits and community activities.

The multidisciplinary approach includes both ventilator management and rehabilitation of chronically ventilator-dependent individuals, paying close attention to nutritional and musculoskeletal issues as well to treating other comorbidities such as tissue trauma, pain, infections, fear, and anxiety. Part of this rehabilitation process often begins at the referring center, based on recommendations made after the CAVC team has assessed the patient. If the referring center is receptive and adequately staffed, many of the initial issues may be tackled while the patient is waiting for transfer to the CAVC unit.

III. The Multidisciplinary Team in the CAVC Unit (7)

A. Physician

A CAVC unit should be led by one or more specialist physicians with experience in ventilation. The physician provides medical leadership and is responsible for the medical assessment and overall management of the patients. Together with the respiratory therapist (RT), the physician is involved in decisions relating to ventilator parameters, interfaces, and airway management. The physician also leads the rapid response team (8) and the cardiac arrest team when on site.

Full-day (24 hours) physician coverage is not essential, providing that experienced respiratory nurses, or in North America, RTs, are on site for 24 hours. If an experienced physician, supported by a knowledgeable team, is available during the day, most of the untoward medical events can be predicted.

The physician works closely with the unit manager, who must have a health care background and provides management leadership in staffing, planning, and implementing strategic and budgetary issues. The other key support person is the clinical coordinator who is responsible for reviewing applications, coordinating assessment at the CAVC unit or at the referring facility, and arranging the transfers to and from other medical or community facilities, as well as consultations with various medical specialties, not always available on site. Although leadership on many issues is by influence rather than authority, the physician carries the ultimate medicolegal responsibility for clinical care and the unit manager carries line responsibility for staff recruitment and performance evaluation.

B. Respiratory Therapist

In North America, RTs provide 24-hour coverage, being recognized as expert in ventilatory support of the patient. In other jurisdictions, this role may be assumed by experienced nurses or physical therapists. They adjust ventilators to provide more portable and friendlier modes for long-term use. They are responsible for airway management and identify the most appropriate tracheotomy tubes (9,10), including requirements for customized tubes, monitoring the need for cuff inflation, and providing adequate humidification for the ventilator circuit. They assess patients for the most appropriate, effective, and comfortable interfaces. They determine the frequency of suctioning for secretion clearance and decide on the use of assisted cough techniques, lung inflation, and the use of in-exsufflation (11).

The RTs are responsible for the leadership of the rapid response and the cardiac arrest teams after official hours and on weekends. All RTs are certified in techniques of advanced life support. Together with the nursing staff, the RTs provide the daily care routine for the tracheotomy tubes, changing them as soon as the stoma is well established. Prior to the patients leaving the unit for outings, the RTs provide the necessary training to family and friends to enable them to safely accompany the patient.

C. Nursing

Nurses skilled in the care of ventilator-dependent patients are responsible for their daily care. The nurse is always with the patient, especially at night, when the nurse may be the only team member to be present on the unit. Patients transferred from ICUs are often frightened and the nurse enables them to express their fears, reassuring them of their safety. Issues related to the ICU syndrome (12) must be addressed with tact and compassion by the nursing staff. Patients require time to appreciate that their requests will be met, even though they do no longer have one to one nursing. The nursing ratio varies from 1:2 to 1:3. Nurses participate in the team assessment of referred patients. At the time of admission, they carry out a second assessment to confirm clinical stability and establish the goals and care plan.

The role of nursing may be enhanced by the presence of a nurse practitioner (NP) experienced in ventilatory care, who can assist with additional training for the nurses, especially in areas such as infection control, wound care, bowel and bladder management, and alternate nutritional approaches, such as enteral feeding tubes or percutaneous intravenous catheters. The NP can also be an excellent liaison between the teams of the CAVC and ICU, both for purposes of patient assessment and for ongoing rehabilitative steps during the waiting period.

D. Physical Therapist

Physical therapist (PT) assesses the functional status of patients on admission, and in partnership with the patient, establishes goals for activities. After a lengthy ICU stay, patients often have extensive muscle wasting and weakness associated with disuse atrophy or myopathy, consequent upon prolonged sedation, toxins, medications, and paralytic agents (13). A program of care is designed to restore strength and function to its fullest potential. Exercises span the spectrum from passive range of motion and simple bed exercises to a comprehensive interval training program. Contractures are especially damaging to mobility, especially among patients who are no longer mobile. The PT also assesses cough effectiveness and together with the RT is responsible for techniques that assist with secretion management.

E. Occupational Therapist

The occupational therapist (OT) assesses activities of daily living and the need for devices to maximize functional independence. For wheelchair-bound patients, the OT assesses the best sitting position and safety for mounting a ventilator on the chair. The OT also teaches patients to safely operate a power wheelchair. A major activity for the OT, especially for patients with severe neuromuscular conditions, is the provision of communication aides. Environmental control systems will facilitate electronic communication through speech, light, and sound controls. Patients will often use computers for business, recreation, and learning. The OTs play a key role in determining the access interface for those who cannot otherwise access a call bell.

F. Speech Language Pathologist

Patients require the ability to maintain communication, whenever possible, by speaking (14). For patients who require cuff inflation for adequate ventilation, for secretion control, or for airway protection, communication can be maintained in writing or through letter boards, the electrolarynx, or computers. The speech language pathologist (SLP) will implement the most appropriate means of communication. Voice-output communications aids may be possible in selected patients and facilitate communication with family members and staff (15). The SLP has an important role in assessing the safety of swallowing (16), which is not generally assessed in the ICU unless there is a suspicion of aspiration. On admission, a swallowing assessment will help avoid aspiration, as well as help to plan optimal nutritional support. High-risk patients with progressive NMD receive ongoing monitoring by the SLP to minimize the risk of swallowing dysfunction.

G. Social Worker

The social worker (SW) assesses family dynamics and the impact of the patient's condition on the family. The SW also assists the family in accessing community support and funding for equipment that can facilitate reincorporation of the patient into the community, or can be used for short stays in the family home. When the caregivers are also the breadwinners, some families will require financial assistance. The SW facilitates outings for patients to go home for holidays, acting as a liaison with home care services that provide the necessary community support.

H. Psychologist

Patients transferred from the ICU often present with features consistent with a posttraumatic stress disorder (17), which might express itself as memory impairment, delusions, panic episodes, and extreme anxiety. The psychologist assists the patient, the family, and the health care providers to address these troublesome symptoms. The psychologist also assists the attending team in dealing with situations of conflict among patients, families, and health care providers. A baseline assessment will often assist in determining which issues are of concern to the patients and prevent unreasonable demands on the health care team. The psychologist must have a good working relationship with a psychiatrist, whose assistance is invaluable in managing patients who develop psychoses or in assessing mental capacity for decision making. This is especially relevant to those who decide to discontinue PMV.

I. Recreational Therapist

Patients who require PMV but who are otherwise medically stable and alert, benefit from engaging in leisure activities. The recreational therapist assesses the patients' inclinations and goals and facilitates their participation in organized activities. Group projects, outings, cooking clubs, and musical groups are just some of the many possible activities that depend only on the imagination and available funding.

J. Clinical Dietitian

Nutritional support is especially important for patients who have spent several weeks or months in an ICU. Malnutrition is commonly associated with prolonged hospitalization (18) and it is aggravated by diminished swallowing, profound dyspnea, and depression. Therefore, all patients are evaluated at baseline for nutritional supplementation. For those who are unable to sustain an adequate oral intake, enteral and sometimes parenteral nutrition may be necessary. For other patients, the advice of the dietitian is invaluable in managing obesity or weight loss and maintaining a healthy weight.

K. Spiritual Advisors

The spiritual needs vary among the different patients and their families. They also vary in any one individual with time. However, there are intense moments in a unit populated by dependant individuals, some of whom are successfully discharged to the community and some of them die. A CAVC unit benefits from the availability of those who can respond to these spiritual needs.

L. Key Consulting Staff

Specialty consultation requirements depend on specific patient issues. However, we consider an ENT specialist, experienced in PMV and in tracheotomy care, to be a great asset to the team. Other key specialties include urology, dermatology, gynecology, general surgery, and ophthalmology.

M. Team Cohesiveness

It is important that the different specialties within the multidisciplinary team attend to issues of communication and respect for each other. Patients can be complex and the environment of ongoing stresses and demands of patients, vulnerable because of their physical dependency, is a challenging one. Clinical practice guidelines, an empathic available manager, and a care coordinator all contribute to enhance the cohesiveness of the team and ultimately the care of the PMV patients. The recruitment and retention of nurses skilled in dealing with patients receiving PMV can be challenging (19). Staff sometimes report inadequate time for completion of essential tasks such as addressing patients' anxieties and providing them with information. The issue of aggressive behavior requires a consistent response from the team.

IV. The Changing Face of the CAVC Unit

Care for ventilator-dependent patients has evolved over the last 20 years to extend the diagnostic categories of patients now considered eligible for PMV. Noninvasive positive pressure ventilation (NIPPV) is an established approach to patients in whom respiratory failure is a consequence of a chronic obstructive pulmonary disease exacerbation (20). There is therefore a diminished likelihood of these patients requiring PMV in the ICU and subsequently being referred to a CAVC unit (21,22). Similarly, patients with TR and obesity hypoventilation are managed with NIPPV (23) and are less frequently referred for CAVC (24,25). Patients receiving bi-level pressure support ventilation, now the most common mode of long-term ventilatory support, do not require the same skill mix as those in a CAVC unit. Therefore, an increasing number of such patients can be admitted to complex continuing care units or skilled nursing facilities.

In parallel with these changing referral patterns, there are increased numbers of patients with progressive degenerative neuromuscular conditions who request PMV, such as those with amyotrophic lateral sclerosis (ALS) and the various types of muscular dystrophy and who have survived into adulthood due to the advances in medical care, including childhood ventilation support.

V. Experience with a CAVC Unit

Our clinical experience with our first 50 patients, admitted over a 15-year period, has been previously reported (7). Subsequently we have extended this experience by the admission of an additional 27 patients. A summary of this experience is illustrative of the evolving role of the CAVC unit.

Of these 77 patients (45 men and 32 women), aged 48 ± 7 years (range 18–79), average length of stay has been 3.1 years (range 1 month to 17 years). Most came from acute care hospitals and 61 directly from ICU. There were five who received NIPPV at home for more than four years, but as a result of their disease progression required invasive ventilation without ventilator free time. Another contributor to their being referred for CAVC was the loss of their main caregiver, to sickness or death, such that they could no longer be managed at home. For 10 patients trained for home ventilation, inadequate home care services prevented their returning to the community. In the absence of this home support, their families were unable to manage the burden of care.

The change in referral patterns is exemplified by 12 patients with spinal cord injury and respiratory failure of whom 10 were admitted prior to 1999. In contrast, of nine patients with ALS, eight have been admitted since 2000 and five are currently "locked in," being totally unable to communicate (Fig. 1).

Despite being admitted for chronic care in the CAVC, prior to 1997, 33% of patients returned to a community environment whereas only 11% of those admitted since 2000 have been able to do so. As patients can less frequently return to the community, the average length of stay is now 4.2 ± 4 years. Insufficient community nurses skilled in dealing with VAIs and insufficient home care funding for equipment have both aggravated this issue. The skilled and experienced multidisciplinary team has ensured that CAVC patients are relatively stable and free of most major complications. In our experience, the most common comorbidity was depression, followed by urinary tract infections (Table 2). In the past year, two patients have required transfer to an acute care facility, for surgery-1 with ALS, for a perforated stomach by the G-tube, and another patient with high spinal cord injury for a partial colonic resection for bowel obstruction. Mortality over the last 20 years has been 29% (22 deaths out of 77 patients), death occurring after a mean length of stay of 5.6 ± 3 years.

VI. Spectrum of Care

In Canada, as in many jurisdictions, the place of the CAVC unit within the spectrum of care of the patient receiving PMV is evolving slowly. For example, a patient at home who

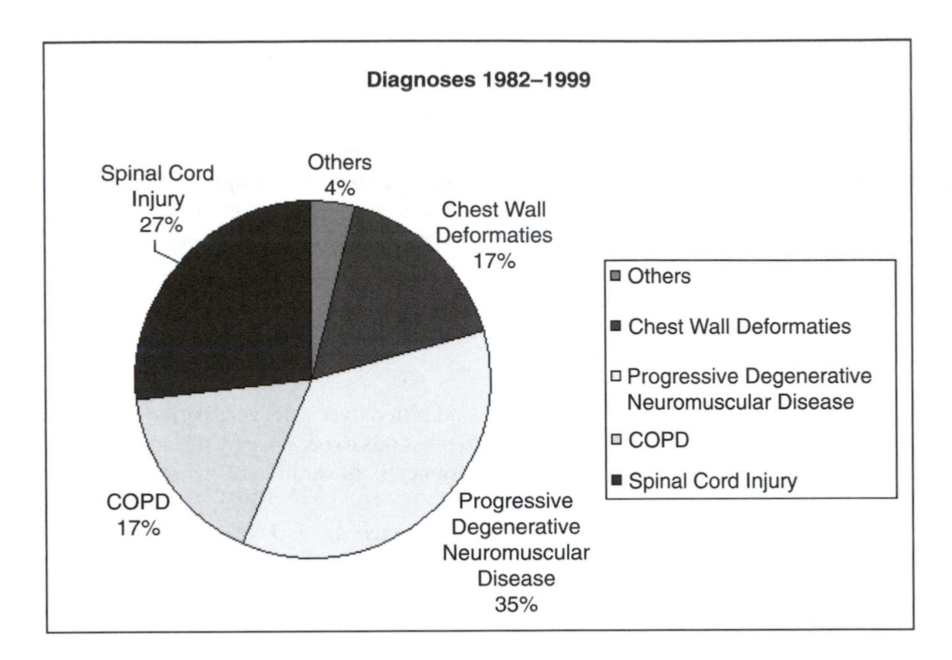

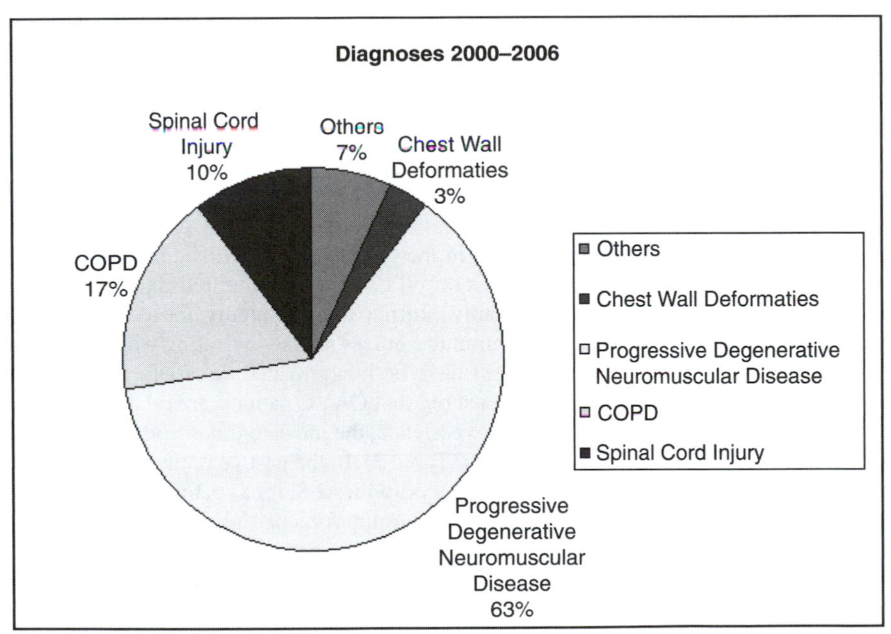

Figure 1 The changing pattern of patients referred for CAVC between 1982 and 1999 compared with 2000–2006.

Table 2 The Major Associated Conditions Among 74 CAVC Patients Admitted Between 1982 and 2006

Associated conditions	Percentage
Depression	26
Urinary tract infection	20
Coronary artery disease	15
Type II diabetes	10
Obesity	7
Seizure disorder	6
Malignancy	3
Cerebrovascular accident	3
Cognitive impairment	3
Others	8

receives invasive positive pressure ventilation and requires an abbreviated admission due to illness is still admitted to an ICU, as invasively ventilated patients cannot be adequately cared for on a general medical ward. A CAVC unit should therefore have sufficient capacity to temporarily admit such patients until their medical situation returns to normal.

Patients who complete home ventilation training usually return home because of a devoted family member who supervises their care. If this supervisor can no longer provide such care, the VAI is often admitted to an ICU or to a CAVC unit. Given that the gap in home care is often temporary, the provision of respite beds within a CAVC unit is an important link in the spectrum of care. Respite beds also support caregiver vacations to avoid burnout. In a prospective study that examined depression, burden, overload, and physical health in caregivers of patients on PMV at home, the authors noted a decline in physical health and a corresponding increase in overload and depression six months after the patient had been discharged (26). In addition, the caregivers of ventilated patients, both in an institution and at home, have higher depression scores than those reported for caregivers for the infirm elderly and persons with Alzheimer's disease (26).

The changes in patient population within the CAVC unit requires structural changes to the facility as the more rehabilitative focus on mentally alert and motivated individuals, driven to achieve their maximal level of functioning is being replaced by totally dependant VAIs who must be moved out of the ICU. Because of this increasing dependency, we have had to adapt rooms to accommodate constant nursing care, or at least enable a system of documenting checking at 15 minutes intervals. Adequate space for palliative care is also necessary.

Palliative care is focused on the relief of symptoms that accompany chronic illness, such as pain, dyspnea, and anxiety (27). Patients receiving PMV often have similar symptoms associated either with their primary diagnosis or with their multiple comorbidities. People unable to exert themselves often experience social isolation and dependency, which leads to depression and frustration. PMV for patients with progressive degenerative NMD, increases life span without impacting on the progression of their underlying disease. The addition of a palliative care service will add value to the patients and their families by providing counseling, education, and overall preparation for end-of-life care. Hypoxia might also impaire cognitive function (28,29) and negatively affect a general sense of invalidity.

As patients with progressive NMD are admitted via the ER to the ICU in acute respiratory failure, it is becoming clear that appropriate chronic disease management for this population should include advanced care directives, in which the patients may indicate their preferences for ventilation and for cardiopulmonary resuscitation. For patients with major impairments who remain on PMV, life satisfaction, as judged by families or health care professionals, underestimates the judgments made by patients regarding their perception of general well-being (30). Therefore, it is important to assess the patients' level of coping directly rather than by surrogate measures.

VII. Special Situations

Some of these situations are mentioned elsewhere in this book in an expanded format. Therefore, we mention only some of the key issues associated with a CAVC unit, including:

A. Tracheotomy-Related Problems

Patients transferred from the ICU often have painful stomas that are chronically colonized or infected with antibiotic-resistant organisms. An antimicrobial drain sponge dressing applied to the stoma is a useful adjunct to the management of these stoma issues (31). Customized tubes are usually required as off-the-shelf tubes are often not adequate for the LTMV patient. The first tracheotomy tube change is done by the physician, often after consulting ENT specialist, especially if there is a history of difficult tracheotomy changes in the ICU. Tubes are changed every four to six weeks by RTs, once it has been established that the changes are straightforward.

Stoma skin integrity is sometimes almost impossible to obtain as the skin of the neck breaks down due to friction, pressure, and moisture of the tracheotomy tube ties. The use of thick dressings to reduce pressure and an absorbent dressing will assist in maintaining dryness and minimize friction. The ties are changed daily or more frequently if necessary. Foam dressings have also been successfully utilized. The risk of tracheobronchial hemorrhage in patients with NMD, especially if they have tracheobronchomalacia or spinal deformities, might be minimized with the use of flexible tracheotomy tubes (32).

B. Psychosocial Issues

Psychological distress in long-term settings is highly prevalent, more so in settings that provide for LTMV. These psychological issues are addressed more comprehensively in Chapter 12 of this book. It is, however, important to provide recreational outlets and home visits for those able to participate.

C. The Locked-in Patient

The locked-in patients, usually with ALS, are a great challenge for the health care professionals. Advanced directives are particularly important. Many patients and their families have unrealistic expectations and are very reluctant to accept disease progression to the stage where communication with the patient is impossible. The team is frustrated by not knowing what the patients' needs are or whether the patient wishes to continue with LTMV.

In our experience, most patients are not appropriately informed about their degenerative disease at the time of their diagnoses, and as a consequence have not been able to make informed decisions regarding their own care.

D. Nutrition

Nutritional assessment upon admission is necessary. Enteral nutrition is preferred in those patients unable to maintain an adequate caloric intake by the oral route. Overfeeding needs to be avoided, and monitoring of the glycemic levels needs to be strict. As many patients experience diarrhea, especially on implementation of enteral feedings, this needs to be aggressively managed (33).

E. Ethical Issues

Life-sustaining treatment decisions should be made in keeping with patients' preferences. In a prospective study published in 1996 about the impact of patient preferences on life-sustaining treatment (34), the Danis et al. reported that the patient's preferences did not determine the use of these treatments. Although life-sustaining treatments increase hospital costs, these higher costs did not flow from patient preferences, but those of the health care team. This study was completed in 1996 and may not reflect today's situation.

VIII. Conclusion

A CAVC unit is the right place for people in need of ventilatory support who do not need to stay in the ICU environment. The success of the CAVC unit, like other clinical units, depends on the training, cohesiveness, and knowledge of the multidisciplinary team. In our experience, a well-established CAVC unit provides a pleasant as well as safe environment, with expertise to promote a rehabilitative approach, conducive to achieving the maximum patient function. The CAVC unit should also have the expertise to assist VAIs to be reintegrated into the community. Stable patients requiring LTMV can reside in a CAVC unit, provided clinical guidelines and appropriate monitoring is available. Such units also serve as a resource for VAIs who can no longer remain in the community.

References

1. MacIntyre NR, Epstein SK, Carson S, et al. Management of patients requiring prolonged mechanical ventilation. Report of a NAMDRC Consensus Conference. Chest 2005; 128:3937–3954.
2. Needham DM, Bronskill SE, Sibbald WJ, et al. Mechanical ventilation in Ontario 1992–2000: incidence, survival and hospital bed utilization of non-cardiac surgery adult patients. Crit Care Med 2004; 32:1504–1509.
3. Sheinhorn D, Chao D, Hassenpflug M, et al. Outcomes in post-ICU mechanical ventilation: a therapist-implemented weaning protocol. Chest 2001; 119:236–242.
4. Robert D, Vitacca M. Ventilatory assistance at home. In: Donner CF, Ambrosino N, Goldstein R, eds. Pulmonary Rehabilitation: Efficacy and Scientific Basis. London: Arnold, 2005:343–352.
5. Young MP, Gooder VJ, Oltermann MH, et al. The impact of a multidisciplinary approach on caring for ventilator-dependent patients. Int J Qual Health Care 1998; 10:15–26.

6. Avendano M, Wijstra P. Chronic ventilatory assistance in the hospital. In: Donner CF, Ambrosino N, Goldstein R, eds. Pulmonary Rehabilitation: Efficacy and Scientific Basis. London: Arnold, 2005:332–342.
7. Wijsktra PJ, Avendano M, Goldstein RS. Chronic assisted ventilatory care (CAVC): a 15 year experience. Chest 2003; 124(3):850–856.
8. Buist MD, Moore GE, Bernard SA, et al. Effects of a medical emergency team on reduction of incidence of and mortality from unexpected cardiac arrests in hospital: preliminary study. BMJ 2002; 324:387–390.
9. Chew JY, Cantrell RW. Tracheostomy. Complications and their management. Arch Otolaryngol 1972; 96:538–545.
10. Meyer M. Iatrogenic tracheobronchial lesions. A report on 13 cases. Thorac Cardiovasc Surg 2001; 49:115–119.
11. Bach JR. Prevention of morbidity and mortality with the use of physical medicine aids. In: Bach J, ed. Pulmonary Rehabilitation: The Obstructive and Paralytic Conditions. Philadelphia: Hanley, Belfus, 1996.
12. McKegney FP. The intensive care syndrome. Conn Med 1966; 30:633–636.
13. Anzueto A. Muscle dysfunction in the intensive care unit. Clin Chest Med 1999; 20:435–452.
14. Manzano JL, Lubillo S, Henriquez D, et al. Verbal communication of ventilator-dependent patients. Crit Care Med 1993; 21:512–517.
15. Happ MB, Kenney Roesch T, Garrett K. Electronic voice-output communication aids for temporarily nonspeaking patients in a medical intensive care unit: a feasibility study. Heart Lung 2004; 33:92–101.
16. Tolep K, Getch KL, Criner GJ. Swallowing dysfunction in patients requiring prolonged mechanical ventilation. Chest 1996; 109:167–172.
17. Jones C, Griffiths RD, Humpris C, et al. Memory delusions and the development of acute posttraumatic stress disorder-related symptoms after intensive care. Crit Care Med 2001; 29:573–580.
18. Souba WW. Nutritional support. N Engl J Med 1997; 336:41–48.
19. Goldman HG. Role expansion in intensive care: survey of nurses' views. Intensive Crit Care Nurs 1999; 15:313–323.
20. British Thoracic Society Standards of Care Committee: BTS Guideline: Non-invasive ventilation in acute respiratory failure. Thorax 2002; 57(3):192–211.
21. Janssens JP, Derivaz S, Breitenstein E, et al. Changing patterns in long-term noninvasive ventilation. A 7 year prospective study in the Geneva Lake area. Chest 2003; 123:67–79.
22. Sanders M, Kern N. Obstructive sleep apnea treated by independently adjusted inspiratory and expiratory positive airway pressures via nasal mask: physiological and clinical implications. Chest 1990; 98:317–324.
23. Strumpf D, Carlisle C, Millman R, et al. An evaluation of the Respironics BiPap bi-level C-Pap device for delivery of assisted ventilation. Respir Care 1990; 35:415–422.
24. Nava S, Ambrosino N, Rubini F, et al. Effects of nasal pressure support ventilation and external PEEP on diaphragmatic activity in patients with severe stable COPD. Chest 1993; 103:143–150.
25. Vitacca M, Naza S, Confalonieri M, et al. The appropriate setting of noninvasive pressure support ventilation in stable COPD patients. Chest 2000; 118:1286–1293.
26. Douglas SL, Daly J. Caregivers of long-term ventilator patients. Chest 2003; 123:1073–1081.
27. Nelson JE. Palliative care of the chronically critically ill patient. Crit Care Clin North Am 2002; 18:659–681.
28. Fix AJ, Golden CJ Daughton D, et al. Neuropsychological deficits among patients with chronic obstructive pulmonary disease. Int J Neurosci 1982; 16:99–105.
29. Carone M, Bertolotti G, Anchisi F, et al. Analysis of factors that characterize health impairment in patients with chronic respiratory failure. Eur Respir J 1999; 13:1293–1300.

30. Bach JR, Tilton MC. Life satisfaction and well-being measures in ventilator assisted individuals with traumatic tetraplegia. Arch Phys Med Rehabil 1994; 75:626–632.
31. Glenda J, Motta, Trigilia D. The effect of an antimicrobial drain sponge dressing on specific bacterial isolates at tracheostomy sites. Ostomy Wound Manage 2005; 51(1):60–66.
32. Iodice FG, Salzano M, Marri M, et al. Tracheobronchial haemorrhage in patients with neuromuscular disorders. Respir Med 2005; 99:1613–1615.
33. Machanick JI, Brett EM. Nutrition and the chronically ill patient. Curr Opin Clin Nutr Metab Care 2005; 8:33–39.
34. Danis M, Mutran E, Garrett J, et al. A prospective study of the impact of patient preferences on life-sustaining treatment and hospital cost. Crit Care Med 1996; 24(11):1811–1817.

17
Indications and Outcomes of Noninvasive Ventilatory Support in Restrictive and Obstructive Disorders

JOÃO C. WINCK
Serviço de Pneumologia, Faculdade de Medicina do Porto, Portugal

ANITA K. SIMONDS
Royal Brompton Hospital, London, U.K.

I. Introduction

The identification of patients eligible for long-term noninvasive ventilation (LTNIV) is a challenging task. Before starting respiratory support, it is essential to ask three main questions: (1) Does the patient have a disease known to cause ventilatory failure? (2) Does the patient have symptoms suggesting hypoventilation? (3) Does the patient have physiological abnormalities confirming hypoventilation? Sometimes, due to disease progression, ventilatory dysfunction increases and ventilatory support must then be adapted accordingly. In this chapter, we will discuss the indications and outcomes of noninvasive ventilatory support in patients with restrictive and obstructive disorders.

II. Indications for Noninvasive Ventilatory Support

A. Disease Categories

A large number of conditions can result in chronic ventilatory failure and patients with these conditions may benefit from home ventilation. Typically, patients with restrictive disorders have decreased compliance of the chest wall, resulting from a thoracic cage deformity or from respiratory muscle involvement (1). In patients with severe obstructive pulmonary disorders, respiratory muscle fatigue and alveolar hypoventilation, especially during sleep, are thought to contribute to respiratory failure (2,3) (Table 1).

It is useful to define the disease category in order to predict the natural history and specific intervention. It is well known that patients with primarily restrictive disorders can have both inspiratory and expiratory muscle weakness, and apart from noninvasive ventilation (NIV), they also need cough assistance (4,5). On the other hand, patients with obstructive disorders rarely need mechanical expiratory aids except when they have a severe infectious exacerbation at which time difficulties in clearing copious secretions can occur (4,6,7).

Some neuromuscular diseases, for example Guillain-Barré syndrome, may only require temporary ventilatory support (8) while others, such as post-polio syndrome require lifelong noninvasive ventilatory support (9). Amyotrophic lateral sclerosis (ALS) is a

Table 1 Indications for Noninvasive Ventilatory Support

Restrictive disorders
Chest wall disorders
Kyphoscoliosis
Thoracoplasty
Fibrothorax
Obesity-hypoventilation syndrome
Stable neuromuscular disorders
Old poliomyelitis
Myopathies
Progressive neuromuscular disorders
Amyotrophic lateral sclerosis
Duchenne muscular dystrophy
Other Neurological Disorders
Cervical Spinal Cord Injury
Phrenic nerve lesions
Obstructive disorders
Chronic obstructive pulmonary disease
Bronchiectasis and cystic fibrosis

disease that can evolve rapidly. If bulbar involvement occurs, noninvasive ventilatory support may be less effective (10).

Since 1993, various guidelines have been proposed for initiating ventilatory support in patients with chronic respiratory failure (3,11–17). Initially, criteria for beginning ventilatory support have relied on abnormal awake blood gases ($Pa_{O_2} < 60$ mmHg and $Pa_{CO_2} \geq 45$ mmHg) or significant nocturnal desaturation, for example, $Sp_{O_2} < 90\%$ for $\geq 20\%$ of the recorded time (11), then on the forced vital capacity (FVC) being <50% predicted (13) or below 1 L (14), or maximum inspiratory pressure less than -30 cmH_2O (3). Recently, more sensitive parameters have included nocturnal $P_{CO_2} \geq 50$ mmHg for more than 50% of the sleep time (14) and a sniff nasal pressure less than -40 cmH_2O (15,18) for assessing the need for ventilatory support.

B. Patient Selection

Symptoms of Nocturnal Hypoventilation

Every consensus statement reinforces the importance of detecting symptoms of nocturnal hypoventilation (3,12–15). However, symptoms may be subtle due to the variability of patient sensitivity and sometimes it is difficult for the patient to establish differences between fatigue, dyspnea, and sleepiness. Therefore, carefully designed questionnaires that assess symptoms systematically may be very useful. Jackson et al. (19) have described a pulmonary symptom scale consisting 14 questions, answered from 1 to 7. Others have used simple questionnaires to evaluate the positive and negative effects of ventilation (20). Although symptom questionnaires are insensitive in identifying patients with sleep-disorderedbreathing (SDB) and nocturnal hypoventilation (19,21), their systematic evaluation is useful in evaluating the response to NIV as compliance with it is strongly correlated with patients' symptoms (22) (Table 2).

Table 2 Symptoms and Signs of Hypoventilation

Symptoms	Signs
Dyspnea on exertion or talking	Tachypnea
Ortopnea	Use of auxiliary respiratory muscles
Frequent nocturnal awakenings	Paradoxical movement of abdomen
Excessive daytime sleepiness	Decreased chest movement
Daytime fatigue	Weak cough
Difficulty clearing secretions	Sweating
Morning headache	Tachycardia
Nocturia	Weight loss
Depression	Confusion, hallucinations, dizziness
Poor appetite	Papilledema
Poor concentration and/or memory	Syncope
	Mouth dryness

Use of rating scales for different symptoms has been also recommended. Dougan et al. (23) developed the motor neurone disease dyspnea rating scale, consisting of 16 questions, each rated on a five-point scale that allows patients with ALS to quantify how dyspnea affects their daily life. This specific questionnaire may be more appropriate for quantifying dyspnea in neuromuscular patients compared with other existing measures, such as the Medical Research Council dyspnea scale (24). Moreover, one of the most commonly used sleepiness scales, the Epworth Sleepiness Scale, may not be as reliable in conditions with such myotonic dystrophy (25).

Physiologic Evaluations

In addition to monitoring symptoms, regular monitoring of respiratory function is essential. The vital capacity (VC) is one of the most reproducible tests for lung function. Although it may not fall below the normal range until there is a 50% reduction in respiratory muscle strength (RMS) (26), its rate of decline can predict survival (27). Opinions vary as to how often pulmonary function should be evaluated. Some clinicians propose that if the VC is > 60% predicted, it should be performed every six months, while if the VC is < 60% predicted, it should be performed at every three to four months (28).

Measurement of the supine VC gives an index of diaphragmatic weakness. A fall >15% indicates diaphragmatic dysfunction and correlates with orthopnea (29); a supine FVC <75% is a sensitive index of reduced transdiaphragmatic pressure (30). Another useful measure is the maximum insufflation capacity (MIC) (31). It is obtained by air stacking consecutively delivered volumes of air from a manual resuscitator or portable volume ventilator, to the maximum volume that the patient can hold with a closed glottis. The patient exhales that volume of air into a spirometer and the maximum values of four or five attempts are recorded (31). The difference between the VC and the MIC is a very good measure of the bulbar function.

The use of peak cough flow (PCF) and peak expiratory flow (PEF) are also useful in monitoring expiratory muscle weakness and bulbar involvement (32,33). When PCF is equal to the PEF, severe bulbar dysfunction takes place (33). Measurement of PCF can be performed with a common portable PEF meter, although it may be overestimated in patients with lower flows (34). PCF should follow a MIC maneuver (35).

A PCF of >270 L/min is required for an adequate cough (36) and a PCF < 160 L/min confers a high risk of pneumonia and respiratory failure (37). Indices of cough strength have been correlated with mortality in ALS (38) and with aspiration status (39). More invasive methods for cough measurement such as cough gastric pressure (cough Pga) may be useful in excluding expiratory muscle weakness in patients with low mouth expiratory pressure (MEP) or with difficulties in performing the MEP maneuver (40). Patients with ALS with a cough Pga < 50 cmH_2O are not able to generate cough spikes (41).

Muscle Strength

Testing for RMS should be obtained periodically. Maximal inspiratory mouth pressure (MIP) values > 80 cmH_2O exclude clinically relevant respiratory muscle weakness (26). A low MIP with a normal MEP suggests isolated diaphragmatic weakness. Sniff nasal inspiratory pressure (SNIP) is more natural and easier to perform maneuver than MIP (42). Values better than −70 cmH_2O for men and better than −60 cmH_2O for women exclude significant inspiratory muscle weakness (43). A SNIP <40 cmH_2O was associated with nocturnal hypoxemia and predicted median survival at six months (43). Chaudri et al. (44) also recommended that patients with SNIP < 30% of predicted are at risk of developing hypercapnia and should have their arterial blood gases (ABG) measured. Some authors advise that in patients with moderate to severe restrictive respiratory defect, the MIP is higher than the SNIP, suggesting that the latter may overestimate the level of inspiratory weakness in this context (45).

Measures of transdiaphragmatic pressure and nonvolitional tests of RMS are more accurate and may be indicated when other tests are difficult to interpret in the context of clinical trials (27).

Blood Gases

When the VC is <50% predicted or MIP is <30% predicted, daytime ABG should be checked (46). Since accurate devices for measuring Pao_2 and $Paco_2$ noninvasively are now available, this is the recommended standard practice. Daytime Sao_2 <95% may be associated with inspiratory or expiratory muscles, or bulbar dysfunction (10). In ALS, when the Sao_2 cannot be normalized by NIV and mechanically assisted cough, a tracheostomy should be performed, if the bulbar dysfunction is severe (10).

End-tidal carbon dioxide tensions ($Petco_2$) (16) can be performed during the day or at night (47,48). Measuring $Petco_2$ with a VC maneuver provides a more accurate estimate of $Paco_2$ and can be very useful for spot checks in hospital or at home (47).

Transcutaneous CO_2 ($TcPco_2$) has been widely used during sleep and after NIV (49–51). $TcPco_2$ measurements require more time and are slightly higher than $Petco_2$ (52–54). As noninvasive methods of CO_2 monitoring are slightly higher than $Paco_2$, a normal reading excludes hypercapnia (26). Recently combined $TcPco_2$–Sao_2 single sensors seem valid in a variety of settings (55–57).

Sleep Studies

Although the incidence of SDB has not been systematically examined in neuromuscular disorders (NMD), many case series have been published in different diseases (58–62). According to Labanowski et al. (58), significant SDB with a respiratory disturbance index >15/hr, occurs in up to 42% of patients with NMD, from 16.7% in early stages of ALS (59) to 57% in Duchenne muscular dystrophy (DMD) (60). The severity, duration, and distribution of muscle weakness in NMDs influence the prevalence of SDB. Ragette et al. (63) noted progression of SDB from rapid eye movement (REM)–related hypopneas to REM-related mixed hypopneas and hypoventilation, followed by both REM and non-REM hypoventilation through to diurnal respiratory failure.

Early respiratory changes in NMDs are often best detected during sleep. Polysomnography (PSG) may be useful in patients with significant daytime sleepiness and suspected nocturnal hypoventilation, especially if the awake $Paco_2$ is borderline or only mildly elevated (27). In a state-of-the-art review, Laghi et al. suggest PSG when abnormalities of spirometry or ABG are first observed (64). Dhand et al. proposed PSG if VC < 40%, $Paco_2$ > 45 mmHg, and base excess (BE) $\geq$ 4 (65). The American Thoracic Society (ATS) consensus statement on the respiratory care of patients with DMD suggests the annual PSG with continuous noninvasive gas monitoring to be the ideal (16). Bourke at al. suggest that the indication for PSG in assessing the need for NIV is unclear in the absence of suspicion of coexistent sleep apnea (66). Others, however, have stressed that PSG is very useful in documenting respiratory failure and subsequently ensuring the efficacy of NIV (67).

As PSG is time-consuming and costly, portable home monitoring has been suggested (68). Greater reductions in Sao_2 may occur at home, as sleep quality may be better (69) (Fig. 1). Investigation of patients with NMD with a simple oximeter during sleep may not be sufficient as an arousal response can be triggered much before a drop in Sao_2 of 3% or more. Night oximetry and Pco_2 monitoring may also provide useful information if PSG is unavailable (16). Many patients with a VC >50% experience nocturnal desaturation (70) and home oximetry can be used as a guide for patients to intensify cough assistance and NIV, thereby avoiding hospitalization (5).

Monitoring of CO_2 during sleep should be part of sleep studies (53,71). Measures include $Petco_2$ at sleep onset, peak $Petco_2$, and duration of $Petco_2$ >50 mmHg expressed as percentage of total sleep time. Measurement of mean as well as maximum $TcPco_2$ is also recommended. Some authors consider an increase in $TcPco_2$ of 3 to 5 mmHg to be relevant (49,52). Normally, $Petco_2$ does not increase significantly during sleep (52). According to Ward et al., nocturnal hypoventilation is defined by a peak $TcPco_2$ >49 mmHg (72), while Ragette et al. suggest a $TcPco_2$ >50 mmHg for >50% sleep time (63).

Although a Cochrane meta-analysis (73) does not recommend the institution of NIV for symptomatic sleep hypopneas, a prospective study from Mellies et al. (74) and a randomized controlled trial by Ward et al. (72) support the indication of NIV for patients with NMD and nocturnal hypercapnia. The consensus conference of the American College of Chest Physicians on MV beyond the ICU recommended that patients who develop symptomatic nocturnal hypercapnia, even in the absence of daytime hypercapnia, are candidates for long-term ventilatory assistance (75).

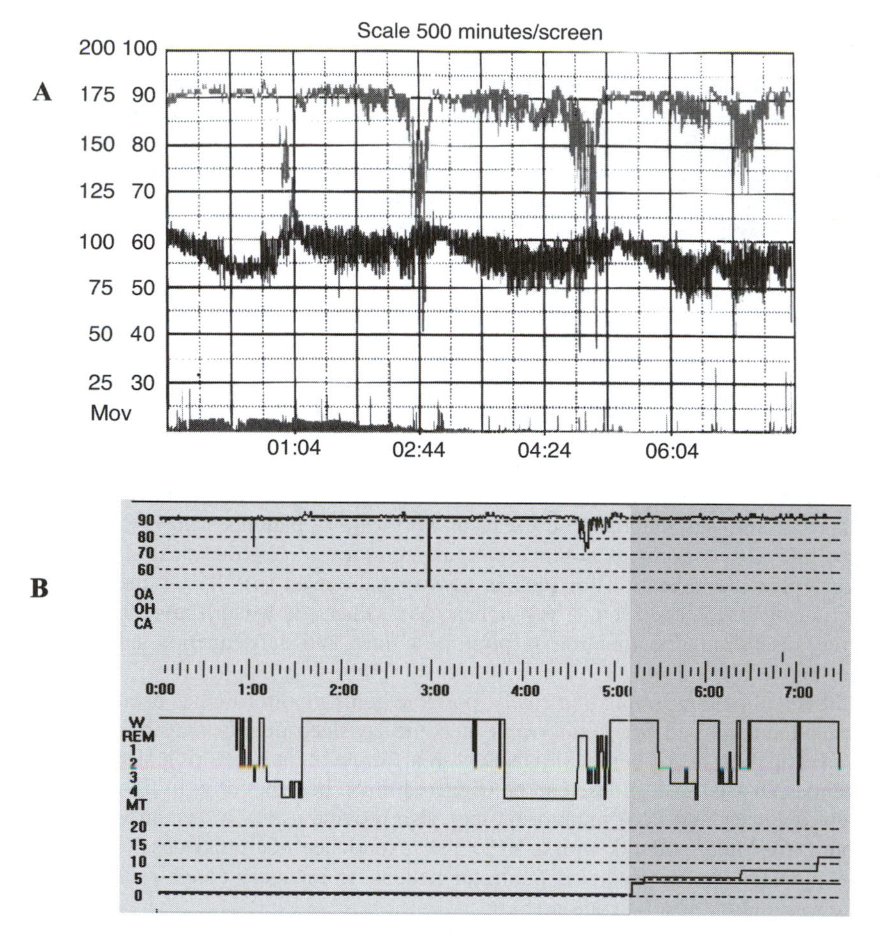

Figure 1 Home oximetry (**A**) and split-night polysomnography (**B**) in an ALS patient with daytime hypercapnia and hypoventilation symptoms.

C. Outcomes

The main goals of NIV are (1) to improve symptoms and physiological measures, (2) to enhance the patient's quality of life, and (3) to improve survival. It is not always possible to reverse the underlying condition, but symptomatic gains and improved lung function may be achieved. Two long-term retrospective studies published in the early 1990s showed significant improvement in nocturnal and diurnal ABG in NIV patients (76,77). Reduction and prevention of respiratory decompensation is also important. Bach et al. have shown that the implementation of an inspiratory and expiratory aids protocol reduced hospitalization and mortality in various NMDs (5,78). Significant gains in quality of life have also been shown (79). Epidemiological studies in Denmark suggest that use of ventilator increased the survival of DMD patients between 1977 and 2001 (80). More recently, randomized controlled trials have shown a clear survival benefit with NIV in ALS patients (81).

III. Noninvasive Ventilatory Support in Restrictive Disorders

The following sections will review the indications for NIV in the most frequent diagnostic categories (Table 1).

A. Chest Wall Disorders

Patients with thoracic restriction (TR) have an increased risk of developing respiratory failure (82). The larger the scoliotic angle, the lower the VC, and the younger the age of scoliosis onset, the greater is the risk (83). In patients who have reached skeletal maturity and have a vital capacity <45% predicted, the risk of developing respiratory failure increases with age (83). Symptoms of cardiorespiratory failure generally appear between the fourth and sixth decade. However, some patients survive into the seventh decade without experiencing problems (84).

Severe TR may induce sleep-related respiratory abnormalities (85) and retrospective long-term studies of nocturnal NIV have shown a better prognosis among those patients, compared to patients with NMD and obstructive disorders (76,77). Prospective studies have demonstrated that NIV improves symptoms, muscle function, and nocturnal gas exchange in patients with daytime hypercapnia and an FVC <50% predicted (86,87). Nocturnal NIV also improves exercise capacity and daytime Pa_{O_2} (88). Data from a large French observational study (89) as well as a recent prospective study (90) have shown that TR patients treated with home mechanical ventilation experience improved survival compared with those treated with oxygen therapy alone. Masa et al. have shown that NIV, but not oxygen, improved nocturnal hypoventilation in seven patients with TR and normal daytime ABGs (91).

Therefore, in symptomatic patients with daytime normocapnia but significant nocturnal desaturation ($Sa_{O_2} < 90\%$ for >10% total sleep time, or mean REM $Sa_{O_2} < 90\%$ and minimum $Sa_{O_2} < 90\%$ or $Sa_{O_2} \leq 88\%$ for 5 consecutive minutes), NIV is warranted (3).

B. Neuromuscular Disorders

NMD can be divided into two groups: stable and progressive. In this chapter, we will discuss two of the more frequently encountered examples in each group. Symptoms are similar to those described previously (Table 2).

Amyotrophic Lateral Sclerosis

ALS is an acquired disorder with a rapidly progressive evolution. Respiratory failure is the principal cause of death (92). Median survival is 32 months from the onset of symptoms and 19 months from diagnosis (93). Despite fears that NIV would delay death without improving quality of life, for some patients with respiratory involvement, NIV has been shown to improve symptoms, quality of life (18,19,94), and survival (81). As ALS patients eventually become quadriplegic, they require a high level of assistance from caregivers (92) and one report suggested that one of the best predictors of the success of NIV was a good caregiver support (95).

It seems reasonable to start NIV in symptomatic patients (Table 2) who have signs of respiratory muscle weakness (FVC <80% predicted or SNIP < 40 cmH_2O) and evidence of nocturnal desaturation or a $Paco_2$ > 49 mmHg (18). Bourke et al. suggested that orthopnea was the most useful criterion for benefit and compliance with NIV (94), and Sivak (96) noted lack of correlation between VC and the success of NIV. In a small prospective study, Jackson et al. (19) suggested that early intervention with NIV, based on nocturnal desaturation (Sao_2 < 90% for 1 min), may improve quality of life.

For most ALS patients, although NIV is initiated at night, it is soon required all day, with the patient becoming totally ventilator dependent (97). If bulbar function is well preserved, continuous NIV using a mouthpiece during the day and an oronasal system at night can be effective. This is the case in 20% of ALS patients who avoid a tracheostomy (10,97,98). However, bulbar muscle dysfunction has a high risk of aspiration as well as poor secretion clearance (97). It carries a worse prognosis (93) and NIV is less well tolerated (99,100). A randomised controlled trial (RCT) reported that patients with moderate to severe bulbar impairment still gained a small improvement in quality of life with NIV (81).

Bulbar muscle dysfunction should be evaluated in all patients with ALS. Apart from rating scales like the ALSFRS (101), one of the best ways to measure muscle dysfunction objectively is by comparing the MIC with the VC and the PEF with the PCF. The wider the gradient, the better the bulbar function (33,35). Bach has shown that in ALS, the ability to generate assisted PCF > 180 L/min and to have a high MIC to VC difference is associated with the capacity to use continuous NIV (36). However, when strictly tailored NIV and mechanically assisted cough do not prevent oxygen desaturation below 95%, aspiration is likely and tracheostomy should be offered (10).

The issue of secretion management is addressed elsewhere in this text. However, mechanically assisted cough is an essential complement of NIV and a key to successful full-time NIV (97).

Duchenne Muscular Dystrophy

DMD is an X-linked recessive pattern of inheritance and affects up to 1 in 3300 males (102). Affected patients typically become wheelchair dependent by the age of 10 to –12 years at which time their VC plateaus. With the development of respiratory muscle weakness and skeletal deformity, the VC starts to fall (103). The patients usually remain asymptomatic until the VC is <450 mL (104). Once the forced expiratory volume in one second (FEV_1) is <40% predicted and the MIP is worse than 30% predicted, the development of hypercapnia is likely and therefore ABG should be measured (105,106). Obstructive sleep apnea occurs commonly among younger children and hypoventilation in older children (107).

Nocturnal NIV is indicated when hypercapnia develops. Vianello and colleagues (108) report a life expectancy of less than one year once diurnal hypercapnia develops. Many studies of NIV in DMD note its effect on increasing survival (103,109,110), which, in one study, increased to a median of 73% at five years (110). In an RCT of normocapnic, asymptomatic, patients with a VC 20–50% predicted, survival did not increase, although use of mask and ventilator was not standardized in this study (111,112) and assisted cough techniques were not included. Some authors suggest that when the VC is <1 L, the five year survival rate is 8% (113), but with secretion clearing aids the 10-year survival can reach 93% (104). Using NIV, up to full time, plus mechanical in-exsufflation guided by home oximetry, Bach and colleagues have extended survival in patients with DMD (78). European reports also recommend NIV for hypercapnic DMD (114).

According to an ATS consensus statement, daytime ventilation should be considered when the awake $Paco_2$ >50 mmHg or when the awake Sao_2 <92% (16). Mouthpiece intermittent positive pressure ventilation (M-IPPV) provides a clear alternative to tracheostomy (115–122). In Europe, M-IPPV is also being used with a simple angled mouthpiece capable of delivering daytime volume-cycled ventilation and extending survival up to seven years in 51% of 42 M-IPPV users (114). As death from cardiomyopathy is significant in DMD, a regular cardiac assessment is needed (123). Of note, although patients with DMD are severely disabled, they still perceive a high quality of life, which does not correlate with physical impairment or the need for NIV (124).

Post-polio Syndrome

Acute paralytic poliomyelitis is still endemic in some countries and vaccine-associated poliomyelitis continues to occur (125). After many years of stability, some patients do deteriorate (126). This "post-polio syndrome" may be characterized by the development of progressive weakness associated with respiratory symptoms among those ventilated during their acute illness (127). Respiratory failure results from thoracic restriction as well as muscle weakness and bulbar involvement (128). Tracheostomy can be avoided with continuous NIV and aggressive mechanical in-exsufflation (128). Retrospective studies of NIV have reported survival rates >90% at five years, making this group the one with the highest benefit (76,129).

C. Spinal Cord Injury

Demographic data forming the U.S. Spinal Cord Injury (SCI) database between 1973 and 2003 show a significant increase in cervical injuries and in ventilator-dependent cases, with 6.8% of SCI patients requiring ventilation on discharge (2000–2003) (130). Most SCI patients who require ventilatory support undergo tracheostomy during their acute hospitalization (131). Despite improvements in SCI medical management, rehospitalization rates associated with respiratory complications remain high (132). Cervical injuries may be higher (C1 and C2) and mid-lower (C3 to C8). The former injuries produce respiratory muscle paralysis, while the latter involve limited expiratory function. Lesions from C3 to C5 significantly compromise inspiration (131). During the 1980s, survival of ventilator-dependent tetraplegic patients ranged from 63% at three years (133) to 33% at five years (134), with only 51% of SCI patients with C3 injury levels able to be weaned (134). Life expectancy was considerably improved in those successfully weaned (135).

Because of their young age, intact mental status, and bulbar musculature, high-level tetraplegic patients are perfect candidates for NIV (136). Patients with lesions below C1 can be managed with NIV, respiratory aids, and manual plus mechanically assisted coughing, provided their assisted PCF > 160 L/min (98).

IV. Noninvasive Ventilatory Support in Obstructive Disorders

A. Chronic Obstructive Pulmonary Disease

Long-term NIV in chronic obstructive pulmonary disease (COPD) remains an area of controversy in the absence of well-designed RCTs, and a European survey (137) noted its heterogeneous use. Case series from the 1990s suggested that COPD patients who developed hypercapnia with long-term oxygen therapy (LTOT) might benefit from NIV, subsequent to which several uncontrolled studies have suggested improvements in ABG and reductions in health care resource utilization (138–140). Results from non-randomized trials have been conflicting (141,142), and two small randomized trials (143,144) showed no improvement. Longer trials, enrolling more hypercapnic patients, may be more likely to show benefit from NIV as acclimatization to this treatment is slower in COPD patients than in those with restrictive disorders.

Casanova et al., in a one-year study (145), randomized 52 COPD patients to standard care or standard care plus NIV with outcomes that included rate of acute exacerbations, hospital admissions, need for intubation and mortality at three, six, and 12 months. Bi-level positive pressure in spontaneous mode was implemented at an expiratory positive airway pressure of 4 cmH_2O and an inspiratory positive airway pressure level of 12 cmH_2O, adjusted to decrease dyspnea and accessory muscle use. Five of the NIV group (total $n = 26$) did not tolerate it and the remainder used it for 6.2 hours per 24 hours, with only a few using it for less than 3 hr/day. One-year survival was similar between groups, as was the number of exacerbations. The breathlessness scores decreased in the NIV group, but only one psychomotor test improved. There was no evidence that the results were better in more hypercapnic patients ($Paco_2 > 7.3$ kPa) or in those who used NIV for >5 hours per 24 hours.

In an Italian multicenter trial (146), 122 stable hypercapnic COPD patients on LTOT for more than six months were randomized to continue LTOT alone, or LTOT plus NIV using a bi-level positive pressure device, over a two-year period. Although dropout rates were similar in both groups and compliance with NIV was impressive at 9 hours per 24 hours, the authors showed only small differences between groups in dyspnea and $Paco_2$.

The studies do, however, suggest that primary end points of number of acute exacerbations and hospital admissions may be a more sensitive measure than mortality. Tuggey et al. (147) examined the economic impact of home NIV in COPD patients with recurrent exacerbations who responded well to NIV during these acute episodes. Good tolerance to home NIV resulted in a cost saving of 11,720 euros (5698–17,743 euros) per patient per year. The number of hospital admissions in the year on NIV compared to the previous year was reduced from five to three and hospital days decreased from a mean (SD) of 78 (51) to 25 (25) ($p = 0.004$), with ICU days falling from 25 to 4 ($p = 0.24$).

Recent Meta-analyses and Systematic Reviews

There have been several systematic reviews and meta-analysis on long-term NIV in COPD (148–150). In the meta-analysis by Wijkstra et al. in 2003 (148), the authors found that three months of NIV in stable COPD patients produced no significant effects on lung function, gas exchange, or sleep efficiency, and a minor increase in Pimax, although there was a suggestion of improvement in six minutes walk as indicated by high upper limit of the confidence limit. There are several RCTs of long-term NIV in stable COPD in progress

Table 3 Pragmatic Selection of COPD Patients for Consideration of Home NIV

- Patients who fail LTOT because of progressive hypercapnia
- Patients with recurrent hypercapnic exacerbations >2/yr responding to acute NIV
- Patients with marked symptomatic nocturnal hypoventilation
- Patients with coexistent obstructive sleep apnea (consider CPAP first)
- Patients with copathology contributing to ventilatory failure, e.g., thoracoplasty, respiratory muscle weakness, morbid obesity

Abbreviations: COPD, chronic obstructive pulmonary disease; NIV, noninvasive ventilation; LTOT, long-term oxygen therapy; CPAP, continuous positive airway pressure.

including a multicenter trial in Germany. For now, some clinicians are using home NIV in selected hypercapnic COPD patients in an attempt to reduce hospital admissions, improve quality of life, and improve dyspnea. Pending results from further RCTS, a pragmatic approach to NIV in COPD is given in Table 3.

Long-term NIV in Cystic Fibrosis

Possible domiciliary indications for NIV in cystic fibrosis (CF) include:

- Physiotherapy adjunct to improve airway clearance of secretions
- Treatment for SDB
- Management of chronic hypercapnic ventilatory failure, including bridging to transplantation and to palliate symptoms

NIV to Improve Airway Clearance

The use of NIV as an adjunct to physiotherapy has been explored in a controlled study (151). In a single session, respiratory rate fell and Sao_2 was higher after physiotherapy using pressure support ventilation compared with control sessions with no respiratory support. Patients reported less fatigue after the NIV-assisted session but the volume of sputum produced did not differ between groups. Holland et al. (152) have also explored the use of NIV during physiotherapy in adult CF patients during an acute exacerbation in a randomized crossover trial. NIV reduced dyspnea and increased mean Sao_2 with no change in sputum weight or FEV_1. In a study of NIV during physiotherapy compared with PEP mask use, Sao_2 improved more with NIV, with patients and physiotherapists finding NIV easier to use.

NIV in SDB in CF

In a group of 32 patients (mean age, 27 years) with FEV_1 36% $\pm$ 10% predicted, Milross et al. (153) noted that morning Pao_2 and evening Po_2 levels were predictive of average minimum Sao_2 overnight. In a small sample, Zinman et al. (154) did not find supplemental oxygen to be of benefit after one year of using it for seven hours per night. Gozal (155) compared nocturnal NIV with LTOT in six patients (mean age, 22 years) with an increase in Pco_2 only seen with oxygen therapy. Milross et al. (156) noted that both NIV and low-flow LTOT improved Sao_2 overnight, particularly during REM sleep, but only NIV reduced the rise in Pco_2 seen in REM.

Home NIV in CF Patients with Ventilatory Failure

Piper et al. (157) used domiciliary NIV for up to 18 months in four CF patients with chronic ventilatory failure who had failed to respond to optimal conventional measures. Using a volume-cycled ventilator, their $Paco_2$ fell, sleep quality improved, and RMS increased. This may suggest at least a stabilizing effect.

Bridging to Transplantation—NIV in End-stage CF

NIV has been used as a means of "bridging" CF patients to heart/lung or lung transplantation. In a retrospective survey, Madden et al. (158) described the use of NIV over a 10-year period in 113 CF patients aged 15 to 44 years with end-stage disease (mean FEV_1, 0.71). Patients were divided into three groups: Group A patients were on the lung transplant waiting list, Group B were being evaluated for transplantation, and Group C were not considered for transplantation either because of contraindications, such as other end organ failure, or refusal to undergo the procedure.

NIV was started for severe respiratory failure Pao_2 6 to 7 kPa, $Paco_2$ 8 to 10 kPa, and a volume-preset ventilator (BromptonPAC™, Smiths, Luton, U.K.) was used. The mean duration of ventilatory support was: Group A 61 (1–600) days, Group B 53 (1–279) days, and Group C 45 (0–379) days. Once patients had stabilized, it was possible to continue the bridge mostly with NIV at home. Survival in NIV users was comparable to less sick nonventilated patients, despite the marked hypercapnia at the start of NIV. There was a significant increase in Pao_2, but $Paco_2$ was unchanged.

CF patients with severe disease are likely to become progressively ventilator dependent, and NIV should always be combined with careful risk management, rapid access to admission for acute exacerbations, and use of palliative care to control symptoms. Many CF patients report that NIV is most effective at relieving symptoms of SDB and assisting physiotherapy, and less effective in reducing dyspnea.

B. Bronchiectasis

A French case series study (77) showed patients with bronchiectasis (mean age, 55 years) had a 48%, three-year probability of continuing NIV. The number of days of hospitalization decreased compared with pre-NIV, but the sample was small. Sixteen percent of NIV recipients with bronchiectasis died of respiratory disease during the three-year study period, a percentage similar to those with COPD. Benhamou et al. (159) examined the long-term outcome of NIV in diffuse bronchiectasis using a comparative case control study. Fourteen cases treated with NIV and LTOT were compared to matched patients using LTOT only. Mean FEV_1 on entry to the study was 700 mL and it was notable that NIV was initiated in most cases at the time of an acute infective exacerbation. Volume preset ventilators were used and long-term compliance was reported as satisfactory in 11 of 14 patients. Compared with the LTOT group, those using the combination of NIV and LTOT spent fewer days in hospital, but there was no significant impact on survival or Pao_2. Median survival was 45 months.

In a U.K. cohort study (76), bronchiectasis patients showed the worst survival of all NIV recipients, with a two-year probability of continuing NIV of <20%. However, lung function and ABG tensions at the initiation of NIV were far worse than in the French series. It is not surprising that patients started on NIV earlier in the course of the disease do better than those in whom NIV is initiated in an end-stage phase. As in CF, individuals with bronchiectasis due to other causes can be successfully bridged to transplantation.

It is clear that the application of long-term NIV in hypercapnic CF and bronchiectasis patients requires further evaluation with outcome measures that include not only lung function and survival but also the use of NIV as a physiotherapy adjunct and its impact on the frequency and severity of infective exacerbations.

References

1. Aldrich TK. The patient at risk of ventilator dependency. Eur Respir J 1989;(suppl 7): 645s–650s.
2. McNicholas WT. Impact of sleep in COPD. Chest 2000; 117(suppl 2):48s–53s.
3. Clinical indications for noninvasive positive pressure ventilation in chronic respiratory failure due to restrictive lung disease, COPD, and nocturnal hypoventilation—a consensus conference report. Chest 1999; 116:521–534.
4. Winck JC, Goncalves MR, Lourenco C, et al. Effects of mechanical insufflation-exsufflation on respiratory parameters for patients with chronic airway secretion encumbrance. Chest 2004; 126:774–780.
5. Bach JR, Ishikawa Y, Kim H. Prevention of pulmonary morbidity for patients with Duchenne muscular dystrophy. Chest 1997; 112:1024–1028.
6. Nava S, Barbarito N, Piaggi G, et al. Physiological response to intrapulmonary percussive ventilation in stable COPD patients. Respir Med 2006; 100:1526–1533.
7. Vargas F, Bui HN, Boyer A, et al. Intrapulmonary percussive ventilation in acute exacerbations of COPD patients with mild respiratory acidosis: a randomized controlled trial [ISRCTN17802078]. Crit Care 2005; 9:R382–R389.
8. Fletcher DD, Lawn ND, Wolter TD, et al. Long-term outcome in patients with Guillain-Barré syndrome requiring mechanical ventilation. Neurology 2000; 54:2311–2315.
9. Bach JR, Alba AS, Shin D. Management alternatives for post-polio respiratory insufficiency. Assisted ventilation by nasal or oral-nasal interface. Am J Phys Med Rehabil 1989; 68(6): 264–271.
10. Bach JR, Bianchi C, Aufiero E. Oximetry and indications for tracheotomy for amyotrophic lateral sclerosis. Chest 2004; 126:1502–1507.
11. Robert D, Willig TN, Leger P, et al. Long-term nasal ventilation in neuromuscular disorders: report of a consensus conference. Eur Respir J 1993; 6:599–606.
12. Rutgers M, Lucassen H, Kesteren RV, et al. Respiratory insufficiency and ventilatory support. 39th ENMC International Workshop, Naarden, European Consortium on Chronic Respiratory Insufficiency. Neuromuscul Disord 1996; 6:431–435.
13. Miller RG, Rosenberg JA, Gelinas DF, et al. Practice parameter: the care of the patient with amyotrophic lateral sclerosis (an evidence-based review): report of the Quality Standards Subcommittee of the American Academy of Neurology: ALS Practice Parameters Task Force. Neurology 1999; 52:1311–1323.
14. Wallgren-Pettersson C, Bushby K, Mellies U, et al. 117th ENMC workshop: ventilatory support in congenital neuromuscular disorders—congenital myopathies, congenital muscular dystrophies, congenital myotonic dystrophy and SMA (II) 4–6 April 2003, Naarden, The Netherlands. Neuromuscul Disord 2004; 14:56–69.
15. Leigh PN, Abrahams S, Al-Chalabi A, et al. The management of motor neurone disease. J Neurol Neurosurg Psychiatry 2003; 74(suppl 4):iv32–iv47.
16. ATS Consensus Statement. Respiratory care of the patients with Duchenne muscular dystrophy. Am J Respir Crit Care Med 2004; 170:456–465.
17. Simonds AK. Recent advances in respiratory care for neuromuscular disease. Chest 2006; 130:1879–1886.

18. Andersen PM, Borasio GD, Dengler R, et al. EFNS task force on management of amyotrophic lateral sclerosis: guidelines for diagnosing and clinical care of patients and relatives. Eur J Neurol 2005; 12:921–938.
19. Jackson CE, Rosenfeld J, Moore DH, et al. A preliminary evaluation of a prospective study of pulmonary function studies and symptoms of hypoventilation in ALS/MND patients. J Neurol Sci 2001; 191:75–78.
20. Butz M, Wollinsky KH, Wiedemuth-Catrinescu U, et al. Longitudinal effects of noninvasive positive-pressure ventilation in patients with amyotrophic lateral sclerosis. Am J Phys Med Rehabil 2003; 82:597–604.
21. Mellies U, Ragette R, Schwake C, et al. Daytime predictors of sleep disordered breathing in children and adolescents with neuromuscular disorders. Neuromuscul Disord 2003; 13:123–128.
22. Jackson CE, Lovitt S, Gowda N, et al. Factors correlated with NPPV use in ALS. Amyotroph Lateral Scler 2006; 7(2):80–85.
23. Dougan CF, Connell CO, Thornton E, et al. Development of a patient-specific dyspnoea questionnaire in motor neurone disease (MND): the MND dyspnoea rating scale (MDRS). J Neurol Sci 2000; 180:86–93.
24. Medical Research Council. Committee on research into chronic bronchitis. Instructions for use of the questionnaire on respiratory symptoms. In: Devon LW, ed. Holman, 1966.
25. Laberge L, Gagnon C, Jean S, et al. Fatigue and daytime sleepiness rating scales in myotonic dystrophy: a study of reliability. J Neurol Neurosurg Psychiatry 2005; 76:1403–1405.
26. Shahrizaila N, Kinnear WJM, Wills AJ. Respiratory involvement in inherited primary muscle conditions. J Neurol Neurosurg Psychiatry 2006; 2006(77):1108–1115.
27. Anonymous. ATS/ERS statement on respiratory muscle testing. Am J Respir Crit Care Med 2002; 166:518–624.
28. Gozal D. Pulmonary manifestations of neuromuscular disease with special reference to Duchenne muscular dystrophy and spinal muscular atrophy. Pediatr Pulmonol 2000; 29:141–150.
29. Varrato J, Siderowf A, Damiano P, et al. Postural change of forced vital capacity predicts some respiratory symptoms in ALS. Neurology 2001; 57:357–359.
30. Lechtzin N, Wiener CM, Shade DM, et al. Spirometry in the supine position improves the detection of diaphragmatic weakness in patients with amyotrophic lateral sclerosis. Chest 2002; 121:436–442.
31. Kang SW, Bach JR. Maximum insufflation capacity. Chest 2000; 118:61–65.
32. Bach JR, Goncalves MR, Paez S, et al. Expiratory flow maneuvers in patients with neuromuscular diseases. Am J Phys Med Rehabil 2006; 85:105–111.
33. Suarez AA, Pessolano FA, Monteiro SG, et al. Peak flow and peak cough flow in the evaluation of expiratory muscle weakness and bulbar impairment in patients with neuromuscular disease. Am J Phys Med Rehabil 2002; 81:506–511.
34. Sancho J, Servera E, Diaz J, et al. Comparison of peak cough flows measured by pneumotachograph and a portable peak flow meter. Am J Phys Med Rehabil 2004; 83:608–612.
35. Kang SW, Bach JR. Maximum insufflation capacity: vital capacity and cough flows in neuromuscular disease. Am J Phys Med Rehabil 2000; 79:222–227.
36. Bach JR. Amyotrophic lateral sclerosis: predictors for prolongation of life by noninvasive respiratory aids. Arch Phys Med Rehabil 1995; 76:828–832.
37. Bach JR, Saporito LR. Criteria for extubation and tracheostomy tube removal for patients with ventilatory failure: a different approach to weaning. Chest 1996; 110:1566–1571.
38. Chaudri MB, Liu C, Hubbard R, et al. Relationship between supramaximal flow during cough and mortality in motor neurone disease. Eur Respir J 2002; 19:434–438.
39. Smith Hammond CA, Goldstein LB, Zajac DJ, et al. Assessment of aspiration risk in stroke patients with quantification of voluntary cough. Neurology 2001; 56:502–506.

40. Man WD, Kyroussis D, Fleming TA, et al. Cough gastric pressure and maximum expiratory mouth pressure in humans. Am J Respir Crit Care Med 2003; 168:714–717.
41. Polkey MI, Lyall RA, Green M, et al. Expiratory muscle function in amyotrophic lateral sclerosis. Am J Respir Crit Care Med 1998; 158:734–741.
42. Fitting J-W, Paillex R, Hirt L, et al. Sniff nasal pressure: a sensitive respiratory test to assess progression of amyotrophic lateral sclerosis. Ann Neurol 1999; 46:887–893.
43. Morgan RK, McNally S, Alexander M, et al. Use of Sniff nasal-inspiratory force to predict survival in amyotrophic lateral sclerosis. Am J Respir Crit Care Med 2005; 171:269–274.
44. Chaudri MB, Liu C, Watson L, et al. Sniff nasal inspiratory pressure as a marker of respiratory function in motor neuron disease. Eur Respir J 2000; 15:539–542.
45. Hart N, Polkey MI, Sharshar T, et al. Limitations of sniff nasal pressure in patients with severe neuromuscular weakness. J Neurol Neurosurg Psychiatry 2003; 74:1685–1687.
46. Perrin C, Unterborn JN, Ambrosio CD, et al. Pulmonary complications in neuromuscular diseases. Muscle Nerve 2004; 29:5–27.
47. Takano Y, Sakamoto O, Kiyofuji C, et al. A comparison of the end-tidal Co_2 measured by portable capnometer and the arterial Pco_2 in spontaneously breathing patients. Respir Med 2003; 97:476–481.
48. Kotterba S, Patzold T, Malin JP, et al. Respiratory monitoring in neuromuscular disease—capnography as an additional tool? Clin Neurol Neurosurg 2001; 103:87–91.
49. Pradal U, Braggion C, Mastella G. Transcutaneous blood gas analysis during sleep and exercise in cystic fibrosis. Pediatr Pulmonol 1990; 8:162–167.
50. Janssens JP, Perrin E, Bennani I, et al. Is continuous transcutaneous monitoring of Pco_2 ($TcPco_2$) over 8 h reliable in adults? Respir Med 2001; 95:331–335.
51. Janssens JP, Howarth-Frey C, Chevrolet JC, et al. Transcutaneous Pco_2 to monitor Noninvasive mechanical ventilation in adults. Assessment of a new transcutaneous Pco_2 device. Chest 1998; 113:768–773.
52. Aittokallio J, Virkki A, Aittokallio T, et al. Non-invasive respiratory monitoring during wakefulness and sleep in pre- and postmenopausal women. Respir Physiol Neurobiol 2006; 150:66–74.
53. Morielli A, Desjardins D, Brouillette RT. Transcutaneous and end-tidal carbon dioxide pressures should be measured during pediatric polysomnography. Am Rev Respir Dis 1993; 148:1599–1604.
54. Cuvelier A, Grigoriu B, Molano LC, et al. Limitations of transcutaneous carbon dioxide measurements for assessing long-term mechanical ventilation. Chest 2005; 127:1744–1748.
55. Heuss LT, Chhajed PN, Schnieper P, et al. Combined pulse oximetry/cutaneous carbon dioxide tension monitoring during colonoscopies: pilot study with a smart ear clip. Digestion 2004; 70:152–158.
56. Bendjelid K, Schutz N, Stotz M, et al. Transcutaneous Pco_2 monitoring in critically ill adults: clinical evaluation of a new sensor. Crit Care Med 2005; 33:2203–2206.
57. Senn O, Clarenbach CF, Kaplan V, et al. Monitoring Carbon Dioxide Tension and arterial oxygen saturation by a single earlobe sensor in patients with critical illness or sleep apnea. Chest 2005; 128:1291–1296.
58. Labanowski M, Schmidt-Nowara W, Guilleminault C. Sleep and neuromuscular disease: frequency of sleep-disordered breathing in a neuromuscular disease clinic population. Neurology 1996; 47:1173–1180.
59. Kimura K, Tachibana N, Kimura J, et al. Sleep-disordered breathing at an early stage of amyotrophic lateral sclerosis. J Neurol Sci 1999; 164:37–43.
60. Khan Y, Heckmatt JZ. Obstructive apnoeas in Duchenne muscular dystrophy. Thorax 1994; 49:157–161.
61. Gilmartin JJ, Cooper BG, Griffiths CJ, et al. Breathing during sleep in patients with myotonic dystrophy and non-myotonic respiratory muscle weakness. Q J Med 1991; 78:21–31.

62. Nicolle MW, Rask S, Koopman WJ, et al. Sleep apnea in patients with myasthenia gravis. Neurology 2006; 67:140–142.
63. Ragette R, Mellies U, Schwake C, et al. Patterns and predictors of sleep disordered breathing in primary myopathies. Thorax 2002; 57:724–728.
64. Laghi F, Tobin MJ. Disorders of the respiratory muscles. Am J Respir Crit Care Med 2003; 168:10–48.
65. Dhand UK, Dhand R. Sleep disorders in neuromuscular diseases. Curr Opin Pulm Med 2006; 12:402–408.
66. Bourke SC, Gibson GJ. Sleep and breathing in neuromuscular disease. Eur Respir J 2002; 19:1194–1201.
67. Lofaso F, Quera-Salva MA. Polysomnography for the management of progressive neuromuscular disorders. Eur Respir J 2002; 19:989–990.
68. Kirk VG, Flemons WW, Adams C, et al. Sleep-disordered breathing in Duchenne muscular dystrophy: a preliminary study of the role of portable monitoring. Pediatr Pulmonol 2000; 29:135–140.
69. Carroll N, Bain RJ, Smith PE, et al. Domiciliary investigation of sleep-related hypoxaemia in Duchenne muscular dystrophy. Eur Respir J 1991; 4:434–440.
70. Elman LB, Siderowf AD, McCluskey LF. Nocturnal oximetry: utility in the respiratory management of amyotrophic lateral sclerosis. Am J Phys Med Rehabil 2003; 82:866–870.
71. ATS Consensus Statement. Standards and indications for cardiopulmonary sleep studies in children. Am J Respir Crit Care Med 1996; 153:866–878.
72. Ward S, Chatwin M, Heather S, et al. Randomised controlled trial of non-invasive ventilation (NIV) for nocturnal hypoventilation in neuromuscular and chest wall disease patients with daytime normocapnia. Thorax 2005; 60:1019–1024.
73. Annane D, Chevrolet JC, Chevret S, et al. Nocturnal mechanical ventilation for chronic hypoventilation in patients with neuromuscular and chest wall disorders. Cochrane Database Syst Rev 2000; (2):CD001941.
74. Mellies U, Ragette R, Dohna Schwake C, et al. Long-term noninvasive ventilation in children and adolescents with neuromuscular disorders. Eur Respir J 2003; 22:631–636.
75. Make BJ, Hill NS, Goldberg AI, et al. Mechanical ventilation beyond the intensive care unit. Report of a consensus conference of the American College of Chest Physicians. Chest 1998; 113(5 suppl):289S–344S.
76. Simonds AK, Elliott MW. Outcome of domiciliary nasal intermittent positive pressure ventilation in restrictive and obstructive disorders. Thorax 1995; 50(6):604–609.
77. Leger P, Bedicam JM, Cornette A, et al. Nasal intermittent positive pressure ventilation. Long-term follow-up in patients with severe chronic respiratory insufficiency. Chest 1994; 105(1): 100–105.
78. Gomez-Merino E, Bach JR. Duchenne muscular dystrophy: prolongation of life by noninvasive ventilation and mechanically assisted coughing. Am J Phys Med Rehabil 2002; 81(6):411–415.
79. Piepers S, Van den Berg J-P, Kalmijn S, et al. Effect of non-invasive ventilation on survival, quality of life, respiratory function and cognition: a review of the literature. Amyotroph Lateral Scler 2006; 7:195–200.
80. Jeppesen J, Green A, Steffensen BF, et al. The Duchenne muscular dystrophy population in Denmark, 1977-2001: prevalence, incidence and survival in relation to the introduction of ventilator use. Neuromuscul Disord 2003; 13:804–812.
81. Bourke SC, Tomlison M, Williams TL, et al. Effects of non-invasive ventilation on survival and quality of life in patients with amyotophic lateral sclerosis: a randomised controlled trial. Lancet Neurol 2006; 5:140–147.
82. Bergofsky FH. Respiratory failure in disorders of the thoracic cage. Am Rev Respir Dis 1979; 119:643–669.

83. Pehrsson K, Bake B, Larsson S, et al. Lung Function in adult idiopathic scoliosis: a 20 year follow up. Thorax 1991; 46:474–478.
84. Rom WN, Miller A. Unexpected longevity in patients with severe kyphoscoliosis. Thorax 1978; 33:106–110.
85. Guilleminault C, Kurland G, Winkle R, et al. Severe kyphoscoliosis, breathing and sleep. The Quasimodo syndrome during sleep. Chest 1981; 79:626–630.
86. Gonzalez C, Ferris G, Diaz J, et al. Kyphoscoliotic ventilatory insufficiency. Effects of Long-term intermittent positive-pressure ventilation. Chest 2003; 124:857–862.
87. Ferris G, Servera-Pieras E, Vergara P, et al. Kyphoscoliosis Ventilatory Insufficiency: noninvasive management outcomes. Am J Phys Med Rehabil 2000; 79:24–29.
88. Fuschillo S, De Felice A, Gaudiosi C, et al. Nocturnal mechanical ventilation improves exercise capacity in kyphoscoliotic patients with respiratory impairment. Monaldi Arch Chest Dis 2003; 59(4):281–286.
89. Chailleux E, Farroux B, Binet F, et al. Predictors of survival in patients receiving domiciliary oxygen therapy of mechanical ventilation. A 10 year analysis of ANTADIR observatory. Chest 1996; 109:741–749.
90. Gustafson T, Franklin KA, Midgren B, et al. Survival of patients with kyphoscoliosis receiving mechanical ventilation or oxygen at home. Chest 2006; 130:1828–1833.
91. Masa JF, Celli BR, Riesco JA, et al. Noninvasive positive pressure ventilation and not oxygen may prevent overt ventilatory failure in patients with chest wall diseases. Chest 1997; 112(1): 207–213.
92. Oppenheimer EA. Amyotrophic lateral sclerosis. Eur Respir Rev 1992; 2:323–329.
93. del Aguila MA, Longstreth WT, McGuire V, et al. Prognosis in amyotrophic lateral sclerosis. Neurology 2003; 60:813–819.
94. Bourke SC, Bullock RE, Williams TL, et al. Noninvasive ventilation in ALS. Indications and effect on quality of life. Neurology 2003; 61:171–177.
95. Cazzolli PA, Oppenheimer EA. Home mechanical ventilation for amyotrophic lateral sclerosis: nasal compared to tracheostomy-intermittent positive pressure ventilation. J Neurol Sci 1996; 139(suppl):123–128.
96. Sivak ED, Shefner JM, Mitsumoto H, et al. The use of non-invasive positive pressure ventilation (NIPPV) in ALS patients. A need for improved determination of intervention timing. Amyotroph Lateral Scler Other Motor Neuron Disord 2001; 2:139–145.
97. Bach JR. Amyotrophic lateral sclerosis. Prolongation of life by noninvasive respiratory aids. Chest 2002; 122:92–98.
98. Bach JR. Continuous noninvasive ventilation for patients with neuromuscular disease and spinal cord injury. Semin Respir Crit Care Med 2002; 23:283–292.
99. Aboussouan LS, Khan SU, Meeker DP, et al. Effect of noninvasive positive -pressure ventilation on survival in amyotrophic lateral sclerosis. Ann Intern Med 1997; 127:450–453.
100. Gruis KL, Brown DL, Schoennemann A, et al. Predictors of Noninvasive ventilation tolerance in patients with amyotrophic lateral sclerosis. Muscle Nerve 2005; 32:808–811.
101. Cederbaum JM, Stambler N. Performance of the Amyotrophic Lateral Sclerosis Functional Rating Scale (ALSFRS) in multicentre clinical trials. J Neurol Sci 1997; 152:51–59.
102. Morton NE, Chung CS. Formal genetics of muscular dystrophy. Am J Hum Genet 1959; 11:360–379.
103. Baydur A, Gilgoff I, Prentice W, et al. Decline in respiratory function and experience with long-term assisted ventilation in advanced Duchenne's muscular dystrophy. Chest 1990; 97:884–889.
104. Bach JR. Management of patients with neuromuscular disease. Philadelphia:Hanley & Belfus, 2004.
105. Hukins CA, Hillman DR. Daytime predictors of sleep hypoventilation in Duchenne muscular dystrophy. Am J Respir Crit Care Med 2000; 161:166–170.

106. Hahn A, Bach JR, Delaubier A, et al. Clinical implications of maximal respiratory pressure determinations for individuals with Duchenne muscular dystrophy. Arch Phys Med Rehabil 1997; 78:1–6.
107. Suresh S, Wales P, Dakin C, et al. Sleep-related breathing disorder in Duchenne muscular dystrophy: disease spectrum in the paediatric population. J Paediatr Child Health 2005; 41:500–503.
108. Vianello A, Bevilacqua M, Salvador V, et al. Long-term nasal intermittent positive pressure ventilation in advanced Duchenne's muscular dystrophy. Chest 1994; 105(2):445–448.
109. Curran FJ, Colbert AP. Ventilator management in Duchenne muscular dystrophy and post-poliomyelitis syndrome: twelve years' experience. Arch Phys Med Rehabil 1989; 70:180–185.
110. Simonds AK, Muntoni F, Heather S, et al. Impact of nasal ventilation on survival in hypercapnic Duchenne muscular dystrophy. Thorax 1998; 53(11):949–952.
111. Raphael JC, Chevret S, Chastang C, Bouvet F. Randomised trial of preventive nasal ventilation in Duchenne muscular dystrophy. French Multicentre Cooperative Group on Home Mechanical Ventilation Assistance in Duchenne de Boulogne Muscular Dystrophy. Lancet 1994; 343 (8913):1600–1604.
112. Muntoni F, Hird M, Simonds AK. Preventive nasal ventilation in Duchenne muscular dystrophy. Lancet 1994; 344:340.
113. Phillips MF, Quinlivan RCM, Edwards RHT, et al. Changes in spirometry over time as a prognostic marker in patients with Duchenne Muscular Dystrophy. Am J Respir Crit Care Med 2001; 164:2191–2194.
114. Toussaint M, Steens M, Wasteels G, et al. Diurnal ventilation via mouthpiece: survival in end-stage Duchenne patients. Eur Respir J 2006; 28:549–555.
115. Alba A, Solomon M, Trainor FS. Management of respiratory insufficiency in spinal cord lesions. In: Proceedings of the 17th Veteran's Administration Spinal Cord Injury Conference, 1969. US Government Printing Office No. 0-436-398 (101), 1971:200–213.
116. Bach JR, Alba AS, Bohatiuk G, et al. Mouth intermittent positive pressure ventilation in the management of postpolio respiratory insufficiency. Chest 1987; 91:859–864.
117. Bach JR, Alba AS. Sleep and nocturnal mouthpiece IPPV efficiency in postpoliomyelitis ventilator users. Chest 1994; 106:1705–1710.
118. Bach JR, S.M. S, Saporito LR. Interfaces for non-invasive intermittent positive pressure ventilatory support in North America. Eur Respir Rev 1993; 3:254–259.
119. Baydur A, Gilgoff I, Prentice W, et al. Decline in respiratory function and experience with long-term assisted ventilation in advanced Duchenne's muscular dystrophy. Chest 1990; 97:884–889.
120. Baydur A, Layne E, Aral H, et al. Long term non-invasive ventilation in the community for patients with musculoskeletal disorders: 46 year experience and review. Thorax 2000; 55(1): 4–11.
121. Boitano LJ, Benditt JO. An evaluation of home volume ventilators that support open-circuit mouthpiece ventilation. Respir Care 2005; 50:1457–1461.
122. McKim DA, LeBlanc C. Maintaining an "Oral Tradition": specific equipment requirements for mouthpiece ventilation instead of tracheostomy for Neuromuscular Disease. Respir Care 2006; 51:297–298.
123. Ishikawa Y, Bach JR, Minami R. Cardioprotection for Duchenne Muscular Dystrophy. Am Heart J 1999; 137:895–902.
124. Kohler M, Clarenbach CF, Boni L, et al. Quality of life, physical disability, and respiratory impairment in Duchenne muscular dystrophy. Am J Respir Crit Care Med 2005; 172: 1032–1036.
125. Howard RS. Poliomyelitis and the postpolio syndrome. BMJ 2005; 330:1314–1318.
126. Jubelt B. Post-Polio Syndrome. Curr Treat Options Neurol 2004; 6(2):87–93.

127. Kidd D, Howard RS, Williams AJ, et al. Late functional deterioration following paralytic poliomyelitis. Q J Med 1997; 90:189–196.
128. Bach JR, Smith WH, Michaels J, et al. Airway secretion clearance by mechanical exsufflation for pot-poliomyelitis ventilator-assisted individuals. Arch Phys Med Rehabil 1993; 74:170–177.
129. Duiverman ML, Bladder G, Meinesz AF, et al. Home mechanical ventilatory support in patients with restrictive ventilatory disorders: a 48-year experience. Respir Med 2006; 100:56–65.
130. Jackson AB, Dijkers M, DeVivo MJ et al. A demographic profile of new traumatic spinal cord injuries: change and stability over 30 years. Arch Phys Med Rehabil 2004; 85:1740–1748.
131. Mansel JK, Norman JR. Respiratory complications and management of spinal cord injuries. Chest 1990; 97:1446–1452.
132. Cardenas DD, Hoffman JM, Kirshblum S, et al. Etiology and incidence of rehospitalization after traumatic spinal cord injury: a multicenter analysis. Arch Phys Med Rehabil 2004; 85: 1757–1763.
133. Splaingard ML, Frates RC, Harrison GM, et al. Home positive-pressure ventilation-twenty years' experience. Chest 1983; 84:376–382.
134. Wicks AB, Menter RR. Long-term outlook in quadriplegic patients with initial ventilator dependency. Chest 1986; 90:406–410.
135. DeVivo MJ, Ivie CS. Life expectancy of ventilator dependent persons with spinal cord injuries. Chest 1995; 108:226–232.
136. Bach JR, Alba A. Noninvasive options for ventilatory support of the traumatic high level quadriplegic patients. Chest 1990; 98:613–619.
137. Lloyd-Owen SJ, Donaldson GC, Ambrosino N, et al. Patterns of home mechanical ventilation use in Europe: results from the Eurovent survey. Eur Respir J 2005; 25:1025–1031.
138. Elliott MW, Simonds AK, Carroll MP, et al. Domiciliary nocturnal nasal intermittent positive pressure ventilation in hypercapnic respiratory failure due to chronic obstructive lung disease: effects on sleep and quality of life. Thorax 1992; 47(5):342–348.
139. Sivasothy P, Smith IE, Shneerson JM. Mask intermittent positive pressure ventilation in chronic hypercapnic respiratory failure due to chronic obstructive pulmonary disease. Eur Respir J 1998; 11(1):34–40.
140. Jones SE, Packham S, Hebden M, et al. Domiciliary nocturnal intermittent positive pressure ventilation in patients with respiratory failure due to severe COPD: long-term follow up and effect on survival. Thorax. 1998; 53:495–498.
141. Meecham Jones DJ, Paul EA, Jones PW, et al. Nasal pressure support ventilation plus oxygen compared with oxygen therapy alone in hypercapnic COPD. Am J Respir Crit Care Med 1995; 152(2):538–544.
142. Lin CC. Comparison between nocturnal nasal positive pressure ventilation combined with oxygen therapy and oxygen monotherapy in patients with severe COPD. Am J Respir Crit Care Med 1996; 154:353–358.
143. Strumpf DA, Millman RP, Carlisle CC, et al. Nocturnal positive-pressure ventilation via nasal mask in patients with severe chronic obstructive pulmonary disease. Am Rev Respir Dis 1991; 144:1234–1239.
144. Gay PC, Hubmayr RD, Stroetz RW. Efficacy of nocturnal nasal ventilation in stable, severe chronic obstructive pulmonary disease during a 3-month controlled trial. Mayo Clin Proc 1996; 71:533–542.
145. Casanova C, Celli BR, Tost L, et al. Long-term controlled trial of nocturnal nasal positive pressure ventilation in patients with severe COPD. Chest 2000; 118:1582–1590.
146. Clini E, Sturani C, Rossi A, et al. The Italian multicentre study on noninvasive ventilation in chronic obstructive pulmonary disease patients. Eur Respir J 2002; 20:529–538.

147. Tuggey JM, Plant PK, Elliott MW. Domiciliary non-invasive ventilation for recurrent acidotic exacerbations of COPD: an economic analysis. Thorax 2003; 58:867–871.
148. Wijkstra PJ, Lacasse Y, Guyatt GH, et al. A meta-analysis of nocturnal noninvasive positive pressure ventilation in patients with stable COPD. Chest 2003; 124(1):337–343.
149. Wijkstra PJ. Non-invasive positive pressure ventilation (NIPPV) in stable patients with chronic obstructive pulmonary disease (COPD). Respir Med 2003; 97:1086–1093.
150. Wijkstra PJ, Lacasse Y, Guyatt GH, et al. Nocturnal non-invasive positive pressure ventilation for stable chronic obstructive pulmonary disease. Cochrane Database Syst Rev 2002;(3): CD002878.
151. Fauroux B, Boule M, Lofaso F, et al. Chest physiotherapy in cystic fibrosis: improved tolerance with nasal pressure support ventilation. Pediatrics 1999; 103:E32.
152. Holland AE, Denehy L, Ntoumenopoulos G, et al. Non-invasive ventilation assists chest physiotherapy in adults with acute exacerbations of cystic fibrosis. Thorax 2003; 58:880–884.
153. Milross MA, Piper AJ, Norman M, et al. Predicting sleep-disordered breathing in patients with cystic fibrosis. Chest 2001; 120:1239–1245.
154. Zinman R, Corey M, Coates AL, et al. Nocturnal home oxygen in the treatment of hypoxemic cystic fibrosis patients. J Pediatr 1989; 114:368–377.
155. Gozal D. Nocturnal ventilatory support in patients with cystic fibrosis: comparison with supplemental oxygen. Eur Respir J 1997; 10:1999–2003.
156. Milross MA, Piper AJ, Norman M, et al. Low-flow oxygen and bilevel ventilatory support: effects on ventilation during sleep in cystic fibrosis. Am J Respir Crit Care Med 2001; 163:129–134.
157. Piper AJ, Parker S, Torzillo PJ, et al. Nocturnal nasal IPPV stabilizes patients with cystic fibrosis and hypercapnic respiratory failure. Chest 1992; 102:846–850.
158. Madden BP, Kariyawasam H, Siddiqi AJ, et al. Noninvasive ventilation in cystic fibrosis patients with acute or chronic respiratory failure. Eur Respir J 2002; 19:310–313.
159. Benhamou D, Muir JF, Raspaud C, et al. Long-term efficiency of home nasal mask ventilation in patients with diffuse bronchiectasis and severe chronic respiratory failure: a case-control study. Chest 1997; 112:1259–1266.

18
Choice of Devices, Ventilators, Interfaces, and Monitors

SUSAN SORTOR LEGER
ResMed Europe, Parc Technologique de Lyon, France

PATRICK LEGER
Laboratoire du sommeil, Service de Pneumologie, Centre Hospitalier Lyon Sud, France

I. Introduction

Successful assisted ventilation depends critically upon adapting mechanical ventilation to the patient's needs. This is particularly true when the noninvasive mode is used, because the patient is conscious and if ventilation is ineffective or uncomfortable, the patient may reject it. In patients with chronic respiratory failure (CRF), noninvasive ventilation (NIV) is performed during sleep and comfort is particularly important if sleep is not to be compromised. An understanding of the technical equipment, in particular the classification and modes of ventilation and the potential problems with each, is crucial, as is the selection of an appropriate interface. This chapter deals with the equipment needs for home mechanical ventilation (HMV), in particular the major ventilator types and modes, interfaces, accessories, and monitoring.

II. Home Mechanical Ventilators

A mechanical ventilator is a machine that can fully or partially substitute for the ventilatory work usually accomplished by the patient's muscles. Understanding the characteristics of ventilators can help make the best choice of equipment for a patient requiring HMV. There is an extensive range of home care ventilators for both pediatric and adult patients. Choosing the machine best adapted for the patient can be a daunting task. A ventilator classification system will help the clinician make this choice. It will also facilitate operating the device and predicting how the ventilator will interact with the patient to support ventilation. We have chosen to use a part of the classification system developed by Chatburn (1) as a basis for describing the different ventilators available today for HMV and for discussing the performance of some of these ventilators.

When providing support, a ventilator can control four primary variables during inspiration: pressure, volume, flow, and time. If a ventilator controls a given variable, then the waveform of this variable during inspiration will ideally remain unchanged from breath to breath regardless of how the load (compliance and resistance) changes (1). Most modern home ventilators are either pressure or flow controllers.

A. Pressure Controllers

Regardless of whether a ventilator uses positive pressure or negative pressure, the transpulmonary pressure gradient determines the tidal volume. A ventilator that is a pressure controller delivers a preset pressure and this variable is unaffected by changes in lung compliance or resistance. A positive pressure ventilator applies pressure inside the chest to expand it using a noninvasive interface, or an artificial airway.

Negative pressure ventilators apply subatmospheric pressure outside the chest to inflate the lungs. The negative pressure causes the chest wall to expand and the pressure difference between the lungs and the atmosphere causes air to flow in.

Table 1 provides a list of the most commonly used pressure controlled ventilators, of which the bi-level devices are the majority.

B. Flow Controllers

If flow is measured and used to deliver a preset volume, then a ventilator is considered to be a flow controller (1). In most of the cases, volume preset ventilation is provided by ventilators that actually measure flow and use flow over time to deliver a preset volume. These machines maintain an approximately constant volume in the face of varying lung mechanics. The most common flow-controlled ventilators are listed in Table 2. As indicated in the table, most of these machines can also provide pressure ventilation.

C. Volume Controllers

More rare today are volume controllers. The distinguishing feature of a volume controller is that it measures directly the volume it delivers. Therefore the only ventilators that qualify as true volume controllers are those whose drive mechanisms allow the direct measure of volume. These machines measure volume change as the displacement of a piston, bellows, or similar mechanism. The few volume-controlled ventilators still available in the market are listed in Table 3. To our knowledge, there are no new volume-controlled ventilators being manufactured.

Once one understands the primary control mechanism of a ventilator, one can examine how a ventilator starts, sustains, and stops inspiration and what it does between inspirations. A ventilator cycle can be broken down into four phases:

- Change from expiration to inspiration
- Inspiration
- Change from inspiration to expiration
- Expiration

In each phase, a particular variable is measured and used to switch from one phase to another. Ventilators are designed to directly control only four possible variables, namely, pressure, volume, flow, or time. During any given inspiration, only one of these variables can be controlled at a time (1). The four phase variables are described in Figure 1.

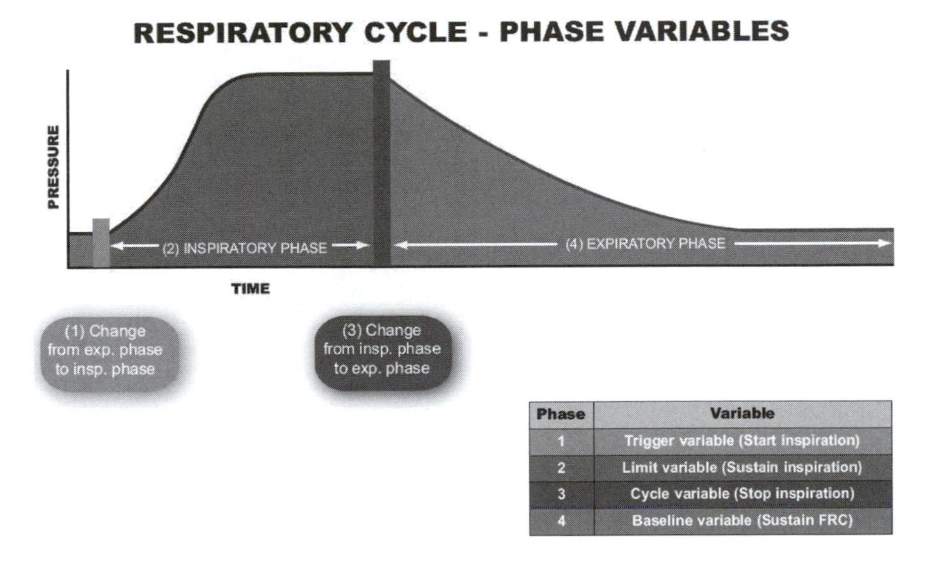

Phase	Variable
1	Trigger variable (Start inspiration)
2	Limit variable (Sustain inspiration)
3	Cycle variable (Stop inspiration)
4	Baseline variable (Sustain FRC)

Figure 1 The phases of the respiratory cycle.

III. Trigger Variables—Change from Expiration to Inspiration

Inspiration is started when one of the trigger variables (pressure, volume, flow, or time) reaches a preset value.

- Time trigger: The ventilator initiates a breath according to a set frequency or time. This is commonly referred to as the backup rate. Knowing the range a ventilator has for a backup rate can be important while choosing a machine, especially for pediatrics.
- Volume, flow, or pressure trigger: The ventilator senses the patient's inspiratory effort in the form of a drop in baseline pressure or an increase in volume or flow.

For ventilators that are pressure, volume, or flow triggered, the patient effort required to trigger inspiration is determined by the ventilator's sensitivity setting. Trigger sensitivity is adjusted by changing the preset value of the trigger variable. Ventilators having a trigger sensitivity adjustment may be more suited for patients with a weak inspiratory effort such as neuromuscular weakness. The trigger variable used for each ventilator is presented as shown in Tables 1 to 3.

Clinicians often wonder if it is better to use a flow- or pressure-based trigger. Several studies have shown that using a flow trigger variable is more sensitive and requires less patient work than using a pressure trigger variable. One in vivo study by Nava using an ICU ventilator showed that in patients with and without chronic obstructive pulmonary disease (COPD), flow triggering was able to significantly reduce the inspiratory effort and delay, compared with pressure triggering (2).

(text continues on page 239)

Table 1 Pressure-controlled Ventilators

Manufacturer and product name	Picture	Inspiratory trigger variable V = multiple sensitivity settings Backup rate min and max	Inspiratory limit variable(s)	Cycle variables V = variable sensitivity settings	Baseline ZEEP = Zero PEEP and use of a valve circuit	Battery I = internal E = external
Pegaso Negavent DA3 Plus		Time	Negative pressure	Time	ZEEP	
Respironics NEV®-100		Time	Negative pressure	Time	ZEEP	
Respironics BiPAP® ST or Harmony		Volume, time 4–30 bpm	Positive pressure	Time, flow	EPAP	E
Respironics BiPAP® Synchrony Note: *AVAPS is not available in every country		Volume, time V 0–30 bpm	Positive pressure with volume security (*AVAPS)	Time, flow	EPAP	E
Tyco Goodknight® 425 ST, Knightstar® 330		Flow, time V 4–25 bpm (425 ST) 3–30 bpm (330 ST)	Positive pressure	Time, flow V	EPAP	E
B&D Electromedical Nippy™ ST		Time, flow 6–60 bpm	Positive pressure	Time, flow	EPAP	E
B&D Electromedical Nippy™ 3		Time, flow V 6–60 bpm	Positive pressure	Time, flow V	ZEEP or EPAP	E

Airox Smart Air® Plus	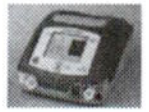	Time, flow V 4–40 bpm	Positive pressure	Time, flow V	EPAP	I, E
Airox Smart Air® ST	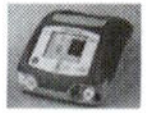	Time, flow V 4–40 bpm	Positive pressure with volume security	Time, flow V	EPAP	E
Weinmann SOMNOvent® ST	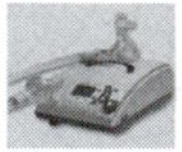	Time, flow V 5–45 bpm	Positive pressure	Time, flow V	EPAP	
Weinmann VENTImotion®	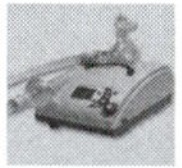	Time, flow V 6–40 bpm	Positive pressure with volume security	Time, flow V	EPAP	I, E
Breas VIVO™ 30	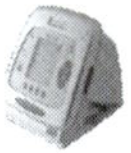	Time, flow V 4–40 bpm	Positive pressure	Time, flow V	EPAP	E
Breas VIVO™ 40	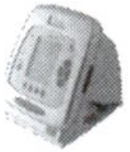	Time, flow V 4–40 bpm	Positive pressure	Time, flow V	EPAP	I, E
ResMed VPAP® III ST Note: Variable trigger and cycle not available in all countries	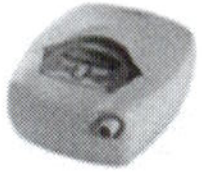	Time, flow V 5–30 bpm	Positive pressure	Time, flow V	EPAP	
ResMed VPAP® III ST A	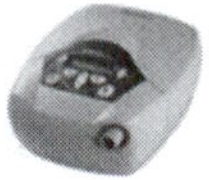	Time, flow V 5–30 bpm	Positive pressure	Time, flow V	EPAP	E
ResMed/Saime VS Integra®	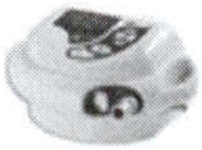	Time, pressure V 5–50 bpm	Positive pressure with volume security	Time, flow V	ZEEP or PEEP	I, E

*AVAPS, average volume-assured pressure support.

Table 2 Flow-controlled Ventilators

Manufacturer and product name	Photo	Inspiratory trigger variable V = multiple sensitivity settings Backup rate min and max	Inspiratory limit variable(s) PP = preprogrammed modes available	Cycle variables V = variable sensitivity settings	Baseline ZEEP = Zero PEEP and use of a valve circuit	Battery I = internal E = external
Tyco Achieva® Portable Vent		Time, flow, pressure V 1–80 bpm	Volume, pressure	Time, flow V	ZEEP, PEEP	I, E
Draeger Carina™ home		Time, flow V 5–50 bpm	Volume, pressure	Flow, time V	ZEEP, PEEP	I, E
ResMed/Saime Elisée 150®		Pressure, time, flow V 2–80 bpm	Volume, positive pressure with volume security, PP	Flow, time V	ZEEP, PEEP	I, E
Airox Legendair®		Time, flow V 6–60 bpm	Volume, pressure with volume security	Time, flow V	ZEEP, PEEP	I, E

Pulmonetic Systems Inc LTV®800, 900, 950[a]	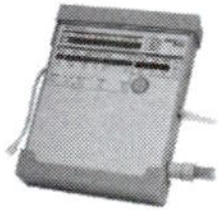	Time, flow, pressure V 0–80 bpm	Volume, pressure	Time, flow V	ZEEP, PEEP	I, E
Respironics PLV® Continuum™	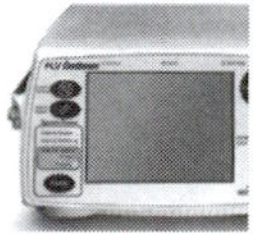	Pressure, time, flow V 0–150 bpm	Volume, pressure, PP	Flow, time V	ZEEP, PEEP	I, E
ResMed/Saime VS Ultra®	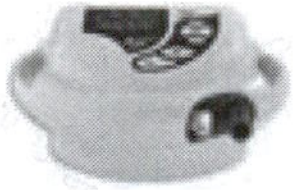	Pressure, time, flow V 0, 5–60 bpm	Volume, pressure with volume security	Flow, time V	ZEEP, PEEP	I, E
Taema Neftis	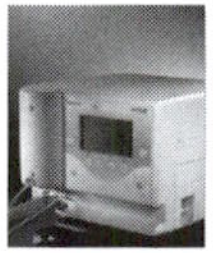	Time, flow V 5–60 bpm	Volume, pressure	Flow, time V	ZEEP, PEEP	

[a]Other models available specifically for pediatric use.

Table 3 Volume Controllers

Manufacturer and product name	Picture	Inspiratory trigger variable V = multiple sensitivity settings Backup rate min and max	Inspiratory limit variable	Cycle variable	Baseline	Battery I = internal E = external
ResMed/Saime Eole®[a]		Time, pressure V 5–90	Volume 50mL–1.55 L	Volume	ZEEP or PEEP	I, E
Respironics PLV®-100, 102[a]		Time, pressure V 2–35	Volume 50 mL–3 L	Volume	ZEEP or PEEP	I, E

[a]Other models available specifically for pediatric use.

A recent bench study comparing home ventilators, in which flow- and pressure-triggered devices were tested, concluded that even though differences existed among machines, all devices required very little triggering effort and had trigger delays <200 milliseconds, with four of the machines having delays of <100 milliseconds. All four machines with trigger delays of <100 milliseconds used flow trigger variables (3).

It is important that inspiration begins in synchrony with the patient's inspiratory effort. Ideally the neural start and the ventilator start of inspiration would be exactly matched (4). However, there are multiple factors that may impact a ventilator's ability to respond to a patient's inspiratory effort. These include:

Trigger delays intrinsic to the design of the ventilator
Leak
Presence of upper airway closure
Presence of intrinsic positive end–expiratory pressure (PEEPi)

The last three factors have a tendency to render the triggering signal difficult or impossible to sense. Missed triggering can be easily identified at the bedside. One simply needs to observe the patient's efforts while listening or observing the inspiration provided by the ventilator. Patient's effort without a response from the ventilator is considered as a missed trigger. This is more frequently observed when the patient sleeps than during awake ventilation. Since observation requires being at the bedside, nocturnal monitoring using polygraphy or polysomnography is an excellent method for documenting these events (Fig. 2). Home-based ventilator monitoring can also be used to help identify triggering problems, with monitoring of leak, rate and AHI (Fig. 3). Patients using assist-only devices may have periods of apnea during sleep, which could impair their ventilation efficacy. Therefore, some form of monitoring should be included if only the assist method of ventilation is chosen.

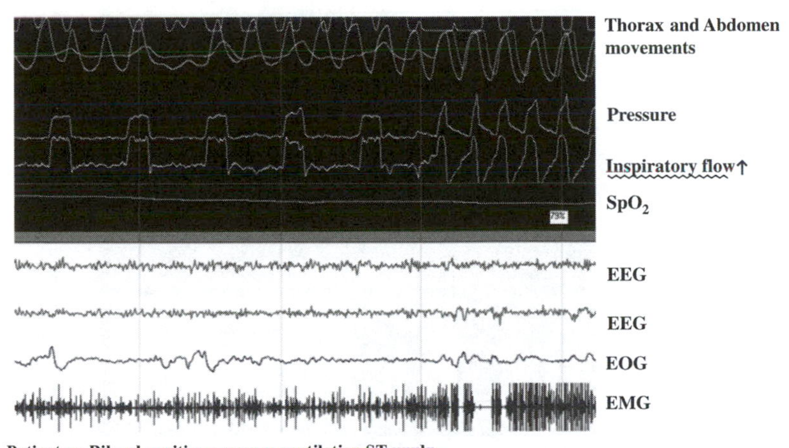

Patient on Bilevel positive pressure ventilation ST mode,
Trigger failure: Breathing at the back-up rate.
Leaks (Inspiratory pressure is low, Duration of inspiration reach the maximum inspiratory time, no decrease in inspiratory flow (leak compensation), no expiratory flow, poor synchronization with time cycled breaths and severe desaturation (79%) during REM sleep. With arousal, patient triggers with re-synchronization occurring.

Figure 2 Respiratory polygraph during ventilation using a bilevel device.

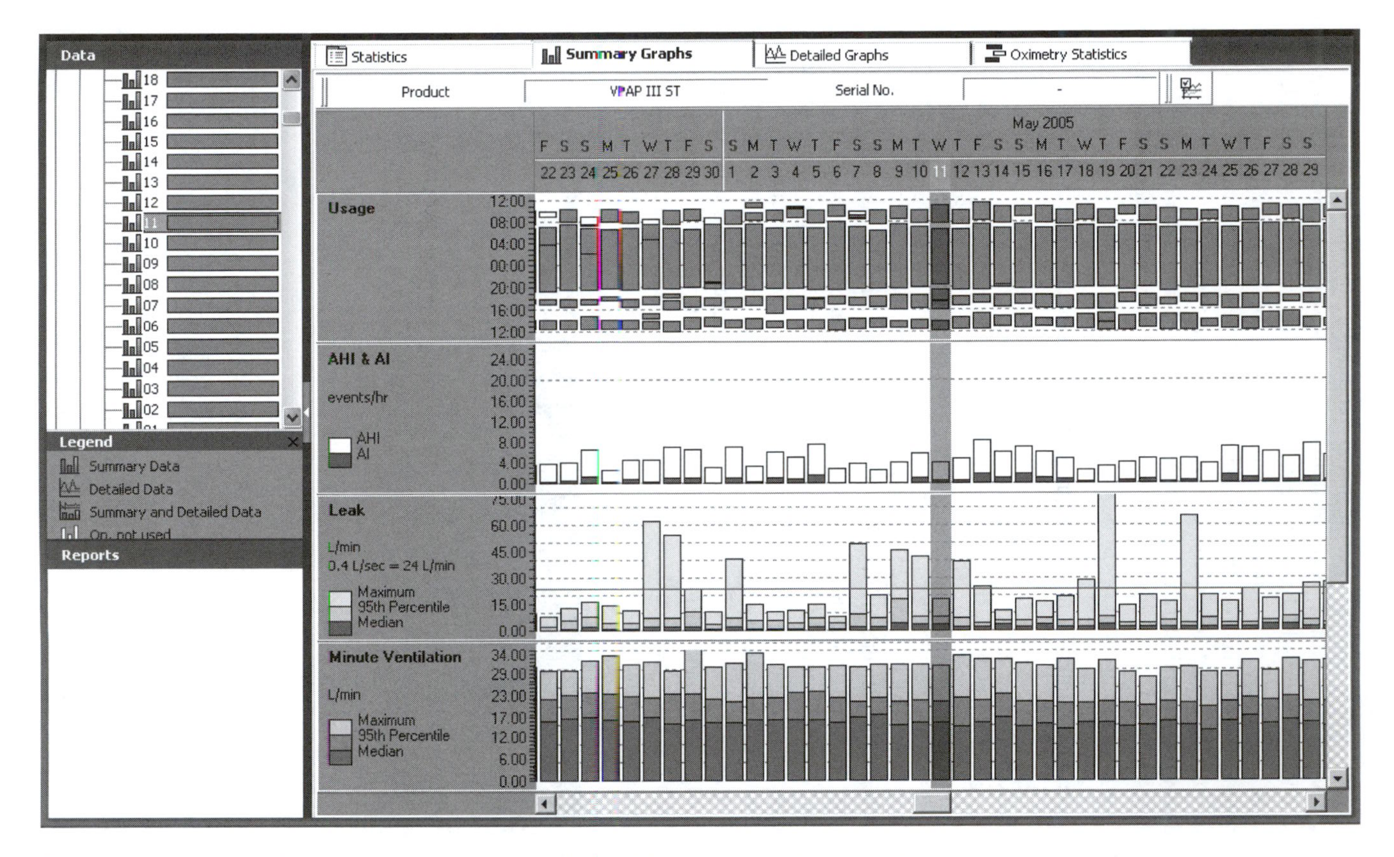

Figure 3 5 weeks of daily monitoring using a bilevel device (VPAP) with the ResMed software program.

There have been limited studies looking at the effect of leakage on triggering. Most modern ventilators compensate for the leak and incorporate algorithms that allow trigger sensitivity to remain good in the face of a leak. This is probably why a recent bench study showed a variable but small effect of leak on triggering times with home ventilators (5). If significant leak is present and thought to interfere with triggering, it should be controlled first before changing trigger sensitivity settings. Leak is easily monitored at home with ventilator-based systems or in the sleep laboratory.

The most significant impact on a patient's ability to trigger a ventilator is the presence of partial or complete upper airway obstruction, which will cause missed or double triggering. This can be easily demonstrated in a sleep study, but can be difficult to identify at home unless apneas and hypopneas are monitored by the ventilator itself.

As home ventilators become more and more sophisticated in their ability to monitor patients, events like missed or double triggering will become easier to identify without requiring laboratory evaluation. When poor triggering is caused by upper airway obstruction, the solution is to increase PEEP rather than change trigger sensitivity. Missed triggering due to hyperinflation in COPD patients may be related to excessive inspiratory pressures, in which case decreasing the pressure support or increasing the expiratory positive airway pressure (EPAP/PEEP) may improve triggering.

In France, most patients receiving HMV only use machines equipped with a backup rate, whereas in some countries, unless it can be shown that a patient is poorly ventilated without a backup rate, an assist-only device is prescribed. We have frequently monitored patients ventilated at home and observed that many of them breathe at the backup rate, regardless of where it is set. There is limited information as to how many patients require a backup rate versus assist-only devices. In one small study, 15% required backup after titration using polysomnography (6).

Increasing the rate is also a strategy for increasing minute ventilation in a passive patient, which could allow the level of pressure support to be maintained at a lower level, limiting mask leak. The range of backup rates available for each ventilator can be found in Tables 1 to 3.

IV. Pressurization

The pressurization phase is the time the machine will use to reach inspiratory pressure. The ability of the ventilator to meet the patient's inspiratory flow demand has mainly been studied in the acute setting where a high-pressure rise time is known to decrease the inspiratory effort (7,8). A recent bench study showed that pressurization characteristics varied considerably among 10 home care ventilators (3). Battisti et al. concluded that some home care ventilators might be limited in patients with high inspiratory demand, those with marked obesity, or those with severe restriction. Depending on the type of home care ventilator, the pressure rise time can be individually adjusted or fixed.

As home care ventilators become smaller in size, their pneumatic performance may be compromised. As rise time settings are often arbitrary numbers, clinicians should ask manufacturers for information on flow performance, as this information is easily available in the form of pressure flow graphs. One should look for the machine's ability to maintain inspiratory pressure stability. Breathing on the machine is also a very good way to evaluate a ventilator's ability to meet inspiratory flow demand.

V. Limit Variable—Sustaining Inspiration

The variable that limits inspiration is the one that attains a constant value before inspiration ends. If one or more variables are not allowed to rise above a preset value during the inspiratory time, it is referred to as a limit variable. This is not necessarily the variable which will end inspiration (1), for example pressure support (PS), where pressure is limited but inspiration is ended by a drop in inspiratory flow.

The most common variable used to sustain inspiration during HMV is pressure. Pressure-limited ventilators are used due to their ability to compensate for leak and to improve patient comfort. Pressure ventilation is easy for clinicians to set and in some modes allows the patient to control their breathing rate and the duration of inspiration. Pressure-limited ventilators are becoming increasingly sophisticated with alarms and batteries, which is allowing them to be increasingly used for more dependent and tracheostomized patients for whom volume ventilation was once the only available option. Although this is no longer the case, there are still significant advantages to using volume-limited ventilation, especially for more dependent patients. Some of these advantages are

- Easier to use with mouthpiece ventilation
- Easier for patients to alter their inspiratory volume by air stacking, which allows variation in speech and improves cough
- Less power and therefore batteries last longer
- In tracheostomized patients, pressure varies with changes in resistance and compliance assuring a certain volume delivery.

There have been several inconclusive studies of patients with CRF comparing volume-targeted with pressure-targeted ventilation (9,10). Given equal efficacy, clinicians can feel comfortable to begin ventilation with the method of their choice. If patients fail to respond or are noncompliant, the other method should be tried. This is especially important for NIV where poor efficacy could lead to the need for a tracheostomy.

Differences between pressure and volume ventilation will soon be much less relevant as flow-controlled ventilators have the ability to deliver both volume and pressure preset ventilation, or a mode combination, such as pressure support with volume security. Ventilators offering this capability incorporate an automatic algorithm, which allows the pressure support to increase over several breaths to achieve a predetermined target volume. Another interesting way to combine pressure and volume modes is to allow the clinician to preprogram different modes of ventilation, giving the patient the ability to switch between these preset modes. This would enable a patient to use a pressure preset mode at night when leaks and airway instability are more frequent and volume ventilation during the day when autonomy and speech are the priorities. Ventilator limit variables are presented in Tables 1 to 3. Machines offering PS with volume security are indicated, and those with the ability to provide preprogram modes are indicated as PP.

VI. Cycle Variable—Ending Inspiration

Inspiration ends when one of the variables (flow, pressure, volume, or time) has reached a preset value (1). Flow and time are the most common variables used to end inspiration for pressure-limited modes and volume and time are the most common variables for volume-limited modes. Most home care ventilators, which provide volume-limited ventilation, would lead one to believe that they are volume cycled. However, they are flow controllers and instead of measuring volume directly, they use inspiratory flow provided over a preset inspiratory time to determine the preset volume. Providing volume preset ventilation in this manner requires setting an inspiratory time and making them time cycled, in contrast to the original volume controllers, which were volume cycled. This may be why some patients using volume-cycled ventilators find it difficult to switch from such ventilators to volume-limited/time-cycled ventilators. This may challenge patients as volume-controlled devices reach the end of their life span, leaving no choice but to switch patients to flow-controlled machines.

In pressure ventilation, most ventilators cycle from inspiration to expiration when inspiratory flow decreases to a predetermined percent of its peak flow or when a preset inspiratory time is reached. It has become increasingly clear that cycling plays an important role in assuring patient-ventilator synchrony (11). This has been quite well studied in pressure support ventilation and several authors have shown that a fixed cycle value can lead to premature cycling in patients with restrictive diseases and delayed cycling in those with obstructive disease (12,13).

In their bench model study, Battisti et al. observed considerable variations in cycling behavior when the 10 ventilators they tested were used at their default cycle settings. Most machines tended to cycle prematurely under normal conditions, with the occurrence of premature cycling increasing with restrictive mechanics. Conversely, under obstructive conditions, most devices exhibited delayed cycling. This general pattern was exacerbated by leakage. Some ventilators were found to be better suited for the obstructive model, others for the restrictive model. Most devices allowed for manual adjustment of cycle sensitivity which they found to completely correct the cycle asynchrony (3). Battisti et al. noted that adjusting the cycle setting on the bench model, where the mechanical conditions are predetermined and fixed, is quite different from adjusting the cycle setting under clinical conditions in which the patient's respiratory mechanics cannot be measured and are likely to change with the magnitude of leaks (11).

Most turbine-based ventilators circumvent some of the cycling problems imposed by leak with algorithms or inspiratory time limits that change expiratory cycle criteria as leak volume changes. It is difficult to assess at home whether these potential solutions maintain or improve synchrony as few home care ventilators can monitor in real time the airway pressure and flow waveforms, which would help the clinician make the assessment. Choosing ventilators with variable cycle sensitivity settings and time limits can significantly improve the clinician's ability to assure good ventilation. These functions are indicated in Tables 1 to 3.

VII. Baseline Variable—Expiration

The variable controlled during the expiratory phase is known as the baseline variable, most commonly, pressure, typically expressed as EPAP or PEEP. It is necessary to have a positive baseline pressure in bi-level devices to assure CO_2 washout. Bi-level devices have also been shown to be effective in managing upper airway collapse, in patients with obstructive sleep apnea and overlap (14). Finally, a positive baseline pressure has been shown to decrease the work of breathing associated with intrinsic PEEP and improve oxygenation (15,16). Some of the indications or advantages of using EPAP or PEEP in home mechanical ventilation are

necessary in bi-level devices to assure CO_2 washout,
splints the upper airway open preventing collapse,
used to increase FRC, to improve gas distribution and oxygenation, and
helps to overcome the work of breathing associated with intrinsic PEEP.

The terms PEEP and EPAP tend to be used interchangeably, but there is a significant difference in the mechanism used to create these pressures. PEEP is created using an exhalation valve and EPAP-like continuous positive airway pressure (CPAP) is created using flow. Ventilator circuits that use exhalation valves have shown significant variation in the resistance to exhalation through the valve. This increased resistance can increase the mean expiratory pressure and the work of breathing (17). Another difference has to do with expiratory pressure stability in the face of a leak. Leak compensation in a bi-level device is equally good during inspiration and expiration, whereas devices using a valved circuit separate these functions, generally providing good leak compensation during inspiration with much less capability during expiration. For this reason, leak usually results in instability or loss of the PEEP pressure. The influence of leak on airway stability, synchronization, work of breathing, or oxygenation remains to be defined.

Only in patient circuits that use an exhalation valve can the baseline pressure return to ambient pressure, known as zero PEEP or ZEEP. The advantage of ZEEP requires study, although it is certainly desirable during daytime ventilation when the upper airway is stable and ventilator energy conservation to preserve battery function is more important than leak compensation. Devices using a valve circuit are indicated in the ventilator table. There are some machines that allow the use of both leak and valve circuits in which case both EPAP and ZEEP are indicated in the Tables 1 to 3.

CO_2 rebreathing has been reported in bi-level ventilators with a single gas delivery circuit and no true exhalation valve (18,19). A recent in vivo study showed that the continual presence of nonintentional leak during NIV provided enough additional CO_2 washout to address this issue (20). However, clinician should remain concerned when using a full-face mask, as the patient is more dependent on the intentional leak rates, which vary significantly.

VIII. Choosing the Right Mode of Ventilation and Adjusting the Settings

A mode of ventilation is a way of communicating an important set of characteristics in only a few words. Once we understand the ventilator control characteristics and how a particular variable is used to switch from one phase of the respiratory cycle to another, modes of ventilation become very easy to understand. For example, when we describe pressure limited modes, we use the cycle criteria to describe

- Pressure support mode: flow cycled
- Pressure control mode: time cycled

The machines that provide pressure-limited ventilation and have time cycling capability can provide the pressure control mode. Those with flow cycling provide pressure support (Tables 1–3).

A. Which Ventilator Mode Is Best Suited for a Particular Patient?

There is no recipe for providing assisted ventilation. The best mode is the one with which the clinician is most comfortable and which the patient tolerates best. Suggested ventilator modes and settings according to etiologies are listed in Table 4. Once a ventilator mode is chosen, the next step is to ensure that it provides adequate ventilation for the patient. We

Table 4 Suggested Ventilator Modes and Settings According to Main Etiologies

Type of disease	Potential challenges encountered during ventilation	Suggested ventilation requirements
Restrictive respiratory disorders	Early cycling	Pressure support with variable cycle sensitivity settings Possibility to fix the inspiratory time or set minimum inspiratory time limits
	Severe restrictive mechanics	Pressure modes with good pressurization, i.e., fast rise time capability Max inspiratory pressures >25 cmH_2O Possibility to fix the inspiratory time or set minimum inspiratory time limits Pressure modes with volume security
	Upper airway obstruction	Stable baseline pressure/EPAP
	Daytime ventilation	Ability to provide zero baseline pressure or ZEEP Possibility to preprogram modes/settings for daytime vs. nighttime ventilation Battery capability Volume ventilation capability
	>16 hr of ventilator use	Secure battery Power failure alarms Possibility to preprogram modes/settings for daytime vs. nighttime ventilation
	Invasive ventilation	Pressure modes with volume security or volume ventilation Alarms Battery if >16 hr dependency
Obstructive lung disease	Late cycling	Maximum inspiratory time limit Minimum inspiratory time <300 msec
	High inspiratory demand	Fast rise time Short trigger delay
	Needs ventilation during exercise	Battery

can ventilate almost any patient with any mode of ventilation if we know how to adjust it properly. Pressure support is the easiest mode to begin NIV as there are few parameters to adjust and most patients tolerate it well. Patients with restrictive diseases may finish inspiration early and those with obstructive diseases may finish later (3). Using a ventilator with variable cycle sensitivity can significantly improve inspiratory cycling in these patients. In some patients, fixing the inspiratory time may be the only way to prevent early or late cycling. Significant leak can also impair proper cycling when using pressure support ventilation. Using a maximum inspiratory time limit will improve synchronization when intermittent leak occurs (Fig. 2). Monitoring and managing leak is very important during NIV. Selecting the best ventilator settings can be a daunting task. The following default settings are recommended for pressure support ventilation.

PS	6–8 cmH_2O
EPAP/PEEP	4 cmH_2O
Rise time	Minimum
Backup rate	Low
Inspiratory trigger	Average or default setting
Expiratory trigger/cycle	Average or default setting

It is recommended to stay with the patient during the initiation of NIV and listen closely to what the patient has to say. On the basis of the feedback from the patient, we have found that the approach described in Figures 4 and 5 can be used to adjust the initial settings used for NIV.

Volume ventilation is often used for patients with a tracheostomy, but can also be very effective for daytime ventilation when using NIV with a mouthpiece (see Figs. 6 and 7). Volume ventilation when used during the day can allow patients to air stack and thus vary

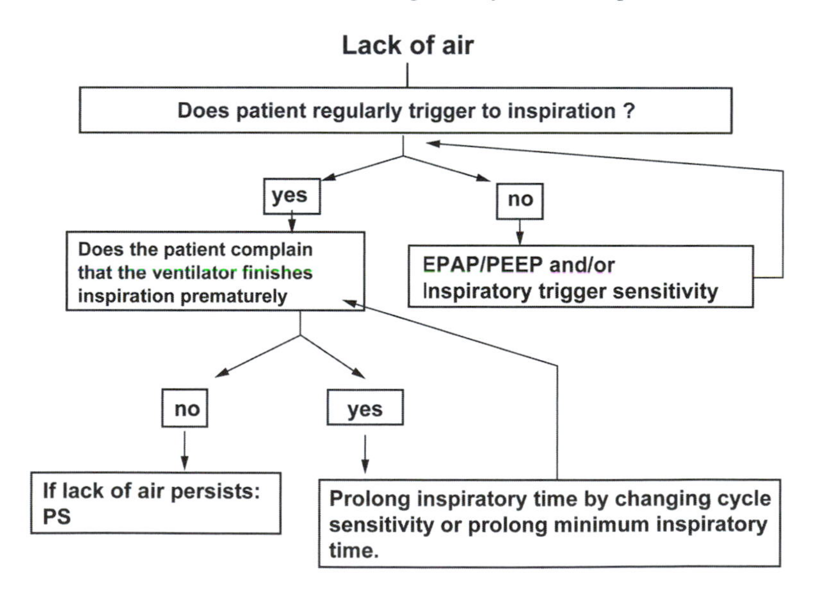

Figure 4 Clinical approach for adjusting initial settings.

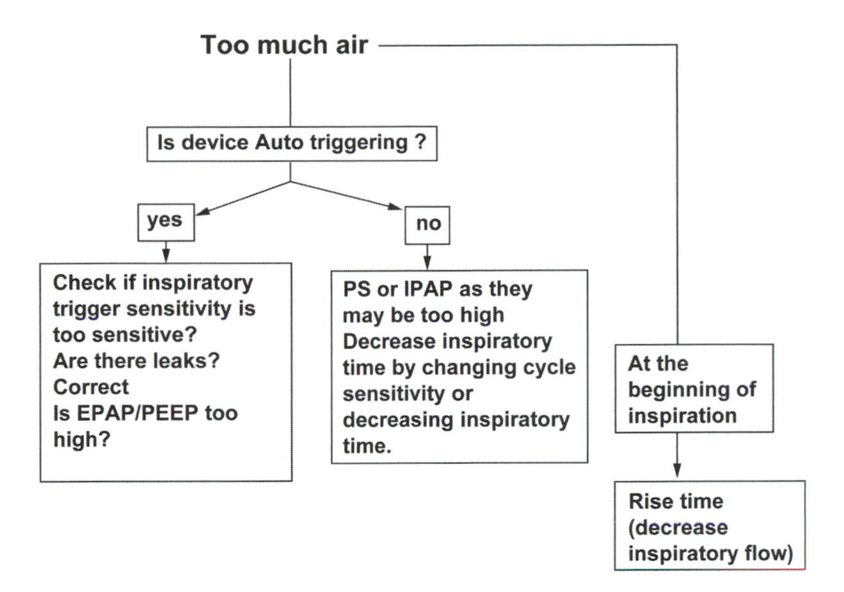

Figure 5 Clinical approach for adjusting initial settings.

their inspiratory volume significantly. Air stacking is the inhalation of several inspiratory tidal volumes without expiration to progressively increase the inspiratory capacity. It improves speech, and more importantly, cough. When using volume ventilation with a mask or an uncuffed tracheostomy tube during sleep, it is important to remember the limitation of this mode for leak compensation. If there is significant leak during sleep, the patient may be

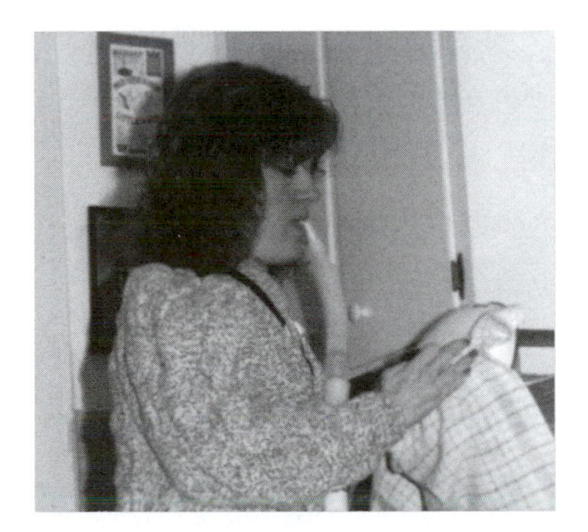

Figure 6 Post-polio patient with severe scoliosis using mouthpiece ventilation during activities of daily living.

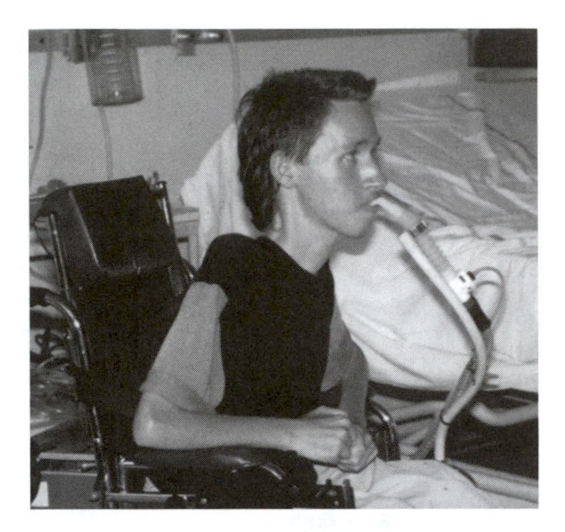

Figure 7 Duchenne muscular dystrophy patient, dependent on noninvasive ventilation using daytime mouthpiece ventilation mounted on his electric wheelchair.

hypoventilated. Although negative pressure ventilation remains an option for NIV, there are few clinicians today comfortable with this mode and few devices are available (21).

Ventilator modes are becoming increasingly sophisticated. Pressure- and flow-controlled ventilators, combined with sophisticated feedback systems, allow the combination of volume- and pressure-limited ventilation. These new modes are based on algorithms, which secure a certain target volume by increasing pressure support over a period of several breaths. Each ventilator has its own unique algorithm to adjust the inspiratory pressure using either inspired or expired volume. Several studies have demonstrated the feasibility of using an algorithm to automatically adjust inspiratory pressure during NIV with effects comparable to those of manually set inspiratory pressures (22–24). The role of these automatic algorithms on the quality of sleep, especially when using "mixed" modes of ventilation, remains to be better defined.

IX. Patient Circuits and Interfaces

A. Circuits

There are three main types of ventilator circuits used for HMV: Single circuits with a leak, single circuits with a valve, and double circuits with a valve. When used with NIV, it is important that the appropriate mask be used. Table 5 summarizes the important points associated with each type of circuit. Circuits with a leak are used for bi-level devices. The intentional leak and CO_2 washout for a given pressure vary significantly depending on the manufacturer and the type of mask. There are many choices of masks for the leak circuit as these masks are also used for CPAP. We have already reviewed the issue of CO_2 washout and concluded that this is not a major concern when using a nasal mask (20). The only type of mask where this might be of clinical concern is with a full-face mask. A full-face mask is

Table 5 Patient Circuits

Leak circuit	Single limb valve circuit	Double limb valve circuit
Leak is usually provided via mask with intentional leak	Non-vented mask required for noninvasive ventilation	Non-vented mask required for noninvasive ventilation
Required with bilevel devices to assure CO_2 washout	CO_2 washout is not an issue as inhalation and exhalation are separated unless dead space is increased	CO_2 washout is not an issue as inhalation and exhalation are separated unless dead space is increased
Must have positive baseline pressure to assure continuous flow and CO_2 washout	Exhalation valve is proximal	Exhalation valve is located at or in the ventilator
Provides good leak compensation during exhalation and stable EPAP pressure	Zero baseline pressure (ZEEP) is possible	Zero baseline pressure (ZEEP) is possible
Exhaled volumes are calculated based on measured inspiratory flow minus leak	Only inspired volumes can be measured	Allows monitoring of exhaled volumes with comparison to inspired volumes
	Variable expiratory resistance depending on exhalation valve	Allows alarms to be set to the exhaled volumes providing greater patient security

often used to manage mouth leak and if there is little mask leak, then CO_2 washout will be dependent on the intentional leak within the mask. The location of the intentional leak within the mask near the bridge of the nose has been shown to improve CO_2 washout (25). There are significant differences in the location and level of intentional leak and this could impair CO_2 washout and ventilation. This information is readily available from the manufacturer and should be reviewed by the clinician.

Circuits using a valve are available as single circuits with the exhalation valve located proximally or as a double circuit with the exhalation valve located at or in the device. The advantage of a double circuit is that it will usually allow the monitoring of exhaled volumes with the ability to set alarms accordingly. Masks used with these circuits are nonvented and there is much less of a selection. One advantage of ventilators that use a valve circuit is the ability to have ZEEP with zero flow during exhalation. This system is probably more comfortable for mouthpiece and daytime ventilation.

B. Interfaces

Nasal masks remain the most commonly used interfaces for NIV. As nocturnal monitoring of leak improves, we are becoming more aware of the propensity for mouth leak during nocturnal ventilation. Mouth leak has been shown to cause dryness and irritation of the upper airway and periods of hypoventilation, dysynchrony, and micro-arousals during sleep (26–28). The use of heated humidification, full-face mask, and chin strap has been shown to decrease these side effects (29). Mouthpiece ventilation is an excellent way to provide daytime ventilation. The mouthpiece is discrete and can be easily mounted on the wheelchair for physically dependent patients. Once installed, patients can use ventilation to the extent they need during the day (Figs. 6 and 7). Tracheostomy is usually reserved for patients with significant upper airway dysfunction or failure of NIV. Unfortunately many patients are tracheostomized during acute respiratory failure and clinicians are wary of removing the tracheostomy once it has been established. Although some patients adapt well to tracheostomy, there are others who benefit from its removal and the use of NIV. Side effects from tracheostomy include increased secretion production, tracheal granulomata, local pain and irritation, decreased ventilator autonomy, and difficulty in vocalization. A safe way to transition a tracheostomy patient to NIV is with the use of a tracheal button, which secures the opening while NIV is established (Figs. 6 and 7).

X. Accessories for HMV

Humidification should be considered for all patients being nocturnally ventilated at home. NIV delivers air at a much higher flow than normal breathing, which may compromise the airway's ability to adequately heat and humidify inspired air (30). One case study reported life-threatening airway obstruction during NIV from inspissated secretions, an adverse event that Wood et al. attributed to inadequate humidification (31). Numerous studies have looked at the benefits of humidification during CPAP but there is little available for NIV. A recent bench study found the NIV using bi-level devices delivers air with low absolute and relative humidity, especially at high inspiratory pressures. The addition of heated humidification markedly improved humidity, the most effective humidification being at the highest hot-plate setting (32). Heated humidification is especially important in the following situations:

Oxygen supplementation
Presence of secretions
Upper airway symptoms
Dry or cold environment

When using heated humidification, water condensation can be minimized by insulating the patient circuit either by covering or by using tubing socks. The insulation can be prepared by the patients using soft insulating material such as fleece.

If required, oxygen is supplemented by adding constant low flow oxygen to the ventilator circuit. When pressure ventilation is used, the presence of leak will significantly decrease the fraction of inspired oxygen (Fio_2) due to leak compensation by the ventilator. This should be considered when titrating oxygen for nocturnal ventilation as it may require a higher liter flow rate compared to that used during the day. Intermittent Spo_2 monitoring should be done at home to ensure that adequate oxygen is provided during sleep. The location of the oxygen source can influence Fio_2 (33). Ventilator modes without leak compensation (i.e. volume mode) can provide a much higher Fio_2 using the same oxygen supply.

Improvements in battery technology have enabled ventilators to use lithium batteries, which provide a longer, more reliable energy source. Volume ventilation has been the gold standard for daytime ventilation, mainly due to the ability to provide auxiliary power using small portable batteries. Ventilators that function with a turbine require a much higher source of energy and until recently the batteries required for even four hours of autonomy were extremely large. As battery and motor technology improve, turbine-based ventilators with internal and external batteries are becoming increasingly available. This will allow the use of smaller and lighter ventilators with more choice of modes for those who require battery backup. Ventilators providing internal and external batteries are indicated in Tables 1 to 3.

XI. Monitoring

Most monitoring of ventilator efficacy occurs in the hospital environment using arterial blood gases and overnight Spo_2. Some centers also incorporated overnight transcutaneous Pco_2. During acute respiratory failure, ventilation is optimized in hospital with real-time monitoring and waveforms. Increasingly elective NIV is being managed with short hospital stays or completely as an outpatient or home procedure. As pressure for hospital beds increases, home-based monitoring will become more important. So what type of monitoring is possible at home?

Most ventilators measure flow volume and pressure as these variables are needed as feedback mechanisms to operate the ventilator. In home care ventilators, these measured variables are not always used to provide sophisticated real-time monitoring. However, with increased data management capabilities, these measures can now be recorded in home care ventilators over a significant period of time with relative ease and little cost. The challenge is to provide this information in a format that can be easily interpreted by the clinician for review. Some examples can be seen in Figures 8 to 10. This is a new science and we are just beginning to learn how to interpret and use this information. Manufacturers are challenged to develop

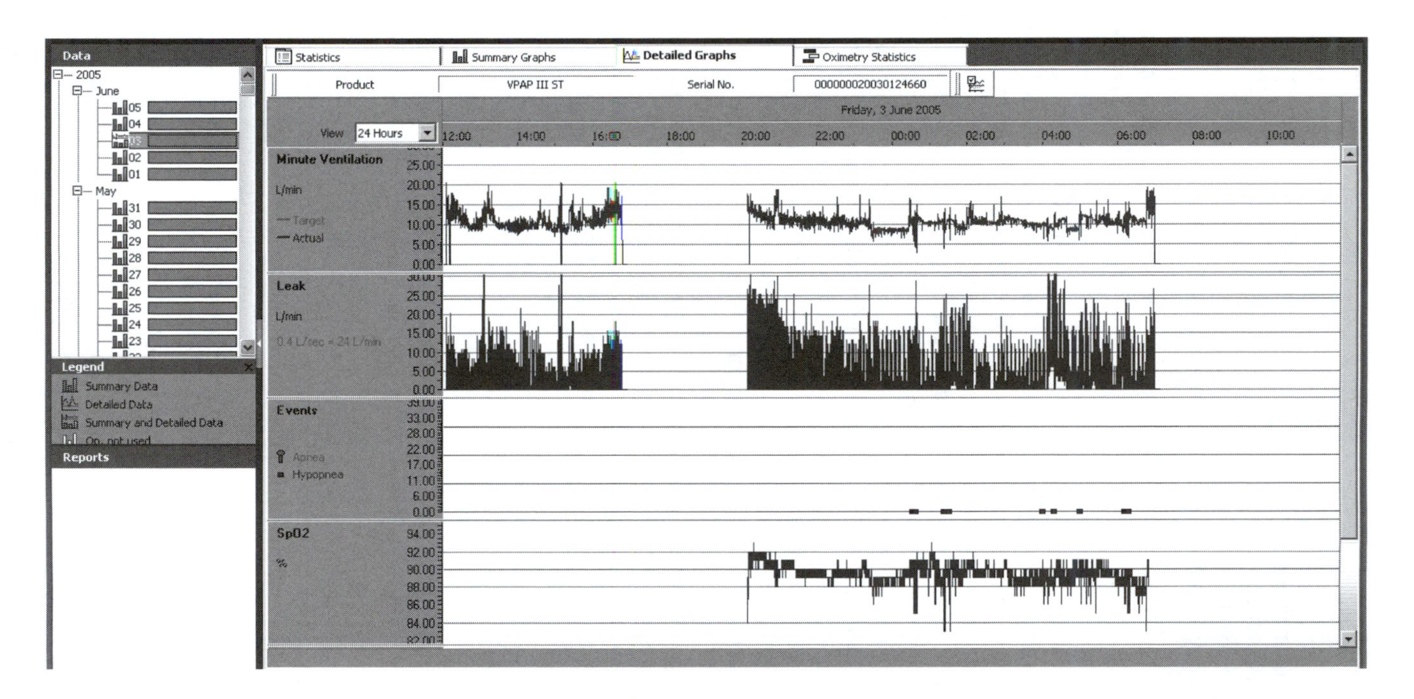

Figure 8 One night of monitoring using ResMed software with a VPAP bilevel device. The top graph shows minute ventilation, middle graph shows unintentional leak, and the bottom graph shows oxygen saturation.

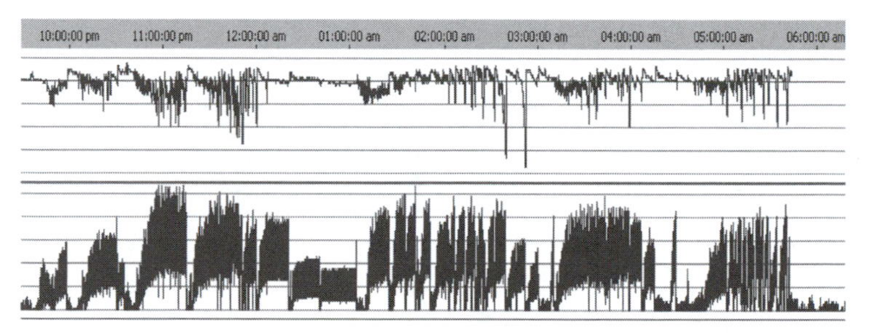

SpO_2 (top) and non-intentional leak (bottom) are provided by ResLink monitoring using VPAP bilevel device by ResMed.

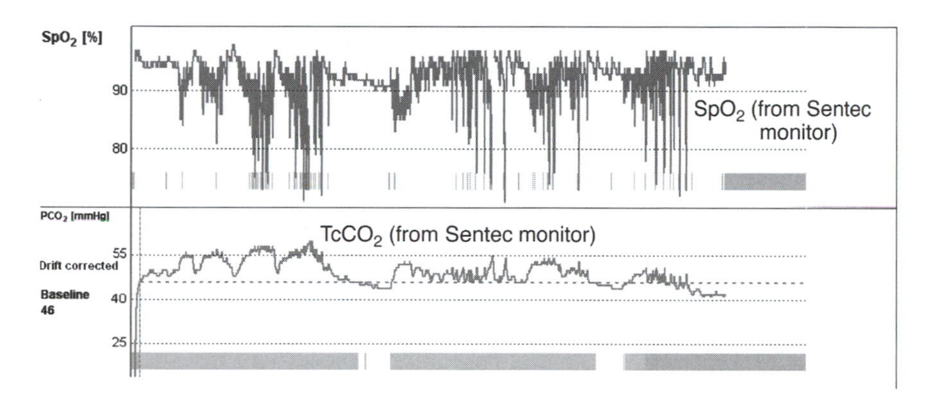

One can see the influence of leak on decreasing SpO_2 and increasing $TcCO_2$.
The correlation with the Sentec and bilevel device are very close.

Figure 9 Transcutaneous CO_2 and SpO_2 using Sentec compared with results from bilevel device.

home monitoring equipments to plot flow and pressure waveforms, as needed, as well as to transfer this information through telemetry.

XII. Conclusion

There is a very substantial choice of ventilators, interfaces, and monitoring systems available for HMV with significant improvements made in these systems in a short period of time (34). Using a classification system to understand how a given ventilator works in general terms, but with enough detail for one particular ventilator to be distinguished from another can help the clinician make the appropriate choice for a particular patient. It can also make it easier to learn the operation of a new device and predict how the ventilator will interact with the patient to support ventilation. As more sophisticated systems for HMV become available, it will be increasingly important to have this foundation in order to select the best mode and settings for a given patient.

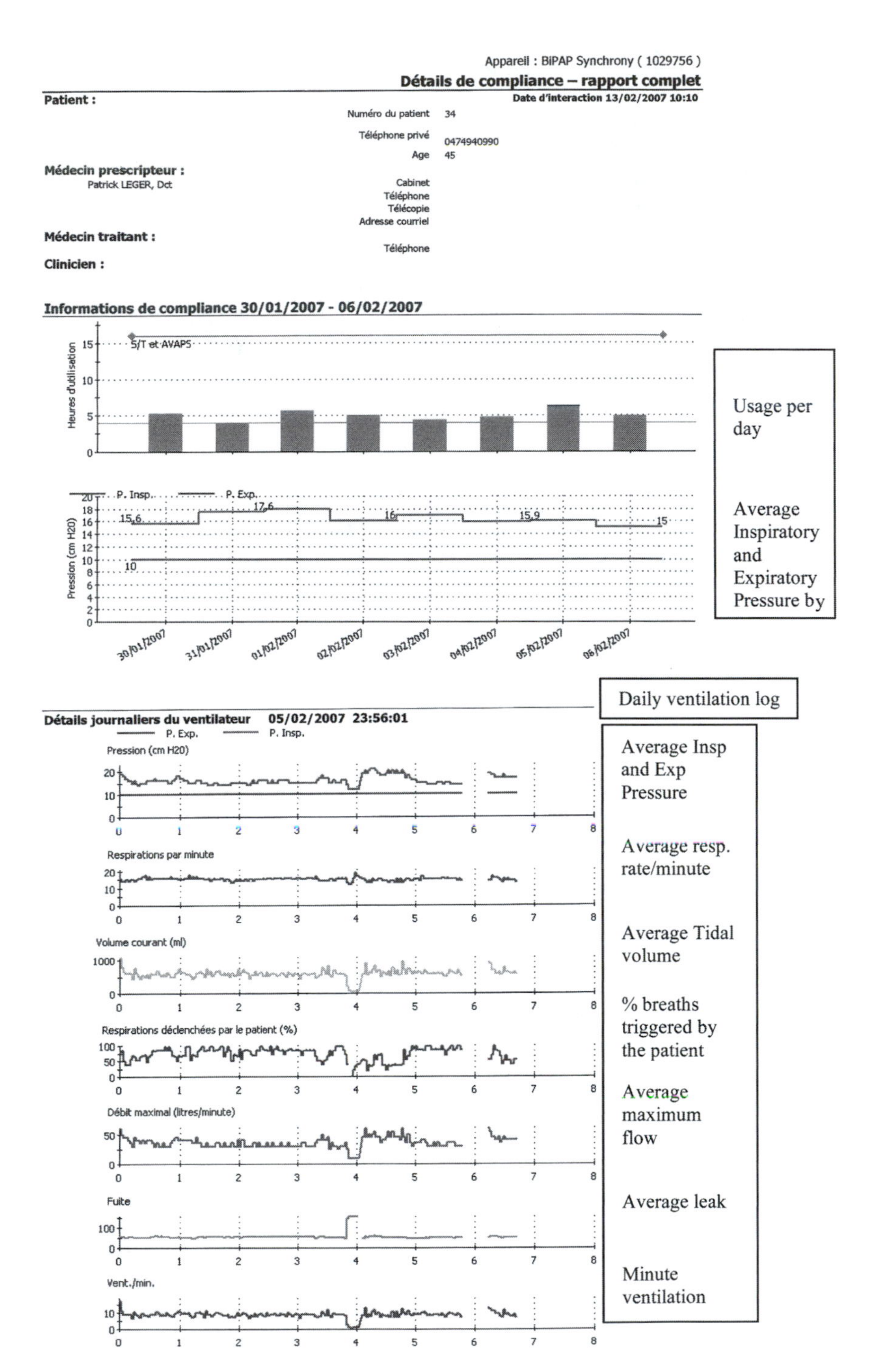

Figure 10 Encore Pro software (Respironics) report from an obesity hypoventilation syndrome patient using bi-level with volume security. *Abbreviation*: AVAPS, average volume-assured pressure support.

References

1. Chatburn RL, Primiano FP. A new system for understanding modes of mechanical ventilation. Respir Care 2001; 46(6):604–212.
2. Nava S, Ambrosino N, Bruschi C, et al. Physiological effects of flow and pressure triggering during non-invasive mechanical ventilation in patients with chronic obstructive pulmonary disease. Thorax 1997; 52:249–254.
3. Battisti A, Tassaux D, Janssens JP, et al. Performance Characteristics of 10 home mechanical ventilators in pressure-support mode: a comparative bench study. Chest 2005; 127:1784–1792.
4. Nava S, Ceriana P. Patient-ventilator interaction during noninvasive positive pressure ventilation. Respir Care Clin N Am 2005; 11:281–293.
5. Stell IM, Paul G, Lee KC, et al. Noninvasive ventilator triggering in chronic obstructive pulmonary disease: a test lung comparison. Am J Respir Crit Care Med 2001; 164:2092–2097.
6. Flynn WE, Piper AJ, Willson GN, et al. Non-invasive ventilatory support: clinical experience with Bi-level pressure preset devices. Proceedings of the Thoracic Society of Australia and New Zealand, March, 1998 (abstr).
7. Bonmarchand G, Chevron V, Chopin C, et al. Increased initial flow rate reduces inspiratory work of breathing during pressure support ventilation in patients with exacerbation of chronic obstructive pulmonary disease. Intensive Care Med 1996; 22:1147–1154.
8. Bonmarchand G, Chevron V, Menard JF, et al. Effects of pressure ramp slope values on the work of breathing during pressure support ventilation in restrictive patients. Crit Care Med 1999; 27:670–671.
9. Restrick LJ, Fox NC, Braid G, et al. Comparison of nasal pressure support ventilation with nasal intermittent positive pressure ventilation in patients with nocturnal hypoventilation. Eur Respir J 1993; 6:364–370.
10. Schonhofer B, Sonnegom M, Haidl P, et al. Comparison of two different modes for noninvasive mechanical ventilation in chronic respiratory failure: volume versus pressure controlled device. Eur Respir J 1997; 10:184–191.
11. Tobin MJ, Jubran A, Laghi F. Patient-ventilator interaction. Am J Respir Crit Care Med 2001; 163:1059–1063.
12. Yamada Y, Du H. Analysis of the mechanisms of expiratory asynchrony in pressure support ventilation: a mathematical approach. J Appl Physiol 2000; 88:2143–2150.
13. Tassaux D, Michotte J, Gainnier M, et al. Expiratory trigger setting in pressure support ventilation: from mathematical model to bedside. Crit Care Med 2004; 32:1844–1850.
14. Sanders MH, Kern N. Obstructive sleep apnea treated by independently adjusted inspiratory and expiratory positive airway pressures via nasal mask. Physiologic and clinical implications. Chest 1990; 98:317–324.
15. Appendini L, Patessio A, Zanaboni S, et al. Physiologic effects of positive end-expiratory pressure and mask pressure support during exacerbations of chronic obstructive pulmonary disease. Am J Respir Crit Care Med 1994; 149:1069–1076.
16. Elliott MW, Simonds AK. Nocturnal assisted ventilation using bilevel positive airway pressure: the effect of expiratory positive airway pressure. Eur Respir J 1995; 8:436–440.
17. Lofaso F, Aslanian P, Richard JC, et al. Expiratory valves used for home devices: experimental and clinical comparison. Eur Resp J 1998; 11:1382–1388.
18. Ferguson GT, Gilmartin M. CO_2 rebreathing during BiPAP ventilatory assistance. Am J Respir Crit Care Med 1995; 151:1126–1135.
19. Lofaso F, Brochard L, Touchard D, et al. Evaluation of carbon dioxide rebreathing during pressure support ventilation with airway management system (BiPAP) devices. Chest 1995; 108:772–778.
20. Hill NS, Carlisle C, Kramer NR. Effect of a nonrebreathing exhalation valve on long-term nasal ventilation using a bilevel device. Chest 2002; 122:84–91.

21. Corrado A, Gorrino M. Long-term negative pressure ventilation. Respir Care Clin 2002; 8:545–557.
22. Battisti A, Tassaux D, Bassin D, et al. Automatic adjustment of noninvasive pressure support with a bilevel home ventilator in patients with acute respiratory failure: a feasibility study. Intensive Care Med 2007; 33(4):632–638.
23. Storre JH, Seuthe B, et al. Average volume-assured pressure support in obesity hypoventilation: a randomized crossover trial. Chest 2006; 130:815–821.
24. Köhler D, Criee CP, Raschke F. Leitlinien zur häuslichen Sauerstoff- und Heimbeatmungstherapie. Pneumologie 1996; 50:927–931.
25. Guilherme P, Schettino P, Kacmarek R, et al. Position of exhalation port and mask design affect the CO_2 rebreathing during noninvasive pressure ventilation. Crit Care Med 2003; 31(8):2178–2182.
26. Meyer TJ, Pressman MR, Benditt J, et al. Air leaking through the mouth during nocturnal nasal ventilation: effect on sleep quality. Sleep 1997; 20(7):561–569.
27. Teschler H, Stampa J, Ragette R, et al. Effect of mouth leak on effectiveness of nasal bilevel ventilatory assistance and sleep architecture. Eur Respir J 1999; 14:1251–1257.
28. Richards GN, Cistulli PA, Ungar RG, et al. Mouth leak with nasal continuous positive airway pressure increases nasal airway resistance. Am J Respir Crit Care Med 1996; 154:182–186.
29. Martins de Araujo MT, Vieira SB, et al. Heated humidification or face mask to prevent upper airway dryness during continuous positive airway pressure therapy. Chest 2000; 117(1):142–147.
30. Lellouche F, Maggiore SM, Deye N, et al. Effect of the humidification device on the work of breathing during noninvasive ventilation. Intensive Care Med 2002; 28(11):1582–1589.
31. Wood KE, Flaten AL, Backes WJ. Inspissated secretions: a life-threatening complication of prolonged noninvasive ventilation. Respir Care 2000; 45(5):491–493.
32. Holland AE, Denehy L, Buchan C, et al. Efficacy of a heated passover humidifier during noninvasive ventilation: a bench study. Respir Care 2007; 52(1):38–44.
33. Schwartz AR, Kacmarek RM, Hess DR. Factors affecting oxygen delivery with bi-level positive airway pressure. Respir Care 2004; 49(3):270–275.
34. Schonhofer B, Sortor-Leger S. Equipment needs for noninvasive mechanical ventilation. Eur Respir J 2002; 20:1029–1036.

19
Training the Home Health Team

JOAN ESCARRABILL
Hospital Universitari de Bellvitge, L'Hospitalet de Llobregat, Barcelona, Spain

ALLEN GOLDBERG
American College of Chest Physicians, Northbrook, Illinois, U.S.A.

I. Introduction

The care of patients with chronic illnesses, especially if they suffer a significant degree of dependence, requires the health care system to adopt a totally different approach. Although professional education is adequate to diagnose and treat acute processes, the focus is on cure, which is based more on the illness than on the patient. Acute care emphasizes hardware, such as high technology and complex facilities, while chronic care emphasizes continuity of care, deliberative models, attention to comfort, and caregiver support. If the acute care strategy is adopted for chronic illnesses, care is partial, fragmented, duplicated, and characterized by poor communication between the hospital and the community (1).

Most chronic illness confronts patients and caregivers with changes in daily life and changes in social relations. They produce disability, often with exacerbations. Medical care is usually continuous and, in the case of the patients with respiratory diseases, is also supported by devices such as oxygen or ventilators (2). Facing the final phases of life is another difficult, added pressure. Most patients with chronic illness require support from a variety of health care professionals, often situated in different health facilities. In the chronic care model, it is crucial to evaluate the patient in a stable situation to establish plans of action for the exacerbations, to promote self-management, and to have a good information system.

The World Health Organization identified several areas in which chronic care must provide effective (3) resources in the community, organization of care (system improvement, leadership, and incentives), effective self-management support, changes in delivery system design by delegation of roles to other professionals, regular follow-up, and decision support tools, such as guidelines and clinical information systems.

An important change in the way we care for patients with chronic illnesses is the intervention of a multidisciplinary team, which is able to answer many individual problems among patients with similar needs. As Wagner emphasized (4), a patient care team is a group of diverse health professionals who communicate regularly with each other about the care of a defined group of patients and participate in that care. The team has both stable members and consultants.

The main aim of the team is to provide care for the patient and the caregiver. The independent living model (5) philosophy summarizes, very well, the priority objectives of the care for patients with chronic illnesses. The person with disabilities should have the same choices and control in his daily life than odd-disabled people and they should have the possibility to live in the community.

To summarize, the key element in the discharge plan for patients with severe chronic illnesses and disabilities is the formation of a health team and the objective to reach the maximum possible level of independence in daily living activities for the patient. The training of the teams and the education of health professionals are crucial. Just as Batavia (6) indicates, small clinical problems cause large inconveniences to the patients with chronic diseases. Moreover, patients with chronic illnesses verify, all too often, that few health care professionals understand the issues of the patient with disabilities.

II. The Actors

The care of patients with chronic illnesses requires interaction among several actors besides the main actor, the patient. A core health care team associated with the hospital will interact with consultants, health authorities, and equipment providers. To guarantee high-quality care of the patient, it is important to train and educate the patient and the caregiver.

A. Health Care Team

In most of the cases, the core team is in the hospital. The specialists who participate in ventilation vary, but tend to include chest physicians, pediatricians, anesthetists, intensivists, respiratory nurses, respiratory therapists, and social workers depending on the characteristic organization of each hospital (7). In most cases, the extended team includes the availability of otolaryngology, neurology, speech therapy, gastroenterology, urology, and a clinical dietician. Teams should be trained in the following (4,8):

- Skills related to home mechanical ventilation (HMV) technology and home care
- Ability to assess the adequacy of caregivers
- Knowledge of community resources
- Capacity to integrate home, outpatient, and hospital care
- Designing of guideline-based care plans that integrate the clinical needs and preferences of the patient
- Behavioral counseling and teaching of self-management
- Expertise in group consultations

The specialized team must include community resources (9). The primary care team of physicians, nurses, and social workers should be invited to actively participate in the care plan as they may be more familiar with the family and the available resources. They are also better able to connect with other nonhealth services like schools, patients' support groups, or recreational centers. The core team should organize communication with the community through periodic meetings, once or twice a year. In most of the cases, especially in complex high dependent patients, a care manager is essential for coordinating the discharge plan (10).

B. Emergency Department

One of the weak points in the care of the ventilator-assisted individuals is the sudden, unexpected visit to the emergency department. These visits cause a lot of anguish and dissatisfaction to the patients, as they are cared for by unknown health professionals who may not have a thorough knowledge of the issues regarding their health. Furthermore, the emergency departments are not usually adapted to the physical needs of the patient with disabilities, so that patients may feel more comfortable in their own wheelchair than on a stretcher. It is dangerous for such a patient to make vital decisions in the heat of the moment. This situation is not infrequent among patients with amyotrophic lateral sclerosis (ALS) who gradually develop respiratory discomfort until they are confronted in the emergency room with a decision as to whether a tracheotomy is appropriate. A much better strategy is to plan the care in order to minimize unplanned emergency department visits. Evaluation of stable patients with ALS improves their survival (11) and avoids unnecessary decisions in the emergency department.

C. Financial Issues and Health Authorities

Financial issues in HMV are important with many of the indirect costs falling on the patient and the family (12). About a third of families of patients on HMV reported burden on their employment, especially if they needed to quit their job or to ask for permission to be away (13). The training of the teams should include an analysis of the burden of HMV on the patient and the caregivers, regarding economic issues and the impact that they may have on the health of both parties. Health authorities vary in their willingness to respond to special cases, but the health team should be prepared to justify the special needs to the health authorities.

D. Providers

Care providers play a crucial role in HMV in most countries. The Eurovent survey showed that, in Europe, ventilator servicing, such as maintenance, repair, delivery of spare parts, and regular surveillance, was carried out mainly by private companies. In some countries like Sweden, ventilator servicing was carried out directly by hospitals. The interaction between servicing companies and the prescriber was poor (14). Another problem was the variety of ventilators that exist in the market, with more than 70 models in Europe for 70% preset pressure and 30% volume ventilation.

It is not possible to know all the existing ventilators in the market. Therefore, the teams should be familiar with a limited number of models which are most available and for which parts can be obtained from the local supplier. The type of ventilator is not necessarily the same for children as for adults. It helps if the teams know the local suppliers so that they can discuss ventilation equipment and accessories. Although it is primarily the responsibility of the health care team, the local supplier can be of great help in detecting potential situations of risk. Cooperation between the health team and the local suppliers should be centered on aspects of quality control, as some patients are not ventilated according to the prescribed guidelines for ventilatory support (15). A detailed study showed that there were limitations in quality control in HMV (16). Alarm malfunctioning was detected with power off in 0.9% devices, disconnection in 18.6%, and obstruction in 5.1% of devices. The study also detected differences between actual, set, and prescribed values of ventilator variables: in 13% of the cases, the differences were >20% and in 4% of the cases they were >30%. The magnitude of error emphasizes the interest in quality control. The training of health team, patients, and caregivers should include the importance of quality control.

E. Caregivers

Caring for people with severe disabilities affects the caregivers physically and psychologically. The caregivers who report strain associated with caregiving have an increased mortality (17). Sleep disturbances, physical strain, restrictions of free time, lifestyle disruption, social isolation, work adjustments, financial burden, and a sense of being overwhelmed, all contribute to the stress on the caregiver (18). Navaie-Waliser et al. (19) showed that one-third of caregivers are in the precarious position of providing high-intensity and continuing care.

In the case of HMV, the burden for the caregiver is even heavier. Tracheostomy causes a substantial amount of caregiver strain, which persists over time. Both patients and caregivers have an ongoing need for information about the disease, in spite of their previous experience (20). Education and support are therefore very important, especially around end-of-life issues. Patients and families should actively participate in life-and-death decisions (21). Sometimes the caregiver is a "hidden client." It is important to take care of the health and the welfare of the caregiver during the visits to the patients with HMV. Training the patient and caregiver should be done without hurry and should include all the aspects related to the care of the patient on HMV, as shown in Table 1.

It is best for the same person to educate the patient and the caregiver to avoid any contradictory interpretations. A checklist facilitates education and prevents oversight. The health care professional should ensure that the caregiver can repeat the information before discharge. Written information is very important to avoid oversight or confusion. Finally, the abilities of the caregiver should be evaluated periodically during outpatient clinic visits.

III. The Interface Between Home and Hospital

The discharge plan should enable transfer of the patient from hospital to home in a comfortable and safe way. Although common elements exist, the discharge plans should be individualized according to the needs of each patient. The health care team should keep in mind the following elements that shape the discharge plan:

- *Severity of the disease*: It is important especially for patients with minimal ventilator free time or tracheostomies.
- *Accessibility to the health team*: Distance determines direct accessibility, and for patients who live far from the hospital, it is difficult to guarantee a direct and an immediate solution in the event of an acute problem. Teams in the community near the patients' house can cover risks if they have a good relationship with the specialized hospital team.
- *Complexity of the care*: It is important especially when the patient requires the intervention of several professionals in the context of a severe disease. The complexity in this case is synonymous with the need for coordination.
- *Time of discharge*: The team should know the resources in the community, to select the best time and date of discharge, avoiding weekends and holidays.
- *Intensity of care*: Home care requires periodic visits to the patient. Hospital at home teams can visit patients once or twice a day and telemedicine is a crucial element in the care of such patients (22).

Table 1 Respiratory Care Education for Patients and Caregivers

The nature of the disease:
Prognosis
Complications
End-of-life issues
Use of the devices:
Settings
Power sources (external batteries)
Identification of the alarm systems
Oxygen attachment
Humidification
Suction units
Routine maintenance of ventilators and masks
Airway management:
Tracheotomy tube changes
Management of tracheal obstruction
Management of tracheal decannulation
Cardiopulmonary resuscitation
Ambu bag (emergency bag)
Assisted cough
Manually
Mechanical (cough assist)
Suctioning
Suctioning equipment
Suctioning technique
Risk management:
Power failure and ventilator malfunction
Accidental disconnection
Circuit obstruction
Mask fit
Tracheotomy blocked, fell out or cannot be replaced.
Communication with the health care team:
General maintenance of the devices and communication with servicing suppliers.
Advice regarding practical arrangements for daily living adaptation: house, work, school, and transport.

Source: Adapted from Refs. 25, 27–29.

- *Caregiver's attitude and skills*: It determines the education plan and the need for informal caregivers, besides the family.
- *Resources*: These should be emphasized and they include suppliers, resources in the community for the activities of daily life, transportation, communication devices, home adaptations and hospice, or other facilities for temporary admission.

The main objectives of the home care team are to promote the independence of the patient, to avoid the social isolation, and to prevent the risks of long stays in the hospital. The structure of the home care plan can be broken down into four elements (23,24): preventive actions and assessment, care related to patient needs, redefinition of care plans and service coordination.

Preventive actions and assessment are related to systematic follow-up, especially just after discharge, including physical, psychosocial, social, and cognitive dimensions. In patients on HMV, it is mandatory to try to solve specific needs like tracheostomy care or acute care during exacerbations. Home visits need a more complete appraisal of the situation in which prolonged mechanical ventilation (PMV) is carried out. The health care professional has more time at patient's home. With more information, it is easier to restructure care plans after the home visit, rather than after consultation in the hospital. Service coordination is very important when several professionals participate in the care of patients on HMV.

Patient and caregiver training at the onset of the HMV is very important. Nevertheless, it is necessary to repeat this training periodically as the patients' needs, the caregiver, or the equipment may change. During home visits, the health care professional should check the learned skills of the patient and the caregiver.

IV. Training According to the Needs and Responsibilities

HMV now has been applied for more than 50 years in some countries, but in western countries, the increment of patients has been progressive, especially during the last 15 years. The Eurovent survey showed that in 2001 there were more than 27,000 HMV patients who were treated in over 480 centers. The study showed wide variations in the patterns of HMV throughout Europe (25). There were large differences in the relative percentage of users in each diagnostic category, in the size of the center, in the percentage of patients with tracheotomy, and in the availability of home care.

Most European centers supervise less than 50 patients. This limits the ventilator experience of the staff. But these small centers can provide the patient greater accessibility. The solution to the dilemma between accessibility and expertise is the creation of networks of centers. The centers with more expertise, technology, and specialists can give support to local centers with less technological resources but who are able to provide closer attention to the patient. Eventually the patient may be transferred from the local center to the center with more technological support for a more complex evaluation, but the routine care is given in the most accessible place. Moreover, in the context of a network the introduction of innovations is easier and permits a more homogeneous dissemination.

In this context, the role of the healthcare coordinator is very important (26), as for each individual, issues such as supervision of the home equipment, or planning of the visits for education, or continued training will improve the quality of life for those receiving PMV.

References

1. DeBusk RF, West JA, Houston Miller N, et al. Chronic disease management. Arch Intern Med 1999; 159; 2739–2742.
2. Wagner EH, Groves T. Care for chronic diseases. BMJ 2002; 325(7370):913–914.
3. World Health Organization. *Innovative care for chronic conditions: building blocks for action.* Geneva: World Health Organization, 2002.
4. Wagner EH. The role of patient care teams in chronic disease management. BMJ 2000; 320:569–571.

5. The Independent Living Institute. Available at: http://www.independentliving.org/. Accessed January 10, 2007.
6. Batavia AI. Accounting for the health-care bill. Lancet 2003; 362:1495–1497.
7. Goldberg AI. Your role in pediatric home ventilation. J Respir Dis 1991; 12:471–480.
8. Boling PA. The physician's role in home health care. New York: Springer, 1997.
9. Goldberg AI. Long-term ventilatory support in the community. Chest 1993; 103:1315–1316.
10. Warren ML, Jarrett C, Senegal R, et al. An interdisciplinary approach to transitioning ventilator-dependent patients to home. J Nurs Care Qual 2004; 19:67–73.
11. Farrero E, Prats E, Povedano M, et al. Survival in amyotrophic lateral sclerosis with home mechanical ventilation: the impact of systematic respiratory assessment and bulbar involvement. Chest 2005; 127:2132–2138.
12. Sevick MA, Kamlet MS, Hoffman LA, et al. Economic cost of home-based care for ventilator-assisted individuals. Chest 1996; 109:1597–1606.
13. Tsara V, Serasli E, Voutsas V, et al. Burden and coping strategies in families of patients under noninvasive home mechanical ventilation. Respiration 2006; 73:61–67.
14. Farre R, Lloyd-Owen SJ, Ambrosino N, et al. Quality control of equipment in home mechanical ventilation: a European survey. Eur Respir J 2005; 26:86–94.
15. Farré R, Giró E, Casolive V, et al. Quality control of mechanical ventilation at the patient's home. Intensive Care Med 2003; 29:484–486.
16. Farré R, Navajas D, Prats E, et al. Performance of mechanical ventilators at the patient's home: a multicentre quality study. Thorax 2006; 61:400–404.
17. Schulz R, Beach SR. Caregiving as a risk factor for mortality: the Caregiver Health Effects Study. JAMA 1999; 282:2215–2219.
18. Koopmanschap MA, van Exel NJA, van den Bis GAM, et al. The desire for support and respite care: preferences of Dutch informal caregivers. Health Policy 2004; 68:309–320.
19. Navaie-Waliser M, Feldman PH, Gould DA, et al. When the caregiver needs care: the plight of vulnerable caregivers. Am J Public Health 2002; 92:409–413.
20. Rossi Ferrario S, Zotti AM, Zaccaria S, et al. Caregiver strain associated with tracheostomy in chronic respiratory failure. Chest 2001; 119:1498–1502.
21. Gilgoff I, Prentice W, Baydur A. Patient and family participation in the management of respiratory failure in Duchenne's muscular dystrophy. Chest 1989; 95:519–524.
22. Miyasaka K, Suzuki Y, Sakai H, et al. Interactive communication in high-technology home care: videophones for pediatric ventilatory care. Pediatrics 1997; 99:E1.
23. Thome B, Dykes AK, Hallberg IR. Home care with regard to definition, care recipients, content and outcome: systematic literature review. J Clin Nurs 2003; 12:860–872.
24. Nett LM, Obrigewith R. Home visiting system and improved quality of life. In: Kira S, Petty TL, eds. Progress in Domiciliary Respiratory Care. Amsterdam: Excerpta Medica, 1994.
25. Lloyd-Owen SJ, Donaldson GC, Ambrosino N, et al. Patterns of home mechanical ventilation use in Europe: results from the Eurovent survey. Eur Respir J 2005; 25:1025–1031.
26. Tearl DK, Cox TJ, Hertzog JH. Hospital discharge of respiratory-technology-dependent children: role of a dedicated respiratory care discharge coordinator. Respir Care 2006; 51:744–749.
27. Simonds AK. Non-invasive Respiratory Support. London: Oxford University Press, 2001.
28. Simonds AK. Risk management of the home ventilator dependent patient. Thorax 2006; 61(5): 369–371.
29. Donner CF, Zaccaria S, Braghiroli A, et al. Organization of home care in patients receiving nocturnal ventilatory support. Eur Respir Mon 1998; 8:320–399.

20
Discharge and Follow-Up

PAULEEN PRATT
Critical Care and Chronic Ventilation Service, University Hospitals of Leicester, NHS Trust, Leicester, U.K.

JOAN ESCARRABILL
Hospital Universitari de Bellvitge, L'Hospitalet de Llobregat, Barcelona, Spain

I. Introduction

The assessment of home discharge and follow-up of the patient with chronic respiratory failure who is medically stable, but requires home mechanical ventilation (HMV), can be complex (1). In the United Kingdom, guidelines are available for pediatric patients (2), but not for adults. Patients considered for HMV vary from the failed-to-wean critical care patients to those with chronic respiratory failure, associated with thoracic restriction disease (TRD), neuromuscular disease (NMD), spinal cord injury (SCI), or chronic obstructive pulmonary disease (COPD). Some commence noninvasive ventilation (NIV) electively after referral to a respiratory specialist. Adequate planning will increase the chances of a successful outcome for the patient, family, and caregivers as well as improve the quality of life of the patient (3). In this chapter, we will discuss the predischarge planning, discharge home, and the follow-up required to achieve successful discharge of the adult ventilated patient (4). There are several barriers to the discharge of children and young people, including the attitude of professionals, the lack of joint commissioning, the lack of ongoing accountability, as well as poor management within health care systems and other partner agencies. These issues are also reflected in the adult population, especially among those ventilated with a tracheostomy. Domiciliary ventilation may be noninvasive or invasive, and ventilation times vary from a few hours at night to total 24-hour ventilation.

The patients' dependence on ventilation must be balanced against the adverse issues related to this dependency and the psychological impact of needing overnight ventilation should not be underestimated when planning for home care (5). (Fig. 1).

II. Predischarge

A. Patient Evaluation

In order to establish the feasibility of home discharge or discharge to a nonacute environment, the following factors should be taken into account.

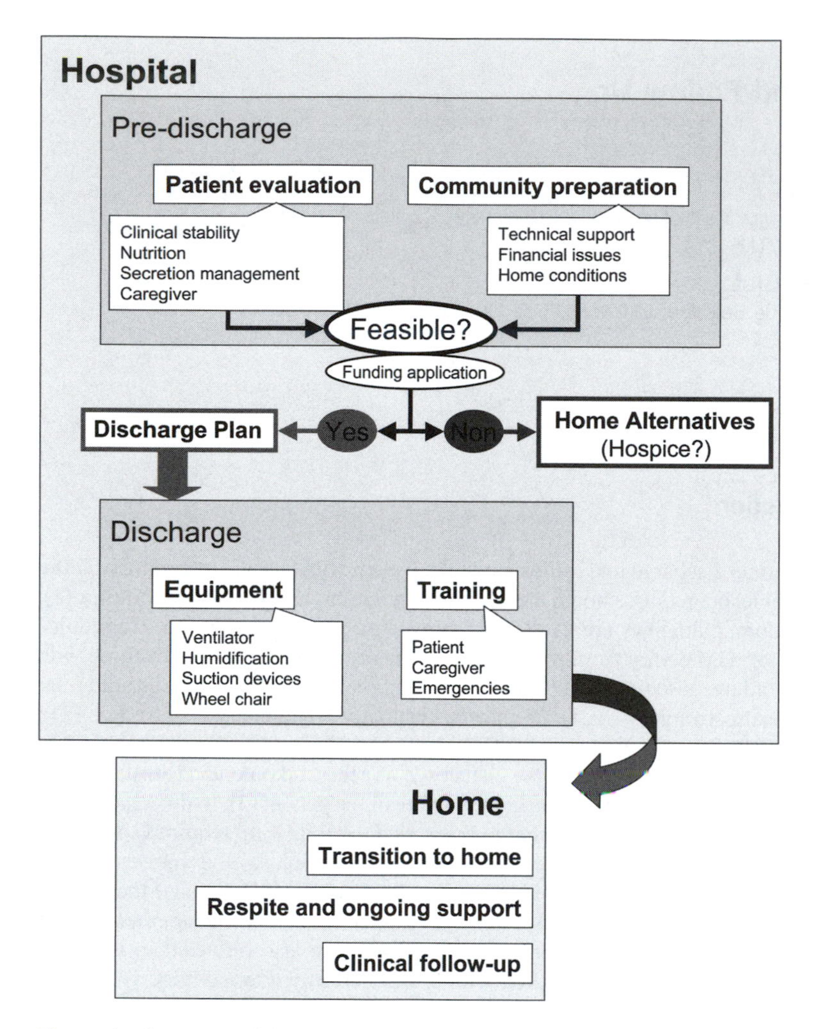

Figure 1 Summary of discharge planning.

Clinical Stability

Both the respiratory system and other comorbidities, especially cardiovascular conditions, should be stable so that ventilator settings and oxygenation no longer require regular medical intervention. The only exception is the patient returning home for end-of-life care, who may be discharged once a palliative care plan is in place.

Nutrition

Adequate nutrition is important. Patients with NIV intermittently are often able to maintain oral intake and some patients, ventilated through a tracheostomy, can also do so provided their swallowing is not impaired. As ventilation can adversely affect swallowing and lead to aspiration (6), patients with bulbar involvement will require swallow assessment and may need placement of a percutaneous endoscopic gastrostomy (PEG) tube.

Secretion Management

Airway secretions must be manageable, with suctioning or mechanically assisted coughing (7). The ability to clear secretions will influence the choice of tracheostomy or the decision to use NIV.

Patient and Family Attitude to Home Care

The patients and caregivers must be motivated for discharge home. Families often underestimate the challenges associated with caring for a ventilated patient at home, particularly those with significant disabilities. It is important that they be aware of the physical and emotional burdens that home ventilation may bring. The home itself may need to be adapted to accommodate the patient's needs of accessibility. Some patients need caregivers to help provide for their needs and companies that specialize in this area are becoming available. The criteria for the assessment of suitability for discharge are summarized in Table 1.

During the evaluation, it will be necessary to establish if the discharge home will be feasible or if an alternate environment for HMV should be considered.

The patient's medical and social requirements should be considered in the light of the actual home conditions, caregiver's attitude and training, distance from the hospital, and availability of technical resources. The team must make a therapeutic alliance with the patient and caregivers if HMV is to be successful, especially in more severely dependent patients. Alternatives to home, such as hospice, long-term care facility, or nursing home can be helpful, whether for a transitional move or for a permanent placement. The aim is to ensure the highest possible level of independence rather than create an acute care environment in the patient's home.

B. Community Preparation

The patient's general practitioner and any community support staff should be involved together with the multidisciplinary team in planning the patient's discharge. If the patient is going home for palliative care, a palliative care consultant and support team should be included.

Table 1 Summary of Criteria for Discharge

Criteria to be met
Ventilation and oxygen needs stable or palliative care plan
Cardiovascular stability or palliative care plan
Patient and family motivated to achieve discharge
Feeding established
Technical resources can be managed at home
Organization of care in the community can be achieved
Funding can be gained for home care package

Health care funding differs among various jurisdictions, even in the same country. The recent Eurovent survey (8) noted wide variations across Europe in users, equipment, and interfaces. In the United Kingdom, nursing care is funded after assessment of the nature, complexity, intensity, and predictability of clinical care needs (9,10).

III. Discharge

A. Equipment

Ventilators

There are over 30 models of ventilators available for home use (11) with inter- and intra-country differences in prescribing and maintenance (12). The care team chooses equipment based on the mode of ventilation, patient mobility, simplicity of use, power and alarm features, as well as maintenance costs. It is advisable to obtain the ventilator before discharge to enable the patient and care team to ensure the most appropriate settings (13). If a patient is dependent on ventilation 24 hours a day, backup power, a backup ventilator, and more rigorous alarms are necessary.

Humidification

Patients receiving noninvasive positive pressure ventilation (NIPPV) have lesser requirements for humidification than those invasively ventilated. Consideration of cuff inflation or deflation will also influence humidification requirements. Humidification involves additional training and a greater risk for patients as well as more maintenance. As several home humidification devices are available, local preferences should be sought. A heat moisture exchanger (HME) offers more flexibility and fewer restrictions for mobility than a heated water bath system (HWB), although a combination (HME-day and HWB-night) may be used for 24-hour ventilation. When assessing HME, the amount of water vapor (in mg/L) should be checked as variations in humidification are significant and the higher the amount of humidification, the better the effect and less the risk of adverse effects.

Suction Devices

Tracheal suctioning may be necessary to assist with secretion clearance. Home suction devices vary in their portability and suction pressures.

Other Equipment

Apart from the basics of ventilation, items such as specialist beds, mattress, home oxygen cylinders, chairs, and a hoist to ensure safe transfer from bed to chair with a minimal number of caregivers, all need to be considered, sourced, and purchased during the planning phase.

Wheel Chair

Mobility is essential to optimize quality of life and ensure that the patient can be mobile. In the United Kingdom, the occupational therapist assesses the patient and orders the wheelchairs, which must also provide a shelf for a portable ventilator.

Disposable Equipment

Funding for disposables, such as ventilator tubing, humidification chambers, suction catheters, etc. must be considered. It is helpful to list all ongoing disposable items to pass on to the general practitioner and community care team in order to ensure that everybody involved has adequate information as to who is responsible for these items, prior to discharge. This will prevent the patient from running out of basic equipment.

B. Training of Family and Caregivers

It is important to work out the individual training needs for family and caregivers including many of the items listed in Table 2. For nocturnal noninvasive ventilation minimal training may be needed, beyond attaching the interface and managing the alarms. However, for those with tracheostomy intermittent positive pressure ventilation (TIPPV) and no ventilator free time, a much more comprehensive training plan is needed, including ventilation care, suctioning, tracheostomy care, plus any other disease-specific care that the patient will need such as feeding, pressure area management, etc.

Trainees must practice suctioning, ventilator tubing changes, tracheostomy changes, and applying interfaces under supervision. Effective training will reduce the risk of readmission to hospital. Good training documentation is also important.

Training of caregivers can increase the anxiety of clinical staff who may not wish to train nonregistered practitioners in "advanced skills" for reasons of risk management and accountability. Issues of staff support, insurance, and liability need to be addressed. Clinical staff need support in handing over care to nonregistered persons and should have an identified senior practitioner to call upon if they have any specific concerns. The caregivers require basic skills to maintain safety at home. It is useful to develop laminated sheets that they can post to remind themselves of simple things such as how to check the humidifier, what different alarms mean, how to set up ventilator tubing with a humidifier, all of which will reassure the patient and their caregivers.

Table 2 Training Plan for Domiciliary Mechanical Ventilation

Items
Care of ventilator, humidifier, and any other equipment
Principles of how the ventilator works and the patient's dependence on this
How to trouble shoot and manage alarms
What power and battery backup in available and how to check that it works
Where to get technical and clinical help
What to do in an emergency if the clinical condition changes
How to assemble, clean, and reset the equipment
How to manage interface (mask, mouthpiece, etc)
How to care for and change a tracheotomy
How to suction or use cough assistance devices

Communication of any risks and actions involved with HMV will ensure that people feel secure in the responsibilities that they are assuming. Funding for educational packages may be necessary and ongoing costs to include many years of life expectancy, as well as an evolving medical condition, need to be planned. Local nurses must be competent in using the ventilator, tracheostomy care, and any other medical considerations as general practitioners and district nurses do not frequently attend such complex patients. A case manager may be required to coordinate care, especially during the initial months of HMV. The patients should receive written information on the equipment and who to call if they have problems. Some patients benefit from partial discharge for a single night or weekend before the final discharge is achieved to gain confidence in the process and to identify any additional areas of concern.

IV. Postdischarge Follow-Up

A. Transition to Home

On the first day after discharge, it is advisable for a home visit to be carried out by an experienced practitioner, ideally the case manager, who is able to troubleshoot and address issues that have occurred in the short span of time since discharge. It is also useful at this point to ensure that the family and patient are well aware of any follow-up referrals that are going to be needed, i.e., referral back to the respiratory physician or to the critical care team dependant on how practice is agreed locally. Technical support may be needed to address any ventilation issues, alarm, or interface problems. The ventilator will need annual servicing. The family must know whom to contact if they have problems with their ventilator, whether they have second machine available, and how to set it up in such a way that it is simple to connect (14).

B. Respite and Ongoing Support

Respite care and ongoing support will optimize the potential for successful home care as the burden of home care can be great (15). Many day centers are not used to taking patients who are ventilated. If a primary caregiver leaves or is unable to cope, the whole family system needs to be reviewed. Respite should be available, and in palliative care patients, a hospice bed may be required. Life expectancy varies and end-of-life issues should respect the patients' wishes. For this to happen, the patient and family should be encouraged to discuss a plan, possibly with the involvement of a palliative care consultant.

C. Readmission Issues

It is important to clarify whether readmission to a critical care environment or any further escalation of treatment is appropriate. This will vary among patients and should respect their wishes as well as the medical indications. Advanced directives for accepting or refusing certain treatments, in the event of a deterioration, must be noted, preferably before discharge home. Therefore, discussions with the family caregivers will help clarify the patient's best interests and their wishes.

Potential for readmission and interventions that are to be delivered in emergency situations should be clarified with the health care teams, in the hospital and the community. In the United Kingdom, there are facilities to register HMV patients with the ambulance service, so that they are aware of the situation if an emergency call is made to that address.

V. Summary

The discharge of patients for HMV is a complex organizational challenge, especially for those with no ventilator free time. A case manager will greatly assist in coordination with health care services and communication with the family and caregivers to ensure a seamless transition from hospital to home. Patients and families require training and should know where to get help after discharge home. Graduated discharge is helpful in addressing any new issues and home visits with a caregiver and a practitioner will build confidence of the family and patient. Patients and family members need to be recognized as individuals as medical and social circumstances vary.

In this chapter, we have highlighted the basic principles of managing the discharge home of the patient who requires prolonged mechanical ventilation. Although this may present major challenges to all concerned, the benefits in health-related quality of life and life expectancy may be substantial. Although some patients do find that the burden of HMV to be very difficult, most adjust with the help of home supports and many go on to achieve the unexpected (16).

There are many useful internet websites available for caregivers and patients. Particularly of use is the Ventilator User Network (www.post-polio.org/ivun).

References

1. Vitacca M, Guerra A, Pizzocaro P, et al. Time consuming of Physicians and Nurses before discharge in patients with chronic respiratory failure submitted to home mechanical ventilation. Rasegna di Patologia dell'Apparto Respiratorio 2005; 20(6):275–283.
2. Elspeth J, Colin W. Core guidelines for the discharge home of the child on long term assisted ventilation in the United Kingdom. Thorax 1998; 53:762–767.
3. Lindahl B, Sandman O, Rasmussen B. Meaning of living at home on a ventilator. Nurs Inq 2003; 10(1):19–27.
4. Noyles J. Barriers that delay children and young people who are dependant on mechanical ventilators from being discharged from hospital. J Clin nurs 2002; 11(1):2–11.
5. Ingadottir T, Jonsdottir H. Technological dependency. The experience of using home ventilators and home oxygen: patients and family perspectives. Scand J Caring Sci 2006; 20(1):18–25.
6. Hales P. Swallowing. In: Russel C, Matta B, eds. Tracheostomy - A Multiprofessional Handbook. London: Greenwich Health care Medical, 2004:187–208.
7. Van Der Schans C, Bach J, Rubin B. Chest physical therapy: mucous mobilising techniques. In: Bach J, ed. Non-invasive Mechanical Ventilation. Philadelphia: Hanley and Belfus Publications, 2002:259–284.
8. Lloyd-Owen SJ, Donaldson GC, Ambrosino N, et al. Patterns of home mechanical ventilation use in Europe: results from the Eurovent survey. Eur Respir J 2005; 25:1025–1031.
9. Department of Health. National Service Framework for Long Term conditions. HMSO 2005.
10. Department of Health. NHS Funding for Long Term Care of Older and Disabled People. Parliamentary and Health Service Ombudsman; HMSO 2002.

11. Farré R, Navajas D, Prats E, et al. Performance of mechanical ventilators at the patient's home: a multicentre quality study. Thorax 2006; 61:400–404.
12. Gonzalex-Bermejo J, Laplanche V, Hussenini F, et al. Evaluation of the user friendliness of 11 home mechanical ventilators. Eur Respir J 2006; 27(6):1236–1243.
13. Farre R, Lloyd-Owen SJ, Ambrosino N, et al. Quality control of equipment in home mechanical ventilation: a European survey. Eur Respir J 2005; 26:86–94.
14. Schonhofer B, Sortor-Leger. Equipment needs for non-invasive mechanical ventilation. Eur Respir J 2002; 20:1029–1036.
15. Douglas S, Daly B. Caregivers of long term ventilator patients: physical and psychological outcomes. Chest 2003; 123:1073–1081.
16. Available at: www.scubadivingdream.com.

21
Health-Related Quality of Life

CLAUDIO F. DONNER
Mondo Medico, Multidisciplinary and Rehabilitation Outpatient Clinic, Borgomanero, Novara, Italy

NICOLINO AMBROSINO
Pulmonary and Respiratory Intensive Care Unit-University Hospital Pisa, Italy and Pulmonary Rehabilitation and Weaning Center, Auxilium Vitae, Volterra (PI), Italy

I. Introduction

When long-term ventilation (via either nasal mask or tracheostomy) is needed, even if only overnight, patients usually have problems in performing the basic activities of daily life such as washing, dressing, and cooking. Consequently, they experience an important physical and psychological handicap that contributes to the high social and economic cost of their condition. Therefore, the effect of therapy on patients' health status and sense of well-being, i.e., their health-related quality of life (HRQL) represents an important outcome of treatment. As the number of patients who survive the intensive care unit (ICU) is increasing, it is becoming more and more evident that their HRQL may be compromised following a critical illness. Almost half of the patients who survive acute respiratory distress syndrome (ARDS) manifest neurocognitive sequelae two years after their illness. Anxiety and depression are commonly noted in this population, whose HRQL is poor (1).

There is limited information on the health status of patients who required immediate ICU admission for acute respiratory failure due to exacerbations of chronic obstructive pulmonary disease (COPD). COPD patients surviving acute or chronic respiratory failure and requiring mechanical ventilation experience a worse perceived health status and cognitive function than stable COPD patients on long-term oxygen therapy (LTOT) who have never previously required ICU admission, although after discharge their health and cognitive status may improve to levels similar to those of stable COPD patients on LTOT (2).

II. Assessment

The terms quality of life (QoL), HRQL, and health status (HS) are often used interchangeably despite the fact that they represent different concepts (3). QoL can be defined as the gap between desires and the degree to which these are achieved. HRQL signifies the effect of disease on this gap. Both QoL and HRQL are subjective indicators of how an individual rates his or her life. HS, on the other hand, measures how a disease impacts on the patient's daily life and well-being, relative to the specific population of similar patients.

III. QoL in Ventilated Patients

Parameters commonly used to measure functional damage or improvement in mechanically ventilated patients correlate poorly with reported impairments of physical function or overall QoL. Therefore they provide an incomplete picture of the patient's HS (4). Although in COPD there is clearly a negative relationship between the spirometric mean values of different patient populations and their QoL, it is well known that within a given study population, this correlation is weak irrespective of the questionnaire used (4–6). There is a growing need for a global estimate of health in patients on long-term home mechanical ventilation, which cannot be inferred from indirect or surrogate measures. An adequate assessment of QoL can only be obtained from the patients themselves by direct measurement using valid, reliable, and interpretable questionnaires.

A. Generic Instruments

Generic questionnaires have been used in patients receiving long-term ventilation to explore HS domains such as emotional functioning, mood changes, activities of daily living, social relationships, and hobbies (7). However, not being designed specifically for respiratory diseases or chronic respiratory failure (CRF), they contain relatively few items of direct relevance to this patient population and many items that are irrelevant.

Medical Outcome Study Questionnaire Short Form 36-item (SF_{36})

The SF_{36} (8) has eight component scores labeled physical function, physical role limitation, bodily pain, general health, vitality, social function, emotional role limitation, mental health, plus a single item on the reported health transition over the last year. Each dimension is scored separately and then transformed to a 0 to 100 scale, with lower scores indicating poorer health. The physical and mental component categories are collapsed to produce two summary scores, the physical component score (PCS) and the mental component score (MCS). The questionnaire takes 5 to 10 minutes to complete and is self-administered.

Simonds and Elliott (9) studied patients with CRF caused by either obstructive or restrictive diseases who required night nasal intermittent positive pressure ventilation (NIPPV). The results, summarized in Figure 1, illustrate that the NIPPV group had a significantly higher impairment in physical function compared to patients with other chronic diseases. General health and mental health were similar to those of patients with other chronic diseases, while physical role limitation and pain were less impaired than in other chronic diseases. Mental health was similar to that of normal subjects.

A comparison of the impact of hypoxia (10) and NIPPV (9) on QoL, as in Figure 2, demonstrates that hypoxic patients have a worse HS than patients requiring overnight mechanical ventilation in terms of their general health, physical function, role limitation due to physical problems, social function, and vitality. This might be attributable to hypoxemia as the hypoxic patients were not on LTOT, whereas those receiving NIPPV had increased arterial oxygen tension (Pa_{O_2}) and reduced arterial carbon dioxide tension (Pa_{CO_2}). Low levels of Pa_{O_2} and high levels of Pa_{CO_2} can negatively affect higher cerebral function, although no differences in mental health have been noted when comparing normal subjects to hypoxic patients and ventilated patients.

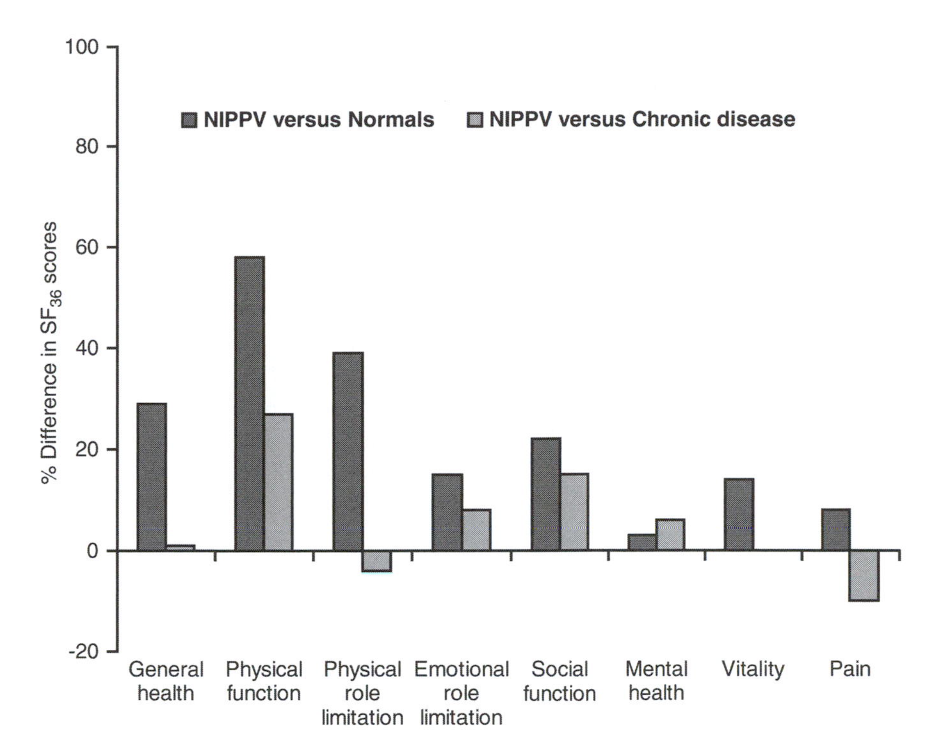

Figure 1 Medical Research Council Short Form Questionnaire (SF_{36}) scores in patients on NIPPV compared with normal subjects (NIPPV vs. normals) and patients with other chronic diseases (NIPPV vs. chronic disease). Positive values indicate a worse quality of life in the NIPPV group. *Abbreviation*: NIPPV, nasal intermittent positive pressure ventilation. *Source*: Modified from Ref. 10.

The SF_{36} was also administered to a group of patients with severe respiratory failure one year after their successful discharge from an ICU (11). All patients had acute or acute on chronic respiratory failure following a chronic pulmonary disease, neuromuscular disorder, chest wall deformity, or sleep apnea with difficult weaning from mechanical ventilation. Despite the very low scores for general health, physical function, and role limitation due to physical problems that were expected given the extreme physical disability, the scores for emotional role limitation, mental health, vitality, and pain did not differ substantially from those of the general population (Fig. 3).

These studies demonstrate that although the SF_{36} is used and is broadly applicable to patients on ventilation, many dimensions of the SF_{36} are too insensitive to differentiate between patients on mechanical ventilation and other conditions.

B. Disease-specific Questionnaires

To increase the level of sensitivity to an impairment in health status, disease-specific questionnaires have been developed. The Chronic Respiratory Questionnaire (CRQ) (12)

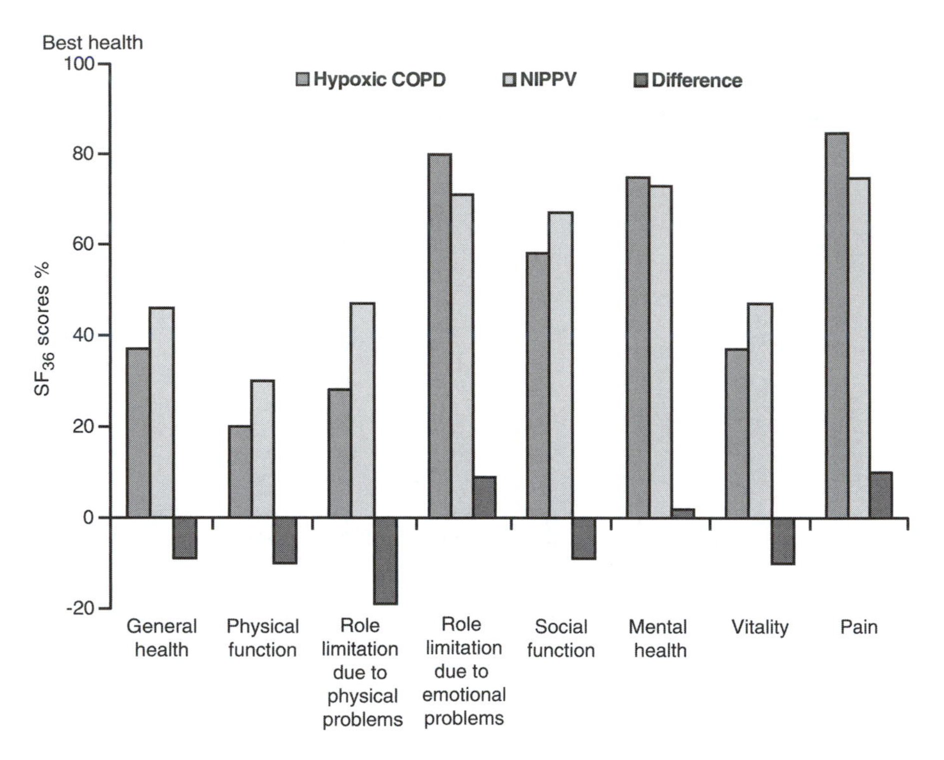

Figure 2 Comparison of Medical Research Council Short Form Questionnaire (SF_{36}) scores in hypoxic patients and in patients on NIPPV. Positive values indicate a worse quality of life in the NIPPV group. *Abbreviations*: COPD, chronic obstructive pulmonary disease; NIPPV, noninvasive positive pressure ventilation. *Source*: Modified from Ref. 26.

and the St. George's Respiratory Questionnaire (SGRQ) (13) are two questionnaires used in severely impaired COPD patients. While the CRQ has been used in patients with forced expiratory volume in 1 second (FEV_1) $\leq$ 39%, its role among those with CRF has not been described (14). In contrast, although the SGRQ was originally designed for patients with asthma or COPD, it has also been used in ventilated COPD patients.

St George's Respiratory Questionnaire

The SGRQ is a self-administered 50-item scale, with 76 weighted responses, grouped into three components: symptoms, a measure of distress due to respiratory symptoms; activity, that causes or is limited by breathlessness; and impacts, a measure of the overall disturbance to daily life and well-being. It takes about 15 minutes to complete. In addition to the component scores, the total score gives a global estimate of the patient's respiratory health. The SGRQ scores range from 0 (best health) to 100 (poorest health). For the total score, a change in score over time of at least 4 points is considered clinically significant (15). The SGRQ is available throughout Europe, North and South America, and versions exist in a number of eastern European and Far Eastern languages.

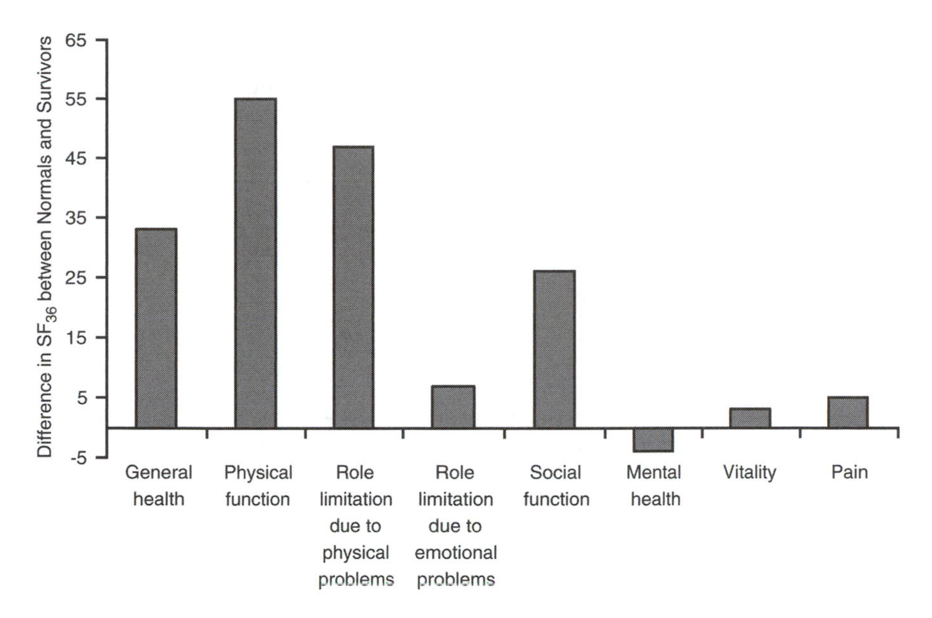

Figure 3 Difference in health status as measured by the Medical Research Council Short Form Questionnaire (SF_{36}) between the normal population and patients surviving 1 year after successful weaning. Positive values indicate a worse quality of life in the group "survivors". *Source*: Modified from Ref. 12.

In patients with COPD and severe hypoxemia, the SGRQ has been correlated with the patient's severity of hypoxemia, a correlation only detectable when using disease-specific questionnaires (16). In fact, this relationship was strong when measured by the SGRQ ($p < 0.01$) and absent with a generic instrument such as the sickness impact profile (SIP). When considering other parameters of health impairment such as the FEV_1 and $Paco_2$, only the degree of hypoxia represented a significant covariate of the SGRQ total score.

In a randomized, crossover study comparing the effects of NIPPV plus LTOT to those of LTOT alone among hypercapnic COPD patients, the SGRQ was sensitive to changes following ventilation (17). QoL with oxygen plus NIPPV was significantly better than with oxygen alone (Fig. 4). During LTOT alone, there was a significant deterioration in the impact and total scores. Conversely, during the NIPPV plus LTOT study period symptoms, impact and total scores improved significantly compared to LTOT alone. The symptom scores also significantly improved over the run-in. Data from this study showed that in severely impaired COPD patients, the combination of LTOT and NIPPV leads to significant improvements in the patients' perceived QoL. It is worth noting that the difference in total score between LTOT alone and LTOT plus NIPPV was nearly 10 units, more than double the minimum clinically significant difference of four units (15).

In another study, investigating the effect of six months' domiciliary NIPPV in 14 hypercapnic COPD patients (18), the SGRQ improved (Fig. 5). Mean baseline scores during the four-week run-in period were very high, reflecting the marked impairment:

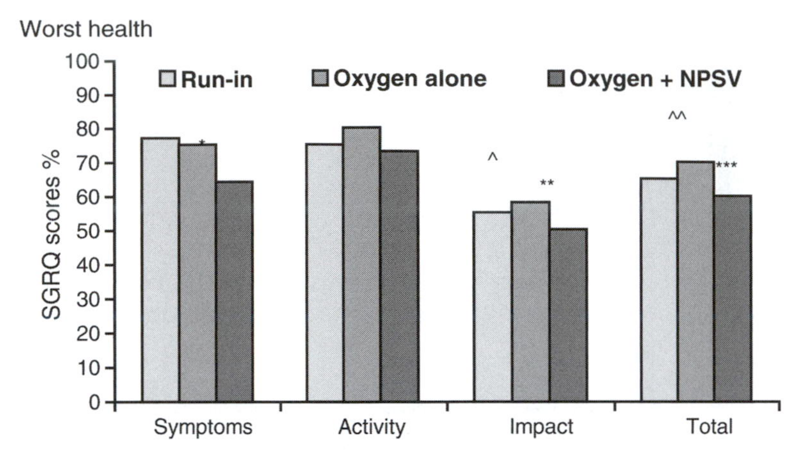

Figure 4 SGRQ scores in 14 patients with hypercapnic chronic obstructive pulmonary disease at baseline, after three months of oxygen therapy alone, and after three months of oxygen therapy plus NPSV. Deteriorated versus run-in, ^$p = 0.01$, ^^$p = 0.03$. Improved versus run-in, +$p = 0.007$. Improved versus oxygen alone, *$p = 0.03$, **$p = 0.002$, ***$p = 0.001$. *Abbreviations*: SGRQ, St. George's Respiratory Questionnaire; NPSV, nasal pressure support ventilation. *Source*: Modified from Ref. 18.

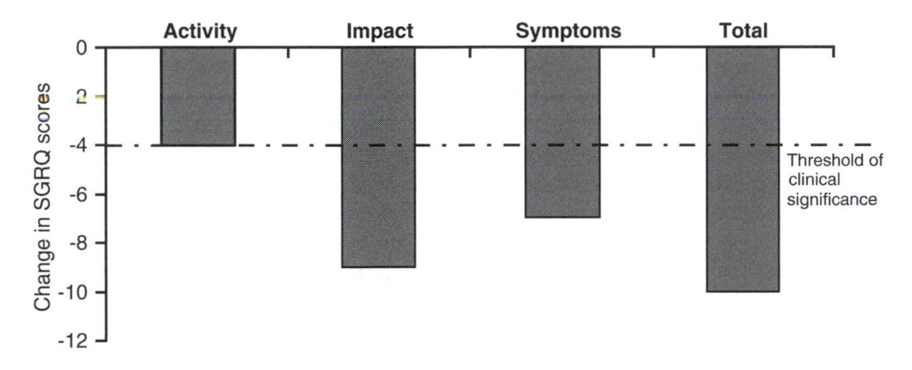

Figure 5 Change in SGRQ scores after six months of nasal intermittent positive pressure ventilation. *Abbreviation*: SGRQ, St. George's Respiratory Questionnaire. *Source*: Modified from Ref. 19.

activity, 69%; impact, 58%; symptoms, 68%; total, 68%. At the end of six months' NIPPV, the improvement was most evident in impact (−9 U) and total (−10 U) scores, in which it was also statistically significant ($p = 0.04$). The improvement in total score was well above the threshold for clinical significance.

Although the SF_{36} and the SGRQ have been used in very severe respiratory patients, neither questionnaire was specifically developed for patients with CRF. These patients may be placed at the very end of the usable scoring range of these questionnaires. Furthermore, CRF can be caused by either obstructive (COPD) or restrictive (kyphoscoliosis, neuromuscular) diseases, but neither the SF_{36} nor SGRQ was designed for them. At present, the only questionnaire specifically designed for CRF is the Maugeri Foundation Respiratory Failure Questionnaire (MRF_{28}) (19).

Maugeri Foundation Respiratory Failure Questionnaire

This 28-item questionnaire was designed to measure health impairment in severe obstructive (COPD) patients or patients with restrictive conditions receiving LTOT or NIPPV. Developed originally in Italy and the United Kingdom and validated for Italian respiratory patients, it has been translated into Czech, English (United Kingdom, United States, Canada), French (Canada, Switzerland) (20), German, Italian, Japanese, Portuguese (Brazil), and Spanish. The MRF_{28} items cover a wide range of areas of life relevant to severe respiratory disease including respiratory and general symptoms, activities, beliefs, attitudes, and expectations relating to ill health, neuropsychological deficits, and social life. The item response option is dichotomous (true or false).

Items are grouped into three specific factors: (*i*) daily activities, i.e., disability in daily life due to breathlessness; (*ii*) cognitive function, i.e., the effect of impaired cognitive function on daily life; (*iii*) invalidity, i.e., the experience of social isolation or dependency on others. Scores range from 0 (best health status) to 100% (worst health status). The MRF_{28} shows that (*i*) it is possible to measure the effect of cognitive dysfunction on the daily life of COPD patients (21,22); (*ii*) the unpleasant effects of respiratory devices often do not correlate with the perception of health (23,24); and (*iii*) most consequences of severe respiratory disease are unrelated to the underlying disease process (25).

The MRF_{28}, which takes 7 to 10 minutes to complete and is self-administered, is able to discriminate between different levels of health impairment better than any other existing questionnaires (19). In particular, its score distribution is wider than that of the SGRQ, SIP, or SF_{36} (Fig. 6). Moreover, in patients with CRF, the MRF_{28} scores are normally distributed and cover the entire range of the questionnaire. In contrast, SGRQ scores cover 76% of its potential range, while SIP and SF_{36} present very narrow interquartile ranges and their score distribution is skewed. This suggests that the MRF_{28} may be a more discriminative instrument for CRF patients than other measures.

To evaluate the long-term reliability of MRF_{28} and its predictive ability for health care utilization, a multinational three-year follow-up study on CRF (Quality of Life Evaluation and Survival Study, QuESS) is underway, involving 73 researchers in nine countries (26). Preliminary data from QuESS show that whereas baseline spirometry, exercise performance, and arterial blood gas analysis are not able to discriminate between patients who will or will not survive, the SGRQ and MRF_{28} are good predictors of mortality in very severe respiratory patients.

A two-year multicenter study (27) examined the effects of NIPPV plus LTOT compared with LTOT alone. In this trial, NIPPV plus LTOT improved $Paco_2$ during oxygen breathing, but survival was similar between treatment groups. After two years, the SGRQ total score, in both groups, showed a slight improvement (4% and 5%) at the limit of clinical significance, mainly because of an improvement in symptoms. Unlike the SGRQ, the MRF_{28} total score showed an improvement only in the NIPPV group. The lack of correlation between the SGRQ and MRF_{28} suggests the need to evaluate QoL using specific instruments for the ventilator-dependent population.

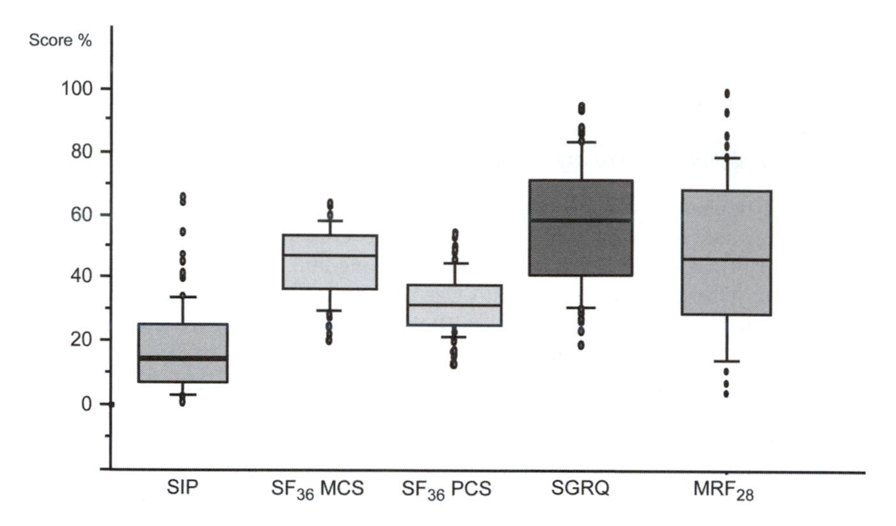

Figure 6 Box plots showing the distribution of scores for the SIP, SF_{36} MCS, SF_{36} PCS, SGRQ, and MRF_{28}. *Abbreviations*: SIP, sickness impact profile; SF_{36} MCS, mental component summary score of the Medical Research Council Short Form Questionnaire; SF_{36} PCS, physical component summary score of the Medical Research Council Short Form Questionnaire; SGRQ, St George's Respiratory Questionnaire total score; MRF_{28}, Maugeri Foundation Respiratory Failure Questionnaire total score. *Source*: Modified from Ref. 26.

C. The Severe Respiratory Insufficiency Questionnaire

Another specific instrument for measuring QoL in ventilated patients is the severe respiratory insufficiency (SRI) questionnaire, developed and tested for its psychometric properties in a multicenter clinical trial that included 226 patients receiving home mechanical ventilation (28). Forty-nine items passed the selection process and were allocated to seven subscales: respiratory complaints, physical functioning, attendant symptoms and sleep, social relationships, anxiety, psychologic well-being, and social functioning. Cronbach's α was >0.7 in all subscales and >0.8 in four of the subscales, indicating high internal consistency. Construct validity by factor analysis indicated one summary scale that accounted for 59.8% of the variance. Concurrent validity was confirmed by correlating subscales of the SRI with the SF_{36} ($0.21 < r < 0.79$). Item-scale correlations revealed a high item discriminant validity. Different diagnostic groups could be discriminated using the SRI. Using this scale, the QoL was ranked as highest in the patients with kyphoscoliosis, followed by neuromuscular diseases, post-tuberculosis respiratory failure, and COPD ($p < 0.05$).

D. QoL in Chronic Respiratory Failure

Most studies on the short- and long-term functional status among survivors of prolonged ventilatory support have been based on patients affected by postoperative, cardiovascular, acute respiratory distress syndrome-related, or trauma diseases (29–33). Studies on the functional status of such patients show conflicting results, with some reporting minimal impairment both in the short and long term (29–31,34) and others noting significant reductions in health status (32,33). In survivors of prolonged mechanical ventilation, the presence of moderate to severe limitations relates more closely to the underlying disease, rather than to the duration of ventilation (30).

Bourke and colleagues (35,36) assessed the effect of NIPPV on QoL and survival in patients with amyotrophic lateral sclerosis (ALS) in a randomized controlled trial. ALS patients were assessed every two months and randomly assigned to NIPPV or standard care if they developed either orthopnea (with MIP <60% predicted) or symptomatic hypercapnia. The QoL outcome measures were the SF_{36} and the symptoms domain of the sleep apnea QoL index. In ALS patients without severe bulbar dysfunction, NIPPV improved survival and maintained QoL. The survival benefit from NIPPV in this group was much greater than that from currently available neuroprotective therapy. In patients with severe bulbar impairment, NIPPV improved sleep-related symptoms, but did not confer a large survival advantage.

In a study of patients with Duchenne muscular dystrophy in which QoL was assessed by the SF_{36}, the questionnaire did not correlate with physical impairment or the need for NIPPV. The surprisingly high QoL experienced by the severely disabled patients in this study should be considered when therapeutic decisions are made (37).

Improvements in QoL, general health perceptions, functional status, and symptoms have been reported from specialist or generalist provided home care to patients with COPD (38). A landmark Canadian trial of self-management education in COPD noted the initial improvements in the impact and activity scales of the SGRQ, with only the impact improvements being maintained at 12 months (39).

An observational cohort study (40) of patients with CRF after long-term mechanical ventilation in the ICU noted that of 87 survivors >6 months, the population included patients with COPD, thoracic restriction, and neuromuscular disorders, as well as various other chronic conditions. The SF_{36} and the SGRQ showed that although physical health was markedly reduced, mental health was only mildly impaired, compared with the general population. QoL was comparable to patients with stable CRF receiving NIPPV who did not need prolonged invasive mechanical ventilation. General QoL was better in patients with restrictive respiratory disease than those with neuromuscular diseases. Neither blood gases nor lung function correlated with QoL.

E. Sexuality

Sexual functioning is affected by chronic illness in many ways and often influences the patient's relationship and satisfaction with their partner. Ibanez et al. (41) evaluated sexual difficulties and changes in communication between male COPD patients in CRF and their wives, using individual semistructured interviews conducted with both parties. The investigators evaluated sexual issues and how they affected the relationship between the couples, the degree of satisfaction with their partner, and the degree of satisfaction with their lives. Some types of sexual problem, such as lack of desire or impotence, were noted in 67% of respondents. Changes in communication as a consequence of the patients' illness were noted by 33% of the wives and sexual changes were noted by 94% of the wives. Wives were significantly less satisfied with the relationship than the husbands because of communication issues. The patients were more satisfied with their partners than with their lives. The study concluded that an important percentage of patients with CRF had sexual difficulties and that such perceptions were linked to the amount of affection between the couple.

Schonhofer et al. (42) evaluated some issues of sexuality in patients with NIPPV. Physiologic data were retrieved from within the six-month period prior to enrolment and the questionnaire focused on sexuality after the initiation of NIPPV. A total of 34.1% of patients were sexually active in comparison to 84% of control subjects. Sexually active patients were younger and had better pulmonary mechanics, gas exchange, and exercise tolerance as well as being mostly married or having a sexual partner. Changes in sexual activity after the initiation of NIPPV varied from: no change (46.3%), to less active (35.8%), more active (12.6%), and increased fantasy (10.5%). Increased fantasy predominated in men. Sexually active patients with NIPPV had sexual intercourse 5.4 ± 4.8 times per month.

F. Quality of Death

As quality of death is an important issue among this patient population and their families, elements of the dying experience are being actively studied by investigators (43), who have characterized the conceptual domains associated with dying and death. The quality of dying and death (QODD) instrument has been developed to evaluate these conceptual domains and is being used by attending physicians, residents, nurses, and family members of patients in the ICU to evaluate the QODD (44). Attending physicians and family members rate the dying experience more positively than do the resident physicians or nurses. Overall, family members of those who died in the ICU had a relatively favorable perception of dying and death, although the quality of end-of-life care was thought to be poor by some. Efforts to measure and improve the QODD will depend on an understanding of these differences in perception, and then determining ways to consider them during the dying process. Future clinical management of the dying process may involve the increased use of such assessment tools.

IV. Conclusion

The impact of CRF on daily life and well-being can be assessed in different ways. It is not possible to predict health status from surrogate measures of lung function, exercise tolerance, or gas exchange, or to predict the health gain by means of physiological measures. Health status can be adequately assessed only through a direct method using valid, reliable, and interpretable QoL instruments. The SGRQ and the MRF_{28} questionnaire are two disease-specific instruments that have been shown to be applicable and reliable in patients receiving long-term ventilation (26).

References

1. Hopkins RO, Weaver LK, Collingridge D, et al. Two-year cognitive, emotional, and quality-of-life outcomes in acute respiratory distress syndrome. Am J Respir Crit Care Med 2005; 171:340–347.
2. Ambrosino N, Bruletti G, Scala V, et al. Cognitive and perceived health status in patients recovering from an acute exacerbation of COPD. A controlled study. Intensive Care Med 2002; 28:170–177.
3. Guyatt GH, Feeny DH, Patrick DL. Measuring health-related quality of life. Ann Intern Med 1993; 118:622–629.

4. Jones PW, Quirk FH, Baveystock CM. Why quality of life measures should be used in the treatment of patients with respiratory illness. Monaldi Arch Chest Dis 1994; 49:79–82.
5. Carone M, Jones PW. Health status ('quality of life'). Eur Respir Mon 2000; 13:22–35.
6. Jones PW. Quality of life: specific problems associated with hypoxaemia. Monaldi Arch Chest Dis 1993; 48:565–573.
7. Randal Curtis J, Martin DP, Martin TR. Patient-assessed health outcomes in chronic lung disease: what are they, how do they help us, and where do we go from here? Am J Respir Crit Care Med 1997; 156:1032–1039.
8. Stewart AL, Hays RD, Ware JE, The MOS short-form general health survey: reliability and validity in a patient population. Med Care 1998; 26:724–732.
9. Simonds AK, Elliot MW. Outcome of domiciliary nasal intermittent positive pressure ventilation in restrictive and obstructive disorders. Thorax 1995; 50:604–609.
10. Crockett AJ, Cranston JM, Moss JR, et al. The MOS SF-36 health survey questionnaire in severe chronic airflow limitation: comparison with the Nottingham Health Profile. Qual Life Res 1996; 5:330–338.
11. Smith IE, Shneerson JM. A progressive care programme for prolonged ventilatory failure: analysis of outcome. Br J Anaesth 1995; 75:399–404.
12. Guyatt GH, Berman LB, Townsend M, et al. A measure of quality of life for clinical trials in chronic lung disease. Thorax 1987; 42:773–778.
13. Jones PW, Quirk FH, Baveystock CM, et al. A self-complete measure for chronic airflow limitation. The St George's Respiratory Questionnaire. Am Rev Respir Dis 1992; 145, 1321–1327.
14. Wegner RE, Jörres RA, Kirsten DK, et al. Factor analysis of exercise capacity, dyspnoea ratings and lung function in patients with severe COPD. Eur Respir J 1994; 7:725–729.
15. Jones PW, Quirk FH, Baveystock CM. The St George's Respiratory Questio"nnaire. Resp Med 1991; 85(suppl B):25–31.
16. Okubadejo AA, Jones PW, Wedzicha JA. Quality of life in patients with chronic obstructive pulmonary disease and severe hypoxaemia. Thorax 1996; 51:44–47.
17. Meecham Jones DJ, Paul EA, Jones PW, et al. Nasal pressure support ventilation plus oxygen compared with oxygen therapy alone in hypercapnic COPD. Am J Respir Crit Care Med 1995; 152:538–544.
18. Perrin C, El Far Y, Vandenbos F, et al. Domiciliary nasal intermittent positive pressure ventilation in severe COPD: effects on lung function and quality of life. Eur Respir J 1997; 10:2835–2839.
19. Carone M, Bertolotti G, Anchisi F, et al. Analysis of factors that characterize health impairment in patients with chronic respiratory failure. Quality of Life in Chronic Respiratory Failure Group. Eur Respir J 1999; 13:1293–1300.
20. Janssens JP, Heritier-Praz A, Carone M, et al. Validity and reliability of a French version of the MRF-28 health-related quality of life questionnaire. Respiration 2004; 71:567–574.
21. Bertolotti G, Carone M, Donner CF, et al. Cognitive dysfunction in the daily life of COPD patients. Am J Respir Crit Care Med 1996; 153:A757.
22. Carone M, Bertolotti G, Zotti AM, et al. Do oxygen therapy and mechanical ventilation have different effects on perceived health in chronic respiratory failure? Eur Respir J 1996; 9 (suppl 23):111s.
23. Carone M, Bertolotti G, Zotti AM, et al. The effect of respiratory devices on perceived health in severe respiratory failure. Am J Respir Crit Care Med 1996; 153(4 pt 2):A754.
24. Carone M, Bertolotti G, Donner CF, et al. Do severe COPD and kyphoscoliosis have different effects on patients' lives? Am J Respir Crit Care Med 1996; 153(4 pt 2):A754.
25. Carone M, Ambrosino N, Bertolotti G, et al., on behalf of the QuESS Group. Quality of Life Evaluation and Survival Study: a 3-year prospective multinational study on patients with chronic respiratory failure. Monaldi Arch Chest Dis 2001; 56:17–22.

26. Carone M, Donner CF. Quality of life and long-term ventilation. Respir Care Clin N Am 2002; 8(3):479–490.
27. Clini E, Sturani C, Viaggi S, et al. The Italian multicentric study on non invasive ventilation in COPD patients. Eur Resp J 2002; 20:529–538.
28. Windisch W, Freidel K, Schucher B, et al. The Severe Respiratory Insufficiency (SRI) Questionnaire: a specific measure of health-related quality of life in patients receiving home mechanical ventilation. J Clin Epidemiol 2003; 56:752–759.
29. Niskanen M, Ruokonen E, Takala J, et al. Quality of life after prolonged intensive care. Crit Care Med 1999; 27:1132–1139.
30. Chatila W, Kreimer DT, Criner GJ. Quality of life in survivors of prolonged mechanical ventilatory support. Crit Care Med 2001; 29:737–774.
31. Lipsett PA, Swoboda SM, Dickerson J, et al. Survival and functional outcome after prolonged intensive care unit stay. Ann Surg 2000; 231:262–268.
32. Schelling G, Stoll C, Vogelmeier C, et al. Pulmonary function and health-related quality of life in a sample of long-term survivors of the acute respiratory distress syndrome. Intensive Care Med 2000; 26:1304–1311.
33. Angus DC, Musthafa AA, Clermont G, et al. Quality adjusted survival in the first year after the acute respiratory distress syndrome. Am J Respir Crit Care Med 2001; 163:1389–1394.
34. Eddleston JM, White P, Guthrie E. Survival, morbidity, and quality of life after discharge from intensive care. Crit Care Med 2000; 28:2293–2299.
35. Bourke SC, Tomlinson M, Williams TL, et al Effects of non-invasive ventilation on survival and quality of life in patients with amyotrophic lateral sclerosis: a randomised controlled trial. Lancet Neurol 2006; 5:140–147.
36. Bourke SC, Bullock RE, Williams TL, et al. Noninvasive ventilation in ALS Indications and effect on quality of life. Neurology 2003; 61:171–177.
37. Kohler M, Clarenbach CF, Böni L, et al. Quality of life, physical disability, and respiratory impairment in Duchenne muscular dystrophy. Am J Respir Crit Care Med 2005; 172:1032–1036.
38. American Thoracic Society. Statement on home care for patients with respiratory disorders. Am J Respir Crit Care Med 2005; 171:1443–1464.
39. Bourbeau J, Julien M, Maltais F, et al. Reduction of hospital utilization in patients with chronic obstructive pulmonary disease. Arch Intern Med 2003; 163:585–591.
40. Euteneuer S, Windisch W, Suchi S, et al. Health-related quality of life in patients with chronic respiratory failure after long-term mechanical ventilation. Respir Med 2006; 100(3):477–486.
41. Ibanez M, Aguilar JJ, Maderal MA, et al. Sexuality in chronic respiratory failure: coincidences and divergences between patient and primary caregiver. Respir Med 2001; 95:975–979.
42. Schonhofer B, Von Sydow K, Bucher T, et al. Sexuality in patients with noninvasive mechanical ventilation due to chronic respiratory failure. Am J Respir Crit Care Med 2001; 164:1612–1617.
43. Heyland DK, Rocker GM, O'Callaghan CJ, et al. Dying in the ICU: perspectives of family members. Chest 2003; 124:392–397.
44. Levy CR, Ely EW, Payne K, et al. Quality of dying and death in two medical ICUs: perceptions of family and clinicians. Chest 2005; 127:1775–1783.

22
Legal and Ethical Issues

DOUGLAS TURNER and PAULEEN PRATT
Critical Care and Chronic Ventilation Service, University Hospitals of Leicester, NHS Trust, Leicester, U.K.

I. Introduction

The ever-increasing availability and use of medical technology has created ethical, legal, and economic dilemmas that were unthinkable only a few years ago. The practice of medical science dictates what is possible, the law of the land dictates what is permissible, and medical, nursing, public, and academic consensus decides what is right and proper. Clinical management that is medically possible, legally permissible, or ethically right may be represented by three different courses of action. This may result in difficulty in clinical decision making.

The purpose of this chapter is to describe some of the legal and ethical issues pertinent to the practice of critical care medicine, in particular, to the management of those patients who are stable but remain ventilator dependent with little prospect of ventilator independence.

The relief of suffering through compassionate and sensitive withholding, or withdrawing life support, has become an essential component of the practice of medicine. Not all patients admitted with life-threatening diseases can be successfully treated, so that critical care support, initiated in good faith and with a reasonable expectation of success, may rapidly become meaningless when all available methods of cure fail to reverse the inexorable course of the disease. At some point, it becomes necessary to limit the level or the duration of an intervention. The difficulty lies in the determination of that time, and when a critical illness may be assumed to have progressed beyond the point where there cannot be any reasonable expectation of recovery.

Doctors have a duty of care to always act in the best interests of the patient. This means offering those treatments where the potential benefits outweigh the burdens or risks associated with treatment and avoiding treatments that are futile or of no benefit to the patient. The difficulty lies in understanding the patient's best interests and avoiding our personal biases in the interpretation of quality of life.

In the United Kingdom, two recent high profile cases, in which there was a difference of opinion as to what constituted "best interests," have highlighted the difficulties in this area. The parents of two children, Charlotte Whyatt and Luke Winston-Jones (1), went to the high court to demand that, in the event of deterioration, their children would be resuscitated and receive advanced respiratory support in an intensive care unit (ICU). This has resulted in much debate, as in both cases the medical decisions were upheld and it was decided that mechanical ventilation and resuscitation was not in the patients' best interests.

It is generally argued that prolonging life is in the best interests of the patient, provided that the treatment is not considered to be excessively burdensome or disproportionate to the expected benefits. Doctors should not strive pointlessly to prolong the dying process with no regard to the patients or the wishes of the patient's representative, the burden of treatment, or an assessment of the effect of treatment on the remaining quality of life for the patient.

Well-intentioned people, including health care workers, have difficulty in making sound moral judgments and it is important that adequate moral justification and reasoning is used. The historical paternalistic view that "the doctor knows best" is outdated and has been widely criticized by both professional and patient groups (2). Many cases are now being referred to the High Court, both within the United Kingdom and internationally. This shift to the judiciary suggests that simple moral codes may be inadequate for finding answers to today's ethical problems.

II. Ethical Theory

An understanding of basic ethical theory is a necessary premise to any valid reasoning process. There may be no single solution to the problems presented in any individual case, but it does not follow that morally unjustified and poorly reasoned answers are beyond valid criticism.

A. Principlism: The Four Principles

Over the past 30 years, the term "principlism" has been used to refer to Beauchamp and Childress' (3) four principles approach to ethical issues.

Principlism and the "four principles with scope" approach to medical ethics is one of the most useful, practical tools to aid decision making in ethical dilemmas within medicine and health care. One significant advantage of this system is its supposed universality. In theory, it is independent of personal philosophy, political beliefs, religion, morality, or life stance. As the principles reflect universally valid norms, they allow intercultural and cross-cultural judgments to be made.

This approach is based on respect for the four prima facie moral principles:

1. *Beneficence*—an obligation to provide benefits and to balance any benefits against the perceived risks.
2. *Non-maleficence*—an obligation to avoid doing harm.
3. *Autonomy*—an obligation to respect the decision-making capacities of autonomous persons.
4. *Justice*—an obligation to consider fairness and equity in the distribution of the benefits. Similar patients with similar diseases should receive comparable treatments. The allocation of expensive, finite resources must consider the effects of this on all the potential recipients.

None of these prima facie moral principles carries any greater weight or has more influence than any of the others. No single one is determinative, although recent rulings suggest the emphasis has shifted to the need for patient autonomy becoming the preeminent principle.

The four principles approach provides a simple, accessible, and culturally neutral approach to ethical issues in health care. "Prima facie" means that the principle is binding unless it conflicts with one of the other principles. If conflict exists, then a choice must be made as to which of the four principles is determinative, i.e., which is the "trumping" principle. Using this system, no single right solution may emerge but the underlying process and reasoning are capable of explanation and justification if challenged.

B. The Application of Principlism

Before the application of the four principles approach to any individual case, it is important that careful, measured consideration is given to six basic precondition questions.

1. *Diagnosis and prognosis.* Clearly a definitive diagnosis is essential as prognostication is likely to be inaccurate if diagnosis is wrong.
2. *Potential for benefit* from proposed intervention, therapy, and support.
3. *Risks* of proposed intervention, therapy, support. Risk of morbidity and mortality.
4. *Burdens* of proposed intervention, therapy, and support. Identifiable burdens include pain, physical discomfort, mental anguish, physiological stress, indignity from dehumanizing interventions, helplessness with loss of independence, prolongation of the dying process, and the wider impact on family and relatives.
5. Level of patient awareness (*competence*).
6. Potential of proposed measures to restore the patient to a way of living he or she would consider as of reasonable *quality*.

It should be apparent from the thorough evaluation of the above conditions that questions 1, 2, and 3 are arguably the prime responsibility of the medical team, while nurses may be in the best position to assess question 4 and the patient or patient representatives can best assess question 6.

If it is clear that recovery from a known diagnosis is extremely unlikely, that benefit is unlikely to accrue from continued support, that such support is likely to prolong dying and involve physical discomfort, mental anguish, or bodily violation, and that survival would result in a quality of life known to be unacceptable to the patient and believed to be unacceptable to all caregivers, then death is in the patient's best interest.

The application of the four principles would be straightforward with no conflicts. Indeed in situations where concordance exists between what the patient wants and what caregivers believe to be in the patient's best interest, rarely result in conflict. In more complex cases, there may be conflict between one or more of the four principles, and in this situation, a judgment must be made as to which principle or principles take precedence. This requires consultation and discussion, which should be an open and inclusive process.

It is not uncommon for conflicts to emerge. Typical examples include:

- The patient who does not possess autonomy like the incompetent, partially incompetent, inaccessible, or insensible patient. Clinical staff should always strive to act in the best interests of patients, but who determines the best interests of an incompetent patient?
- The patient who makes "bad choices" and refuses therapy or support, which the caregivers feel is overwhelmingly in the patient's best interests, or insists on therapy or support that caregivers consider to be of no benefit.

- Respecting one patient's autonomy results in harm to another more deserving patient.
- If there exists a very fine balance between risks, benefits, and burdens.

It is not possible to cover all potential eventualities. We describe one possible, pragmatic "process approach" to the application of the four principles.

III. Pragmatic Process for Application of the Four Principles

The relief of suffering through sensitive and compassionate withholding or withdrawal of life support has become an essential component of the practice of critical care medicine. In one survey conducted between 1987 and 1993, deaths in the ICUs that followed the withdrawal of life support increased from 51% to 90% (4).

There is a point where all would agree that intensive care has moved beyond the realm of beneficence, but there is a wide, gray area in which opinion is bound to differ. This transition from the need for restorative to the need for palliative care may be gradual or sudden and is often sensed by the nursing caregivers and relatives, before medical staff.

If an intensivist is faced with a situation where intensive therapy has failed, thought should be given to limitation or withdrawal of that therapy, as futile treatment deprives the patient of a good death.

Decisions on treatment limitation and withdrawal must be discussed with all medical and nonmedical health care providers directly involved in the patient's care. It is the intensivist's responsibility to be certain that a consensus exists. A judgment that a treatment is inadvisable can be made only after all relevant viewpoints have been considered. Withdrawal or limitation of treatment should, where possible, be initiated with unanimous agreement of the clinical team and the family.

Families sometimes agree among themselves that a treatment should be terminated so as to prevent further suffering. However, they may be reluctant to broach the subject with health care professionals for fear of their being considered unduly pessimistic or lacking in concern for their ill relative. Once the subject is broached, the family may express their feelings with conviction and relief. The family must be spared the belief that they were responsible for the death of a loved one. Under these circumstances, death can be accepted and allowed to occur in surroundings of tranquility and dignity. It is far preferable for the patient and family to experience death under these circumstances, often with the family present, than their being ushered from the room during futile, last minute attempts to resuscitate. All involved must appreciate that it is not a right to impose death, but a right to choose a course of action that will fail to avert death.

If a clinician believes that a patient is suffering and death is inevitable, then the best interests of the patient would be to end this suffering. This is unlawful in many countries and defined as euthanasia. However, the withdrawal of futile interventions is accepted morally and legally if death is inevitable. No clinician can be forced into giving a treatment that they believe is futile and not in the patient's best interest, provided it is based on clinical issues and not resource allocation. Beauchamp and Childress note that the delivery of futile care may be confused with showing "commitment to care." The following principles should apply to decisions that involve withholding or withdrawing life support.

Treatment Limitation and Withdrawal of Support Protocol

- There must be sound clinical grounds for believing that continued support is not in the patient's best interests and this must be justifiable if challenged by a "responsible body of medical opinion." A second medical expert opinion is mandatory.
- Medical and nursing consensus is essential.
- Any previously expressed wish of the patient should be sought, considered, and respected.
- Agreement of the relatives should be sought unless it is considered inappropriate to burden relatives with a share of the responsibility. Such agreement or the reason for lack of such agreement should be documented in the patient's notes.
- Limitation decisions may be generic, e.g., do not escalate (DNE), or more specific. For example, it may be decided that the following are inappropriate cardiopulmonary resuscitation (CPR), renal replacement therapy, inotropes, reventilation, reintubation etc. The classical do-not-resuscitate (DNR) order should be abandoned, as it is too nonspecific. More specific instructions are preferable, e.g., "not for CPR in the event of cardiac arrest," "not for reintubation" etc. Such instructions must be explicitly and contemporaneously documented in the patient's notes.
- Withdrawal decisions should be specific, e.g., withdraw ventilation, oxygen, inotropes, etc. All such decisions must be documented explicitly and contemporaneously in the patient's notes.
- Once a limitation or a withdrawal of treatment decision has been made, the most senior clinician and nurse should have a sensitive discussion with the patient's relatives or representatives to make them aware of the proposed course of action and get their implicit understanding and agreement.
- The plan for withdrawal must take into account that any medical intervention where the doctor's primary intention is to end the patient's life is contrary to medical ethics and unlawful. The primary motivation for terminal sedation must be to relieve suffering and not to hasten death.
- Prior to the institution of a withdrawal of treatment decision, the details of the plan must be clear to all caregivers.
- The institution of withdrawal decisions must be done in a gradual, sensitive way that is acceptable to the relatives and all caregivers.
- Every effort should be made to provide a private, dignified, and peaceful death. Prevention of physical discomfort and mental anguish is a paramount consideration.

While most treatment limitation and withdrawal decisions are made openly, with the explicit agreement of all relevant parties, relatives may disagree with the medical and nursing consensus concerning the limitation or withdrawal of life support (5). Such sentiments may be related to dissatisfaction with care, deeply held religious beliefs, cultural mores, a futile hope for a miracle, or the inability to "let go" of a loved one. It is necessary to know the rationale for their refusing to agree with limitation or withdrawal decisions in order for logical and compassionate reasons to be put forward that may allow them to reconsider their decision. Both relatives and caregivers must feel that they have properly and completely discharged their moral responsibility to the patient. All those involved must feel that they have not let the patient down at a time when the patient is unable to express an opinion.

It is, therefore, imperative that such predicaments are handled with a sensitive and human touch. It is particularly important that a paternalistic approach is not adopted as this often inflames the situation. Insistence that treatment limitation decisions will be imposed and once documented will be irrevocable totally disregards the wishes of relatives and must be avoided. A suggested protocol for such situations is as follows:

- Avoid paternalism and agree to respect the wishes of relatives.
- Relatives must believe that the ICU team has their best interests at heart.
- Pressure on beds must be excluded from the equation.
- Speak at regular intervals to close relatives, the patient's nurse, and referring clinician.
- On each occasion discuss their hopes for the patient. Reinforce the view that the medical and nursing staffs are of the opinion that meaningful recovery is extremely unlikely.
- Tactfully assert that continuing treatment is depriving the patient of a peaceful and dignified death, and that the burden of treatment far outweighs the benefit of a few more days of life on a ventilator.
- Stress that the transition from restorative to palliative care is an active process that puts emphasis on preventing physical discomfort and mental anguish, while maintaining human dignity and family privacy.
- Request that the second opinion from the intensivist who agreed with the decision to limit or withdraw support is available to the relatives to reinforce the caregivers' sentiments.
- If the relatives' opinion remains steadfast despite all due processes having been allowed, and if the opinion of all caregivers is that continued treatment is not in the patient's best interests, a case conference should be called with clinical, legal, and family representatives. The purpose of the meeting is to consider the hospital's view on propriety, the risk of taking a view contrary to the patient's relatives, and to consider an application to request involvement of the judiciary.
- Some organization may have clinical ethics committees who can also advise and support in this difficult scenario.

The above approaches were designed for acutely ill patients with multiple organ failure, who required invasive multisystem support. Although patients with isolated respiratory failure, who require long-term ventilation, differ in a number of respects, the importance of an open, inclusive, and measured decision-making process cannot be overemphasized. Notwithstanding that their long-term prognosis is related to the underlying etiology, there is increasing evidence that ventilation, even in degenerative respiratory conditions, can extend life that is of good quality (6,7). Such patients fall broadly within the following three groups:

1. Quadriplegia and respiratory quadriplegia
2. Progressive or stable neuromuscular conditions
3. Chronic ventilatory failure secondary to chronic respiratory disease or skeletal deformity

The same four principles approach remains valid when applied to patients who are fully competent, with a stable, nonprogressive condition, such as respiratory quadriplegia, requiring a permanent tracheostomy and ventilatory support. It can be argued that in such circumstances, ventilatory support is beneficent (preserves life), non-maleficent (prevents death), and fair and equitable (resource costs not disproportionate). As long as continued support is consistent with the patient's wishes it would seem warranted. A serious ethical dilemma exists if such a patient demands discontinuation of ventilatory support as it could be argued that such a course of action would be inhumane in a conscious, sentient individual and that the primary intention of this act would be to end the patient's life. This is discussed further in a later section.

IV. Living Wills and Patient Autonomy

Many people fear that if they become unable to express their wishes, they may be exposed to therapies to prolong life that they would reject if able to do so. This inability to express their wishes amounts to a loss of autonomy and although relatives can communicate the patient's expressed wishes, they have little standing in the legal sense as they cannot consent or refuse treatment on behalf of anyone else. Most health care professionals will ask family members about a patient's expressed wishes, even though this holds no legal standing in most jurisdictions. For this reason, we have seen the emergence of living wills and advance directives. Patients, while well and legally competent, draw up these documents to clarify their wishes in the event of serious illness or degenerative disease.

An advance directive is a legal document that informs the care providers as to which treatments and supports the signatory does not wish to receive, if they become incompetent or unable to express their wishes.

There are two types of advance directive. The individuals may simply state their specific wishes, or alternatively may grant a named person the right to execute a "continuing Power of Attorney." This person can then legally make decisions for the patient if the patient is judged incompetent. The legal system in England accepts the use of living wills and, in general, they are upheld if they clearly state the grounds on which they are made and defined specifically the treatments being refused. They must be in writing, signed, and witnessed. It is accepted that basic care, such as pain relief and hygiene needs, cannot be refused. Brazier (8) highlights the potential risks and difficulties of living wills and particularly the situation in which a named person given a "Power of Attorney," who in old age becomes incapable of making these difficult choices, or even misuses the power invested in them.

Living wills go some way to protecting patient autonomy. In the case of *Malette v. Shulman* (9) in the United States, a physician was found guilty of disregarding patient autonomy when he administered a blood transfusion, in an emergency situation, to a Jehovah's Witness, who had left clear written instruction of her wishes even if this led to her death.

V. Patient Request for Treatment Withdrawal or Terminal Wean

When considering commencement or continuation of mechanical ventilation, the potential benefits, risks, and burdens of this support should be considered, taking into account the patient's wishes (respect for autonomy). The patient already receiving chronic ventilation, who presents issues of continuing or withdrawing treatment, does so within the context of euthanasia.

It is useful to distinguish between euthanasia performed by killing the patient (active euthanasia) and that performed by omitting to prolong the patient's life (passive euthanasia). It is also important to distinguish between euthanasia that is voluntary (patient autonomously requests death), nonvoluntary (patient unable competently to give consent), and involuntary (competent but have their views on the matter paternalistically disregarded).

In euthanasia, the primary objective is the death of the patient and the ethical argument is that if death is considered to be in the patient's best interests, it represents a moral, good choice. The withdrawing or withholding of life-prolonging treatment in the critical care setting is not motivated by bringing about death, but by protecting the patient from the burden of futile treatment, thus allowing palliation (relief of pain and mental anguish). Many would consider that the relevant test to distinguish "passive euthanasia" from humane palliation would be to ask the question "if the patient does not die, have the clinicians succeeded in their goal?" In the case of passive euthanasia, the answer will be "no." In the case of withdrawing and withholding treatment because it would be burdensome or harmful, the clinician will have succeeded even if the patient survives.

All acts that have the primary aim and intention of bringing about death are illegal in the United Kingdom at this present time, even if they are judged to be in the patient's best interests. However, passive euthanasia, such as withholding and withdrawing treatments, are legally permissible; even though they are likely to result in death, as long as the primary intention is to protect the patient from burden and harm.

Much debate has occurred as to whether passive euthanasia is euthanasia at all. Garrad and Wilkinson (10) note that although active euthanasia is ethically unacceptable, omission of prolonging treatments is somehow justified morally. The law seems to support this view in some ways.

A relevant example is of Miss B (11), a woman who was deemed to be competent, was receiving long-term invasive mechanical ventilation, and requested the clinical staff to remove her from the ventilator. Although the staff refused, the courts decided that to continue mechanical ventilation against her wishes was unlawful and that she was competent to refuse this treatment, even if it led to her death. There was legal acceptance that it was permissible to allow her to end her life and that to continue with a treatment against her wishes was an assault. This has been described as legally sanctioned ethical homicide, assisted suicide, and active euthanasia.

There are few legal precedents and clarity is lacking. Some clinicians will have difficulty in performing an act that they feel is not right and proper even if deemed by the courts to be legally permissible. In the case of Miss B, she was moved to a different hospital for her terminal wean. There is, of course, no sound reason why judicial decisions are any more cogent on matters of ethical principle than those of academics or practicing clinicians. However, any consideration of the moral basis of clinical practice must take account of judicial determinations. Local policies should be drawn up for the management of a terminal wean to take account of comfort and dignity of the patient, ethical values of the staff, and the practicalities of the process.

Understanding the primary intention and gaining consent for withholding or withdrawing care in the competent patient is a vital step. We need to be certain that the patient is fully informed of all options, including what might be achieved through palliative care, whether discharge home might be possible, and the magnitude of the burden of ongoing treatment. To wish to die to avoid being a burden seems wrong and ethically unjustifiable, until the situation is fully explored and the patient fully informed regarding the options for ongoing care and the support available for the patient and the family.

VI. Chronic Ventilatory Failure

Patients with quadriplegia, muscular dystrophy, and post polio survive for many years (12) without making huge demands on health care resources. It is important that the patient's judgment of "quality of life" is given more emphasis than notions perceived by the caregivers (13,14).

If the "four principles" approach is applied to patients with progressive neurological diseases, the arguments for the beneficence, non-maleficence, and distributive justice for invasive ventilatory support are far from compelling. The interests of patients with such progressive diseases are not always best served by offering invasive ventilatory support, although the use of noninvasive support is well recognized (15). It is best to identify patients at high risk of developing chronic respiratory failure so that they can be referred to a ventilation service in advance of an acute deterioration. At this time, their views and options can be planned with the involvement of their families.

Patients with thoracic restriction or advanced parenchymal diseases, who develop respiratory failure, represent a heterogeneous group. For such patients, nocturnal noninvasive ventilation is the preferred alternative. The results are very encouraging among those with stable thoracic restriction and less clear among those with advanced parenchymal diseases. The development of specialized facilities for long-term ventilation is described elsewhere in this book.

VII. Conclusions

The four principles approach is suggested as a useful vehicle for the ethical dilemmas associated with medical practice. The challenge for the practicing physician is to determine the right and proper course of action when there is conflict between two or more of these fundamental principles. The importance of a transparent, inclusive, and contemporaneously documented process for such decision making cannot be overemphasized. Advances in medical technology, combined with an informed, vociferous public, ready to seek legal redress for perceived and actual wrongs, means that referral to the judiciary will become more commonplace. When moral codes and beliefs between the health care professionals and the patients are in concordance, acceptable ethical decisions are easier. However, patients and clinical staff may have different priorities in their decision making.

In patients with chronic respiratory failure where long-term mechanical ventilation is a feasible option, early identification and a full explanation with active patient participation of all possible options is essential. Patients can then be assisted in making informed choices, and be supported in these choices by their families and their clinical teams.

References

1. The Ethox Centre, Department of Public Health and Primary Health Care, University of Oxford, www.ethox.org.uk
2. Savulescu J. Rational non-interventional paternalism: why doctors ought to make judgements of what is best for their patients. J Med Ethics 1995; 21(6):327–331.
3. Beauchamp TL, Childress JF. Principles of Biomedical Ethics. 5th ed. York and Oxford: Oxford University Press, 2001.
4. Prendergast TJ, Luce JM. Increasing incidence of witholding and withdrawal of life support from the critically ill. Am J Respir Crit Care Med 1997; 155(1): 15–20.
5. BBC News. Doctors win right to let baby die. Available at: http://news.bbc.co.uk/1/hi/wales/north_west/3764938.stm. Accessed October 22, 2004.
6. Windisch W, Freidel K, Schucher B, et al. Evaluation of health related quality of life using the MOS 36 short form health status survey in patients receiving non-invasive positive pressure ventilation. Intensive Care Med 2003; 29(4):615–621.
7. Markstrom A, Sundell K, Lysdahl M, et al. Quality of life evaluation of patients with neuromuscular and skeletal diseases treated with non-invasive home mechanical ventilation. Chest 2002; 122(5):1695–1700.
8. Brazier M. Medicine Patients and the Law. 3rd ed. London: Penguin Books, 2003.
9. Malette v. Shulman, 72 OR2d 417 (Ontarion CA 1990).
10. Garrard E, Wilkinson S. Passive euthanasia J Med Ethics 2005; 31:64–68.
11. Ms B v. NHS Hospital, EWHC 429 (2002).
12. Lloyd-Owen SJ, Donaldson GC, Ambrosino N, et al. Patterns of home mechanical ventilation use in Europe: results from the Eurovent study. Eur Resp J 2005; 25:1025–1031.
13. Hardart MK, Burns JP, Truonq RD. Respiratory support in spinal muscular atrophy–type I: a survey of physician practices and attitudes. Pediatrics 2002; 110:e24.
14. Bach JR, Campagnolo DI, Hoeman S. Life satisfaction of individuals with Duchenne muscular dystrophy using long-term mechanical ventilatory support. Am J Phys Med Rehabil 1991, 70(3): 129–35.
15. Duiverman M, Bladder G, Meinesz A, et al. Home Mechanical ventilation support in patients with restrictive ventilatory disorders: a 48 year experience. Respir Med 2006; 100:56–65.

23
Pharmacological Treatment for Patients with Chronic Respiratory Failure

GERHARD LAIER-GROENEVELD
Evangelisches und Johanniterkrankenhaus Oberhausen, Medizinische Klinik II, Lungen-und Bronchialheilkunde, Oberhausen, Germany

I. Introduction

Most patients, requiring ongoing ventilation, present either with an acute exacerbation experiencing an acute increase in symptoms, or through the gradual progression of their disease without any clearly detectable event. Hypercapnic ventilatory failure is the primary indication for mechanical ventilation as it reflects insufficiency of the ventilatory pump, or of ventilatory drive in coping with the ventilatory load. Hypoxia, consequent on underlying lung disease, may also contribute to ventilatory failure.

Acute exacerbations superimposed on advanced chronic disease require the effective administration of noninvasive ventilation (NIV) to improve morbidity and mortality. NIV should also enable a steady improvement in spontaneous ventilatory capacity. A decrease in partial pressure of carbon dioxide in arterial blood ($Paco_2$) during ventilation and subsequently during unassisted respiration is the best indicator of effective NIV (1,2).

Adjunctive pharmacological therapies, aimed primarily at the cardio-respiratory system, will have a modest role initially, but as the disease becomes more chronic, there is a reduction in the potential for medications to contribute substantially. Therefore, although medications are prescribed in an attempt to optimize performance, it is important to do so in a way that minimizes the possibility of detrimental effects that can occur, for example, from corticosteroids or short-acting beta agonists. The following comments highlight some of the adjunctive therapies for the ventilated patient.

II. Bronchodilators for COPD

Chronic obstructive pulmonary disease (COPD), because of its high prevalence, is frequently the cause of or a major contributor to respiratory failure. COPD is also a common comorbid diagnosis among patients with severe community-acquired pneumonia, who develop respiratory failure. COPD indicators include a chronic history of smoking, age over 55 years, a history of wheezing, and evidence of expiratory flow limitation with hypercapnia (3). Pulmonary function tests are important in characterizing airflow limitation in patients with COPD who are being considered for NIV. Although COPD is characterized by airflow limitation that is only partially reversible, most patients with COPD will show some degree of reversibility, especially as they recover from an exacerbation (4).

Airway obstruction impairs respiration by limiting expiratory flow, so that it cannot be increased in response to increased ventilatory demand. Ventilation must occur at a higher volume and frequency, resulting in increased inspiratory muscle activity. Early airway closure promotes dynamic hyperinflation and increases intrinsic positive end-expiratory pressure (PEEP). Therefore, the inspiratory muscles are exposed to an increased load at the onset of inspiration to overcome intrinsic PEEP until inspiratory flow occurs. If bronchodilatation can be achieved, improved lung emptying by decreasing the intrinsic PEEP will unload the inspiratory muscles. Therefore, in obstructive disorders, bronchodilators act mainly through improved airflow, enhancing inspiratory capacity, diminishing hyperinflation, and allowing respiration at a better length tension relationship of the respiratory muscles. Their direct action on the respiratory muscles themselves is considered to be minor (5,6).

The regular use of long-acting beta agonists (LABA) by metered dose inhaler twice daily (formoterol or salmeterol), as well as short-acting beta agonists (SABA) (salbutamol or terbutaline) 1–2 puffs on demand, are the first choice. Alternatively, the short-acting anticholinergic (SAAC) ipratropium four times daily, or, the long-acting anticholinergic (LAAC) tiotropium once daily are used as maintenance therapy, with short-acting bronchodilators as necessary. Recent guidelines suggest that in moderate and severe disease, both LABAs and LAACs should be used in combination (7). Both are also available by nebulization for patients with more acute obstruction. Patients vary in their responses to beta agonists and anticholinergics, some responding immediately and others only after repeated administration. Therefore, an aggressive trial of combination of bronchodilators should be performed in COPD subjects presenting with ventilatory failure.

Theophyllines can also have a beneficial effect as bronchodilators in patients with COPD. However, they are associated with dose-related adverse effects that include nausea, vomiting, seizures, or arrhythmias. They also interact with a long list of other medications, including antibiotics. Blood levels of 8–15 mg/L are recommended, with much of the therapeutic effects occurring at the lower blood levels. Although theophyllines are still used as adjunctive therapy in addition to long-acting bronchodilators, they are considered to have only a small effect in advanced COPD.

III. Corticosteroids (COPD)

Corticosteroids are effective through their anti-inflammatory properties and the more acute the exacerbation, the more they are of benefit. There is general agreement that short course of corticosteroids increases the rate of recovery from acute exacerbations (8–10). They may be started intravenously, if necessary, and then continued orally as soon as the patient is able to swallow safely. A short course of corticosteroids may also be of benefit in chronically obstructed COPD patients. The optimum duration is not known, although 10–14 days of therapy is commonly prescribed. Dosage is usually tapered over this time, the exact schedule varying with the clinician's experience and practice location.

Large doses of oral steroids have similar effects as moderate doses. Prednisolone in doses of 25–50 mg once or twice a day have been used effectively in acute exacerbations and are therefore part of standard therapy in some jurisdictions. Higher doses are less effective in chronic COPD and can be harmful if administered for longer periods of time as the risks of fluid retention, diabetes, osteoporosis, etc. are greatly increased. Five days of 25–50 mg of prednisolone, rapidly tapered, in response to the patient's improving dyspnea, is used by many clinicians. The corticosteroid is withdrawn completely by 14 days. If the patients have used corticosteroids for longer periods, a more gradual return to their maintenance dose is required to prevent corticosteroid-induced adrenal insufficiency. Inhaled corticosteroids have little or no role in COPD patients requiring NIV. Their role is more long-term in an attempt to reduce exacerbation frequency, and to improve health-related quality of life (11,12).

COPD sometimes occurs concomitantly with other disorders, such as scoliosis, fibrosis, or post-tuberculosis sequelae. A short course of corticosteroids can still be useful during acute infective exacerbations with prompt tapering as recovery occurs.

IV. Oxygen Therapy (Neuromuscular Diseases)

In the absence of any associated airways disease, patients with neuromuscular diseases (NMD) who receive NIV will usually not require supplemental oxygen, as their lungs are not grossly impaired (13,14). When hypoxemia does occur, it may relate to ventilation-perfusion imbalance associated with peripheral atelectasis or to the accumulation of secretions. The process of ventilatory support will assist the management of any peripheral atelectasis. Specific measures such as physical therapy, with or without suctioning, mechanical aids, or occasionally bronchoscopy may be necessary to remove secretions. It is unusual for NMD patients to require long-term oxygen therapy (LTOT) once they are effectively ventilated, especially if NIV has restored them to a normal $PaCO_2$ while breathing spontaneously. When LTOT is required, it can be provided at home using concentrator, liquid, or cylinder modalities. For ambulatory use, liquid oxygen and lightweight cylinders have been used as well as the more recently developed portable concentrators.

V. Antibiotics

Repeated or prolonged antibiotic therapy bears the risk of diarrhea, enterocolitis, and the development of antibiotic resistance (15). Colonization of the tracheobronchial tree with microorganisms is not indicative of invasive infection. Antibiotic therapy should therefore be used with care. In COPD, *Haemophilus influenzae*, *Streptococcus pneumoniae*, and *Moraxella catarrhalis* may be responsible for up to 50% of acute exacerbations. With more severe disease or among hospitalized patients, gram-negative bacteria such as *Pseudomonas aeruginosa* are frequently found. Therefore, antibiotic regimens that take into consideration the patient location as well as the most likely infecting agents are used for COPD patients receiving NIV, either at home or in hospital. Nosocomial infections are less frequent among patients receiving NIV than among invasively ventilated patients. Many exacerbations are triggered by viral infections, which are sometimes followed by bacterial bronchitis. Early antibiotic therapy is not necessary at this stage in the absence of pneumonic infiltration. For NIV patients without COPD, respiratory exacerbations are managed with broad spectrum antibiotics.

VI. Cardiac Dysfunction

Right heart failure is commonly associated with acute or chronic respiratory failure and bilateral edema, pleural effusions, and fluid accumulation in the pre-sacral area make it easy to recognize. The hormone "Pro BNP" is a helpful marker of heart failure. Management of heart failure is mainly comprised of fluid restriction and diuretics, in addition to adequate ventilation, treatment of hypoxia, and treatment of infections unless other contributing causes of heart failure are identified. As coronary artery disease is common, left heart failure may coexist with ventilatory failure even during NIV. Echocardiography is of value in this population as the management of heart failure depends on the predominant cause and whether the effects are mainly on the left or right ventricle.

VII. Secretions

Secretion clearance is addressed in detail elsewhere in the text. However, physical therapy and careful hydration are the cornerstones of management. Mucupurulent secretions are often noted in acute respiratory failure. Administration of acetylcysteine 600 mg/day will decrease sputum viscosity but its value in NIV patients has been less well studied. In patients with NMD, manually assisted coughing, air stacking, and mechanical devices can all be used in patients with a facial mask. On rare occasions, bronchial lavage under local anesthesia can be carried out during NIV. Secretion clearance reduces the ventilation pressures required to overcome the impedance to airflow.

VIII. Body Positioning

Body positioning is important in patients receiving NIV as the accessory muscles of respiration are generally less effective in the recumbent patient. Coughing is also more effective in an upright position. Body positioning is important for patients ventilated invasively, especially when sedated, as the supine position promotes reflux and aspiration of gastric contents.

IX. Mobilization

NIV enables the patient to remain relatively mobile during an exacerbation. Adequate mobility is important to prevent stiffness and contractures, muscular atrophy, and functional deterioration. Once immobility or neuropathy occurs, it is a slow and difficult recovery. Walking aids and possibly muscle stimulators will increase the mobility of patients receiving ventilatory support (16).

X. Aspiration in Tracheotomized Patients

In the ICU, tracheal tubes are inflated to prevent air leakage during mechanical ventilation as well as to avoid aspiration from impaired swallowing. Aspiration of small amounts of secretions into the trachea is not uncommon, even with cuffed tracheostomy tubes. However, nutritional contents may be aspirated in tracheotomized patients, especially if they have discoordinated swallowing as in patients with NMD. These aspirations will inevitably enter the lower airways, as their passage has not been prevented by a tracheal cuff. They sometimes require removal by bronchoscopy, but are best dealt with by regular suctioning and frequent tracheostomy tube changes or inner cannula changes depending on the type of tracheostomy tube used. Patients who aspirate consistently will require alternate approaches to feeding.

Selection of the appropriate size of cannula is mandatory for a good seal around the stoma as even moderate air leaks will reduce the effectiveness of speech. Ventilation should be sufficient to maintain the $PaCO_2$ in a safe range, if not in a normal range, with slightly higher ventilator settings to compensate for any leak. These settings should be monitored over time, especially at night, to ensure that ventilation is effective. A one-way speaking valve may also assist patients.

XI. Summary

In summary, whereas for obvious reasons the immediate focus in patients with ventilatory failure is the prompt initiation of effective mechanical ventilatory support, it is also necessary for the health care professional to be mindful of the management of other aspects of their care, such as bronchodilators, steroids, antibiotics, and oxygen as well as issues such as secretion clearance, positioning, mobilization, and the potential for aspiration, especially among those patients ventilated through a tracheostomy. Many of these points are amplified elsewhere in this text.

References

1. Schucher B, Laier-Groeneveld G, Huettemann U, et al. Effects of intermittent self-ventilation on ventilatory drive and respiratory pump function. Med Klin (Munich) 1995; 90(1 suppl 1):13–16.
2. Windisch W, Kostić S, Dreher M, et al. Outcome of patients with stable COPD receiving controlled noninvasive positive pressure ventilation aimed at a maximal reduction of Pa(CO2). Chest 2005; 128(2):657–662.
3. Rennard SI, Calverly PMA. Bronchodilaters in chronic obstructive pulmonary disease. In: Sifiakas NM, ed. Management of chronic obstructive pulmonary disease. Eur Respir Mon 2006; 38:266–280.
4. Anthonisen NR, Lindgren PG, Tashkin DP, et al. Bronchodilator response in the lung health study over 11 years. Eur Respir J 2005; 26:45–51.
5. Murciano D, Aubier M, Lecocguic Y, et al. Effects of theophylline on diaphragmatic strength and fatigue in patients with chronic obstructive pulmonary disease. N Engl J Med 1984; 311(6): 349–353.
6. Uzuki M, Yamakage M, Fujimura N, et al. Direct inotropic effect of the beta-2 receptor agonist terbutaline on impaired diaphragmatic contractility in septic rats. Heart Lung 2007; 36(2):140–147.
7. Global Strategy for the Diagnosis, Management and Prevention of COPD, Global Initiative for Chronic Obstructive Lung Disease (GOLD) 2006. Available at: http://www.goldcopd.org.
8. Siafakas NM, Vermeire P, Pride NB, et al. Optimal assessment and management of chronic obstructive pulmonary disease (COPD). The European Respiratory Society Task Force. Eur Respir J 1995; 8:1398–1420.

9. Celli BR, MacNee W. ATS/ERS Task Force. Standards for the diagnosis and treatment of patients with COPD: a summary of the ATS/ERS position paper. Eur Respir J 2004; 23:932–946.
10. Singh JM, Palda VA, Stanbrook MB, et al. Corticosteroid therapy for patients with acute exacerbations of COPD: a systematic review. Arch Intern Med 2002; 162:2527–2536.
11. Cazzola M. Single inhaler budesonide/formoterol in exacerbations of chronic obstructive pulmonary disease. Pulm Pharmacol Ther 2006; 19:79–89.
12. Fein A, Fein AM. Management of acute exacerbations in chronic obstructive pulmonary disease. Curr Opin Pulm Med 2000; 6:122–126.
13. Ries AL, Bauldoff GS, Carlin BW, et al. Long pulmonary rehabilitation: Joint ACCP/AACVPR Evidence-Based Clinical Practice Guidelines. Chest 2007; 131(5 suppl):4S–42S.
14. Nonoyama ML, Brooks D, Lacasse Y, et al. Oxygen therapy during exercise training in chronic obstructive pulmonary disease. Cochrane Database Syst Rev 2007; (2):CD005372.
15. Roede BM, Bresser P, El Moussaoui R, et al. Three vs. 10 days of amoxycillin-clavulanic acid for type 1 acute exacerbations of chronic obstructive pulmonary disease: a randomised, double-blind study. Clin Microbiol Infect 2007; 13(3):284–290.
16. Crisafulli E, Costi S, De Blasio F, et al. Effects of a walking aid in COPD patients receiving oxygen therapy. Chest 2007; 131(4):1068–1074.

24
Patient-Ventilator Interfaces for Invasive and Noninvasive Ventilation

PAOLO NAVALESI
Intensive Care Unit, Università del Piemonte Orientale "A. Avogadro", Azienda Ospedaliera "Maggiore della Carità", Novara, Italy

ANNALISA CARLUCCI
Pulmonary Rehabilitation and Respiratory Intensive Care, Fondazione S. Maugeri-IRCCS, Pavia, Italy

PAMELA FRIGERIO
Azienda Ospedaliera Niguarda Ca' Granda, Milano, Italy

I. Introduction

Most patients receiving long-term domiciliary ventilation (LTDV) are ventilated with positive pressure ventilators, either invasively through a tracheostomy, or noninvasively, using masks or other interfaces. There is much less interest today in the use of negative pressure ventilators, such as the poncho-wrap and cuirass, or in abdominal displacement ventilators such as the pneumobelt or rocking bed. In the last 15 years the use of noninvasive ventilation (NIV) has progressively increased, extending the indications for LTDV to many categories of patients. The many advantages of NIV over invasive positive pressure ventilation (IPPV) include ease of use, fewer complications, avoidance of the unpleasant side effects of a tracheostomy (1,2), improved comfort (3), and reduced cost (4).

Bach and colleagues reported on the use of NIV to treat 257 patients with severe chronic respiratory failure and intact bulbar function (3). NIV was used for approximately 10 years with 144 patients receiving NIV > 20 hr/day. Sixty-seven patients were successfully switched to NIV from IPPV. In a subsequent retrospective observational study, Bach noted that the hospitalization rate and days in hospital for 24 patients with Duchenne's muscular dystrophy (DMD) treated with NIV and cough assistance was significantly lower than for 22 DMD patients treated with invasive ventilation (5). NIV has also been applied for up to 24 hr/day over several months in patients with amyotrophic lateral sclerosis (6).

Nevertheless, IPPV is preferred for most patients who require continuous support and in those unable to protect their upper airway, as well as those who tolerate NIV poorly (7). A recent study suggested that some patients with restrictive thoracic disease (RTD) who received IPPV, enjoyed a better quality of life than those receiving NIV (8). Therefore, the choice of ventilation strategy should consider the preference of the patient and the caregiver as well as the environment (7).

II. Invasive Ventilatory Assistance

Patients receiving IPPV represent a small fraction of the patients receiving domiciliary ventilation. In a recent European survey, they comprised 13% of those ventilated at home, representing 24%, 8%, and 5%, respectively, of patients with neuromuscular disease (NMD), parenchymal disease, and RTD, respectively (9). Selection and management of tracheostomy tubes for IPPV must maximize the patients' ability to speak and swallow (7).

A. Tracheostomy Tubes

The choice of size, shape, and composition of the tube should be individualized. Tracheostomy tubes and cannulae for home use are made of plastic or silicon. Silicone tubes are more flexible than PVC tubes and may offer a better fit. To allow for connection to the ventilator, the tube must extend at least 2 to 3 cm beyond the stoma, but should be situated no closer than 2 cm from the carina. The tube curvature should be such that the tube is in the center of the tracheal lumen rather than impinging on the tracheal wall—to avoid damage to the tracheal wall and to avoid problems with ventilation, comfort, and speech.

The cuffed tube has a soft balloon at the distal end, which is inflated to prevent air leaks through the upper airway. Low-pressure, high-volume cuffs are preferred for long-term use to reduce the risk of damaging the tracheal mucosa (10,11). When the cuff is deflated, air may be able to flow around the tube allowing vocalization. Vocalization can be further enhanced by the use of speaking valves, which are one-way valves that close during exhalation and remain open during inhalation. These valves differ in their opening pressure resistance and therefore vary in the added work of breathing (12). If speaking valves are used with cuffed tubes, the cuff must always be deflated. Some patients with NMD can be ventilated through a cuffless tracheostomy tube, which may enable speech (13–16). A small number of patients speak with the assistance of a "talking tracheostomy tube," which utilizes an external gas source, entering the airway above the cuff. This group of patients is limited by the economics of providing a pressurized gas source.

Dependent upon the curvature, cuffed and cuffless tubes may have an inner cannula, which is either reusable or disposable. It can easily be removed for cleaning or if secretions block the airway.

Fenestrated tubes are designed to allow increased airflow to the upper airway for vocalization, but they are too frequently incorrectly positioned and the fenestration may promote the growth of granulation tissue. An unfenestrated inner cannula must be inserted to ventilate and to suction the patient's airway.

B. Complications of Tracheostomy

Tracheostomy complications differ with the time course of ventilation. Early complications include hemorrhage (1), stomal infection (17), and to a lesser extent, pneumothorax, pneumomediastinum, and subcutaneous emphysema (1). Granulation tissue is a late complication that may lead to tracheal obstruction and bleeding (10). Tracheal stenosis occurs as a consequence of excessive cuff inflation pressure (18). Pressures >30 mmHg occlude the capillary flow (19). Bacterial colonization may contribute to cartilage necrosis and tracheal malacia (2,20). One of the most dramatic complications of tracheostomy is massive hemorrhage from erosion of the innominate artery (21). Although uncommon, this complication has been reported in patients with DMD (22). Tracheo-esophageal fistula is also a rare complication of tracheostomy (2,23).

III. Noninvasive Ventilation

NIV is often an effective treatment for patients with acute respiratory failure, especially when secondary to exacerbation of chronic obstructive pulmonary disease (COPD) (24). NIV is also utilized for long-term ventilation (LTV) of patients with chronic respiratory failure due to thoracic restriction or NMD. It is used less frequently for COPD as there is only limited evidence of its long-term effectiveness in this condition (25). In stable patients, NIV is affected by the type of interface used (26).

A. Noninvasive Interfaces

The choice of the interface plays an important role in the application of NIV. It affects patient tolerance, a major determinant for the success of NIV (27). Each interface has advantages and disadvantages that should be considered on an individual basis. The ideal characteristics of the mask and the system of fixation are summarized in Tables 1 and 2.

Table 1 Ideal Characteristics of the Mask

Good stability
Nontraumatic
Soft contour
Light weight
Leak free
Long lasting
Nondeformable
Made of hypoallergenic material
Low resistance to airflow
Reduced dead space
Anti-asphyxia valve (oro-nasal mask).
Swivel connector with 360° rotation
Inexpensive
Easy to clean

Table 2 Ideal Characteristics of the Fixation System

Stable
Easy to apply and remove
Quick release system
Nontraumatic
Light and soft
Made of transpiring material
Rewashable

Mouthpiece

The use of a mouthpiece for LTV has been described in patients with NMD (3). Bach has used mouthpiece ventilation for up to 24 hr/day in patients with NMD, provided they had adequate bulbar function (3). Mouthpieces are commercially available in different types and sizes and different degrees of flexion, to meet patient comfort and improve tolerance to NIV. Custom-fitted mouthpieces are also available. They reduce the risk of orthodontic problems that sometimes follow long-term mouth ventilation. With mouth ventilation the gums should be regularly monitored for sores (28). Nasal plugs or nose clips are used for patients who experience significant nasal leaks during sleep (28,29).

Nasal and Oro-nasal (facial) Masks

Nasal and oro-nasal masks are available in multiple pediatric and adult sizes. Many masks are composed of a soft surface (cushion or flail) in direct contact with the patient and a stiff, transparent shell. These two parts can be either glued in a single piece or hooked to each other. The part directly in contact with the patient's skin is latex free and is made from soft, malleable plastic or silicone material. An inner lip or a dual-wall cushion helps achieve a tighter seal. The external shell is made from a more rigid plastic or silicone material. The shell includes the points of attachment or prongs to anchor the headgear. The more points of attachment to the headgear, the higher the probability of a stable fit. When positioned peripherally, prongs allow for a more uniform distribution of pressure on the face and less movement of the mask during the inspiratory phase. Dual pressure ports can be used for oxygen administration and pressure checks. Most masks have bleed holes in their shell to avoid rebreathing. Often, the shells of oro-nasal masks include an anti-asphyxia valve that automatically opens in case of loss of pressure. Masks must be able to be rapidly released in the event of an emergency.

Other Nasal Interfaces

- Small nasal interfaces, sometimes named mini-masks, have the advantage of not exerting pressure over the bridge of the nose. The bulk of the mask is minimized to reduce the sense of claustrophobia and to reduce airflow leakage up to the eyes. The patient may also wear glasses during ventilator use.
- External nasal masks are attached around the nasal pinna, thereby assuring minimal facial contact and no pressure on the bridge of the nose.
- Nasal pillows or prongs consist of soft rubber pledgets that are directly inserted into the nostrils. Nasal pillows can be as effective as face masks in reducing Pa_{CO_2} (26). These pillows are available in multiple sizes.
- Total full-face masks seal around the whole facial perimeter, including the chin, eyes, and forehead. They eliminate the risk of skin breakdown on the bridge of the nose.
- The helmet consists of a transparent PVC hood secured by two armpit braces at two hooks (one anterior and the other posterior) on a metallic ring that joins the helmet with a soft collar. The helmet was designed to deliver a precise, inspired oxygen fraction during hyperbaric oxygen therapy but has recently been utilized for NIV in acute patients, on a short-term basis. Helmets are not suited for LTMV.

Physiologic Aspects of Mask Selection

Air leaks may reduce the efficiency of NIV, reducing tolerance for ventilation by increasing patient-ventilator dyssynchrony through loss of triggering sensitivity. By interfering with ventilator on and off cycling, leaks may promote frequent arousals leading to sleep fragmentation (30,31). During pressure-targeted ventilation, air leaks compromise the use of flow triggering, causing the ventilator to auto-cycle. They also interfere with off cycling, hindering the achievement of the inspiration termination criteria (32). In patients with NMD and hypercapnic respiratory failure, the air leaks during nocturnal NIV are associated with persisting daytime hypercapnia (33).

Air leak dynamics and mask mechanics during NIV have been evaluated by Schettino et al. (34), who calculated the pressure determining the adhesion of the mask to the skin ($P_{mask\text{-}occl}$) as the difference between the pressure fitting the mask against the face ($P_{mask\text{-}fit}$), assessed as the pressure inside the cushion and the airway pressure (P_{aw}). An abrupt increase in the rate of the air leak occurred when $P_{mask\text{-}occl}$ approached zero, while for values >2 cmH_2O, the leak was negligible and nearly constant. Accordingly, to increase $P_{mask\text{-}occl}$ and reduce the air leak, one may either increase $P_{mask\text{-}fit}$, by tightening the headgear, or decrease P_{aw}, by reducing the pressure applied by the ventilator. With the former approach, if $P_{mask\text{-}fit}$ equals or exceeds skin capillary pressure, tissue perfusion is hampered, which leads to skin sores that discourage the use of NIV (29,35).

Improved alveolar ventilation may be partly compromised by an increase in the dynamic dead space (VD_{dyn}), derived from the physiologic dead space (VD_{phys}) plus the dead space of the apparatus (VD_{ap}). Whereas the physiologic dead space is influenced by the tidal volume, the dead space of the apparatus is a fixed consequence of the internal volume of the interface. Differences in flow pattern and pressure waveform associated with the machine and mode of ventilation, also affect the dead space of the apparatus. Saatci et al. (36) noted that during spontaneous breathing, a face mask increased VD_{dyn} from 32% to 42% of tidal volume (VT) above VD_{phys}. Positive pressure during the expiratory phase reduced VD_{dyn} close to VD_{phys}, while inspiratory pressure support without positive end-expiratory pressure decreased VD_{dyn} from 42% to 39% of VT, i.e., VD_{dyn} remained higher than VD_{phys}. When the exhalation port was placed close to the nasal bridge, VD_{dyn} was lower than VD_{phys} as a consequence of a beneficial flow path that decreased VD_{dyn} (from 42% to 28% of VT), in the presence of an expiratory positive pressure.

The site of the exhalation port affects CO_2 rebreathing (37,38) with more effective CO_2 clearing when the exhalation port is located within the oro-nasal mask.

Clinical Aspects

Oro-nasal masks are used more frequently in an acute setting, while the nasal masks are commonly utilized for long-term management (Fig. 1) (39,40). Navalesi et al. noted that patients with stable chronic respiratory failure tolerated NIV better when using a nasal mask, compared with an oro-nasal mask or nasal pillows (26). Nasal interfaces reduce the sense of claustrophobia, minimize the complications of vomiting, and do not impede expectoration, verbal communication, or oral intake (41) but have the disadvantage of allowing intermittent or continuous oral leaks.

Oro-nasal masks may be preferred, in the presence of significant mouth breathing. Moreover, the improvement in arterial blood gases is less (26) and slower (35) with the

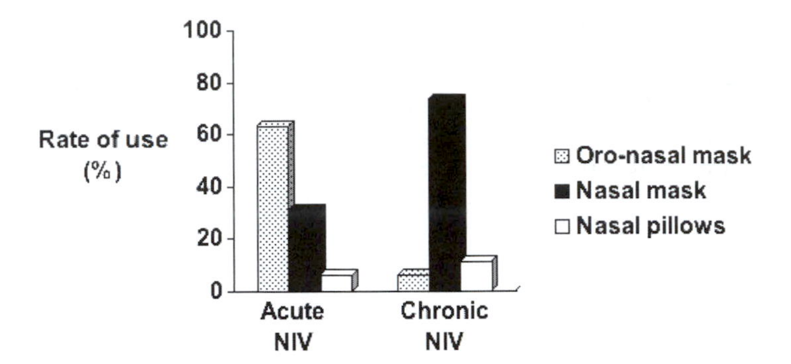

Figure 1 Rate of use of three different noninvasive interfaces (oro-nasal mask, nasal mask, nasal pillows), as reported by the studies where noninvasive ventilation was utilized to treat acute (*left*) and chronic (*right*) patients. The oro-nasal mask is the interface of choice in patients with acute or acute on chronic ventilatory failure, while it is less commonly employed for domiciliary treatment of stable chronic ventilatory failure. The nasal mask is preferred for long-term treatment of chronic patients. *Source*: From Refs. 39 and 40.

nasal mask than with the oro-nasal mask. Edentulous patients have smaller mouth leaks with oro-nasal masks than with nasal masks (42). To reduce nocturnal mouth leaks a chin strap may be used (33), although this is of limited effectiveness as it only promotes jaw closure but does not seal the oral cavity. Mouth leaks diminish as patients acclimate to NIV (28). In some patients, the positive pressure applied to the airway during sleep may elevate the soft palate and the base of the tongue enough to avoid excessive air leakage (28). Some patients with minimal leakage during wakefulness have consistent leaks during sleep and in others, leaks are reduced during sleep (28). Oro-nasal masks are preferred for patients with increased nasal resistance. They are as effective as nasal masks in delivering NIV to patients with nocturnal hypoventilation syndromes (43).

Masks can cause conjunctival irritation, oral dryness, and skin lesions on the bridge of the nose, which may vary from erythema to ulceration (44). Firm, even pressure over the entire mask is sufficient for a good seal, and excessive pressure should be avoided. Skin breakdown can be minimized by choosing the right mask shape and size (45) using forehead spacers, rotating interfaces, and applying a semipermeable polyurethane film dressing to any initial abrasions.

IV. Conclusions

Home ventilation is preferentially delivered noninvasively by positive pressure ventilators. Ease of use, reduced cost, and fewer interface complications have extended the utilization of long-term mechanical ventilation to increasing numbers of patients, although invasive ventilation is still preferred for most patients who require continuous ventilatory assistance. Choosing the correct interface is important to the long-term success of domiciliary ventilation. As a wide variety of interfaces are available, knowledge of their advantages and side effects is important in selecting the best fit for any particular individual.

References

1. Myers EN, Carrau RL. Early complications of tracheotomy. Incidence and management. Clin Chest Med 1991; 12:589–595.
2. Wood DE, Mathisen DJ. Late complications of tracheotomy. Clin Chest Med 1991; 12:597–609.
3. Bach JR, Alba AS, Saporito LR. Intermittent positive pressure ventilation via the mouth as an alternative to tracheostomy for 257 ventilator users. Chest 1993; 103:174–182.
4. Bach JR, Intintola P, Alba AS, et al. The ventilator-assisted individual. Cost analysis of institutionalization vs rehabilitation and in-home management. Chest 1992; 101:26–30.
5. Bach JR, Rajaraman R, Ballanger F, et al. Neuromuscular ventilatory insufficiency: effect of home mechanical ventilator use v oxygen therapy on pneumonia and hospitalization rates. Am J Phys Med Rehabil 1998; 77:8–19.
6. Cazzolli PA, Oppenheimer EA. Home mechanical ventilation for amyotrophic lateral sclerosis: nasal compared to tracheostomy-intermittent positive pressure ventilation. J Neurol Sci 1996; 139 suppl:123–128.
7. Clinical indications for noninvasive positive pressure ventilation in chronic respiratory failure due to restrictive lung disease, COPD, and nocturnal hypoventilation—a consensus conference report. Chest 1999; 116:521–534.
8. Markstrom A, Sundell K, Lysdahl M, et al. Quality-of-life evaluation of patients with neuromuscular and skeletal diseases treated with noninvasive and invasive home mechanical ventilation. Chest 2002; 122:1695–1700.
9. Lloyd-Owen SJ, Donaldson GC, Ambrosino N, et al. Patterns of home mechanical ventilation use in Europe: results from the Eurovent survey. Eur Respir J 2005; 25:1025–1031.
10. Yaremchuk K. Regular tracheostomy tube changes to prevent formation of granulation tissue. Laryngoscope 2003; 113:1–10.
11. Braz JR, Navarro LH, Takata IH, et al. Endotracheal tube cuff pressure: need for precise measurement. Sao Paulo Med J 1999; 117:243–247.
12. Prigent H, Orlikowski D, Blumen MB, et al. Characteristics of tracheostomy phonation valves. Eur Respir J 2006; 27:992–996.
13. Gregoretti C, Squadrone V, Fogliati C, et al. Trans-tracheal open ventilation in acute respiratory failure secondary to severe COPD exacerbation. Am J Respir Crit Care Med 2006; 173:877–881.
14. Bach JR, Alba AS. Tracheostomy ventilation. A study of efficacy with deflated cuffs and cuffless tubes. Chest 1990; 97:679–683.
15. Nomori H, Ishihara T. Pressure-controlled ventilation via a mini-tracheostomy tube for patients with neuromuscular disease. Neurology 2000; 55:698–702.
16. Gregoretti C, Olivieri C, Navalesi P. Physiologic comparison between conventional mechanical ventilation and transtracheal open ventilation in acute traumatic quadriplegic patients. Crit Care Med 2005; 33:1114–1118.
17. Watanakunakorn C. Successful novel drainage treatment of mediastinal abscess complicating tracheostomy. Chest 1989; 96:946–948.
18. Andrews MJ, Pearson FG. Incidence and pathogenesis of tracheal injury following cuffed tube tracheostomy with assisted ventilation: analysis of a two-year prospective study. Ann Surg 1971; 173:249–263.
19. Weymuller EA Jr., Bishop MJ, Fink BR, et al. Quantification of intralaryngeal pressure exerted by endotracheal tubes. Ann Otol Rhinol Laryngol 1983; 92:444–447.
20. Cooper JD, Grillo HC. Experimental production and prevention of injury due to cuffed tracheal tubes. Surg Gynecol Obstet 1969; 129:1235–1241.
21. Scalise P, Prunk SR, Healy D, et al. The Incidence of tracheoarterial fistula in patients with chronic tracheostomy tubes: A retrospective study of 544 patients in a long-term care facility. Chest 2005; 128:3906–3909.

22. Saito T, Sawabata N, Matsumura T, et al. Tracheo-arterial fistula in tracheostomy patients with Duchenne muscular dystrophy. Brain Dev 2006; 28:223–227.
23. Harley HR. Ulcerative tracheo-oesophageal fistula during treatment by tracheostomy and intermittent positive pressure ventilation. Thorax 1972; 27:338–352.
24. Taylor SJC, Candy B, Bryar RM, et al. Effectiveness of innovations in nurse led chronic disease management for patients with chronic obstructive pulmonary disease: systematic review of evidence. BMJ 2005; 331:485.
25. Meyer TJ, Hill NS. Noninvasive positive pressure ventilation to treat respiratory failure. Ann Intern Med 1994; 120:760–770.
26. Navalesi P, Fanfulla F, Frigerio P, et al. Physiologic evaluation of noninvasive mechanical ventilation delivered with three types of masks in patients with chronic hypercapnic respiratory failure. Crit Care Med 2000; 28:1785–1790.
27. Carlucci A, Richard JC, Wysocki M, et al. Noninvasive versus conventional mechanical ventilation. An epidemiologic survey. Am J Respir Crit Care Med 2001; 163:874–880.
28. Kacmarek RM, Malhotra A. Equipment Required for Home Mechanical Ventilation. 2nd ed. New York: McGraw-Hill, 2006.
29. Mehta S, Hill NS. Noninvasive ventilation. Am J Respir Crit Care Med 2001; 163:540–577.
30. Meyer TJ, Pressman MR, Benditt J, et al. Air leaking through the mouth during nocturnal nasal ventilation: effect on sleep quality. Sleep 1997; 20:561–569.
31. Bach JR, Robert D, Leger P, et al. Sleep fragmentation in kyphoscoliotic individuals with alveolar hypoventilation treated by NIPPV. Chest 1995; 107:1552–1558.
32. Mehta S, McCool FD, Hill NS. Leak compensation in positive pressure ventilators: a lung model study. Eur Respir J 2001; 17:259–267.
33. Gonzalez J, Sharshar T, Hart N, et al. Air leaks during mechanical ventilation as a cause of persistent hypercapnia in neuromuscular disorders. Intensive Care Med 2003; 29:596–602.
34. Schettino GP, Tucci MR, Sousa R, et al. Mask mechanics and leak dynamics during noninvasive pressure support ventilation: a bench study. Intensive Care Med 2001; 27:1887–1891.
35. Meduri GU, Turner RE, Abou-Shala N, et al. Noninvasive positive pressure ventilation via face mask. First-line intervention in patients with acute hypercapnic and hypoxemic respiratory failure. Chest 1996; 109:179–193.
36. Saatci E, Miller DM, Stell IM, et al. Dynamic dead space in face masks used with noninvasive ventilators: a lung model study. Eur Respir J 2004; 23:129–135.
37. Schettino GP, Chatmongkolchart S, Hess DR, et al. Position of exhalation port and mask design affect CO_2 rebreathing during noninvasive positive pressure ventilation. Crit Care Med 2003; 31:2178–2182.
38. Ferguson GT, Gilmartin M. CO_2 rebreathing during BiPAP ventilatory assistance. Am J Respir Crit Care Med 1995; 151:1126–1135.
39. Schonhofer B, Sortor-Leger S. Equipment needs for noninvasive mechanical ventilation. Eur Respir J 2002; 20:1029–1036.
40. Elliott MW. The interface: crucial for successful noninvasive ventilation. Eur Respir J 2004; 23:7–8.
41. Meduri G, Spencer S. Noninvasive mechanical ventilation in the acute setting. Technical aspects, monitoring and choice of interface. Eur Respir Mon 2001:106–124.
42. Richards GN, Cistulli PA, Ungar RG, et al. Mouth leak with nasal continuous positive airway pressure increases nasal airway resistance. Am J Respir Crit Care Med 1996; 154:182–186.
43. Willson GN, Piper AJ, Norman M, et al. Nasal versus full face mask for noninvasive ventilation in chronic respiratory failure. Eur Respir J 2004; 23:605–609.
44. Hill NS. Complications of noninvasive ventilation. Respir Care 2000; 45:480–481.
45. Gregoretti C, Confalonieri M, Navalesi P, et al. Evaluation of patient skin breakdown and comfort with a new face mask for non-invasive ventilation: a multi-center study. Intensive Care Med 2002; 28:278–284.

25
Tracheostomy Weaning from Longer Term Ventilation

DOUGLAS A. MCKIM
University of Ottawa, Ottawa, Ontario, Canada

J. AFONSO ROCHA
Hospital da Senhora da Oliveira-Guimaraes, Guimaraes, Portugal

I. Introduction

Many lives are saved in critically ill patients by the introduction of an endotracheal tube (ETT) and mechanical ventilation. Most patients are capable of weaning from such invasive support once the acute process has resolved. Approximately 10% to 24% (1,2) are unable to wean from endotracheal intubation and require the surgical placement of a tracheostomy. Although timing of tracheostomy placement is controversial, a tracheostomy may offer advantages over more prolonged intubation (3).

General indications for tracheostomy placement include (*i*) upper airway obstruction, (*ii*) invasive mechanical ventilation (IV), (*iii*) airway clearance, (*iv*) airway protection, and rarely (*v*) obstructive sleep apnea. Engoren et al. (1) demonstrated that those able to wean from tracheostomy support, whether during or after hospital admission, had an improved survival rate. Whether this is a reflection of a less severe underlying condition or whether the tracheostomy itself portends a worse outcome is uncertain. Tracheostomy weaning is often conducted outside of acute care hospitals and therefore this skill is not limited to those who work in intensive care settings.

Tracheostomy tubes are associated with long-term complications, particularly related to cuff inflation (4). As this population has already failed endotracheal weaning, they must be approached in a systematic way to optimize the likelihood of success. Ceriana et al. have suggested a decision tree to help with this process (5).

Some studies suggest that liberation from mechanical ventilation is a requirement for decannulation (6), but this precludes the provision of noninvasive ventilation (NIV) as part of decannulation and may be impossible for some patients who could otherwise be decannulated. Other reports recognize that decannulation may proceed to NIV 24 hours a day without the requirement of an artificial airway (7) provided bulbar function is adequate and airway clearance is achieved (8).

In this chapter we will discuss recommendations from the literature regarding decannulation as well as our personal clinical experience. We will comment on the pathophysiology of ventilator dependence, the determination of candidates for weaning from ventilation and tracheostomy, and a stepwise approach to decannulation. Lastly, we will discuss the choices of noninvasive ventilatory supports and techniques that clinicians may utilize, such as lung volume recruitment (LVR), assisted coughing and mechanical airway clearance.

II. Pathophysiology of Ventilator Dependence

The most common causes of failure to wean include chronic obstructive pulmonary disease (COPD) exacerbations, neuromuscular diseases, hypoxic respiratory failure, post surgical complications (2), and heart failure. Weaning from the tracheostomy must consider the balance of respiratory muscle function and work of breathing. The work of breathing is determined by ventilatory demand, compliance of the lungs and chest wall, airway resistance, and intrinsic positive end-expiratory pressure ($PEEP_i$). Adequacy of ventilatory drive and neuromechanical output can be assessed from the respiratory rate, airway occlusion pressure at 100 milliseconds ($P_{0.1}$), maximum inspiratory pressure (MIP), and maximum voluntary ventilation (MVV).

Chest wall compliance may be reduced in kyphoscoliosis, fibrothorax, or spinal cord injury and lung compliance may be reduced in pulmonary edema, pulmonary fibrosis, and acute respiratory distress syndrome (ARDS) and COPD in the presence of hyperinflation. Airway secretions or bronchoconstriction may contribute to increased airway resistance. Respiratory drive and muscle function may be compromised by anesthetics, sedation, coma, or hypercapnia, and muscle dysfunction may occur in the presence of malnutrition, hypophosphatemia, disuse atrophy, sepsis, myopathies, or limited oxygen delivery (9). The factors that led to a tracheostomy must be optimized prior to decannulation.

Patients with neuromuscular disease present a combination of inspiratory muscle weakness, expiratory muscle weakness, and increased work of breathing from progressive stiffness of the lungs and chest wall. Inspiratory muscle weakness results in a progressive reduction in lung volumes, such as tidal volume and vital capacity (10–13). Prolonged restriction of movement of ribcage joints and soft tissues and the lung itself results in the substitution of normal loose collagen for contracted dense collagen. As a result, there is decreased lung-chest wall compliance and increased dynamic elastance, both contributing to amplify the elastic and resistive load imposed on the already weakened respiratory muscles. In an attempt to reduce perceived respiratory effort, the response is early interruption of inspiration, truncating tidal volume, and increasing respiratory rate. This rapid, shallow breathing pattern increases the ratio of physiologic dead space to tidal volume (V_D/V_t), which further reduces chest mobility and CO_2 clearance.

There is an important distinction between dependence on an *artificial airway* and *mechanical ventilation*, which can be provided noninvasively (9). The requirement for an artificial airway may reflect bulbar impairment as, in those with adequate bulbar function, noninvasive ventilation will sustain adequate ventilation even with very limited respiratory muscle function. Therefore, tracheostomized patients with preserved bulbar control can undergo decannulation. Airway secretions are important determinants of dependence on mechanical ventilation through an artificial airway, and aspiration pneumonia may result from an impaired level of consciousness, poor bulbar function, or inability to cough effectively. Such issues must be addressed by airway clearance techniques, prior to decannulation.

III. Candidacy for Weaning and Decannulation

Mechanical ventilation is associated with several complications including respiratory muscle weakness, ventilator-induced lung injury, trauma to the upper airway, and ventilator-associated pneumonia (14,15). Therefore, minimizing the duration of invasive ventilatory support should be a clinical priority. The application of standardized protocols positively influences weaning outcomes (5,14,16) and reduces the duration of the weaning phase, the length of ventilatory support, the length of stay in the ICU, and ventilator-associated complications (5,17,18).

Tracheostomy is the preferred long-term artificial airway (19,20) as it is associated with improved comfort, phonation, and oral nutrition, compared with endotracheal intubation, as well as earlier discharge from the ICU (19,21,22). Tracheostomy improves secretion management and LVR and enables manually or mechanically assisted coughing. The more favorable ventilatory profile through reduced dead space, airway resistance, and reduced hyperinflation, reduces the work of breathing and may also facilitate weaning (23–26).

The term "weaning" encompasses two different stages with specific requirements: (*i*) discontinuation of invasive ventilation and (*ii*) removal of the artificial airway (Fig. 1). The first step is to assess the potential to discontinue invasive ventilation either to autonomous breathing or to NIV support. If the patient fulfills the necessary criteria, a formal spontaneous breathing test (SBT) is performed. If successful, the patient can then be disconnected from the ventilator, or in case of a failed SBT transitioned to NIV. The next step includes removal of the artificial airway, provided secretion management or upper airway obstruction is not an issue.

A. Step 1: Discontinuation from Invasive Ventilation

As the underlying condition improves, there should be daily assessment of the potential for discontinuing invasive ventilation. Criteria include adequate mentation, absence of fever or anemia, cessation of neuromuscular-blocking agents and sedatives, hemodynamic stability, correction of electrolyte and metabolic disorders, and adequate oxygenation (5,14–17, 27,28) (Fig. 1). After these criteria are met an SBT should be considered.

Weaning failure increases the risk of myocardial ischemia, left ventricular dysfunction, and pulmonary hypertension (27,29). In a prospective cohort study, Epstein et al. (30) evaluated medical outcomes of 42 patients reintubated after an unsuccessful extubation attempt. They noted an increase in mortality, duration of ICU and hospital stay, dependence on ventilatory support, and requirements for long-term care among these patients. Predicting failure to wean has been disappointing (15,27,31), especially among patients with neuromuscular disease who often perform better than expected (13,32).

Predictive measurements (Fig. 1) can be made while the patient is receiving ventilatory support or during a brief period of spontaneous breathing. Vallverdu et al. (33) analyzed weaning indexes in 257 patients undergoing a two-hour T-piece breathing trial, who met standard weaning criteria. Using discriminant analysis, the best predictors of successful weaning for the whole population were days of ventilation before weaning, frequency to tidal volume ratio, maximum inspiratory and expiratory pressure, airway occlusion pressure, and vital capacity. The highest rate of reintubation was in neurological patients, in whom secretion clearance by coughing, as reflected in the MEP, was a useful factor in decision making.

Meade et al. (31) noted that the best predictors of successful extubation were respiratory rate <38 breaths/min (sensitivity, 88%; specificity, 47%), rapid shallow breathing index <105 breaths/L/min (sensitivity, 65–96%; specificity, 0–73%), and $P_{0.1}/P_{Imax}$ <0.09 (sensitivity, 69%; specificity, 96%). Except for the maximal occlusion pressure most parameters achieved

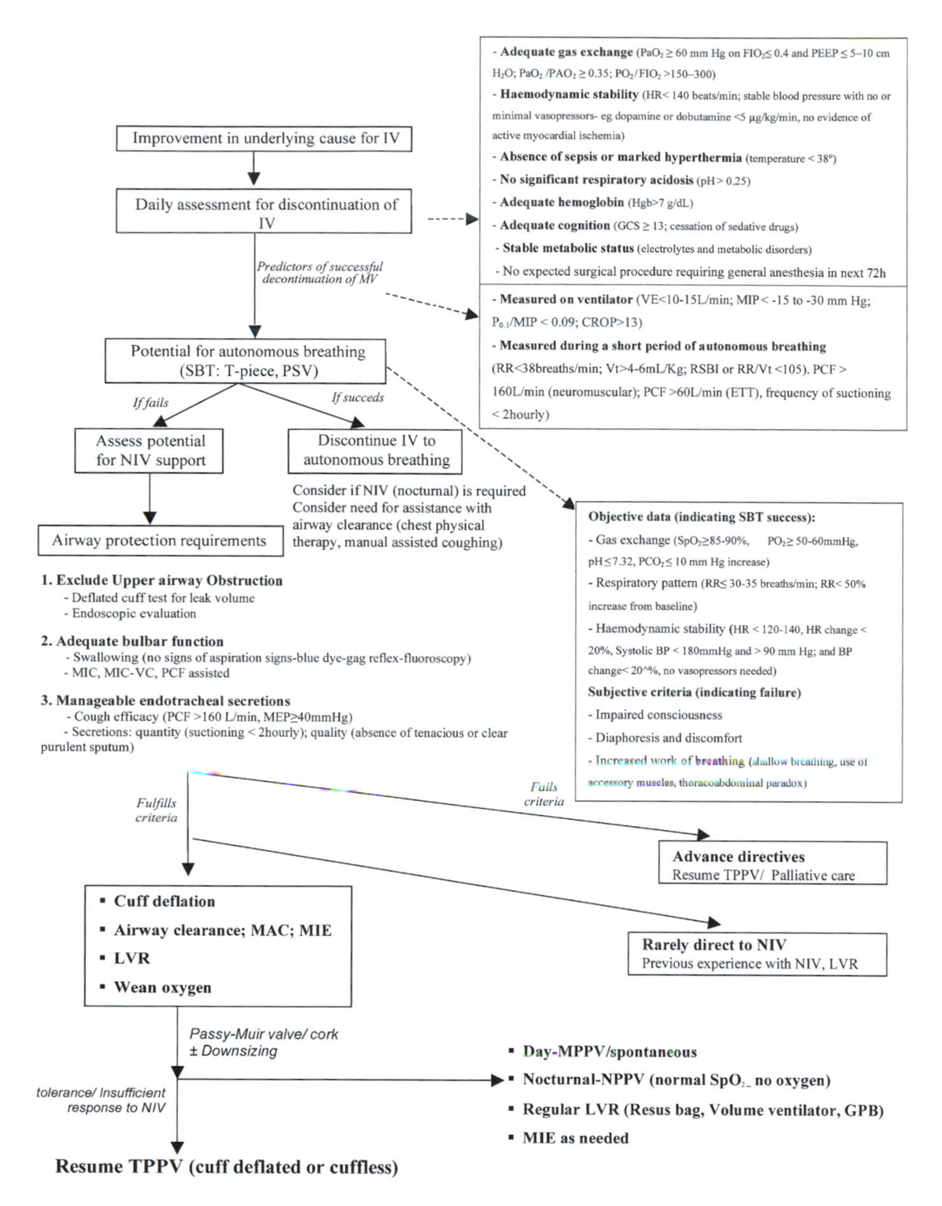

Figure 1 Stepwise approach to weaning and decannulation from invasive ventilation. *Abbreviations*: Pa_{O_2}, partial pressure of oxygen in arterial blood; F_{IO_2}, fractional concentration of oxygen in inspired gas; PEEP, positive end-expiration pressure; P_{AO_2}, alveolar oxygen partial pressure; HR, heart rate; VE, minute ventilation; MIP (=P_{Imax}), maximum inspiratory pressure; $P_{0.1}$, airway occlusion pressure; CROP, compliance, rate, oxygenation, and pressure index; RR(f), respiratory rate; V_t, tidal volume; RSBI (f/V_t), rapid shallow breathing index; PCF, peak cough flow; ETT, endotracheal tube; Sp_{O_2}, pulse oximetry; BP, blood pressure; VF, videofluoroscopy; MIC, maximum insufflation capacity; MEP, maximum expiratory pressure; LVR, lung volume recruitment; TPPV, tracheostomy positive pressure ventilation; NIV, noninvasive ventilation; MAC, manually assisted coughing; MIE, mechanical in-exsufflation; MPPV, mouthpiece positive pressure ventilation; NPPV, nasal positive pressure ventilation.

a high sensitivity but a low specificity (27,31), resulting in under-selection of patients for weaning trials, who might otherwise be able to tolerate discontinuation of invasive ventilation.

Psychological, nonrespiratory factors are important in weaning failure and ventilatory dependence (15). Frequent communication between health care professionals, patients, and their families minimizes stress, increases cooperation, and improves weaning outcomes (34). Airway protection parameters, such as cough reflex in response to suctioning (17), cough strength [maximum expiratory pressure, peak cough flow (PCF)], and magnitude of endotracheal secretions, including quantitative and qualitative properties of sputum, are strong predictors of extubation and decannulation outcomes (13,17,35).

A well-conducted SBT provides important information regarding the adequacy of the ventilatory system (15). The actual method used—low levels of continuous positive airway pressure (CPAP) (5 cmH_2O), pressure support ventilation (PSV) (5–7 cmH_2O), or a simple "T-piece"—does not affect the outcome (36). Proponents of CPAP suggest that it counteracts expiratory airway collapse, reducing dynamic hyperinflation and $PEEP_i$ in COPD (37). Spontaneous breathing for 120 minutes is no more predictive than for 30 minutes (38) in terms of respiratory pattern, oxygenation, hemodynamic stability, and patient comfort (Fig. 1). Ability to tolerate an SBT is associated with a weaning success of at least 77% (15). For patients unable to do so, clinicians should try to treat any contributors to weaning failure, focusing on unloading respiratory muscles, optimizing comfort, and avoiding complications.

Weaning can be assisted with stable support techniques, which include multiple daily T-piece trials alternating with periods of ventilatory support, and techniques of progressively reducing ventilatory support such as synchronized intermittent mandatory ventilation (SIMV) and PSV. Prospective randomized trials of daily T-piece trials, PSV, or SIMV among intubated patients (39) favor T-piece and PSV approaches over SIMV. There is no evidence that more recent modes of ventilation further improve weaning outcomes (40).

NIV is used during weaning as it provides inspiratory support and external PEEP which will rest respiratory muscles, reducing the amplitude of negative intrathoracic pressure, improving left ventricular function (41), and respiratory pattern (16). NIV decreases the risk of artificial airway-associated pneumonia (42), allows earlier resumption of oral feeding and speech, enables easier warming and humidification of air, improves glottic function to assist cough, and increases patient comfort. Burns and colleagues, in a systematic review (43) of NIV compared with traditional weaning, noted that NIV was associated with lower mortality, reduced ICU and hospital length of stay, and total duration of mechanical support.

For NIV use, patients must have an adequate bulbar function, patent upper airways, and an adequate cognitive state. NIV also provides inspiratory support for LVR and cough-assisting techniques. It delays tracheostomy, reduces respiratory complications, hospitalizations, and improves survival (13,32,44,45). Together with volume recruitment maneuvers and cough-assisting techniques, NIV hastens weaning even in neuromuscular disease when there is no measurable vital capacity (13,32). Patients with amyotrophic lateral sclerosis, Duchenne's muscular dystrophy, and spinal cord injury are able to maintain 24-hour NIV using a mask at night and a mouthpiece during the day (32).

Adjunctive Techniques

Individuals with thoracic restriction, neuromuscular conditions, and spinal cord injury benefit from adjunctive techniques for volume recruitment and secretion clearance. In fact, the failure to satisfy traditional weaning criteria does not necessarily predict an inability to tolerate decannulation, although the ability for such patients to protect their airways is critical (18).

LVR will augment lung volumes provided there is no decrease in chest wall or parenchymal compliance. This physical technique pioneered in the polio era uses positive pressure through a mouthpiece to provide adequate ventilation. Sequential breaths can be "stacked," using the glottis as an expiratory check valve, to achieve vital capacities close to normal. Bach refers to this as the maximum insufflation capacity (MIC) (10). Periodic full inflations improve lung and chest wall compliance and reduce the work of breathing (11,12), cough capacity, and airway clearance (Fig. 2). Volume recruitment may be approached using a handheld resuscitation bag to achieve adequate volume and also an adequate PCF (>160 L/min) with or without a manually assisted cough.

Adjunctive techniques help offset some of the loads imposed on already weakened respiratory muscles (46). However, good oropharyngeal and laryngeal muscle strength and

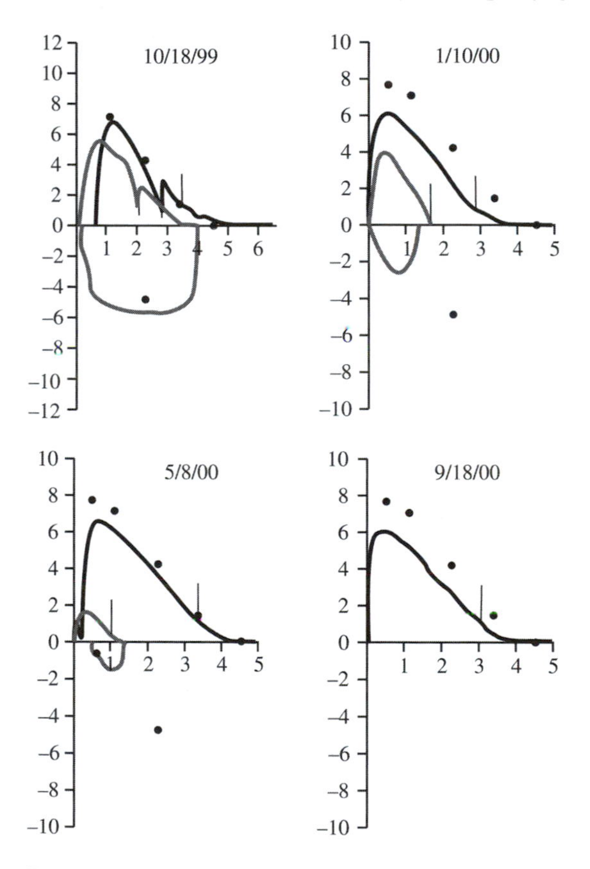

Figure 2 Lung volume recruitment. Flow volume loops. The MIC is maintained (higher expired flow) in a patient with ALS over a period of one year despite complete loss of measurable, spontaneous (lower flow) respiratory muscle function. *Abbreviations*: MIC, maximum insufflation capacity; ALS, amyotrophic lateral sclerosis.

coordination are necessary for glottic control, without which expiratory flow and PCF cannot be improved (47). Since the maximum insufflation capacity-vital capacity (MIC-VC) difference and PCF correlate with bulbar function, they are used as indicators of patients' ability to be managed noninvasively. Volume recruitment should not be used in patients with impaired consciousness, recent hemoptysis, pneumothorax, recent lung surgery, severe airflow obstruction, or increased intracranial pressure. In our opinion, to reduce the risk of barotrauma, volume recruitment should not be performed through a tracheostomy tube with the cuff inflated (48).

The ability to generate a PCF, whether unassisted or manually assisted, >160 L/min is considered critical for successful extubation and adequacy of long-term NIV. The threshold criteria are higher for elective, noninvasive respiratory management, noninvasive ventilation, volume recruitment, and assisted coughing of neuromuscular ventilatory failure (49). Intubated patients with a PCF $\leq$60 L/min (measured through the ETT) have a fivefold reduction in successful extubation and are up to 19 times more likely to die in hospital (35).

For patients with an inadequate cough, the mechanical insufflator-exsufflator [(MIE) Cough Assist^{TM}] is designed to mimic a physiologic cough. Insufflation applies positive pressure to the airway, followed by immediate negative pressure exsufflation, sometimes coupled with an abdominal thrust. Bach (50) evaluated PCF in 46 neuromuscular patients and found increases in PCF from unassisted (1.81 ± 1.03 L/sec), assisted with LVR alone (3.37 ± 1.07 L/sec), LVR with abdominal thrust (4.27 ± 1.29 L/sec), or MIE (7.47 ± 1.02 L/sec), respectively. The effectiveness of MIE depends on upper airway patency during exsufflation, and it may not be effective with impaired glottic closure in patients with a PCF <2.7 L/sec (51). Furthermore, it may have no advantage over manually assisted cough if the manually assisted PCF >4 L/sec (51). MIE is effective through an endotracheal and especially a tracheostomy tube with the cuff inflated (13). It is more effective and preferred by patients compared with endotracheal suctioning for maintaining SaO_2 >95%, increasing MIP, decreasing airway resistance and work of breathing (52).

The suggested protocol is five cycles followed by 20 to 30 seconds rest, repeated as necessary to control dyspnea, secretions, and oxygenation. In a lung model, optimal exsufflation flow was achieved with pressures of ±40 cmH_2O, insufflation and exsufflation times of three and two seconds, respectively (53), although these pressures may be inadequate during infectious exacerbations or in patients with decreased chest wall compliance, in whom pressures as high as ±70 cmH_2O have been effective (54).

Although generally safe, the same precautions are advised for MIE as with volume recruitment (recent hemoptysis, pneumothorax, emphysema, etc.). The benefit of MIE in COPD is minimal (55).

B. Step 2: Stepwise Decannulation

To Spontaneous Ventilation

The patients who required a tracheostomy may subsequently manage spontaneous ventilation with improvements in their underlying condition and respiratory muscle strength and endurance. Resolution of dynamic hyperinflation also improves the length-tension relationships of the inspiratory muscles (56). Strengthening of the upper extremities or the inspiratory muscles has provided mixed results (57,58).

Tracheostomy mask trials may begin at 10 to 20 minutes twice daily being balanced with ventilatory support, especially overnight (59,60). Some patients may only require nocturnal support. Oxygen supplementation is associated with a worse long-term prognosis in neuromuscular disease (61). Endoscopic examination of the upper airway is recommended if upper airway compromise is suspected (21). Trials of cuff deflation should proceed in the absence of significant aspiration. As tolerance increases a Passy-Muir valve can be added to enhance the ability to cough by utilizing the glottis (Fig. 1).

Closure of the tracheostomy with a gloved digit will help determine tolerance for corking, the next level in weaning. If well tolerated, a cork or cap can replace the Passy-Muir valve during wakefulness. Daytime naps are useful and can be monitored noninvasively as they mimic overnight sleep. After several nights without significant symptoms or desaturation, the tracheostomy can be decannulated. A full respiratory polysomnogram is not necessary unless sleep disordered breathing or marked desaturation persists.

To Noninvasive Ventilation

The elective application of NIV, even 24-hour support, to patients with progressive neuromuscular disease is well accepted. It can be electively provided to fully informed patients to prevent unnecessary emergency and critical care admissions. In contrast, chronic ventilatory support in COPD only applies to a small number of patients (62,63). As such the following recommendations are for neuromuscular patients without intrinsic lung disease.

The application of 24-hour NIV to patients weaning from tracheostomy requires good bulbar function and airway clearance. Removal of the tracheostomy tube (Fig. 1) must involve cuff deflation to ensure volume recruitment and mouth positive pressure ventilation. Otherwise, MIE only can be used to optimize airway clearance. Patients already able to perform LVR with a handheld resuscitation bag, a volume ventilator, or through glossopharyngeal breathing (GPB) are very likely to be successfully extubated directly to noninvasive ventilation. The speech and language pathologist will assess the oral-motor and reflex functions of the airway as well as the degree of communication and cooperation. A blue dye test or videofluroscopy will exclude aspiration (64). We generally do not downsize the tracheostomy tube as it results in significant leak at the stoma and prevents the generation of pressure necessary for LVR.

If cuff deflation is complicated by sialorrhea anticholinergic medications, such as scopolamine, glycopyrrolate, or amitriptyline may be used. Sublingual, 1% ophthalmic atropine, 1 to 4 drops up to q.i.d. is also effective (65), unless narrow angle closure glaucoma is present.

Prior to cuff deflation it is preferable to switch to a home volume ventilator set for patient's comfort and adequate minute ventilation, with note taken of the peak airway pressure (P_{AW}). Suctioning through the mouth and through the tracheostomy is necessary. With the cuff deflated, brief suctioning or use of the MIE may also be necessary. The P_{AW} falls as the cuff is deflated, so the delivered volume should be increased to reach the previously observed P_{AW}. Respiratory rate may need to be increased temporarily to improve patient comfort. Glottic function may require a few days to recover. SaO_2 should be maintained at $>90\%$.

Once cuff deflation is tolerated comfortably, a Passy-Muir valve (PMV) should be added in-line, directly onto or close to the tracheostomy. Progressive hyperinflation from upper airway obstruction must be excluded. While adjusting the tidal volume and respiratory rate to comfort, the patient is encouraged to perform LVR. The inspired volume is then exhaled through the mouth. Both the spontaneous VC and the MIC can be measured through the mouth. The number of breaths stacked and therefore the volume recruited is gradually increased, limited only by glottic function and the high pressure setting on the ventilator. The latter, which is usually set at approximately 40 cmH_2O, should be increased to at least 50 cmH_2O. In our practice, outpatients using chair-mounted ventilators and mouth intermittent positive pressure ventilation (MPPV) commonly have their high pressure alarms set to 60 to 70 cmH_2O in order to accommodate LVR.

The patient who has mastered both LVR and ventilation with the PMV in-line with the ventilator tubing and has sufficient oral-motor function can be trained to use a mouthpiece to replace the tracheostomy (66). This mouthpiece is held in place with the teeth and lips. Volumes for tidal breathing and LVR can then be obtained from the ventilator through the mouthpiece or with a resuscitation bag (Fig. 3A). The MIC generated either by MPPV or with the PMV in-line with the tubing can also be utilized to generate a more normal cough flow and augment airway clearance. The MIE may also be employed both through the tracheostomy and through a full-face mask after decannulation. MPPV can be maintained during all waking hours and the PMV replaced by a cork as tolerated.

In patients with little or no ventilator-free breathing time, daytime ventilation is maintained and nocturnal support is added with a bi-level system or a volume ventilator. For volume ventilation, specific masks without whisper swivels or exhalation ports are required. Full-face masks should be avoided if possible in patients without upper extremity function, as they may be unable to remove the mask urgently. A comfortable mask is selected and ventilatory parameters are set to approximate the daytime minute ventilation. Although nocturnal ventilation is normally slightly below that of the awake individual, equivalent levels of ventilation may eliminate ventilator triggering and provide more complete respiratory muscle rest.

During a ventilation trial the patient is encouraged to nap while being monitored (Fig. 3B). Prior to decannulation, ventilation is provided around a corked tracheostomy tube. The patient then proceeds to overnight NPPV with oximetry monitoring. For some patients, bi-level

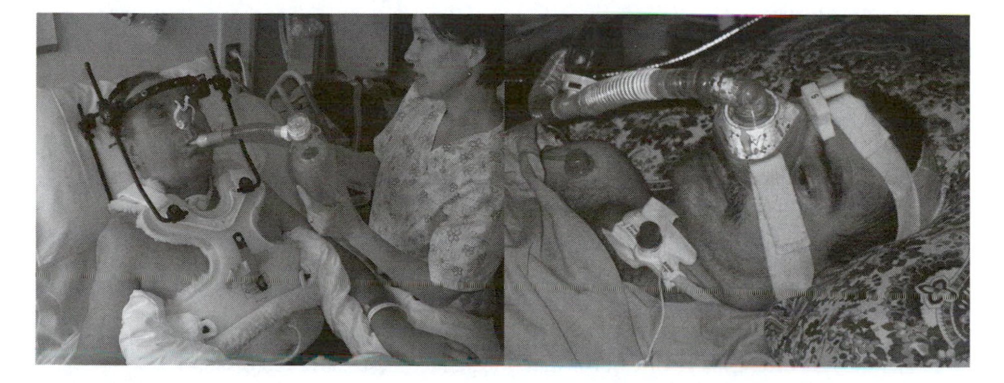

Figure 3 (**A**) An LVR using a resuscitation bag in spinal cord injury around tracheostomy tube. (**B**) Ventilation trial with volume ventilation around a corked tracheostomy tube. *Abbreviation*: LVR, lung volume recruitment.

ventilation with expiratory positive airway pressure (EPAP) may be necessary to treat the upper airway obstruction. A full respiratory polysomnogram is also useful to titrate ventilatory support.

Once the patient can use daytime and nocturnal ventilatory supports, with PCFs >160 L/min, they can safely be decannulated and an occlusive dressing applied as the stoma will require a few days to close. LVR techniques should be continued indefinitely to optimize lung and chest wall compliance and to maintain adequate airway clearance. This preventive approach will reduce the likelihood that the patient will require invasive support again.

References

1. Engoren M, Engoren CA, Buderer NF. Hospital and long-term outcome after tracheostomy for respiratory failure. Chest 2004; 125:220–227.
2. Esteban A, Anzueto A, Alia I. How is mechanical ventilation employed in the intensive care unit? An international utilization review. AMJRCCM 2000; 161:1450–1458.
3. Rumbak MJ, Newton M, Truncale T, et al. A prospective, randomized, study comparing early percutaneous dilational tracheotomy to prolonged translaryngeal intubation (delayed tracheotomy) in critically ill medical patients. Crit Care Med 2004; 32(8):1689–1694.
4. Bach JR, Alba AS. Tracheostomy ventilation: study of efficacy of deflated cuffs and cuffless tubes. Chest 1990; 97:679–683.
5. Ceriana P, Carlucci A, Navalesi P, et al. Weaning from tracheotomy in long-term mechanically ventilated patients: feasibility of a decisional flowchart and clinical outcome. Intensive Care Med 2003; 29(5):845–848.
6. Heffner JE. The technique of weaning from tracheostomy. Criteria for weaning; practical measures to prevent failure. J Crit Illn 1995; 10(10):729–733.
7. Bach JR, Goncalves M. Ventilator weaning by lung expansion and decannulation. Am J Phys Med Rehabil 2004; 83(7):560–568.
8. Goodenberger DM, Couser JI Jr., May JJ. Successful discontinuation of ventilation via tracheostomy by substitution of nasal positive pressure ventilation. Chest 1992; 102(4):1277–1279.
9. Jubran A, Tobin MJ. Pathophysiologic basis of acute respiratory distress in patients who fail a trial of weaning from mechanical ventilation. Am J Respir Crit Care Med 1997; 155(3):906–915.
10. Bach JR, Kang SW. Disorders of ventilation: weakness, stiffness, and mobilization. Chest 2000; 117(2):301–303.
11. Sinha R, Bergofsky EH. Prolonged alteration of lung mechanics in kyphoscoliosis by positive pressure hyperinflation. Am Rev Respir Dis 1972; 106(1):47–57.
12. Lechtzin N, Shade D, Clawson L, et al. Supramaximal inflation improves lung compliance in subjects with amyotrophic lateral sclerosis. Chest 2006; 129(5):1322–1329.
13. Bach JR, Saporito LR. Criteria for extubation and tracheostomy tube removal for patients with ventilatory failure. A different approach to weaning. Chest 1996; 110(6):1566–1571.
14. Ferrer M, Bernadich O, Nava S, et al. Noninvasive ventilation after intubation and mechanical ventilation. Eur Respir J 2002; 19(5):959–965.
15. MacIntyre NR, Cook DJ, Ely EW Jr., et al., American College of Chest Physicians, American Association for Respiratory Care, American College of Critical Care Medicine. Evidence-based guidelines for weaning and discontinuing ventilatory support: a collective task force facilitated by the American College of Chest Physicians; the American Association for Respiratory Care; and the American College of Critical Care Medicine. Chest 2001; 120(6 suppl):375S–379S.
16. Ferrer M, Bernadich O, Alarcon A, et al. Noninvasive ventilation during weaning from mechanical ventilation. Clin Pulm Med 2002; 9(5):279–283.

17. Walsh TS, Dodds S, McArdle F. Evaluation of simple criteria to predict successful weaning from mechanical ventilation in intensive care patients. Br J Anaesth 2004; 92(6):793–799.
18. Scheinhorn DJ, Chao DC, Stearn-Hassenpflug M, et al. Outcomes of post-ICU mechanical ventilation: a therapist-implemented weaning protocol. Chest 2001; 119(1):236–242, 19.
19. Hsu CL, Chen KY, Chang CH, et al. Timing of tracheostomy as a determinant of weaning success in critically ill patients: a retrospective study. Crit Care 2005; 9:R46–R53.
20. Heffner JE. Timing of tracheostomy in mechanically ventilated patients. Am Rev Respir Dis 1993; 147:768–771.
21. Heffner JE, Hess D. Tracheostomy management in the chronically ventilated patient. Clin Chest Med 2001; 22(1):55–69.
22. Diehl JL, El Atrous S, Touchard D, et al. Changes in the work of breathing induced by tracheotomy in ventilator-dependent patients. Am J Respir Crit Care Med 1999; 159:383–388.
23. Pierson DJ. Tracheostomy and weaning. Respir Care 2005; 50(4):526–533.
24. Chadda K, Louis B, Benaïssa L, et al. Physiological effects of decannulation in tracheostomized patients. Intensive Care Med 2002; 28(12):1761–1767.
25. Epstein SK. Anatomy and physiology of tracheostomy. Respir Care 2005; 50(4):476–482.
26. Hussey JD, Bishop MJ. Pressures required to move gas through the native airway in the presence of a fenestrated vs a nonfenestrated tracheostomy tube. Chest 1996; 110(2):494–497.
27. Goldstone J. The pulmonary physician in critical care. 10: difficult weaning. Thorax 2002; 57 (11):986–991.
28. Lessard MR, Brochard LJ. Weaning from ventilatory support. Clin Chest Med 1996; 17(3): 475–489.
29. Srivastava S, Chatila W, Amoateng-Adjepong Y. Myocardial ischemia and weaning failure in patients with coronary artery disease: an update. Crit Care Med 1999; 27(10):2109–2112.
30. Epstein SK, Ciubotaru RL, Wong JB. Effect of failed extubation on the outcome of mechanical ventilation. Chest 1997; 112(1):186–192.
31. Meade M, Guyatt G, Cook D, et al. Predicting success in weaning from mechanical ventilation. Chest 2001; 120:400–424.
32. Bach JR, Alba AS, Saporito LR. Intermittent positive pressure ventilation via the mouth as an alternative to tracheostomy for 257 ventilator users. Chest 1993; 103:174–182.
33. Vallverdu I, Calaf N, Subirana M. Clinical characteristics, respiratory functional parameters, and outcome of a two-hour T-piece trial in patients weaning from mechanical ventilation. Am J Respir Crit Care Med 1998; 158(6):1855–1862.
34. Blackwood B. The art and science of predicting patient readiness for weaning from mechanical ventilation. Int J Nurs Stud 2000; 37(2):145–151.
35. Smina M, Salam A, Khamiees M, et al. Cough peak flows and extubation outcomes. Chest 2003; 124(1):262–268.
36. Hess D. Ventilator modes used in weaning. Chest 2001; 120:474S–476S.
37. Petrof BJ, Legare M, Goldberg P. Continuous positive airway pressure reduces work of breathing and dyspnea during weaning from mechanical ventilation in severe chronic obstructive pulmonary disease. Am Rev Respir Dis 1990; 141(2):281–289.
38. Esteban A, Alia I, Tobin MJ, et al. Effect of spontaneous breathing trial duration on outcome of attempts to discontinue mechanical ventilation. Spanish Lung Failure Collaborative Group. Am J Respir Crit Care Med. 1999; 159(2):512–518.
39. Esteban A, Frutos F, Tobin MJ, et al. A comparison of four methods of weaning patients from mechanical ventilation. Spanish Lung Failure Collaborative Group. N Engl J Med 1995; 332:345–350.
40. Hess D. Ventilator modes used in weaning. Chest 2001; 120(6 suppl):474S–476S.
41. Appendini L, Patessio A, Zanaboni S. Physiologic effects of positive end-expiratory pressure and mask pressure support during exacerbations of chronic obstructive pulmonary disease. Am J Respir Crit Care Med 1994; 149(5):1069–1076.

42. Hess DR. Noninvasive positive-pressure ventilation and ventilator-associated pneumonia. Respir Care 2005; 50(7):924–929, discussion 929–931.
43. Burns KEA, Adhikari NKJ, Meade MO. Noninvasive positive pressure ventilation as a weaning strategy for intubated adults with respiratory failure. Cochrane Database Syst Rev 2003, Issue 4. Art. No.: CD004127. DOI: 10.1002/14651858.CD004127.
44. Bach JR, Ishikawa Y, Kim H. Prevention of pulmonary morbidity for patients with Duchenne muscular dystrophy. Chest 1997; 112:1024–1028.
45. Kang SW, Bach JR. Maximum insufflation capacity. Chest 2000; 118(1):61–65.
46. Misuri G, Lanini B, Gigliotti F. Mechanism of CO_2 retention in patients with neuromuscular disease. Chest 2000; 117:447–453.
47. Bach JR, Bianchi C, Aufiero E. Oximetry and indications for tracheotomy for amyotrophic lateral sclerosis. Chest 2004; 126:1502–1507.
48. The Ottawa Hospital. Respiratory therapy policy and procedure mechanical insufflation-exsufflation for paralytic/restrictive disorders. Available at: http://www.irrd.ca/education/policy/mie-policy.pdf.
49. Tzeng AC, Bach JR. Prevention of pulmonary morbidity for patients with neuromuscular disease. Chest 2000; 118; 1390–1396.
50. Bach JR. Mechanical insufflation-exsufflation. Comparison of peak expiratory flows with manually assisted and unassisted coughing techniques. Chest 1993; 104(5):1553–1562.
51. Sancho J, Servera E, Diaz J. Efficacy of mechanical insufflation-exsufflation in medically stable patients with amyotrophic lateral sclerosis. Chest 2004; 125:1400–1405.
52. Sancho J, Servera E, Vergara P, et al. Mechanical insufflation-exsufflation vs. tracheal suctioning via tracheostomy tubes for patients with amyotrophic lateral sclerosis: a pilot study. Am J Phys Med Rehabil 2003; 82:750–753.
53. Gómez-Merino E, Sancho J, Marín J, et al. Mechanical insufflation-exsufflation pressure, volume, and flow relationships and the adequacy of the manufacturer's guidelines. Am J Phys Med Rehabil 2002; 81:579–583.
54. Sancho J, Servera E, Marín J, et al. Effect of lung mechanics on mechanically assisted flows and volumes. Am J Phys Med Rehabil 2004; 83:698–703.
55. Winck JC, Gonçalves MR, Lourenço C, et al. Effects of mechanical insufflation-exsufflation on respiratory parameters for patients with chronic airway secretion encumbrance. Chest 2004; 126:774–780.
56. Schols AM, Slangen J, Volovics L. Weight loss is a reversible factor in the prognosis of chronic obstructive pulmonary disease. Am J Respir Crit Care Med 1998; 157(6 pt 1):1791–1797.
57. McCool FD, Tzelepis GE. Inspiratory muscle training in the patient with neuromuscular disease. Phys Ther 1995; 75(11):1006–1014.
58. Martin AD, Davenport PD, Franceschi AC. Use of inspiratory muscle strength training to facilitate ventilator weaning: a series of 10 consecutive patients. Chest 2002; 122(1): 192–196.
59. White JE, Drinnan MJ, Smithson AJ, et al. Respiratory muscle activity and oxygenation during sleep in patients with muscle weakness. Eur Respir J 1995, 8; 807–814.
60. Johnson MW, Remmers JE. Accessory muscle activity during sleep in patients with chronic obstructive pulmonary disease. J Appl Physiol 1984, 57; 1011–1017.
61. Bach JR, Rajaraman R, Ballanger F, et al. Neuromuscular ventilatory insufficiency: effect of home mechanical ventilator use v oxygen therapy on pneumonia and hospitalization rates. Am J Phys Med Rehabil 1998; 77(1):8–19.
62. Rossi A. Noninvasive ventilation has not been shown to be ineffective in stable COPD. Am J Respir Crit Care Med 2000; 161(3 pt 1):688–689.
63. Tuggey JM, Plant PK, Elliott MW. Domiciliary noninvasive ventilation for recurrent acidotic exacerbations of COPD: an economic analysis. Thorax 2003; 58: 867–871.

64. Peruzzi WT, Logemann JA, Currie D, et al. Assessment of aspiration in patients with tracheostomies: comparison of the bedside colored dye assessment with videofluoroscopic examination. Respir Care 2001; 46(3):243–247.
65. Hyson HC, Johnson AM, Jog MS. Sublingual atropine for sialorrhea secondary to parkinsonism: a pilot study. Mov Disord 2002; 17(6):1318–1320.
66. Boitano LJ, Benditt JO. An evaluation of home volume ventilators that support open-circuit mouthpiece ventilation. Respir Care 2005; 50(11):1457–1461.

26
Communication Alternatives

MIGUEL DIVO
Caritas St. Elizabeth's Medical Center, Tufts University School of Medicine, Boston, Massachusetts, U.S.A.
ELIZABETH GARTNER and SUZANNE SCINTO
West Park Healthcare Centre, Toronto, Ontario, Canada

I. Introduction

Communication is the exchange of information between individuals by means of speech, writing, or a common system of signs and gestures. The development of this complex system of communication has helped humans survive, express ideas, and emotions, and negotiate with one another. In mechanically ventilated (MV) patients, the ability to relate to others on a day-to-day basis is profoundly limited if communication needs are not addressed (1). Even the most basic communication needs include the ability to request, refuse, interact socially, and exchange information (2).

In the MV population, if speech is interrupted by the inflated cuff of the endotracheal tube, expressing one's needs is dependent on nonvocal intuitive alternatives, such as gesturing, writing, or pointing to alphabet, and picture boards (3). These alternative ways of communication are compromised by the severity of the medical condition, the level of sedation, and sometimes by the use of restraints during periods of confusion (3). The ability of the MV patient to communicate is also limited by health care providers' lack of training in alternative communication skills, as well as patients' inability to use conventional means of communication, such as writing (4,5). Failure to understand their patients creates frustration that results in healthcare providers avoiding interaction with their patients (4,5). Consequently, MV patients experience feelings of panic, insecurity, social isolation, and loss of control, which may result in depression and self-seclusion (3,6–8).

Since communication is necessary for so many aspects of life, it is essential to enable MV patients to do so as effectively as possible. In this chapter we outline the necessary considerations for restoring, augmenting, or providing alternative communication methods for MV patients.

II. Restoring and Augmenting Communication

A. Considerations for Evaluation

Communication is both a receptive and expressive exchange of information from one person to another. In order to optimize communication, an understanding of the following interdependent processes is necessary.

1. The sensory-receptive process involves auditory, visual, and tactile functions. Sensory inputs are processed in the brain at the occipital cortex (visual reception), at the temporal cortex (auditory reception), and at the somatosensory cortex (tactile reception) (Fig. 1a–c).
2. The analysis-association process involves the processing of auditory, visual, and tactile stimuli into meaningful ideas known as semantics. This stimuli processing occurs in the cerebral cortex at the posterior portion of the dominant hemisphere's superior temporal gyrus, known as Wernicke's association area (Fig. 1d).
3. Words are selected (syntax and pragmatics) in the prefrontal and premotor region of the cortex, 95% of the time in the left hemisphere, known as Broca's speech area. (Fig. 1e)
4. The cognitive process involves attention, memory, sequencing, problem solving, and executive functioning.
5. The motor control or expressive language process involves vocalization, writing, gestures, and gross or fine motor movement. Motor control is initiated in the contralateral motor cortex (Fig. 1f,g), and then transmitted to the cerebellum, basal ganglia, and peripheral nervous system, culminating in a muscle group to elicit an action.

By understanding the anatomic and physiologic components of communication, the clinician can perform a bedside evaluation, including a review of the medical history, a cognitive assessment using, for example, the mini mental status exam (9), and comprehensive physical examination with particular attention to any neurological lesions as well as the type of mechanical ventilation. This evaluation is contextualized, taking into consideration the patients' developmental and cultural aspects of language and communication, their physical and social environments such as being at home versus in an institution, and familiar versus unfamiliar communication partners (10). Communication is seen as a dynamic process which varies throughout the patient's life (Fig. 2).

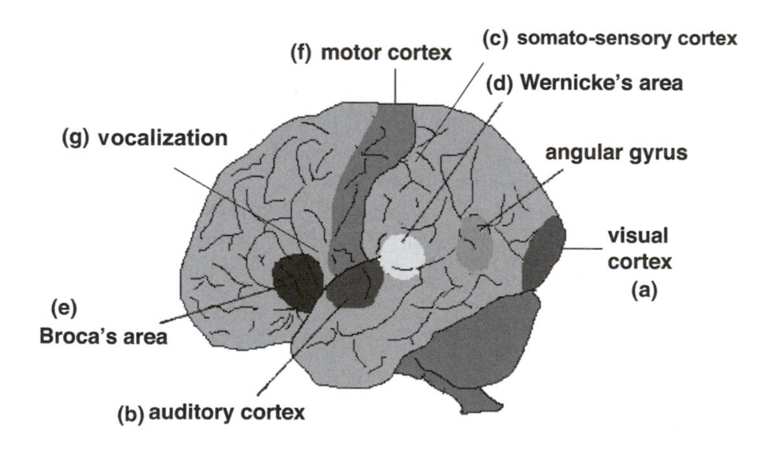

Figure 1 Map of brain cortex, indicating communication and speech functions.

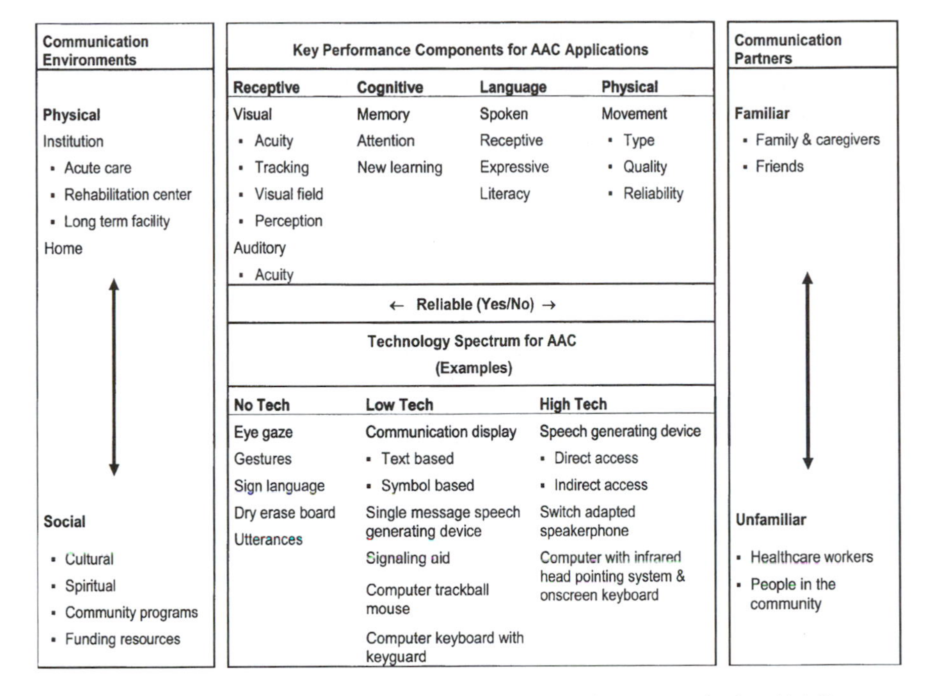

Figure 2 Dynamic relation of the augmentive and alternative communication (AAC) systems.

This initial screen assists the clinician in requesting specialty consultations that will guide communication options, according to the patient's current and future needs. In addition to the respiratory medicine specialist, the consultants may include an occupational therapist, a speech-language pathologist, a physical therapist, a respiratory therapist, a social worker, and a biomedical technologist.

III. Communication Modalities in the MV Patient

Communication modalities for MV patients may be divided into two broad categories.

1. *Ventilator-supported speech*—the restoration of speech while the patient remains on mechanical ventilation.
2. *Augmentative and alternative communication*—any communication approach that either supplements or replaces the individual's speech or writing.

Factors that influence the most appropriate communication methods depend on the acuity of the respiratory failure—during an acute intensive care unit episode or for long-term mechanical ventilation? the communication status—does the patient have the ability to speak, write, or use communication aids? functional abilities—does the patient produce reliable and consistent movement? Other factors include the cost, funding resources, patient preference, and skills of the communication partner.

A. Ventilator-Supported Speech

In the initial days of intubation, gestures, eye blinking, writing, and pointing are more intuitive and appropriate since the endotracheal tube has disabled speech. In patients requiring long-term invasive positive pressure ventilation, one advantage of replacing the endotracheal tube with a tracheostomy tube is the liberation of the pharynx, larynx, and upper airway. The tracheostomy tube may decrease discomfort, reduce the need for sedation, and reduce the use of restraints with the potential to restore speech and swallowing (11–13). In an international ICU survey, tracheostomy tube placement was performed for a median of 11 days of invasive ventilation (14). Therefore the initial attempt to restore speech tends to occur two to three weeks after the initial intubation.

The basic step to restore speech begins with suctioning secretions pooled above the tracheostomy tube cuff, recognizing that the subglottic space below the chords and above the cuff may be virtually inaccessible to the caregiver. The cuff is then deflated to create a channel for air to flow to the larynx and cause the vocal folds to vibrate once again. At this time careful suctioning is used to clear the remaining secretions. As most ventilators are designed to work as closed systems, i.e. without leakage, the success of this technique depends on careful patient selection and some ventilator adjustments to improve voice quality and prevent unnecessary triggering of the ventilator's alarm.

Patient Selection

Careful patient selection prevents unsafe levels of alveolar hypoventilation with subsequent hypoxemia and hypercapnea, especially if the tidal volume leakage is >20%. Any compensatory increase in respiratory rate and shortened expiratory time, attributable to the air leakage, may aggravate dynamic hyperinflation, especially among patients with airflow obstruction (15). Ventilator-supported speech has been reported in patients with neuromuscular diseases (NMD) and intact bulbar function (16–19). The physiologic characteristics that enable this population to tolerate ventilator-supported speech include little or no decrease in chest wall or lung compliance and the absence of airflow obstruction. Therefore, patients with NMD may be ventilated with a deflated or cuffless tracheostomy tube accepting the modest compromise in alveolar ventilation (16,20–22). Patient populations, such as those with chronic obstructive pulmonary disease may be able to tolerate cuff deflation for short periods provided there is adequate supervision.

Ventilator Adjustments

Common problems observed with ventilator-supported speech include short sentences, long awkward pauses, fluctuating speech volume, and poor voice quality (17). Voice quality and volume are a function of tracheal pressure (19). Tracheal pressure elevation is required to produce a pressure gradient to promote airflow across the vocal cords in order to produce sound. In nonmechanically ventilated subjects, tracheal pressure is kept relatively constant during exhalation, at 5 to 10 cmH_2O (18,23,24), while in MV patients, there is a sudden rise during inhalation followed by a sudden fall in pressure when the expiratory valve opens. Consequently, speech with the cuff down technique is mostly produced during inhalation and less on exhalation (Fig. 3a). In order to improve voice quality, tracheal pressure should be maintained in the positive range and as constant as possible throughout most of the respiratory cycle (Fig. 3b).

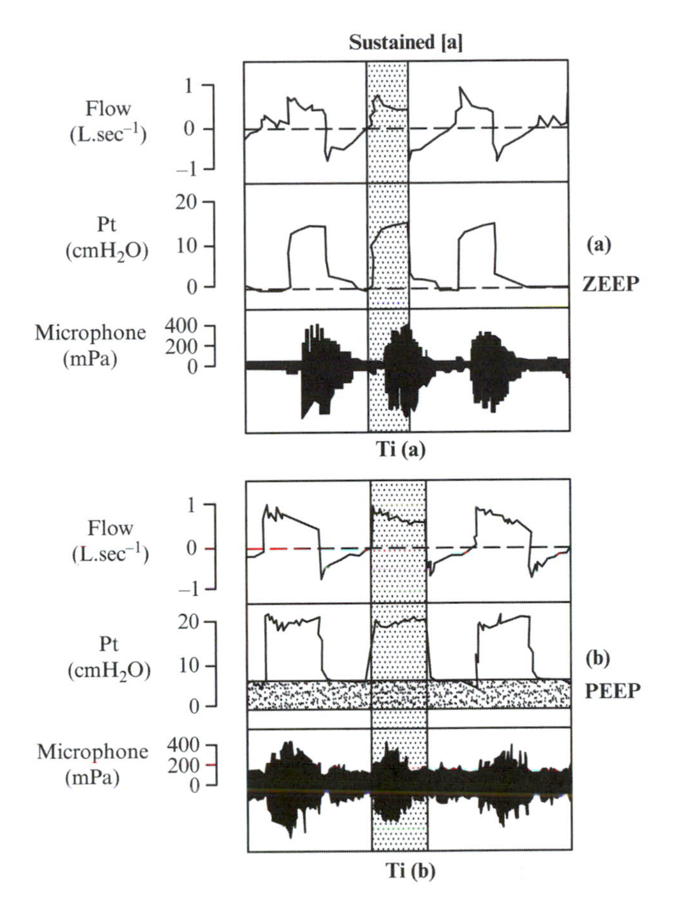

Figure 3 Simultaneous recording of voice, P_T, and flow in ventilator-supported speech. (**a**) and (**b**) demonstrate the effect of prolonging t_i and adding PEEP on the P_T curve, resulting in prolonged sentences, duration, and amplitude. Note that t_i (**a**) $<$ t_i (**b**) and that P_T is positive during exhalation in (**b**). *Abbreviations*: P_T, tracheal pressure; t_i, inspiratory time; PEEP, positive end-expiratory pressure; ZEEP, zero end-expiratory pressure. *Source*: Modified from Ref. 19.

This can be accomplished by

1. increasing inspiratory time (Ti),
2. applying positive end-expiratory pressure (PEEP) or by using an in-line one-way valve (25), and
3. ensuring a relatively low impedance leak channel to enable the exhalatory flow to reach the vocal cords.

In the first condition inspiratory time can be increased by augmenting the tidal volume and decreasing inspiratory flow in the volume-controlled modes of mechanical ventilation (17). In pressure-support mode, inspiratory time can be prolonged by the delay in reaching the target inspiratory flow as a consequence of the intentional air leak (19).

Cycling from inhalation to exhalation in the pressure-support mode is dependent on reaching a percentage—usually 25% of the peak inspiratory flow (PIF) achieved at the set pressure support. In some modern ventilators, these cycling criteria can be manually adjusted to 5–55% of the PIF. This addition can further help to prolong inspiratory time by decreasing the target percentage.

The second condition requires the addition of positive pressure throughout the exhalation phase (PEEP). This positive pressure is applied to the exhalation HMB of the ventilator, changing the pressure gradient there by diverting gas through the vocal cords. Applying PEEP from 5 to 10 cmH_2O will maintain a positive tracheal pressure during exhalation and therefore extend speech into this phase (Fig. 3b). Combining PEEP with the previous maneuvers has an additive effect, which results in longer sentences, shorter awkward pauses, and less volume fluctuations (17,19) (Fig. 4). However, due to the intentional air leak, the set PEEP cannot be maintained, resulting in a drop in airway pressure that may be erroneously interpreted by the ventilator as a triggered breath. As this can result in autocycling, the triggering mode should be set on pressure trigger and the sensitivity adjusted accordingly. Some modern ventilators have introduced an automatic leak compensation feature in which the microprocessor will automatically adjust the bias flow to compensate for the air leak. This feature prevents autocycling and maintains constant positive tracheal pressure during exhalation.

The third condition is the creation of an effective and adjustable air leak channel during tracheostomy cuff deflation. An effective channel has a lower impedance compared to the tracheostomy tube and exhalation HMB, in order to allow airflow to reach the vocal cords. If the impedance is too high, exhaled volume is diverted to the tracheostomy tube

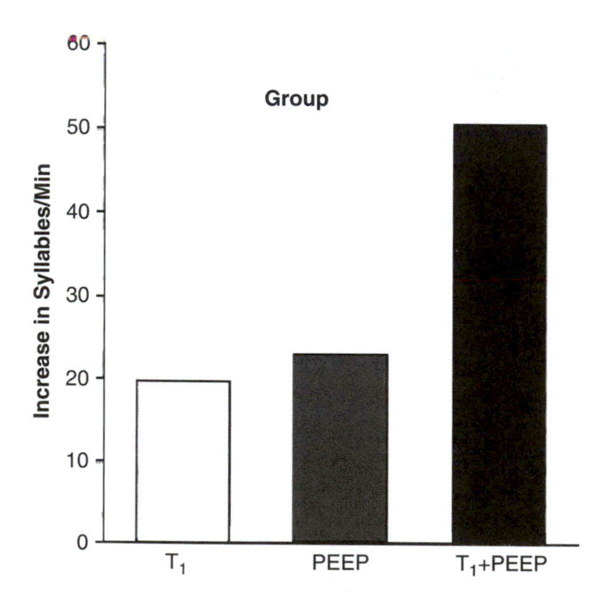

Figure 4 Changes in speaking rate (syllables per minute) at baseline and after lengthening T_i, applying PEEP and adding both interventions. *Abbreviations*: T_i, inspiratory time; PEEP, positive end-expiratory pressure. *Source*: From Ref. 17.

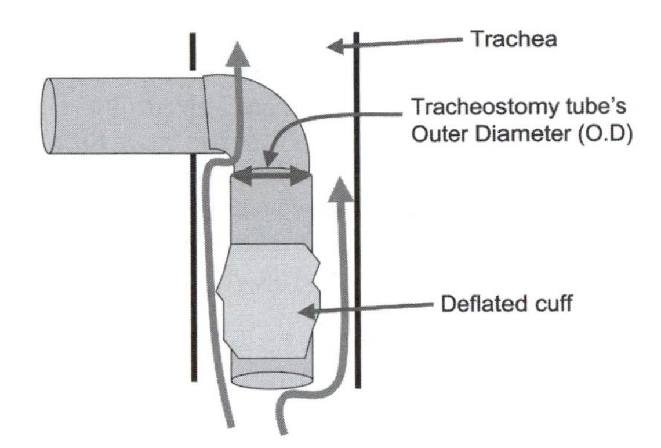

Figure 5 Relationship between tracheal diameter and tracheostomy tube sizing in order to allow speech.

and to the expiratory limb of the ventilator circuit and speech is only produced during inhalation.

The channel's impedance is mainly affected by the tracheal diameter in relation to the outer diameter of the tracheostomy tube and the added resistance of the volume of the deflated floppy cuff (Fig. 5).

Appropriate selection of a tracheostomy tube in relation to the patient's tracheal size and anatomy can impact the first two variables. The normal trachea has a coronal diameter of 13 to 25 mm in men and 10 to 21 mm in women and a sagittal diameter of 13 to 27 mm in men and 10 to 23 mm in women (26,27). In normal subjects, the tracheal mean cross-sectional area changes dynamically on average 35% from end inspiration (average area = 280 mm^2) to end expiration (average area = 178 mm^2) (26,27). Different tracheostomy tube manufacturers produce models with the same inner diameter (ID), but dissimilar outer diameter (OD) and shaft length, so attention should be placed on the three main dimensions when selecting a tube: ID, OD, and shaft length. Regarding the added diameter by the deflated cuff, some models (Bivona® TTS™, Smiths Medical International Limited, Kent, U.K.) offer a low profile tight to the shaft cuff which has the benefits of a cuffed tube while adding little dimension to the OD of the shaft when deflated.

Another alternative to improve airflow to the larynx and overcome the limitations of the reduced OD-to-tracheal wall area is the use of a fenestrated tracheostomy tube. Fenestrated tubes have single or multiple openings located on the outer curve of the shaft. When the nonfenestrated inner cannula is removed, the fenestrations facilitate airflow from the tube's lumen into the larynx, reducing airflow resistance. The effectiveness of this design has only been proven in vitro (28); however, in vivo, the fenestrations may be occluded by the posterior membrane of the trachea or obstructed by granulation tissue growing into the orifice blocking gas flow, and inducing hemorrhage (29).

Cuff Down with Speaking Valve

If the patient's voice quality is compromised, for example, by reduced volume or duration of vocalization despite increasing inspiratory time and adjusting the PEEP, a one-way valve provides a way for ventilated patients to produce speech, provided subglottic airway obstruction is ruled out (25). The cuff down, one-way valve technique improves speech throughout the expiratory phase by blocking airflow through the expiratory limb of the ventilator circuit. This technique is both effective and tolerated by patients (25). The aerodynamic characteristics of the various speaking valves have been characterized (30,31). Inspiratory resistance through speaking valves is 2.5 $cmH_2O/L/sec$ at a flow rate of 0.5 L/sec (30,31). The valve must be configured within the circuit to avoid the addition of dead space and to enable adequate humidification by ensuring that it does not prevent flow to a heat and moisture exchanger. If airflow cannot be detected when the cuff is deflated, despite appropriate tracheostomy sizing, endoscopic evaluation of the upper airway is warranted (32).

B. Nonverbal Communication Alternatives for the MV Patient

When assessing for an augmentative or alternative communication (AAC) system, the patient's communication needs, functional abilities, and environments must be considered (Fig. 2). The patient may need face-to-face communication, written communication, or telecommunication. The patient's functional abilities will determine their access and use of the AAC system. Therefore, the occupational therapist must identify the most reliable and consistent movements that the patient can reproduce. The speech-language pathologist evaluates how language is best represented within the communication system, i.e. traditional orthography for patients with intact language and functional literacy versus symbol based systems. The level of technology must be congruent with the communication partners and the environment. For instance, requesting medical care from a nurse while lying in a hospital bed differs from having a social conversation with a friend while sitting in a wheelchair at home. In a hospital setting where efficient communication is essential, low-technology solutions might be a better fit with the environment. A single switch used to activate the nurse call system and a symbol-based communication board quickly notifies caregivers and identifies needs, respectively. In the community setting, more sophisticated technology enables the patient to communicate fully. A high-tech, speech-generating device attached to a power wheelchair enables the user to communicate within or outside of the home.

Since communication depends on the partner as well as the environment, more than one communication system or strategy may be required. A familiar communication partner readily understands the communicator's utterances and gestures, such that efficient communication may not require technology. Conversely, an unfamiliar communication partner relies on more detailed messages, often dependant on sophisticated technology. A range of communicative strategies broadens opportunities for communication leading to enhanced quality of life. The prescription process of AAC systems should also consider cost. Various organizations, such as private healthcare insurance, social assistance government programs, diagnosis-specific societies, and charitable foundations, might assist with AAC system funding.

IV. Conclusion

The ability to communicate ensures that basic needs are met, preserves autonomy, and is a means of survival and safety. The inability of MV patients to communicate has the potential to result in anxiety, loss of control, and social isolation. If natural speech cannot be restored, then it is necessary to use methods that supplement or replace natural speech. For this purpose, an understanding of the anatomy of speech and language is essential. Ventilator-supported speech requires careful patient selection for those who can tolerate cuff deflation without significant alveolar hypoventilation. Ventilator-supported speech can be achieved by cuff deflation alone or by cuff deflation and the use of a one-way speaking valve. Ventilator settings and tracheostomy tube selection each contributes to intelligible phonation. However, in the absence of intelligible speech, AAC strategies will assist ventilated patients in communicating in different environments and with a variety of communication partners. AAC strategies include no-tech, low-tech and high-tech options.

References

1. Combes A, Costa MA, Trouillet JL, et al. Morbidity, mortality, and quality-of-life outcomes of patients requiring $\geq$ 14 days of mechanical ventilation. Crit Care Med 2003; 31(5):1373–1381.
2. Rowland C. Communication matrix www.designtolearn.com 2004 last accessed, 06/2006.
3. Menzel LK. Factors related to the emotional responses of intubated patients being unable to speak. Heart Lung 1998; 27(4):245–252.
4. Hall DS. Interactions between nurses and patients on ventilators. Am J Crit Care 1996; 5(4): 293–297.
5. Salyer J, Stuart BJ. Nurse-patient interaction in the intensive care unit. Heart Lung 1985; 14(1): 20–24.
6. Bergbom-Engberg I, Haljamae H. Assessment of patients' experience of discomforts during respirator therapy. Crit Care Med 1989; 17(10):1068–1072.
7. Happ MB. Communicating with mechanically ventilated patients: state of the science. AACN Clin Issues 2001; 12(2):247–258.
8. Pennock BE, Crawshaw L, Maher T, et al. Distressful events in the ICU as perceived by patients recovering from coronary artery bypass surgery. Heart Lung 1994; 23(4):323–327.
9. Folstein MF, Folstein SE, McHugh PR. "Mini-mental state". A practical method for grading the cognitive state of patients, for the clinician. J Psychiatr Res 1975; 12(3):189–198.
10. Townsend E. Enabling Occupation: An occupational therapy perspective. Ottawa, Ontario: CAOT Publications ACE, 2002.
11. Astrachan DI, Kirchner JC, Goodwin WJ Jr. Prolonged intubation versus tracheotomy: complications, practical and psychological considerations. Laryngoscope 1988; 98(11):1165–1169.
12. Heffner JE. Tracheotomy application and timing. Clin Chest Med 2003; 24(3):389–398.
13. Nieszkowska A, Combes A, Luyt CE, et al. Impact of tracheotomy on sedative administration, sedation level, and comfort of mechanically ventilated intensive care unit patients. Crit Care Med 2005; 33(11):2527–2533.
14. Esteban A, Anzueto A, Alia I, et al. How is mechanical ventilation employed in the intensive care unit? An international utilization review. Am J Respir Crit Care Med 2000; 161(5):1450–1458.
15. Hess DR. Facilitating speech in the patient with a tracheostomy. Respir Care 2005; 50(4):519–525.
16. Bach JR, Alba AS. Tracheostomy ventilation. A study of efficacy with deflated cuffs and cuffless tubes. Chest 1990; 97(3):679–683.
17. Hoit JD, Banzett RB, Lohmeier HL, et al. Clinical ventilator adjustments that improve speech. Chest 2003; 124(4):1512–1521.
18. Hoit JD, Shea SA, Banzett RB. Speech production during mechanical ventilation in tracheostomized individuals. J Speech Hear Res 1994; 37(1):53–63.
19. Prigent H, Samuel C, Louis B, et al. Comparative effects of two ventilatory modes on speech in tracheostomized patients with neuromuscular disease. Am J Respir Crit Care Med 15 2003; 167(2):114–119.
20. Bloch-Salisbury E, Shea SA, Brown R, et al. Air hunger induced by acute increase in P_{CO_2} adapts to chronic elevation of P_{CO_2} in ventilated humans. J Appl Physiol 1996; 81(2):949–956.
21. Bloch-Salisbury E, Spengler CM, Brown R, et al. Self-control and external control of mechanical ventilation give equal air hunger relief. Am J Respir Crit Care Med 1998; 157(2):415–420.

22. Shea SA, Hoit JD, Banzett RB. Competition between gas exchange and speech production in ventilated subjects. Biol Psychol 1998; 49(1–2):9–27.
23. Hoit JD, Hixon TJ. Body type and speech breathing. J Speech Hear Res 1986; 29(3):313–324.
24. Hoit JD, Solomon NP, Hixon TJ. Effect of lung volume on voice onset time (VOT). J Speech Hear Res 1993; 36(3):516–520.
25. Manzano JL, Lubillo S, Henriquez D, et al. Verbal communication of ventilator-dependent patients. Crit Care Med 1993; 21(4):512–517.
26. Breatnach E, Abbott GC, Fraser RG. Dimensions of the normal human trachea. AJR Am J Roentgenol 1984; 142(5):903–906.
27. Stern EJ, Graham CM, Webb WR, et al. Normal trachea during forced expiration: dynamic CT measurements. Radiology 1993; 187(1):27–31.
28. Hussey JD, Bishop MJ. Pressures required to move gas through the native airway in the presence of a fenestrated vs a nonfenestrated tracheostomy tube. Chest 1996; 110(2):494–497.
29. Siddharth P, Mazzarella L. Granuloma associated with fenestrated tracheostomy tubes. Am J Surg 1985; 150(2):279–280.
30. Fornataro-Clerici L, Zajac DJ. Aerodynamic characteristics of tracheostomy speaking valves. J Speech Hear Res 1993; 36(3):529–532.
31. Zajac DJ, Fornataro-Clerici L, Roop TA. Aerodynamic characteristics of tracheostomy speaking valves: an updated report. J Speech Lang Hear Res 1999; 42(1):92–100.
32. Rumbak MJ, Graves AE, Scott MP, et al. Tracheostomy tube occlusion protocol predicts significant tracheal obstruction to air flow in patients requiring prolonged mechanical ventilation. Crit Care Med 1997; 25(3):413–417.

27
Electrophrenic Respiration

RACHEL HEFT
West Park Healthcare Centre, Toronto, Ontario, Canada

ROGER S. GOLDSTEIN
West Park Healthcare Centre, University of Toronto, Toronto, Ontario, Canada

I. Introduction

Electrophrenic respiration was developed in 1948 by Sarnoff et al. (1) who reported successful ventilation among dogs, cats, rabbits, and monkeys when electrodes were attached directly to their phrenic nerves. In these studies they were able to achieve minute ventilation and blood gases comparable to those measured during periods of unassisted ventilation, noting the relationship between the applied voltage and the resultant respiratory volumes. In these animals electrophrenic respiration could maintain satisfactory blood gases for up to 22 hours (1). Since diaphragmatic stimulator implant surgery was developed for chronic ventilatory support in 1968, several thousand patients worldwide have benefited from its use (2). In 1973 Glenn and colleagues first reported on the effectiveness of diaphragmatic pacing among patients with quadriplegia and those with chronic alveolar hypoventilation (3). Commercially available systems are currently accessible from three sources worldwide—Avery Biomedical Devices™ in the United States, Atrotech™ in Finland, and MedImplant™ in Austria. The only system approved for use by the FDA is the Avery Biomedical Devices system. At present this company is following 300 patients, 200 of whom are residents of the United States and 17 of whom are based in Canada. This number is small when considering that in the United States 4% of the annual 10,000 new spinal injury patients require mechanical ventilation (4) and that quadriplegia is not the only indication for phrenic pacing.

Phrenic nerve pacers can provide full or partial ventilatory support among patients with central hypoventilation or spinal cord injury (SCI), who might then be able to avoid the restrictions imposed by invasive or noninvasive positive pressure mechanical ventilation (NIPPV). The entire system weighs half a kilogram and can easily be carried in a small pouch. Patient portability and independence are both enhanced, as is self-confidence. The pacers provide ventilation by stimulating the phrenic nerves, causing the diaphragm to contract and thereby creating a pressure gradient, as with normal physiologic ventilation. This approach to ventilation also avoids airway irritation by pressurized inspiratory flow, decreased venous return, and barotrauma, each of which has been associated with positive pressure ventilation (PPV). Some degree of upper airway obstruction is frequently associated with phrenic nerve pacing, as the usual upper airway stabilizers and dilators do not precede inspiration as in the normal respiratory cycle. However, provided that the upper airway obstruction is not severe, tracheal decannulation may still be an option for some patients. The principle of pacing is straightforward and should not prevent the patient being discharged to a community setting, provided appropriate supports for their underlying condition are in place.

II. Patient Selection

Careful patient selection is important if diaphragmatic pacing is to be effective. The main indications are SCI above C_3, central alveolar hypoventilation, which may be idiopathic or secondary to brain stem injury, or other conditions that affect daytime or nocturnal ventilatory control. Whereas patients with high SCI require 24-hour ventilation, those with hypoventilation may only require support for part of this cycle.

Patients with healthy lungs and good diaphragmatic and phrenic nerve function are selected for diaphragmatic pacing. Contraindications include restrictive parenchymal or chest wall conditions, progressive neuromuscular conditions that affect the diaphragm or phrenic nerves, and medical instability. Although nerve grafting involving anastamoses of the intercostal nerve and the distal phrenic nerve has been described, it is an added complication, which requires thoracic surgery in association with pacer implantation.

A transcutaneous phrenic nerve stimulator is used to test the diaphragmatic response to phrenic nerve stimulation. The normal phrenic nerve conduction time is 5.5 to 8.4 milliseconds (5). Conduction time and the diaphragmatic response to phrenic nerve stimulation can also be measured with an electromyogram or by fluoroscopy. However, false negatives do occur, especially among patients dependent on PPV who may have developed partial atrophy of the diaphragm. Post-trauma complications such as autonomic dysreflexia can also reduce the effects of pacing, and therefore it is recommended that an appropriate waiting period be observed prior to consideration of pacing. This waiting period varies from patient to patient (6). Some patients have been paced within months of becoming quadriplegic, while in others it may take years. It is also important for patients and caregivers to be motivated and able to self-direct care or actually manage care if community living is an option. Pacing is initiated 28 days after phrenic nerve electrode and subcutaneous receiver implantation, to ensure that local edema has subsided and electrode attachment is well established.

III. The Pacer System

The pacer system is composed of four components (Fig. 1), two external and two internal. The external transmitter generates the stimulus signal that comprises a series of high-frequency impulses. These impulses travel along one or two antennae, depending on whether pacing is unilateral or bilateral, attached to the transmitter at one end and taped to the patients' skin. The antennae are situated in the skin immediately over the surgically implanted receivers. The internal receivers (Fig. 2) are implanted in a subcutaneous pocket, usually in the chest, where they can easily be palpated through the skin. These receivers are attached to the electrodes (Figs. 3 and 4), which are surgically fixed around the phrenic nerve. Therefore, the stimulus generated by the transmitter travels along the antennae, through the skin to the receiver, along the electrodes, and down the phrenic nerve, resulting in diaphragmatic contraction.

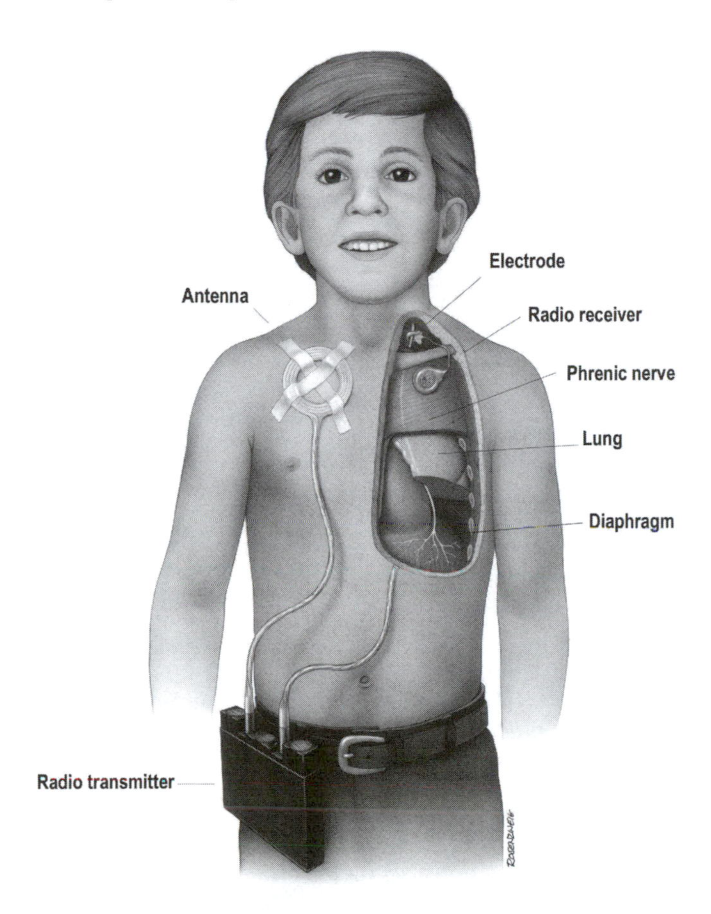

Figure 1 Representation of a bilateral pacing system. Note the following components—transmitter, antenna, receiver, and electrode. *Source*: From Avery Biomedical Devices.

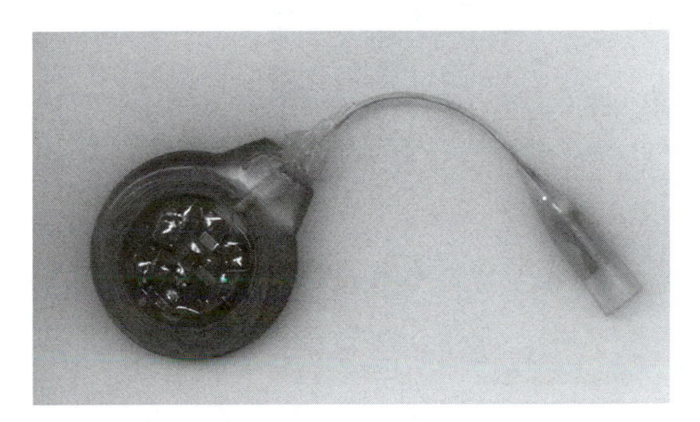

Figure 2 Photograph of monopolar receiver. This disk shaped device contains the electronic circuitry embedded in epoxy resin and coated with silicone rubber. The electrical connector is attached to the phrenic nerve electrode. *Source*: From Avery Biomedical Devices.

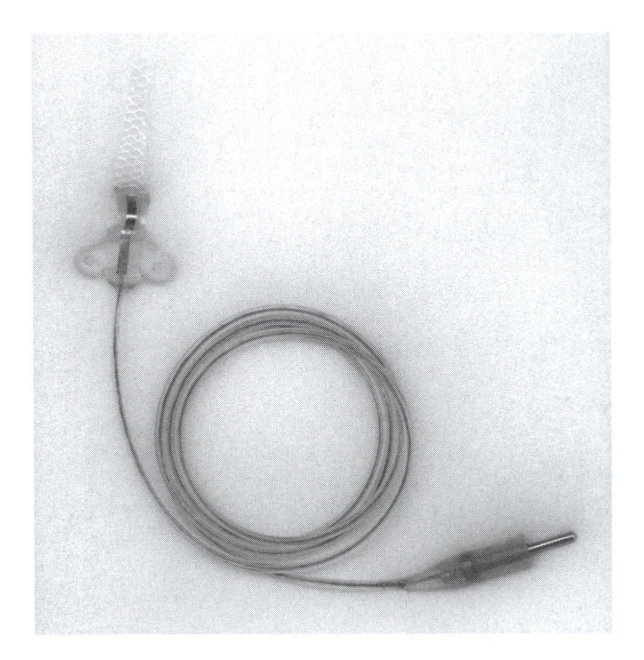

Figure 3 Photograph of monopolar electrode. This electrode is composed of highly flexible stainless steel fibers, insulated by silicone rubber, with a platinum nerve contact on one end and a connector that mates with the receiver. *Source*: From Avery Biomedical Devices.

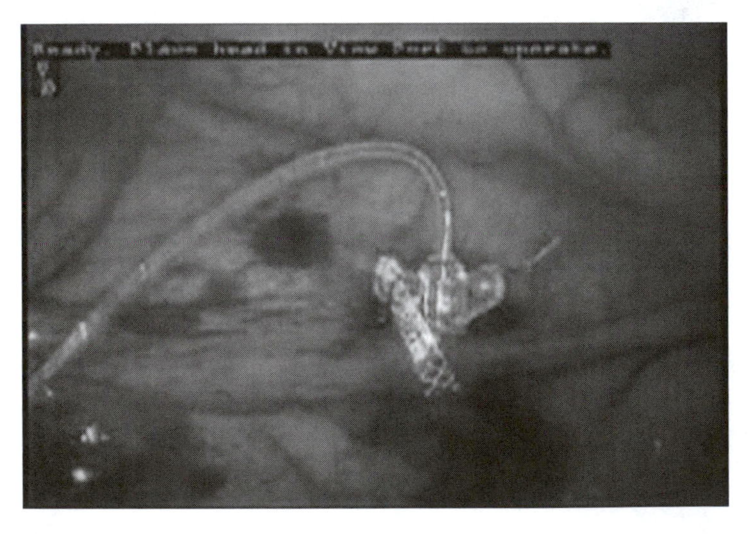

Figure 4 Photograph of monopolar electrode attached to phrenic nerve. *Source*: From Avery Biomedical Devices.

IV. Settings

In the Avery system, the pacer transmitter unit is powered by 9-V batteries. The Mark IV™ transmitter has a battery indicator light, which flashes on inspiration. The battery indicator will stop flashing as the power is reduced to a critical level, approximately 24 to 36 hours in advance of loss of transmitter output. In the latest transmitter model, there is an additional circuit that maintains transmitter output as voltage decreases, so that there is no effect on ventilation; however, in older models, as battery output decreases, so does the stimulus output and consequently the ventilation. Therefore, battery maintenance must occur on a regular schedule.

The patient or the caregiver can alter the main control of amplitude. Externally placed amplitude dials determine the strength of the impulses. Each "breath" consists of a series of pulses that recruit nerve fibers, causing the diaphragm to contract. Increasing the amplitude increases the voltage output and therefore the strength of the diaphragmatic contraction, which translates into tidal volume. There is no exact correlation between the numbers on the dial and the voltage output, i.e., a setting of 1.54 does not represent 1.54 V and this 1.54 setting on two different units may not necessarily deliver the same voltage. However, the numbers are relevant in tracking the same patient over time. The initial setting determination is established with the patient supine. It is important that other factors such as infection, abdominal distention, pressure sores, or urinary retention not be present. Each hemidiaphragm is assessed independently to determine the lowest amplitude required for diaphragmatic excursion. If the first pulse does not elicit a response, the amplitude is further increased. When both minimal amplitudes are combined a starting tidal volume is obtained, and the clinician can then fine-tune ventilation from measures of gas exchange, from breath sounds, and from patient comfort. For quadriplegic patients placed in the sitting position, an abdominal binder may help achieve higher volumes by increasing the curvatures of the diaphragm and by stabilizing the anterior abdominal wall. Setting changes for other positions or conditions are carefully recorded, and the patient is provided with written instructions for pacer management.

The respiratory rate control may be located externally or internally—in both cases, the factory preset rate is 12 breaths per minute (bpm). This rate can easily be adjusted by the clinician through the transmitter control box. The combination of rate and tidal volume will determine the minute volume. This can be titrated to achieve adequate carbon dioxide and oxygen saturation levels as well as patient comfort.

The remaining settings are internal and require slightly more advanced technology for adjustments. The inspiratory time is factory preset at 1.3 seconds. This represents the total time for inspiration and may be adjusted to alter the inspiratory to expiratory ratio, for patients requiring high respiratory rates or to increase patient comfort.

The pulse interval is factory preset at 50 milliseconds and represents the distance from the beginning of each pulse to the next within the pulse train. This period may be lengthened in order to decrease the number of pulses during inspiration. Increasing the pulse interval will decrease the total number of pulses delivered within the inspiratory time. This "dropping" of extra pulses will decrease unnecessary electrical stimulation of the phrenic nerve and diaphragm.

The slope is factory preset at zero, i.e., all of the pulses in the pulse train are of the same amplitude. Changes in slope will change the pattern of nerve fiber recruitment and may result in a smoother and more comfortable contraction.

The last of the internal settings is the pulse width (each individual pulse in the train is set at 150 microseconds). For patients experiencing fatigue, modification of the impulses and amplitudes will result in more successful conditioning.

Settings are patient specific, and diaphragmatic contraction should be obtained with the least amount of electrical stimulation. Therefore, rate and amplitude are adjusted to maximize patient comfort as well as gas exchange. Internal settings are usually left at their factory preset values unless there is problem with comfort or sustained ventilation. Setting requirements may change over time, and therefore annual reassessments of amplitude requirements are recommended. Some patients may be paced for 24 hours, while others can only tolerate eight hours. Some patients keep well for many years until a system component becomes dysfunctional. In others, frequent changes are required to alleviate dyspnea or to compensate for position changes. In our experience 24-hour paced ventilation has been sustained for 32 years.

V. Troubleshooting

In addition to the patient's history, regular evaluation of tidal volume, frequency, and gas exchange will enable identification of malfunction. A reduction in tidal volume necessitates checking the amplitude, battery, antenna placement, transmitter, and receiver. With the Avery system, a trans-telephonic message (TTM) to the manufacturer will assist in diagnosing any issues with the transmitter or the internal components. TTMs may be sent by the patients, on a routine basis, from home. The clinical team should be cognizant that infections and pressure sores, especially among quadriplegic patients, may cause altered responses to pacing.

Less frequently, local infections, scar tissue, or fluid around the receiver can impair pacing effectiveness. If receiver migration has occurred or if the internal components require repair or replacement, then surgical exploration may be required. Dysfunctional phrenic nerve conduction or diaphragmatic responses are sometimes reversible.

VI. Safety Issues

As with any life support equipment, patient safety is essential. Current systems do not include alarms that would indicate apnea or hypoventilation and rely on low battery voltage indicators. External apnea monitors are an option, although many patients refuse to use them.

VII. Glossopharyngeal Breathing

Decannulated patients, or those in whom tracheostomy can be corked, should be taught glossopharyngeal breathing (GPB), also known as "frog breathing." It entails gulping boluses of air, each of which is then pushed into the trachea using the base of the tongue. Through this method, patients may sustain adequate ventilation for many hours. Training is initially time consuming, but experienced patients can maintain above-average tidal volumes for many hours or can stack volumes of more than 2 L, a useful approach to aid in secretion clearance. The capability to employ an alternative method of ventilation will assist in patient safety and independence. Backup ventilation—preferably with a volume ventilator, for invasive or noninvasive support—should be provided, as should a manual resuscitation device.

Patient and caregiver education is part of safe pacing. It should include operational information, equipment maintenance, basic troubleshooting, community support systems, and appropriate responses to respiratory infections, respiratory distress, and respiratory arrest. Paced patients require a respiratory specialist and a registered respiratory therapist or respiratory nurse experienced in pacing. Technical support from the manufacturer is always available for ongoing support. Regular monitoring and adjustments will have a positive influence on sustained use of pacing technology. The effective use of pacing can make an important contribution to the quality of life of quadriplegic patients or those with disorders of central respiratory control.

VIII. Clinical Examples

The following case examples illustrate clinical issues associated with diaphragmatic pacing.

A. Case 1: Primary Alveolar Hypoventilation—The Need for Annual Assessment

Ms. X is a 48-year-old woman who was diagnosed with primary alveolar hypoventilation at the age of 15. Following many episodes of hypoxemia, she developed pulmonary hypertension and secondary polycythemia. Her spontaneous tidal volumes were highly erratic, fluctuating from 100 to 700 cc on a breath-to-breath basis. If she thought carefully about it, she could maintain her breathing, for example, in the shower; however, if she forgot she would turn blue and lose consciousness. Diaphragmatic pacers were implanted in 1975 for daytime use. At night her pacers were turned off, and she was ventilated noninvasively using a volume ventilator, equipped with appropriate alarms. She was stable for many years, living and working full time in the community. Her pacers were replaced in 1991 as part of routine maintenance. Annual visits have noted satisfactory gas exchange day and night while breathing room air. Day ventilation was provided with diaphragmatic pacers; amplitude, right 2.10 to 2.73, left 3.2 to 4.1; rate 12 bpm to yield tidal volumes of 600 to 800 cc; Sa_{O_2} 96%; and P_{CO_2} 35 to 51 mmHg. Night ventilation, was provided with assist control volume ventilation, via nasal mask; tidal volume of 600 cc, respiratory rate 12 bpm, Sa_{O_2} 90–99%, and P_{CO_2} 36 to 53 mmHg.

In 2002 her left receiver failed and was replaced. In 2005 her ventilation status deteriorated, and she was noted to have nocturnal Sa_{O_2} of 81–98% with a mean of 91% and P_{CO_2} of 60 to 81 mmHg with a mean of 72 mmHg. A loose transmitter battery wire had affected her daytime pacing. Her daytime ventilatory failure was sufficient to elevate her nighttime P_{CO_2}. She had not sensed the ventilatory failure, which was noted at the time of annual evaluation. The wire was repaired, and four days later her nocturnal P_{CO_2} had fallen to 51 to 62 mmHg, mean 55 mmHg, and her Sa_{O_2} had improved to 88–99%, mean 92%.

This patient with primary alveolar hypoventilation did not sense her underlying respiratory failure—either initially, when she would turn blue and lose consciousness, or subsequently, when, after many years of stability, a pacing wire failed.

B. Case 2: High SCI—Augmenting Ventilation by GBP

Mr. X is a 44-year-old man who at 18 years became quadriplegic when he sustained a C_1 SCI, subsequent to a diving accident. His ventilation was maintained for 24 hr/day, using diaphragmatic pacers implanted six months following his accident. Initially he was paced on the right side during the day and the left side at night. His airway was suctioned through a tracheostomy tube. Backup ventilation was established with a portable volume ventilator.

He was also taught GPB increasing his endurance to eight hours, to maintain an alternate method of ventilation and to augment tidal volumes, for secretion clearance, while his tracheostomy tube was corked. With this enhanced ventilatory independence, he returned to live in the community, first to a transitional living center and subsequently to an attendant care facility.

Maintenance for his pacers over the years included left sided receiver relocation from upper chest to lower rib cage (1985), right sided receiver replacement (1985) and relocation (1986). His paced nocturnal Sao_2 was 90–97% and his Pco_2 was 36 to 46 mmHg.

In 1995 he requested tracheal decannulation, which occurred without problems. Volume ventilation with nasal pillows was established as a backup. He remains in the community, works and goes on vacation, enjoying good health. On two occasions he required out patient chest physiotherapy and in-exsufflation to assist with secretion clearance, associated with a lower respiratory infection. On these occasions, he was not satisfied that his secretions were being cleared completely by his manual resuscitator assisted cough or by GPB.

Despite the impairment of a high SCI, diaphragmatic pacing together with GPB enabled this patient to live independently and to be decannulated. He could manage his secretions effectively, with the exception of two outpatient visits for secretion clearance, during lower respiratory infections.

C. Case 3: SCI and Long Term Diaphragmatic Pacing

Ms. X received bilateral diaphragmatic pacers at the age of 18, following a diving accident in which she sustained a C_1 quadriplegia. She was paced 24 hr/day for 32 years. Shortly after implantation surgery, she learned GPB and was decannulated after breath stacking up to 2.5 L. A few years later, she moved to a transitional living center and then to an attendant care facility in the community. She used a van, as a consultant, to demonstrate equipment for the disabled and became an acknowledged mouth painter, regularly spending time with others recently paralyzed.

She had minimal maintenance issues for many years, with the exception of transmitter replacements. Her tidal volumes ranged from 450 to 700 cc on minimal amplitude settings (right 2.4 and left 2.5) and a respiratory rate of 12 bpm, to maintain blood gases within the normal range. Routine follow-up phrenic nerve studies showed that conduction time on both sides and the diaphragmatic response to phrenic nerve stimulation was normal.

In 2003 she required surgery unrelated to her respiratory condition. Postoperatively she required intubation and ventilation. When she resumed pacer ventilation, her pacers were turned up to much higher amplitudes, to "promote" better ventilation. However, her tidal volumes remained low at 320 to 350 cc and during her recovery she used manual ventilation and GPB frequently, to provide comfort, by increasing her volumes to 650 cc. Repeat phrenic nerve conduction studies showed that the left phrenic nerve was not discharging, and it was feared that after 30 years of pacing the nerve had become dysfunctional. Nocturnal nasal volume ventilation was implemented to provide ventilatory support while resting the phrenic nerves at night. During the day she used them only for short periods, being ventilated by GPB and by NIPPV. Within two months her pacing volumes improved dramatically and subsequent nerve conduction studies showed that full bilateral phrenic nerve responses were again present.

This very stable individual, paced for more than 30 years, was managed perioperatively by a team with no pacemaker experience. The inappropriate increase in amplitude did not substantially increase tidal volumes but did create phrenic nerve dysfunction. The situation was reversed by resting the nerves and fortunately full recovery occurred.

Diaphragmatic pacing is a viable alternative to PPV for a small number of carefully selected patients, with SCI or central hypoventilation. Regular assessments by an experienced clinical team, backup ventilation, GPB, effective secretion management, and appropriate education will enable these complex patients to enjoy increased independence and an improved quality of life.

References

1. Sarnoff SJ, Hardenbergh E, Whittenberger JL. Electrophrenic respiration. Am J Physiol 1948; 155(1):1–9.
2. Avery Biomedical Devices. Instruction Manual—Implanted Breathing Pacemaker System, 2004.
3. Glenn WWL, Holcomb WG, Hogan J, et al. Diaphragm pacing by radiofrequency transmission in the treatment of chronic ventilatory insufficiency. J Thorac Cardiovasc Surg 1973; 66(4):505–520.
4. Onders RP, Aiyar H, Mortimer T. Characterization of the human diaphragm muscle with respect to the phrenic nerve motor points for diaphragmatic pacing. Am Surg 2004; 70:241–247.
5. Dumitru D, Amato AA, Zwarts, MJ. Electrodiagnostic Medicine. 2nd ed. Philadelphia: Hanley & Belfus Inc., 2002.
6. Adams RD, Maurice V, Ropper AH. Principles of Neurology. 6th ed. New York: McGraw-Hill, 1997.

28
Secretion Management

MIGUEL R. GONÇALVES
Pulmonary Medicine Department, Intensive Care and Emergency Department, University Hospital S. João, Porto, Portugal

I. Introduction

In healthy individuals, mucociliary clearance and cough mechanisms are normally effective and efficient for defense on secretion encumbrance, but may become ineffective if these systems malfunction and in the presence of excessive bronchial secretions. Mucus secretion and clearance are extremely important for airway integrity and pulmonary defense. It has been estimated that mucus secretion volume is between 10 and 100 mL/day in healthy subjects (1).

Mucus is transported from the lower respiratory tract into the pharynx by airflow and mucociliary clearance. Overload of normal secretion or mucociliary clearance impairs pulmonary function and increases the risk of infection. When there is extensive ciliary damage and secretion encumbrance, coughing becomes critically important for airway hygiene (2). Airflow-dependent clearance can also be increased by moving secretions from the periphery of the lung to the more proximal airways, where greater secretion depth and higher expiratory airflow can improve expectoration. This is why cough is generally incorporated into most chest physical therapy techniques (3).

Cough and expectoration of mucus are the best-known symptoms in patients with pulmonary impairment disorders. Airway clearance may be impaired in disorders associated with abnormal cough mechanics, altered mucus rheology, altered mucociliary clearance, or structural airway defects. A variety of interventions are used to enhance airway clearance with the goal of improving lung mechanics and gas exchange, and preventing atelectasis and infection (4).

Techniques for augmenting the normal mucociliary clearance and cough efficacy have been used for many years to treat patients with respiratory disorders from different etiologies. In the recent years, new technologies and more advanced techniques have been developed to be more comfortable and effective for the majority of patients. Postural drainage (PD) with manual chest percussion and shaking has, in most parts of the world, been replaced by more independent and effective techniques such as the active cycle of breathing, autogenic drainage, R-C Cornet®, Flutter®, positive expiratory pressure mask, high frequency chest wall oscillation (HFCWO), intrapulmonary percussive ventilation (IPV), and mechanical insufflation-exsufflation (MI-E) (2). The evidence in support of these techniques is variable and the literature is confusing and sometimes conflicting, regarding the clinical indication for each technique. This fact may be related to the intensity, duration, and frequency being different between physiotherapists in different parts of the world, and have changed over the years (5).

The effective elimination of airway mucus and other debris is one of the most important factor that permits successful use of chronic and acute ventilation support (noninvasive and invasive) for patients with either ventilatory or oxygenation impairment. In ventilatory dependent patients, the goals of intervention are to maintain lung compliance and normal alveolar ventilation at all times and to maximize cough flows for adequate bronchopulmonary secretion clearance (6).

In patients primarily afflicted with ventilatory impairment, 90% of the episodes of respiratory failure are a result of the inability to effectively clear airway mucus during intercurrent chest colds (7). Although the use of respiratory muscle aids is the single most important intervention for eliminating airway secretions for patients with inspiratory and expiratory muscle weakness, as for normal coughing these aids may not adequately expulse secretions from the very small peripheral airways, more than six divisions from the trachea, the flows that they create may not be sufficient to secretions that are obstructing the smaller airways (8). In these situations, as well as for patients with severe bulbar muscle dysfunction who aspirate upper airway secretions, it is important to consider other methods to gradually move mucus and airway debris. Moreover, it has been demonstrated that in acute episodes of respiratory failure, morbidity and mortality can be avoided without hospitalization with a correct and effective secretion management protocol (9).

II. Physiological Basis for Mucus Hypersecretion and Transport from the Lower Respiratory Tract

Healthy human lungs are protected against inhaled dust particles and microorganisms by the continuous production of mucus and by the transport of deposited particles and mucus to the oropharynx. Airway mucus is a viscoelastic gel containing water, carbohydrates, proteins, and lipids and it is transported from the lower respiratory tract into the pharynx by airflow and mucociliary clearance. Airway mucus is produced throughout the bronchial tree by serous cells, goblet or mucus cells. The depth and composition of mucus depend on secretion from airway glands, goblet cell discharge, and active ion transport across surface epithelium (1,10).

The transport of secretions (mainly carried out via ciliary movement) depends on mechanical vectors in which the positive forces oppose those of inertia and friction. Because fluids are involved, the most important frictional forces are determined by rheological characteristics, interface surface tension, and adhesion between the secretions themselves and the epithelium (11,12).

The relation between the viscosity and elasticity of the secretions is one of the determining factors in transport velocity. If the gel phase is in practice the only one really transported, the sol phase creates a low-resistance milieu where the cilia can beat, an environment that is essential for transport in the direction of the upper airways. One of the most important rheological properties of mucus is viscosity. Viscosity is resistance to flow and represents the capacity of a material to absorb energy while it moves. Elasticity is the capacity to store the energy used to move or deform material. The ratio between viscosity and elasticity appears to be an important determinant of the transport rate (6,10). Mucus transport by ciliary beating is influenced by the viscoelastic and surface properties of the mucus. Theoretical models suggest that a decrease in the ratio of viscosity to elasticity can result in an increase in mucociliary transport (13).

Patients who have bronchorrhea are unable to clear secretions effectively. Mucociliary clearance is more sensitive to high levels of viscosity, although high levels of elasticity may also impede ciliary transport. Cough transportability is less dependent on viscosity. Preliminary studies suggest that for mucus with similar degrees of tenacity, cough transportability is increased with greater mucus viscosity (3).

At any point on the bronchial tree, the transport surface is determined by the inside diameter and the number of airways at this level. Moving from the center toward the periphery, diameters decrease, but the number of airways increases exponentially so that the transport surface decreases proportionally. As a result, the transporting surface of the airways decreases from the peripheral to the central airways. Accumulation of mucus in the central airways is normally countered by the higher mucus transport rate centrally than peripherally, and possibly by a greater reabsorption of watery constituents centrally.

The small transport surface in the main airways (which could lead to the accumulation of secretions) is compensated in normal subjects by greater velocity related to higher ciliary beat frequency. The most important transport mechanism of mucus in the bronchial tree is mucociliary transport. This movement takes place by coordinated activity of cilia that cover the bronchial surface of the airways. Ciliated cells are found in the airways from the trachea to the terminal bronchioles. Each cell contains about 200 cilia, all of which end in little claws. The cilia beat in the direction of the oropharynx with a frequency of about 8 to 15 Hz. The claws of the cilia reach the mucus gel layer and push this layer towards the oropharynx. The recovery beat in the direction of the bronchioles takes place only in the periciliary sol layer. The cilia normally move the mucus at 1 mm/min in smaller airways and at up to 2 cm/min in the trachea (1,4,6).

Longer cilia should be able to clear mucus faster because they can generate a greater forward velocity. In smaller airways the cilia are generally shorter and fewer in number than in the large bronchi, and even though the cilia beat frequency may be comparable, the rate of momentum transfer to the mucus is proportionately less.

Acute and chronic airway inflammation can also lead to acquired ciliary dysfunction and to sloughing of the ciliated epithelium, with disruption of the mucociliary elevator. With chronic airway inflammation the cilia can be damaged, making it even more difficult to clear the secretions.

III. Impairment of Mucus Elimination and Clinical Indications for Airway Clearance Techniques

In normal conditions, secretion production is small and voluntary coughing is unproductive. However, when disease is present (such as in acute bronchitis), the molecular components change, production increases considerably, and sputum is formed from mucus, inflammatory cells, cell debris, and bacteria. Disruption of normal secretion or mucociliary clearance impairs pulmonary function and lung defense and increases risk of infection (14). However, it is not clear whether hypersecretion is only a marker of inflammation or a cause of pathological changes. There is even some evidence that stasis of mucus protects against inhaled material (15).

When there is extensive ciliary damage and mucus hypersecretion, airflow-dependent mucus clearance such as cough becomes critically important for airway hygiene. As a result of mucus production increase and poor ciliary response related to inflammation, ciliary clearing ceases to be capable of maintaining airway permeability, and coughing must take on a greater role in expelling excess secretions (16). In lung diseases characterized by mucus hypersecretion and impaired airway clearance, the excess mucus is largely expectorated by coughing. Effective cough depends on high gas flow and intrathoracic pressures to enhance mucus removal (17). Cough is ineffective when respiratory muscles are weak or when mucus adheres to the airway wall.

Severe mucus plugging in the peripheral airways may have an effect on lung volume, such as the residual volume to total lung capacity ratio or trapped gas volume. A smaller amount of mucus, not completely obstructing the airways, may have an effect on forced expiratory flow variables (5,16,18).

For patients with chronic airways disease, mucus stasis can contribute to bronchial obstruction and chronic expectoration can be a physically and socially disabling problem. Mucus retention can also cause pathological changes in the lungs and is thought to contribute to the progression of airways disease. It is, therefore, not surprising that for patients with chronic airways disease, mucus hypersecretion has been associated with increased mortality (19) and it is thought to contribute to the development of respiratory tract infections.

Mucus clearance and bronchial hygiene are often decreased in patients with airways diseases, such as asthma, chronic obstructive pulmonary disease (COPD), and cystic fibrosis (CF), as well as in patients with neuromuscular disorders and consequent dysfunctional cough or glottic control.

A. Patients with Airways Diseases

Stasis of mucus in the airways may contribute to bronchial obstruction in patients with chronic bronchitis and also in patients experiencing an acute asthmatic episode. Mucus retention can cause pathological changes in the lungs and is thought to contribute to the progression of airways disease.

In asthmatic patients, the most common symptoms are dyspnea and bronchospasm than can usually be reversed with bronchodilatation therapy that probably has no effect on mucus clearance transport (20). Hypersecretion is usually present in the acute episodes of asthma and normally mucus transport is impaired due to reduction of ciliary activity (21). Mucus hypersecretion and changes in the rheological or surface properties of mucus may also cause reduction of ciliary activity (6). In these patients, mucus transport can be recovered or remain reduced, despite favorable changes in mucus viscoelasticity after an exacerbation.

In patients with COPD there is a persistent and permanent dyspnea and airway obstruction, with incomplete reversibility with therapy. Normally, in these patients, the mucociliary transport is not so impaired, until an acute exacerbation occurs. During an acute exacerbation of COPD, hypersecretion is usually present and may be induced by bacterial infections. Secretion encumbrance and ineffectiveness of airway clearance is associated with failure of noninvasive ventilation (NIV), whereas endotraqueal intubation and mechanical ventilation is necessary in acute exacerbations of COPD. The duration of mechanical ventilation was correlated with hospital mortality (22).

CF is a relatively common, inherited, life-limiting disorder. The major clinical manifestations of CF respiratory disease are retention of sputum, reduced exercise capacity, pulmonary function impairment, and breathlessness (23).

Genetic defect causes abnormal mucus secretion in the airways, potentially leading to airway obstruction and mucus plugging. This blockage predisposes the airways to infection and inflammation, which in turn promote further mucus secretion. Persistent infection and inflammation within the lungs are the major contributory factors to airway damage and the progressive loss of respiratory function. Although bronchial mucus is considered to be a bigger problem in CF than in COPD, the rheological characteristics of CF sputum are comparable to those of sputum from chronic bronchitis patients (6,24).

Treatment methods, which improve mucus clearance, are considered essential in optimizing the respiratory status and reducing the progression of lung disease. Physical therapy involves a range of interventions (including airway clearance and physical training), which have an overall aim of reducing progression of CF respiratory disease. Many different airway clearance techniques are available, but, in general, their goal is to reduce disease progression by augmenting the normal mucociliary clearance mechanism of the lungs and facilitating expectoration (25).

B. Patients with Neuromuscular Disorders

Airway mucus elimination can be impaired by factors external to the lungs and airways. When mucociliary clearing fails and coughing is indispensable for bronchial clearance, the effectiveness in eliminating secretions is determined by the amount of flow generated in the expulsive phase. These factors depend on the linear velocity of gas flow, the diameter of the segment, and dynamic compression, and they are manifested basically in the peak cough flow (PCF) (26).

In NMD there is a progressive decrease in vital capacity (VC), which is mainly related to muscle weakness. The lung volume changes that appear in some NMD patients are attributable to a combination of muscle weakness and alterations of the mechanical properties of the lungs and the chest wall (27). In NMD three factors may affect lung compliance in such cases: the presence of subclinical and heterogeneous alveolar collapses, the generalized increase of superficial alveolar tension in consequence of low-volume ventilation, and the shortening and hardening of the elastic fibers of the lung because of sustained absence of "stretching" of the parenchyma (12,28).

If these muscles are weak, they do not manage to completely insufflate the lungs and thus are also unable to generate an adequate PCF. Changes in the ability to cough, understood as the inability to expel secretions effectively or finding it difficult to do so, may precede alterations in alveolar ventilation and places patients at risk for atelectasis, mucus plugging, and pneumonia. Such alterations are the main cause of morbidity and mortality in patients with NMD (9). Paradoxically, the problem of managing secretions has received little attention in the care of NMD patients.

Along with hypoventilation, these alterations represent the most important problem from the patient's point of view (29). Severe bulbar dysfunction and glottic dysfunction most commonly occur in patients with amyotrophic lateral sclerosis (ALS), spinal muscle atrophy type 1, and the pseudobulbar palsy of central nervous system etiology (30). Inability to close the glottis and vocal cords results in complete loss of the ability to cough and swallow.

Difficulty in swallowing liquids may result in the pooling of saliva and mucus in the pharynx, especially in the valleculae (wedge-shaped space formed by the base of the tongue and the epiglottis) and the pyriform sinuses (space formed on each side between the inferior pharyngeal constrictor and the thyroid cartilage). This accumulation results in the perception of excessive pharyngeal secretions, similar to postnasal drip (31).

IV. Patient Evaluation or Monitoring for Clinical Decision Making

The respiratory patient evaluation includes a survey for symptoms of chronic and/or acute alveolar hypoventilation, medical history, physical examination, cough evaluation, and simple pulmonary function tests. Measurement of mucous transport through the bronchial tree by radiolabeled tracers is a technique that has been used above all to study mucociliary clearance, as well as the measurement of the volume of expectorated mucous (32).

Respiratory physiotherapy interventions can be evaluated using different outcome variables, such as bronchial mucus transport measurement, measurement of the amount of expectorated mucus, pulmonary function, medication use, frequency of acute exacerbations and quality of life (2,5,33).

A. Medical History

The hypoventilation situation can vary depending on a patient's medical history (COPD, asthma, CF, NMD) and the phase in which the patient's condition is evaluated. At the positive end of the continuum will be patients who consider their cough to be satisfactory and productive. At the negative end will be those who are unable to generate even minimal coughing, either in cases of acute bronchial disease or after minor aspirations of food fragments. This situation of "loss of control" is evident both for patients and for those around them and should be considered a potential emergency (4,8,9,12).

In evaluating the circumstances related to cough effectiveness, it is useful (because of its prognostic value) to look for altered articulation of words or swallowing (both being expressions of bulbar dysfunction), as well as changes in speaking volume (related to the strength of the thoracic muscles). The ability to perform a Valsalva maneuver shows the ability to close the upper airways, which is essential both for effective spontaneous coughing and manually assisted cough maneuvers (34). An especially dangerous situation arises with the association of altered swallowing and the absence of effective cough, with risk of death by suffocation or aspiration pneumonia (35–38). On the other hand, patients with NMD or paralyzed diaphragms who breathe to a large degree with accessory breathing or abdominal muscles, or those whose diaphragms are too weak when supine to move the abdominal contents to ventilate the lungs can have much lower VC and less breathing tolerance when supine. They may also occasionally have reduced chest expansion with abdominal retractions during inspiration, which is also related to cough impairment.

B. Physical Examination

Patient examination findings depend on the particular moment in the course of the disease. In the initial phases, the range of ventilatory movements is satisfactory, the cough maneuver is normal, the mucus production is low, and the subject is able to carry out the Valsalva maneuver. Respiratory stability starts to be at risk when ventilatory mechanics symptoms occur. The patient is observed for paradoxical breathing. Typically, patients with spinal cord injuries and childhood onset myopathies have very weak intercostal muscles and breathe predominantly with their diaphragms. Their chest wall volumes decrease during inspiration. Small ventilatory movements are performed with great participation of the accessory muscles and coughing efforts that are unproductive. This is a reflection of great suffering due to the feeling of dyspnea and mucous accumulation (7,39–41). Lung auscultation reveals the existence of abundant secretions and lack of effective mobility.

Oxygen saturation (Sao_2) and end-tidal CO_2 ($Etco_2$) measurements are very important to access ventilatory impairment. Routine arterial blood gas analyses are not justified for these patients. Pain from the arterial stick causes hyperventilation and can cause falsely low CO_2 tensions. A single glimpse at Pao_2 and Sao_2 is much less useful as a guide for assisted ventilation and airway secretion elimination than is continuous Sao_2 monitoring. If the Sao_2 baseline is found to be below 95%, the patient is asked to increase breathing effort. If this effort normalizes Sao_2, then the low baseline Sao_2 is usually in large part due to underventilation. When increasing or normalizing alveolar ventilation does not normalize Sao_2, severe ventilation-perfusion and secretion accumulation is present (9,42).

The efficacy of end-tidal CO_2 and transcutaneous CO_2 measurements are extremely close for older children and adults. With currently available sensors, the latter has been shown to correlate extremely well with $Paco_2$. Although both can be accurate in assessing stable $Paco_2$ during mechanical ventilation, both can underestimate increases in hypercapnia and can be an optimal evaluation for therapy (19,43,44).

C. Pulmonary Function and Cough Tests

Evaluation of physiotherapy interventions only with pulmonary function tests appears to be inadequate for significant conclusions. However, it is known that mucus retention has a strong impact on pulmonary function and gas exchange. Severe mucus retention can cause an acute decrease in VC, forced VC, flow rates, as well as Sao_2. Patients with severe airway obstruction have more difficulties expectorating mucus. Patients with ineffective cough and low VCs are in extreme respiratory distress in the presence of secretion accumulation. A correct evaluation of pulmonary function and cough parameters may predict a successful respiratory physiotherapy treatment.

A spirometer is used to measure VC in sitting, recumbent, and sidelying positions. The spirometer is also used to measure the maximal insufflation capacity (MIC) for patients with VCs at least 30% less than predicted normal levels, who are trained in air stacking (45). Usually a manual resuscitator is used for the patient to air stack via a mouthpiece for the MIC measurements (Fig. 1).

Unassisted PCF is measured by having the patient cough as hard as possible through a peak flow meter. The PCF is then measured with the patient coughing from a maximally air stacked volume (the MIC) (Fig. 2). The patient coughs via an oronasal interface if there is a tendency for insufflated air to leak out of the nose. Finally, (fully) assisted PCF is measured from the MIC with an abdominal thrust timed to glottic opening (Fig. 3). The most important PCF measurement is usually the latter because it is the manually assisted cough that the patient must often use to clear airway secretions to avoid respiratory failure. The inability to generate a PCF greater than 2.7 L/sec even when MIC exceeds 1 L, generally indicates the existence of fixed upper airway obstruction or significant bulbar impairment, with hypopharyngeal collapse during mechanical assistance to aid cough (46–48).

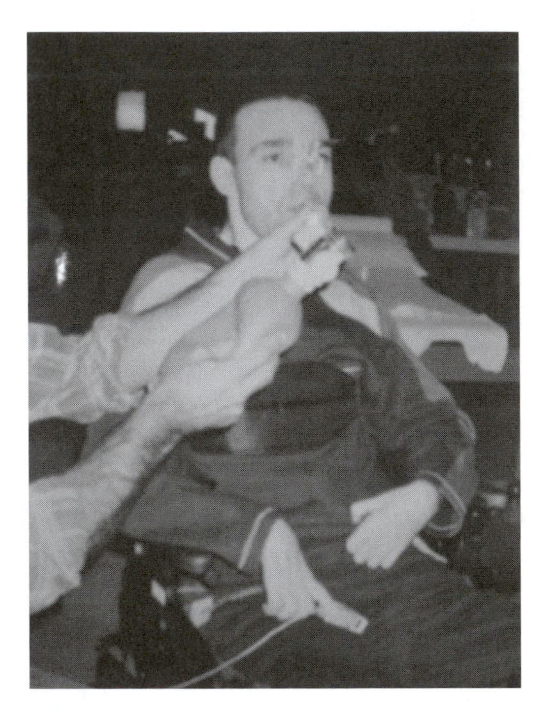

Figure 1 Air stacking with manual resuscitator via a mouthpiece in a high spinal cord patient with low vital capacity and suboptimal peak cough flow.

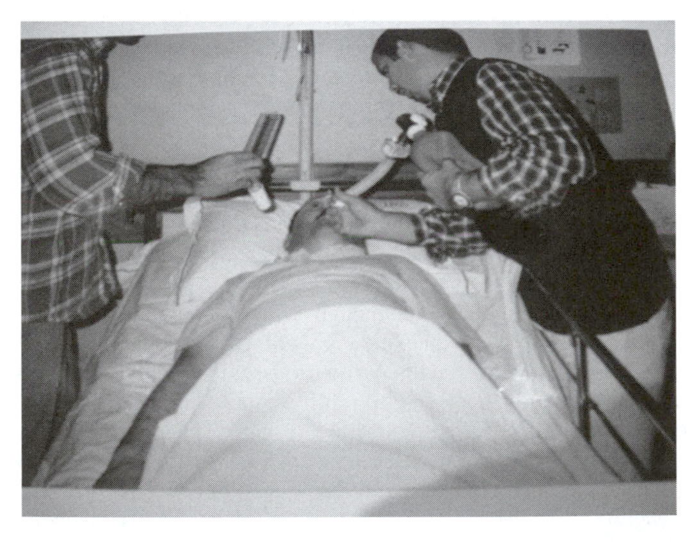

Figure 2 PCF measured from the maximally air stacked volume (MIC) in supine position in a neuromuscular patient. *Abbreviations*: PCF, peak cough flow; MIC, maximum insufflation capacity.

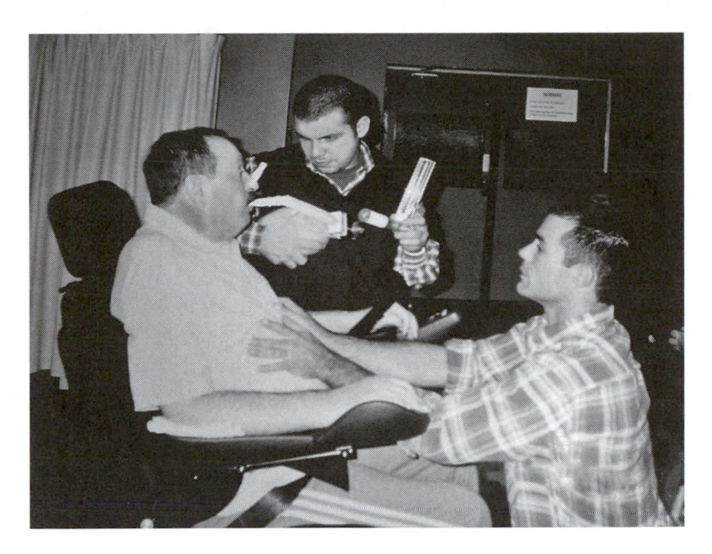

Figure 3 PCF measured from the MIC with an abdominal thrust timed to glottic opening in a sitting position in neuromuscular patient. *Abbreviations*: PCF, peak cough flow; MIC, maximum insufflation capacity.

V. Control of Mucus and Airway Clearance Techniques

Techniques for controlling and assisting the mobilization of secretions from the airways have long been advocated for use in the patient with impairment in mucociliary clearance or an ineffective cough mechanism. The goals of this therapy are to reduce airway obstruction, improve mucociliary clearance and ventilation, and optimize gas exchange.

Approaches to preventing airway secretion retention include pharmacotherapy to reduce mucus hypersecretion or to liquefy secretions, and the application of chest physiotherapy (CPT) techniques. (CPT) can be defined as the external application of a combination of forces to increase mucus transport that include PD, special breathing exercises, manual chest vibration and percussion, autonomous instrumental techniques, and manually assisted coughing.

Research studying the results of airway clearance is often difficult to evaluate because the components of a given treatment have not been standardized. Availability of equipment or education about a technique, as well as cultural differences in its application, confound the results. CPT does not appear to benefit patients during recovery from acute exacerbations of COPD or pneumonia. These conditions are characterized by interstitial pathology, which cannot be influenced by physical interventions in the airways (16,22,49). Further studies are needed to identify the patients, and more circumstances, who are at risk from complications or adverse effects of CPT.

A. Positioning and Postural Drainage

PD is a passive technique in which the patient is placed in positions that allow the broncho-pulmonary tree to be drained with the assistance of gravity. Positioning the patient to enable gravity to assist the flow of bronchial secretions from the airways has been a standard treatment for some time in patients with retained secretions (2,50). Knowledge of the anatomy of the tracheobronchial tree is vital for an effective treatment. Each lobe to be drained must be aligned so that gravity can mobilize the secretion progression to the upper airways. It is probably most effective when there are relatively large quantities of mucus with low adhesiveness. Different positions have been described for draining the large bronchi. Localization of airway mucus is essential. The goal is to vertically position the secretion encumbered bronchi for a sufficient period of time, generally about 20 minutes, to drain it. The time required probably depends on the quantity of mucus, its viscoelasticity, and its adhesiveness. The combination of PD with breathing techniques and manual CPT (Fig. 4) increases the effectiveness of airway clearance in patients with different etiologies. Gravity-assisted positions will facilitate the clearance of secretions in patients with abnormalities of the cilia, for example, primary ciliary dyskinesia, and the drainage of secretions from open abscess cavities, but their clinical effectiveness in other conditions like COPD is still questioned (51).

PD positioning can affect ventilation, perfusion, and Sao_2 in both obstructive and restrictive disorders, and many patients with primarily ventilatory impairment have less and often no breath volumes in various PD positions. Positioning can also place the patient at risk for skin and cardiac complications, cerebral blood flow or intracranial pressure changes, and for gastroesophageal reflux (6,52).

B. Breathing Control Techniques

Breathing control techniques include autonomous breathing exercises like forced and deep expirations, and diaphragmatic breathing to optimize airway mucus clearance.

One of the techniques described as the most efficient in mucus clearance is the active cycle of breathing technique (ACBT) (2). The ACBT consists of repeated cycles of three

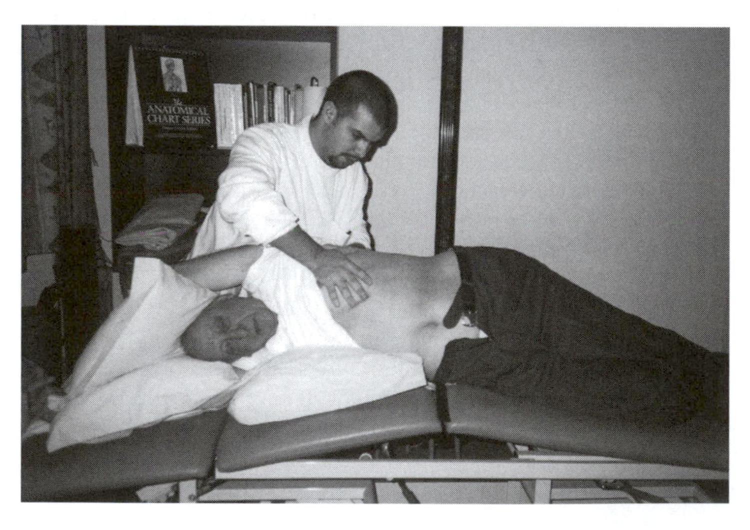

Figure 4 Manual chest physiotherapy applied in a postural drainage position in an airway disease patient.

ventilatory phases: breathing control (tidal breathing at the patient's own rate and depth, encouraging use of the lower chest with relaxation of the upper chest and shoulders); thoracic expansion exercises (deep breathing exercises emphasizing inspiration with or without breath hold, expiration is quiet and relaxed); and the forced expiration technique (one or two huffs combined with periods of breathing control). Huffing to low lung volumes will assist in mobilizing and clearing the more peripherally situated secretions and, when secretions have reached the larger and proximal upper airways, a huff or cough from a high lung volume can be used to clear them (18,53). The concept of the equal pressure point explains the mechanism of the effectiveness of huffing in airway clearance. The period of breathing control is essential between the huffing phases to prevent bronchospasm. In patients with asthma, CF, and chronic airflow limitation, there is no evidence of any increase in airflow obstruction. The ACBT technique may be performed by a patient independent of a caregiver, but it has also been shown to be equally effective with assistance (33).

Another breathing control technique that is widely used is autogenic drainage (2,53). This technique is based on breathing at different lung volumes and expiration is used to move the mucus. The aim is to maximize expiratory flow. Breathing at low-lung volume, in the individual patient, is used to mobilize more peripherally situated mucus. Breathing around the individual's tidal volume is said to collect mucus in the middle range, and with breathing around high-lung volumes, expectoration of secretions from the central airways is promoted. When sufficient mucus has reached the upper airways, it may be cleared by a cough. The regimen is adapted for the individual.

Autogenic drainage uses diaphragmatic breathing to mobilize secretions by varying expiratory airflow. It consists of three phases: breathing at low-lung volumes to "unstick" the peripheral secretions, breathing at low- to mid-lung volume (tidal volume) to collect the mucus in the middle airways, and breathing at mid- to high-lung volumes to evacuate the mucus from the central airways (2). The method of using this breathing technique has been modified according to different protocols. The Belgian and German models are the ones that are used more in clinical practice.

These kind of breathing control exercises like ACBT and autogenic drainage are not indicated in severe ventilatory dependent patient that are in an assist-controlled mechanical ventilation mode, however it may be used during weaning protocols.

In resume, inspiratory breathing exercises coupled with mobilization and body positioning are used to increase lung volumes and improve ventilation. They can promote relaxation and reduce anxiety. Expiratory breathing techniques with an open glottis (a huff) or with a closed glottis (a cough) are used to increase expiratory flow rates and, thus, enhance airway clearance. Forced expiratory maneuvers should be used with caution in patients with bronchospasm to avoid exacerbation of spasm, or cardiac dysfunction.

C. Manual Chest Physical Therapy Techniques

Approaches to preventing retention of airway secretions include the use of medication to reduce mucus hypersecretion or to liquefy secretions, and the facilitation of mucus mobilization. To complement this objective, CPT techniques are shown to be very effective in preventing pulmonary complications in infant and adult patients with bronchopulmonary secretion accumulation. The principles of manual CPT techniques consist in the application of external forces in the thoracic cage that have direct effect on mucus mobilization.

Manual chest percussion, sometimes referred to as chest clapping, is very well known in the respiratory physiotherapy community and it consists in manual application of rhythmic clapping with cupped hands to the ventral, lateral, and dorsal side of the thorax of the patient at a frequency of approximately 3 to 6 Hz. It is often applied in PD positions and used for 10- to 20-minute treatment sessions whenever there is auscultatory or oximetry evidence of airway secretion retention.

Some authors demonstrated an increase in airflow obstruction when chest clapping was included in an airway clearance regimen (54). Chest clapping has also been shown to cause an increase in hypoxemia, but when short periods of chest clapping have been combined with three or four thoracic expansion exercises, no fall in oxygen saturation has been seen (2). Some patients with severe lung disease demonstrate oxygen desaturation with self-chest clapping. This may be due to the work of the additional upper limb activity. On the basis of three randomized, controlled trials of CPT and one observational study, manual chest percussion as applied by physical or respiratory therapists is ineffective and perhaps even detrimental in the treatment of patients with acute exacerbations of COPD (55).

Another manual chest physical therapy technique is vibration. Vibration is a sustained cocontraction of the upper extremities of a caregiver to produce a vibratory force that is transmitted to the thorax over an involved lung segment. Vibration is applied throughout exhalation concurrently with mild compression of the patient's chest wall. Vibration is proposed to enhance mucociliary transport from the peripheral of the lung fields to the larger airways. Since vibration is used in conjunction with PD (Fig. 5) and percussion, many studies do not isolate the effects of vibration from the other components.

Manual thoracic techniques are effective in removing pulmonary secretions, facilitating inspiration, and improving alveolar ventilation. Guidebooks have been published that demonstrate the hand placements and thrusting techniques in children and adults (56).

D. Instrumental Techniques for Mucus Mobilization

Methods of promoting airway clearance using specific devices have been included in most respiratory therapy programs. Such methods use devices to promote special breathing

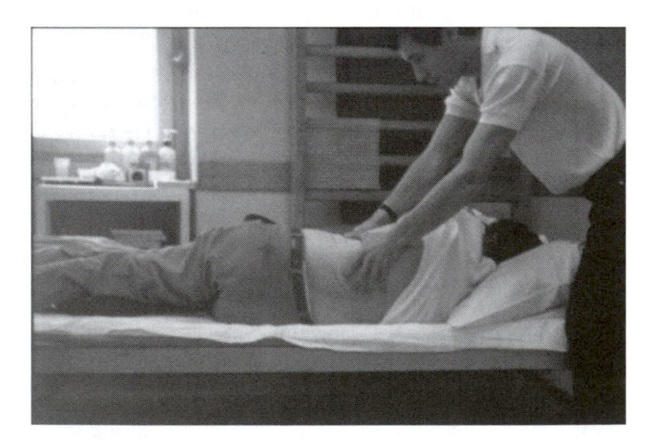

Figure 5 Manual chest vibration used in conjunction with postural drainage in an airway disease patient.

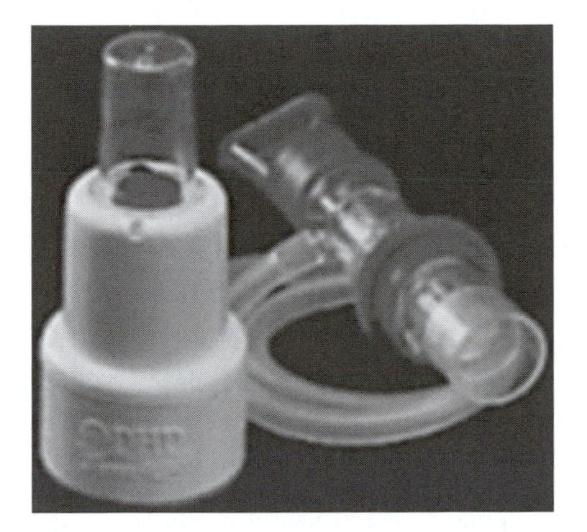

Figure 6 PEP device with a mouthpiece. *Abbreviation*: PEP, positive expiratory pressure.

patterns like the positive expiratory pressure (PEP) breathing, the flutter breathing, and the cornet breathing.

The development and utilization of PEP breathing came about in the 1980s in Denmark and is now widely used in Europe with increasing acceptance in North America. Application of PEP breathing is based on the hypothesis that mucus in peripheral small airways is more effectively mobilized by coughing or forced expirations, if alveolar pressure and volume behind mucus plugs are increased. PEP is usually applied by breathing through a facemask or a mouthpiece with an inspiratory tube containing a one-way valve, and an expiratory tube containing a variable expiratory resistance (Fig. 6). It results in PEP throughout expiration (2,6,57).

A manometer is inserted into the system between the valve and the resistance to monitor the pressure. This pressure should be 10 ± 20 cmH_2O at mid-expiration. Tidal breathing, with a slightly active expiration, is used and lung volume is retained at a raised level by avoiding complete expiration. The forced expiration technique is used to clear the secretions that are mobilized. The duration and frequency of treatment are adapted for each individual. PEP increases the pressure gradient between the open and closed alveoli, thus tending to maintain alveoli patency. It increases the functional residual capacity (FRC). This reduces the resistance in collateral and small airways.

High or low pressure PEP may be prescribed. The prescription for high pressure PEP requires the patient to perform forced VC maneuvers through the range of expiratory resistances with the mask connected to a spirometer. The possible benefit of PEP and high pressure PEP on mucus transport remains to be proven. However, PEP is useful when there are indications to at least temporarily increase lung volume.

Flutter breathing is a combination of PEP and air column oscillation applied at the mouth. It is an inexpensive means of oscillating the air column in conjunction with providing PEP. The patient expires through a small pipe shaped device called Flutter VRP1®. The expiratory opening of the pipe is closed by a small stainless steel ball.

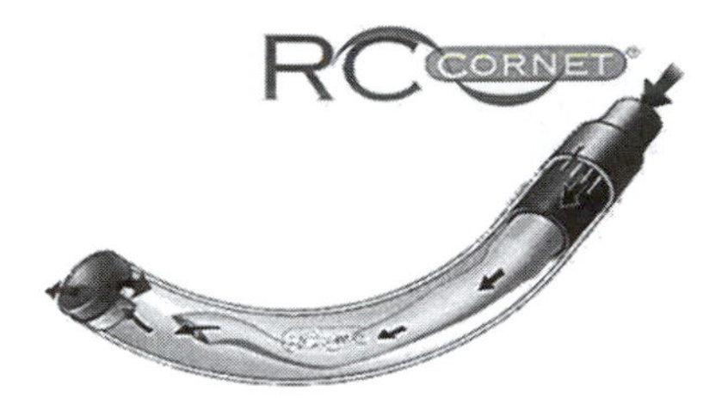

Figure 7 RC Cornet® device.

During expiration the stainless steel ball is pushed upward, producing aPEP, and falls downward again, producing an interruption of the expiratory flow. The mucus mobilizing effect is thought to be due to both a widening of the airways due to the increased expiratory pressure and the occurrence of airflow oscillations due to the oscillating ball (58). In addition, intermittent airflow accelerations are produced by the same ball movements.

This device helps to loosen secretions, which are mobilized to the central airways and cleared by deep exhalations through the device with the aid of subsequent coughing and/or huffing (59). Carefully controlled studies need to be conducted before this technique can be widely recommended.

Another device that follows the same physiological principles of the flutter device is the RC Cornet®. This device is a curved plastic tube containing a flexible latex-free valve-hose (Fig. 7). During expiration through the Cornet, a PEP and oscillatory vibration of the air within the airways are generated. It can be used in any position, as it is independent of gravitational forces. The flow, pressure, and frequency of the oscillations can be adjusted to suit the individual patient. Just as with the flutter, secretions mobilized to the central airways are cleared by coughing or huffing.

The effect of these three techniques on sputum viscoelasticity is very important and evident in clinical practice. Studies show that the viscoelasticity was significantly lower following treatment with these devices. It is hypothesized that this reduction would improve mucociliary and cough clearability, but it is interesting to note that there are no studies that compare the differences between the regimens in the quantity of sputum expectorated during the treatment sessions.

E. Manually Assisted Coughing Techniques

Cough is the primary defense mechanism against foreign bodies in the lower airways. Any stimulation of the pharyngeal, laryngeal, tracheal, or bronchial receptors can create a cough. When this mechanism is not functioning correctly, mucus restraint will occur as bronchial obstruction. This problem may be due to the fact that the subject is incapable of a deep inspiration, or glottis closure, or rising intra-abdominal and intrathoracic pressure.

An effective cough is based on expiratory muscle force capable of producing effective PCFs. The PCF is a routine measure in the evaluation of neuromuscular patients (60), and clinical investigations suggest that it should be used in spinal cord patients as well (61,62).

An effective PCF requires a pulmonary inspiration or insufflations until 85–90% of the VC is reached, and the generation of high intrathoracic pressure so as to expel 2.3–2.5 L of air at a PCF of 6–20 L/sec. For an effective cough to occur, the PCF must be higher than 270 L/min (12). Kang and Bach (63) also proved that the PCF value could be even higher if it is performed through the MIC. The MIC is related to the pulmonary compliance and with the pharyngeal and oropharyngeal muscle function. After a deep inspiration, the subject makes an apnea and receives an extra air volume (through a manual resuscitator or volume ventilator) via a mouthpiece or nasal interface. This extra air volume will produce the lung distension, allowing a cough at a higher volume, and therefore prove more effective.

Another aspect to consider beyond deep inspiration is the inspiratory apnea, assured through the glottic function. The deep inspiration stretches the airways, and increases the contraction force of the expiratory muscles as well as the retraction force of the lung parenchyma; the inspiratory apnea (with glottic closure) facilitates the airway distribution to the most peripheral areas of the lung and increases intrathoracic pressure.

The patient with partial or complete abdominal muscle paralysis is unable to produce an effective cough. The abdominal thrust is an assisted coughing technique that consists of the association of two techniques: the costophrenic compression and the Heimlich maneuver. The combination of deep lung insufflations to the MIC followed by the manually assisted cough with abdominal thrust (Fig. 8) has been shown to increase significantly PCF's values in restrictive patients (47,64).

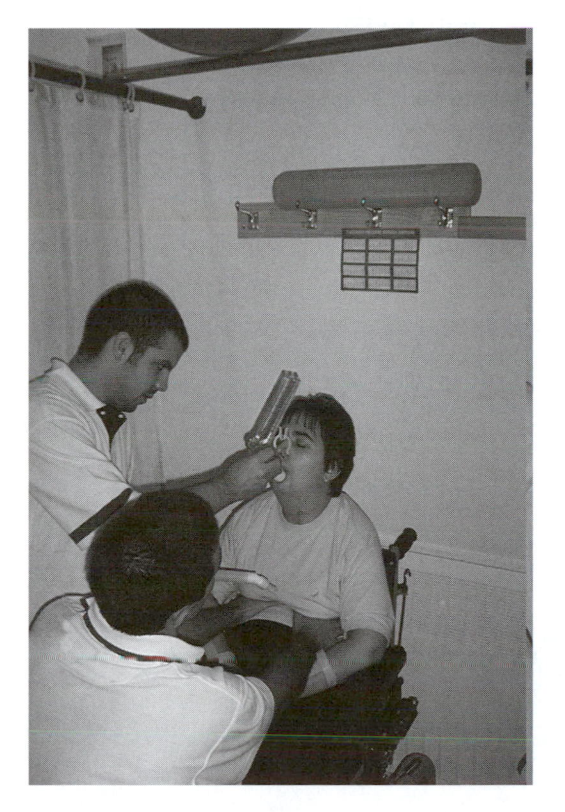

Figure 8 Manually assisted cough with abdominal thrust to measure PCF in sitting position. *Abbreviation*: PCF, peak cough flow.

Although an optimal insufflation followed by an abdominal thrust provides the greatest increase in PCF, PCF can also be significantly increased by providing only a maximal insufflation or by providing only an abdominal thrust without a preceding maximal insufflation. Interestingly, PCF values are significantly increased more by the maximal insufflation than by the abdominal thrust (65,66).

Manually assisted coughing and MIC maneuver require a cooperative patient, good coordination between the patient and the caregiver, adequate physical effort, and often frequent application by the family caregiver (Figs. 9 and 10). It is usually ineffective in

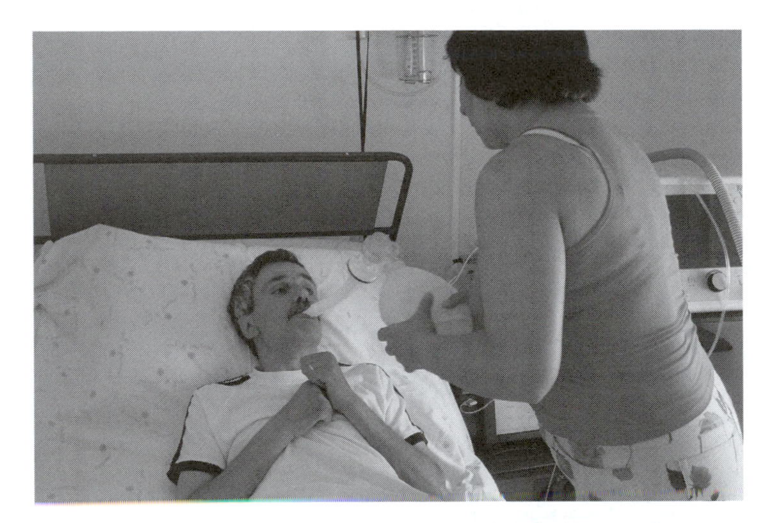

Figure 9 Air stacking and manually assisted cough in a patient with neuromuscular disease, performed by the family caregiver.

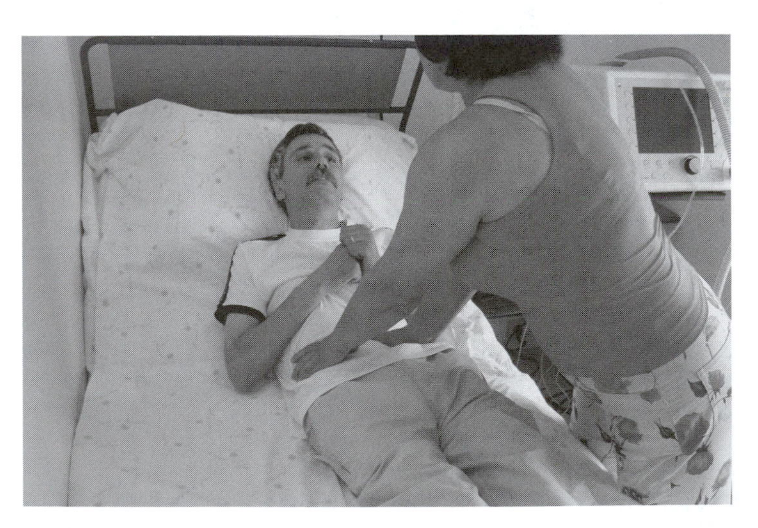

Figure 10 Air stacking and manually assisted cough in a patient with neuromuscular disease, performed by the family caregiver.

the presence of severe scoliosis because of a combination of restricted lung capacity and the inability to effect diaphragm movement by abdominal thrusting because of severe rib cage and diaphragm deformity.

Abdominal compressions should not be used for 1 to 1.5 hours following a meal, however, chest compressions can be used to augment PCF. Chest thrusting techniques must be performed with caution in the case of an osteoporotic rib cage. Unfortunately, since it is not widely taught to health care professionals, manually assisted coughing is underutilized (67).

VI. Mechanical Respiratory Muscle Aids for Secretion Management

Respiratory muscle aids for secretion management are devices and techniques that involve mechanical application of forces to the body or intermittent pressure changes to the airway to assist in expiratory muscle function and airway mucus clearance. The devices that act on the body include HFCWO that create atmospheric pressure changes with oscillations around the thorax and abdomen, intrapulmonary percussive ventilators that create a rapid frequency adjusted for internal percussion for mucus progression to the large airways, and insufflation-exsufflation devices that apply force and pressure changes directly to the airway to assist the expiratory muscles for cough augmentation and the inspiratory muscles for lung expansion.

A. Mechanical Insufflation-Exsufflation

In 1951, Barach et al. described an exsufflator attachment for iron lungs (68). The device used a vacuum cleaner motor with a 5-inch solenoid valve attachment to an iron lung portal. With the valve closed, the motor developed a negative intratank pressure of −40 mmHg. At peak negative pressure the valve opened, triggering a return to atmospheric pressure in 0.06 seconds and causing a passive exsufflation. This mechanism increased PCF by 45% for six ventilator supported poliomyelitis patients. An additional increase was obtained by timing an abdominal compression with valve opening. These techniques were sufficiently effective for the investigators to report that the exsufflation produced by this device "completely replaced bronchoscopy as a means of keeping the airway clear of thick tenacious secretions" (69,70). These investigations led to the construction and implementation of an exsufflation-with-negative pressure device called a "Cof-flator" that initiated the concept of (MI-E) for secretion clearance. Then, in 1995, an automatically cycling device became available. In 2001, it was renamed the "Cough-Assist™".

Mechanical insufflator-exsufflators (Cough-Assist, J. H. Emerson Co., Cambridge, Massachusettes, U.S.A.) deliver deep insufflations (at positive pressures of 30 to 50 cmH_2O) followed immediately by deep exsufflations (at negative pressures of –30 to –50 cmH_2O). The insufflation and exsufflation pressures and delivery times are independently adjustable (71). With an inspiratory time of two seconds and an expiratory time of three seconds, there exists a very good correlation between the pressures used and the flows obtained (72).

Except after a meal, an abdominal thrust is applied in conjunction with the insufflation-exsufflation mechanically assisted coughing (MAC) (66). MI-E can be provided via an oronasal mask (Fig. 11), a simple mouthpiece, or via a translaryngeal or tracheostomy tube. When delivered via the latter, the cuff, when present, should be inflated (73).

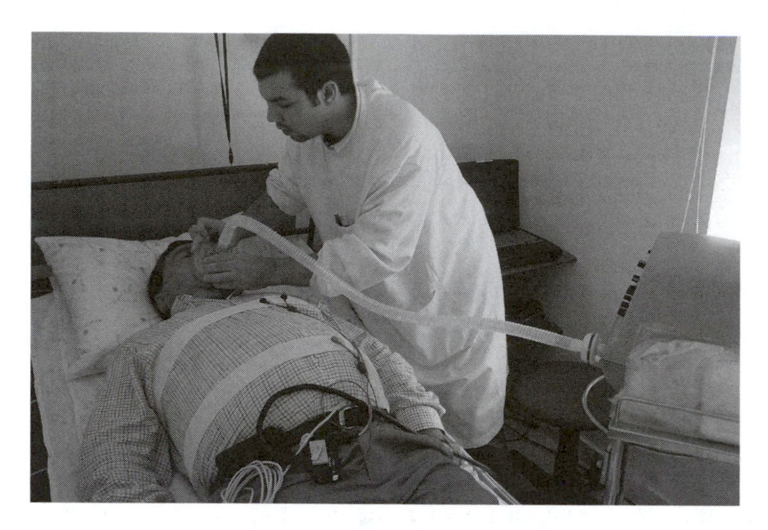

Figure 11 Mechanical insufflation-exsufflation provided via an oral-nasal mask in a monitorized patient with neuromuscular disease.

MI-E applied with an oronasal mask can generate PCFs greater than 2.7 L/sec in motor neuron disease patients, with the exception of those with very acute bulbar dysfunction (74), in whom there exists great instability of the upper airways (48). If, in normal subjects, the sudden application of negative pressure at this level produces reflex activation of the genioglossus to maintain permeability, in those patients with diminished strength and speed of the pharyngeal muscles there will be obstruction during the expiratory phase (12).

The Cough-Assist can be manually or automatically cycled. Manual cycling facilitates caregiver-patient coordination of inspiration and expiration with insufflation and exsufflation, but it requires hands to deliver an abdominal thrust, to hold the mask on the patient, and to cycle the machine. One treatment consists of about five cycles of MI–E or MAC followed by a short period of normal breathing or ventilator use to avoid hyperventilation. Insufflation and exsufflation pressures are almost always from +35 cmH_2O to +60 cmH_2O to –35 cmH_2O to –60 cmH_2O. Most patients use 35 cmH_2O to 45 cmH_2O pressures for insufflations and exsufflations. In experimental models, +40 cmH_2O to –40 cmH_2O pressures have been shown to provide maximum forced deflation VCs and flows (46,65,72). Multiple treatments are given in one sitting until no further secretions are expulsed, and any secretion or mucus induced desaturations are reversed. Use can be required as frequently as every few minutes round the clock during chest infections. Although no medications are usually required for effective MI-E in neuromuscular ventilator users, liquefaction of sputum using heated aerosol treatments may facilitate exsufflation when secretions are inspissated.

The use of MI-E via the upper airway can be effective for children as young as 11 months of age. Patients this young can become accustomed to MI-E and permit its effective use by not crying or closing their glottises. Between two and one-half and five years of age most children become able to cooperate and cough on queue with MI-E. Exsufflation-timed abdominal thrusts are also used for infants (75,76).

Whether via the upper airway or via indwelling airway tubes, routine airway suctioning misses the left main stem bronchus about 90% of the time. MI-E, on the other hand, provides the same exsufflation flows in both left and right airways without the discomfort or airway trauma of tracheal suctioning and it can be effective when suctioning is not. Patients almost invariably prefer MI-E to suctioning for comfort and effectiveness and they also find it to be less tiring (77,78).

When mucous plugs are eliminated in acute episodes in ventilated neuromuscular patients, MI–E may attain 300% improvement in VC as well as normalization of oxygen saturation (35). Contraindications of the technique include previous barotrauma, the existence of bullae, emphysema, or bronchial hyperreactivity (79). There continue to be no publications contradicting the reports of effectiveness or describing significant complications of MI-E. Even when used following abdominal surgery, and following extensive chest wall surgery no disruption of recently sutured wounds was noted (80,81). Secondary effects, such as pneumothorax, aspiration, or coughing up blood, are reduced considerably by treating the mentioned contraindications. On the other hand, gurgling noises and abdominal distension are rare and can be eliminated by lowering the insufflation pressure. The significant increase of forced expiratory flows in periods immediately following post-exsufflation indicates that MI–E does not provoke obstruction of the airways. As patients with spinal shock can present bradycardias, MI–E should be carried out cautiously with gradual increase in pressures, or premedication with anticholinergics (82). In patients with very low VC who have not previously received maximum insufflations, the use of high pressures may cause thoracic muscle discomfort; thus, progressive increase is also indicated.

The use of MI–E has been demonstrated to be very important in extubating NMD patients following general anesthesia, despite their lack of any breathing tolerance, and managing them with NIV (8,9,60). It is also permitted to avoid intubation or to quickly extubate NMD patients in acute ventilatory failure with no breathing tolerance and profuse airway secretions due to intercurrent chest infections (37,83,84). MI–E in a protocol with manually assisted coughing, oximetry feedback, and home use of noninvasive intermittent positive pressure ventilation was shown to effectively decrease hospitalizations and respiratory complications, and mortality for patients with NMD (7,85).

B. Intrapulmonary Percussive Ventilation

The intrapulmonary percussive ventilator (Percussionaire™, Breas Medical, Inc) (Fig. 12) is an airway clearance device that simultaneously delivers aerosolized solution and intrathoracic percussion. This modified method of intermittent positive pressure breathing imposes high-frequency minibursts of gas (at 50–550 cycles/min) on the patient's own respiration. This creates a global effect of internal percussion of the lungs, which could promote clearance of the peripheral bronchial tree. The percussions (subtidal volume) are delivered continuously through a sliding air-entrainment device (called Phasitron) powered by compressed gas at 20–40 psi. The high frequency gas pulses expand the lungs, vibrate and enlarge the airways, and deliver gas into distal lung units beyond accumulated mucus (51,53,86). Treatment with IPV is titrated for patient comfort and visible thoracic movement.

The patient initiates the flow of gas, and during inspiration the pulsatile flow results in an internal percussion. Interruption of the inspiratory flow allows for passive expiration. This technique has been shown to be as effective as a standard CPT and to assist mucus

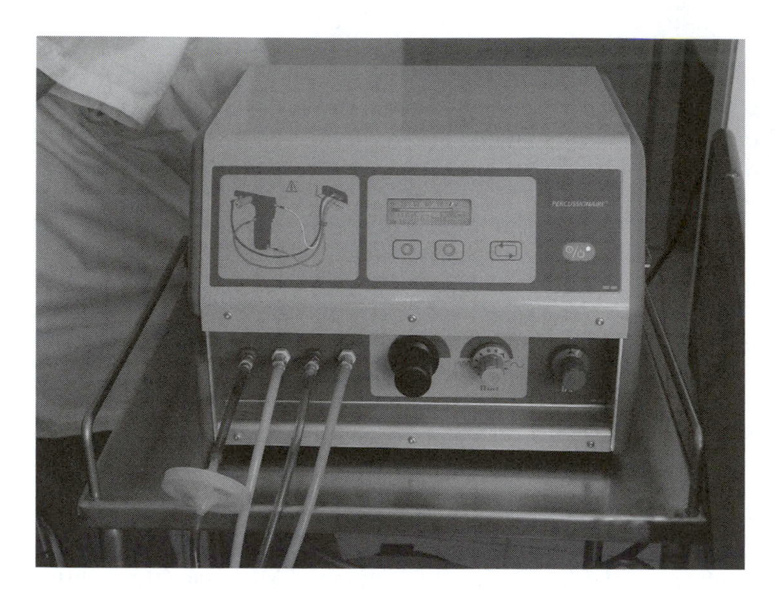

Figure 12 Intrapulmonary percussive ventilator (Percussionaire™, Breas Medical, Inc., Glen Burnie, Maryland, U.S.A.).

clearance in patients with secretion encumbrance arising from different etiologies, such as CF (87), acute exacerbations of COPD (88), and Duchenne muscle dystrophy (86).

IPV can be delivered through a mouthpiece, a facial mask, and also through a endotraqueal and tracheostomy tube (89). The primary aims of this technique are to reduce secretion viscosity, promote deep lung recruitment, improve gas exchange, deliver a vascular "massage," and protect the airway against barotrauma. The main contraindication is the presence of diffuse alveolar hemorrhage with homodynamic instability. Relative contraindications include active or recent gross hemoptysis, pulmonary embolism, subcutaneous emphysema, bronchopleural fistula, esophageal surgery, recent spinal infusion, spinal anesthesia or acute spinal injury, presence of a transvenous or subcutaneous pacemaker, increased intracranial pressures, uncontrolled hypertension, suspected or confirmed pulmonary tuberculosis, bronchospasm, empyema or large pleural effusion, and acute cardiogenic pulmonary edema.

C. High-frequency Chest Wall Oscillation

In 1939, it was recognized that alveolar ventilation and blood circulation could be assisted by rapidly alternating negative and positive pressure under a chest shell. J. H. Emerson developed the first high-frequency chest wall oscillation jacket, the Ucyclist–B Vest, to facilitate bronchial secretion clearance, in the early 1950s, but he provided oscillation only during part of the breathing cycle. Barach described use of a similar unit by patients with chronic bronchial asthma and emphysema in 1966 (90).

During high-frequency chest wall oscillation (HFCWO), positive pressure air pulses are applied to the chest wall. Oscillation and vibration can be applied externally to the chest wall or abdomen by rapidly oscillating pressure changes in a vest (ThAIRapy Vest™, American Biosystems, Inc., St. Paul, Minnesota, U.S.A.), or by cycling oscillating pressures

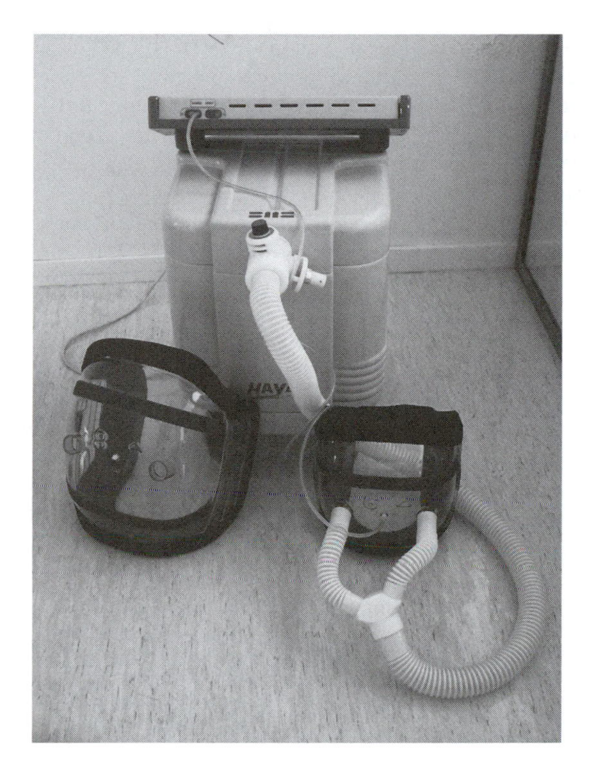

Figure 13 High-frequency chest wall oscillation through a chest shell (Hayek™ oscillator, Breasy Medical Equipment Inc., Stamford, Connecticut, U.S.A.).

under a chest shell (Hayek™ oscillator, Breasy Medical Equipment Inc., Stanford, CN) (Fig. 13). The ThAIRapy Vest™ provides oscillation at 5 to 25 Hz. Mechanical vibration is performed at frequencies up to 40 Hz. Vibration is applied during the entire breathing cycle or during expiration only. The adjustable inspiration to expiration ratio of the Hayek oscillator permits asymmetric inspiratory and expiratory pressure changes (e.g., +3 to −6 cmH_2O), which favor higher exsufflation flow velocities to mobilize secretions. Baseline pressures can be set at negative, atmospheric, or positive values thus commencing oscillation above, at, or below the FRC (6,91).

The ThAIRapy Vest™ is constructed to fit over the entire thorax and should extend to the top of the thigh when the patient is sitting upright. The pressure control setting should be adjusted to either the high or the low setting according to patient comfort. The average length of time spent in each treatment session will vary according to patient tolerance, amount, and consistency of secretions and the phase of the patient's illness (acute or chronic) (51). Simultaneous use of aerosolized medication or saline is recommended throughout the treatment. This humidifies the air to counteract the drying effect of the increased airflow (88).

HFCWO may act like a physical mucolytic, reducing both the spinability and viscoelasticity of mucus and enhancing clearance by coughing (6,53,92). HFCWO has demonstrated efficacy in assisting mucus clearance in patients with disorders associated with mucus hypersecretion, but has preserved muscle function such as in CF (92). HFCWO is an external noninvasive respiratory modality proven effective in mobilizing airway secretions from the small peripheral airways, and in improving mucus rheology in patients with CF, and has become an important modality in the airway clearance techniques of this group of patients (24,93,94). High-frequency oscillation to the airways has also been reported to increase mucus transport in healthy subjects (95).

These beneficial effects on both mucus clearance and clinical parameters are not so evident in other groups of patients such as in those with COPD. Moreover, side effects of percussion and vibration include increasing obstruction to airflow for patients with COPD (49,96,97). The proven value of HFCWO in patients with relatively normal mucus composition and characteristics but with neuromuscular weakness is still under investigation, especially as a long-term treatment modality. In one study, the addition of HFCWO to randomly selected patients with ALS failed to achieve any significant clinical benefits in relation to the time of death (survival days). In addition, HFCWO failed to modify the rate of decline in forced vital capacity, given the progressive nature of this chronic neurodegenerative disease process. There were no significant differences concerning the frequency of atelectasis, pneumonia and number of hospitalizations for a respiratory related abnormality, or requirement for tracheostomy and mechanical ventilation (91).

Contraindications for HFCWO are mostly the same as for IPV, plus head or neck injury not yet stabilized, burns, open wounds, infection or recent thoracic skin grafts, osteoporosis, osteomyelitis, coagulopathy, rib fracture, lung contusion, distended abdomen, and chest wall pain (6,93).

VII. Conclusion

Hypersecretion, reduced mucus transport, and airflow obstruction are impairments, while chronic coughing and expectoration of mucus or dyspnea can limit the patient in daily or recreational activities and can therefore be classified as disabilities. The impact of secretion clearance appears to be a strong one in the improvement of the patient's quality of life, since it has direct influence on the improvement of symptoms related to secretion encumbrance.

There continues to be widespread debate as to which airway clearance regimen should be used and when. In most comparisons, bronchial hygiene physical therapy produced no significant effects on pulmonary function, apart from clearing sputum in COPD and in bronchiectasis. There is not enough evidence to support or refute the use of bronchial hygiene physical therapy in people with COPD and bronchiectasis (49). However, there is strong evidence that supports the use of respiratory physical therapy techniques for secretion clearance in NMD to improve quality of life and survival (9,60,98,99).

If one or more of these techniques are proven to be significantly more effective and efficient, consideration would still have to be given to the technique to which a particular patient will adhere and, in today's world, to cost implications. Long-term studies (1 $\pm$ 4 years) are very much harder to set up and very expensive, but necessary to increase understanding of airway clearance. Efficacy studies should be performed in homogeneous groups of patients with well-described characteristics in terms of age, sex, diagnosis, baseline pulmonary function tests, and, if possible, compliance characteristics. The effects of secretion clearance techniques are probably determined by special characteristics of subgroups characterized by lung mechanics, bronchial hyperreactivity, rheological properties of mucus, and localization of mucus in the bronchial tree (6,53).

So, in conclusion, in patients with ventilatory impairment, NIV is a very efficient technique in respiratory management; however, in the majority of the cases, secretions are excessive and NIV alone is likely to fail. The role of respiratory physiotherapy in these cases is crucial and should be based on the principles and goals of intervention described in this chapter to permit an efficient treatment while the patient is hospitalized, and prevent hospitalizations when the patient is at home, where family members must be trained to provide the treatment and maintain the achievement of the therapeutic goals, and therefore maximize the potential of pulmonary rehabilitation.

References

1. Rubin BK. Physiology of airway mucus clearance. Respir Care 2002; 47(7):761–768.
2. Pryor JA. Physiotherapy for airway clearance in adults. Eur Respir J 1999; 14(6):1418–1424.
3. Zahm JM, King M, Duvivier C, et al. Role of simulated repetitive coughing in mucus clearance. Eur Respir J 1991; 4(3):311–315.
4. McCool FD, Rosen MJ. Nonpharmacologic airway clearance therapies: ACCP evidence-based clinical practice guidelines. Chest 2006; 129(suppl 1):250S–259S.
5. van der Schans CP, Postma DS, Koeter GH, et al. Physiotherapy and bronchial mucus transport. Eur Respir J 1999; 13(6):1477–1486.
6. Van der Schans C, Bach J, Rubin BK. Chest physical therapy: mucus-mobilization techniques. In: Bach JR, ed. Noninvasive Mechanical Ventilation. 1st ed. Philadelphia: Hanley & Belfus Inc., 2002:259–284.
7. Bach JR. Prevention of morbidity and mortality with the use of physical medicine aids: the obstructive and paralytic conditions. In: Bach JR, ed. Pulmonary Rehabilitation. Philadelphia: Hanley & Belfus Inc., 1996:303–329.
8. Gomez-Merino E, Bach JR. Duchenne muscular dystrophy: prolongation of life by noninvasive respiratory muscle aids. Am J Phys Med Rehabil 2002; 81:411–415.
9. Tzeng AC, Bach JR. Prevention of pulmonary morbidity for patients with neurosmucular disease. Chest 2000; 118:1390–1396.
10. Rubin EM, Scantlen GE, Chapman GA, et al. Effect of chest wall oscillation on mucus clearance: comparison of two vibrators. Pediatr Pulmonol 1989; 6(2):122–126.
11. Wolkove N, Baltzan MA Jr., Kamel H, et al. A randomized trial to evaluate the sustained efficacy of a mucus clearance device in ambulatory patients with chronic obstructive pulmonary disease. Can Respir J 2004; 11(8):567–572.
12. Servera E, Sancho J, Zafra MJ. Cough and neuromuscular diseases. Noninvasive airway secretion management. Arch Bronconeumol 2003; 39(9):418–427.
13. King M, Zahm JM, Pierrot D, et al. The role of mucus gel viscosity, spinnability, and adhesive properties in clearance by simulated cough. Biorheology 1989; 26(4):737–745.
14. Wolkove N, Kamel H, Rotaple M, et al. Use of a mucus clearance device enhances the bronchodilator response in patients with stable COPD. Chest 2002; 121(3):702–707.
15. Olseni L, Midgren B, Wollmer P. Mucus clearance at rest and during exercise in patients with bronchial hypersecretion. Scand J Rehabil Med 1992; 24(1):61–64.
16. van der Schans CP, Piers DA, Beekhuis H, et al. Effect of forced expirations on mucus clearance in patients with chronic airflow obstruction: effect of lung recoil pressure. Thorax 1990; 45(8):623–627.
17. Bennett WD, Foster WM, Chapman WF. Cough-enhanced mucus clearance in the normal lung. J Appl Physiol 1990; 69(5):1670–1675.

18. Pryor JA, Webber BA, Hodson BA, et al. Evaluation of the forced expiration technique as an adjunct to postural drainage in treatment of cystic fibrosis. BMJ 1979; 2(6187):417–418.
19. American Thoracic Society. Standards for the Diagnosis and Care of Patients with Chronic Obstructive Pulmonary Disease. Am J Respir Crit Care Med 1995; 152(5 pt 2):S77–S121.
20. Clarke SW, Pavia D. Lung mucus production and mucociliary clearance: methods of assessment. Br J Clin Pharmacol 1980; 9(6):537–546.
21. Hondras MA, Linde K, Jones AP. Manual therapy for asthma. Cochrane Database Syst Rev 2000; (2):CD001002.
22. Plant PK, Owen JL, Elliot MW. Non-invasive ventilation in acute exacerbations of chronic obstructive pulmonary disease: long term survival and predictors of in-hospital outcome. Thorax 2001; 56:708–712.
23. Webber BA, Pryor JA. Respiratory physiotherapy for cystic fibrosis. J Pediatr 1989; 115(1): 167–168.
24. van der Schans C, Prasad A, Main E. Chest physiotherapy compared to no chest physiotherapy for cystic fibrosis. Cochrane Database Syst Rev 2000; (2):CD001401.
25. Bradley JM, Moran FM, Elborn JS. Evidence for physical therapies (airway clearance and physical training) in cystic fibrosis: an overview of five Cochrane systematic reviews. Respir Med 2006; 100(2):191–201.
26. Sancho J, Servera E, Diaz J, et al. Comparison of peak cough flows measured by pneumotachograph and a portable peak flow meter. Am J Phys Med Rehabil 2004; 83(8):608–612.
27. Schneerson JM, Simonds AK. Noninvasive ventilation for chest wall and neuromuscular disorders. Eur Respir J 2002; 20(2):480–487.
28. Bach J R, Zhitnikov S. The management of neuromuscular ventilatory failure. Semin Pediatr Neurol 1998; 5(2):92–105.
29. Bach JR, Campagnolo DI, Hoeman S. Life satisfaction of individuals with Duchenne muscular dystrophy using long-term mechanical ventilatory support. Am J Phys Med Rehabil 1991; 70(3): 129–135.
30. Chaudri MB, Liu C, Hubbard R, et al. Relationship between supramaximal flow during cough and mortality in motor neurone disease. Eur Respir J 2002; 19(3):434–438.
31. Elman LB, Dubin RM, Kelley M, et al. Management of oropharyngeal and tracheobronchial secretions in patients with neurologic disease. J Palliat Med 2005; 8(6):1150–1159.
32. King M. Physiology of mucus clearance. Paediatr Respir Rev 2006; 7(suppl 1):S212–S214.
33. Pryor JA, Webber BA, Hodson ME. Effect of chest physiotherapy on oxygen saturation in patients with cystic fibrosis. Thorax 1990; 45(1):77.
34. Lahrmann H, Wild M, Zdrahal F, et al. Expiratory muscle weakness and assisted cough in ALS. Amyotroph Lateral Scler Other Motor Neuron Disord 2003; 4(1):49–51.
35. Servera E, Sancho J, Gomez-Merino E, et al. Non-invasive management of an acute chest infection for a patient with ALS. J Neurol Sci 2003; 209(1–2):111–113.
36. Servera E, Gomez-Merino E, Perez E. Home mechanical ventilation in amyotrophic lateral sclerosis patients is not always a problem. Chest 2000; 117(3):924.
37. Bach JR, Saporito LR. Criteria for successful extubation and tracheostomy tube removal for patients with respiratory failure. Chest 1996; 110(6):1566–1571.
38. Bach JR. Amyotrophic lateral sclerosis: prolongation of life by noninvasive muscle aids. Chest 2002; 122(1):92–98.
39. Bach JR. Introduction to rehabilitation of neuromuscular disorders. Semin Neurol 1995; 15(1): 1–5.
40. Bach J. Noninvasive Mechanical Ventilation. Philadephia: Hanley & Belfus, 2002.
41. Dean E. Clinical decision making in the management of the late sequelae of poliomyelitis. Phys Ther 1991; 71(10):752–761.
42. Bach JR, Bianchi C, Aufiero E. Oximetry and indications for tracheotomy for amyotrophic lateral sclerosis. Chest 2004; 126(5):1502–1507.

43. Ishikawa Y, Bach JR. Nocturnal respiratory failure as an indication of noninvasive ventilation in the patient with neuromuscular disease. Respiration 1998; 65(3):226.
44. Bach J. Home mechanical ventilation for neuromuscular ventilatory failure: conventional approaches and their outcomes. Bach JR, ed. Noninvasive Mechanical Ventilation. Philadelphia: Hanley & Belfus, 2002:103–128.
45. Kang SW, Bach JR. Maximum insufflation capacity. Chest 2000; 118(1):61–65.
46. Sancho J, Servera E, Marin J, et al. Effect of lung mechanics on mechanically assisted flows and volumes. Am J Phys Med Rehabil 2004; 83(9):698–703.
47. Bach JR, Goncalves MR, Paez S, et al. Expiratory flow maneuvers in patients with neuromuscular diseases. Am J Phys Med Rehabil 2006; 85(2):105–111.
48. Sancho J, Servera E, Diaz J, et al. Efficacy of mechanical insufflation-exsufflation in medically stable patients with amyotrophic lateral sclerosis. Chest 2004; 125(4):1400–1405.
49. Jones AP, Rowe BH. Bronchopulmonary hygiene physical therapy for chronic obstructive pulmonary disease and bronchiectasis. Cochrane Database Syst Rev 2000; (2):CD000045.
50. Ross J, Dean E, Abboud RT. The effect of postural drainage positioning on ventilation homogeneity in healthy subjects. Phys Ther 1992; 72(11):794–799.
51. Langenderfer B. Alternatives to percussion and postural drainage. A review of mucus clearance therapies: percussion and postural drainage, autogenic drainage, positive expiratory pressure, flutter valve, intrapulmonary percussive ventilation, and high-frequency chest compression with the ThAIRapy Vest. J Cardiopulm Rehabil 1998; 18(4):283–289.
52. Oldenburg FA Jr., Dolovich MB, Montgomery JM, et al. Effects of postural drainage, exercise, and cough on mucus clearance in chronic bronchitis. Am Rev Respir Dis 1979; 120(4):739–745.
53. Hess DR. The evidence for secretion clearance techniques. Respir Care 2001; 46(11):1276–1293.
54. Wolmer P, Ursing K, Midgren B, et al. Inefficiency of chest percussion in the physical therapy of chronic bronchitis. Eur J Respir Dis 1985; 66(4):233–239.
55. Bach PB, Brown C, Gelfand SE, et al. Management of acute exacerbations of chronic obstructive pulmonary disease: a summary and appraisal of published evidence. Ann Intern Med 2001; 134(7):600–620.
56. Hubert J. 1989. Mobilisations du Thorax. Les edicions Medicales et Paramedicales de Charleroi, Montignies-sur-Sambre, Belgium.
57. Lannefors L, Wollmer P. Mucus clearance with three chest physiotherapy regimes in cystic fibrosis: a comparison between postural drainage, PEP and physical exercise. Eur Respir J 1992; 5(6):748–753.
58. Konstan MW, Stern RC, Doershuk CF. Efficacy of the Flutter device for airway mucus clearance in patients with cystic fibrosis. J Pediatr 1994; 124(5 pt 1):689–693.
59. Pryor JA, Webber BA, Hodson ME, et al. The Flutter VRP1 as an adjunct to chest physiotherapy in cystic fibrosis. Respir Med 1994; 88(9):677–681.
60. Bach JR, Ishikawa Y, Kim H. Prevention of the pulmonary morbidity for patients with Duchenne muscular dystrophy. Chest 1997; 112:1024–1028.
61. Bach JR, Alba AS. Noninvasive options for ventilatory support of the traumatic high level quadriplegic patient. Chest 1990; 98(3):613–619.
62. Bach JR. New approaches in the rehabilitation of the traumatic high level quadriplegic. Am J Phys Med Rehabil 1991; 70(1):13–9.
63. Kang SW, Bach JR. Maximum insufflation capacity: vital capacity and cough flows in neuromuscular disease. Am J Phys Med Rehabil 2000; 79(3):222–227.
64. Sivasothy P, Brown L, Smith I E, et al. 2001. Effects of manually assisted cough and mechanical insufflation on cough flow of normal subjects, patients with chronic obstructive pulmonary disease (COPD), and patients with respiratory muscle weakness. Thorax 56:438–444.
65. Bach JR. Mechanical insufflation-exsufflation: comparison of peak expiratory flows with manually assisted and unassisted coughing techniques. Chest 1993; 104(5):1553–1562.
66. Bach JR. Don't forget the abdominal thrust. Chest 2004; 126(4):1389–1390.

67. Bach JR, Chaudhry SS. Standards of care in MDA clinics. Muscular dystrophy association. Am J Phys Med Rehabil 2000; 79(2):193–196.
68. Barach AL, Beck GJ, Bickerman HA, et al. Mechanical coughing: studies on physical methods of producing high velocity flow rates during the expiratory cycle. Trans Assoc Am Physicians 1951; 64:360–363.
69. Beck GJ, Scarrone LA. Physiological effects of exsufflation with negative pressure (E.W.N.P.). Dis Chest 1956; 29(1):1–16.
70. Barach AL, GJ Beck. Exsufflation with negative pressure: physiologic and clinical studies in poliomyelitis, bronchial asthma, pulmonary emphysema and bronchiectasis. Arch Intern Med 1954; 93(6):825–841.
71. Winck JC, Gonçalves MR, Lourenço C, et al. Effects of mechanical insufflation-exsufflation on respiratory parameters for patients with chronic airway secretion encumbrance. Chest 2004; 126(3):774–780.
72. Gomez-Merino E, Sancho J, Marin E, et al. Mechanical insufflation-exsufflation: pressure, volume, and flow relationships and the adequacy of the manufacturer's guidelines. Am J Phys Med Rehabil 2002; 81(8):579–583.
73. Bach JR, Smith WH, Michaels J, et al. Airway secretion clearance by mechanical exsufflation for post-poliomyelitis ventilator-assisted individuals. Arch Phys Med Rehab 1993; 74(2):170–177.
74. Farrero E, Prats E, Povedano M, et al. Survival in amyotrophic lateral sclerosis with home mechanical ventilation: the impact of systematic respiratory assessment and bulbar involvement. Chest 2005; 127(6):2132–2138.
75. Bach JR, Niranjan V, Weaver B. Spinal muscular atrophy type 1: a noninvasive respiratory management approach. Chest 2000; 117:1100–1105.
76. Niranjan V, Bach JR. Noninvasive management of pediatric neuromuscular ventilatory failure. Crit Care Med 1998; 26(12):2061–2065.
77. Garstang SV, Kirshblum SC, Wood KE. Patient preference for in-exsufflation for secretion management with spinal cord injury. J Spinal Cord Med 2000; 23(2):80–85.
78. Sancho J, Servera E, Vergara P, et al. Mechanical insufflation-exsufflation vs. tracheal suctioning via tracheostomy tubes for patients with amyotrophic lateral sclerosis: a pilot study. Am J Phys Med Rehabil 2003; 82(10):750–753.
79. Whitney J, Harden B, Keilty S. Assisted cough: a new technique. Physiotherapy 2002; 88(4): 201–207.
80. Williams EK, Holaday DA. The use of exsufflation with negative pressure in postoperative patients. Am J Surg 1955; 90(4):637–640.
81. Marchant WA, Fox R. Postoperative use of a Cough Assist device in avoiding prolonged intubation. Br J Anaesth 2002; 89(4):644–647.
82. Bach JR. Cough in SCI patients. Arch Phys Med Rehabil 1994; 75(5):610.
83. Vianello AC, Arcaro A, Gallan G, et al. Mechanical insufflation-exsufflaton improves outcomes for neuromuscular disease patients with respiratory tract infections. Am J Phys Med Rehabil 2005; 84(2):83–88.
84. Servera E, Sancho J, Zafra MJ, et al. Alternatives to endotracheal intubation for patients with neuromuscular diseases. Am J Phys Med Rehabil 2005; 84(11):851–857.
85. Bach J, Goncalves M. Ventilatory weaning by lung expansion and decanulation. Am J Phys Med Rehabil 2004; 83:560–568.
86. Toussaint M, De Win H, Steens M, et al. Effect of intrapulmonary percussive ventilation on mucus clearance in duchenne muscular dystrophy patients: a preliminary report. Respir Care 2003; 48(10):940–947.
87. Varekojis SM, Douce FH, Flucke FH, et al. A comparison of the therapeutic effectiveness of and preference for postural drainage and percussion, intrapulmonary percussive ventilation, and

high-frequency chest wall compression in hospitalized cystic fibrosis patients. Respir Care 2003; 48(1):24–28.
88. Vargas FH, Bui N, Boyer A, et al. Intrapulmonary percussive ventilation in acute exacerbations of COPD patients with mild respiratory acidosis: a randomized controlled trial [ISRCTN17802078]. Crit Care 2005; 9(4):R382–R389.
89. Trawoger R, Kolobow T, Cereda M, et al. Clearance of mucus from endotracheal tubes during intratracheal pulmonary ventilation. Anesthesiology 1997; 86(6):1367–1374.
90. Bach JR. A historical perspective on the use of noninvasive ventilatory support alternatives. Respir Care Clin N Am 1996; 2(2):161–181.
91. Chaisson KM, Walsh S, Simmons Z, et al. A clinical pilot study: high frequency chest wall oscillation airway clearance in patients with amyotrophic lateral sclerosis. Amyotroph Lateral Scler 2006; 7(2):107–111.
92. Hansen LG, Warwick WJ, Hansen KL. Mucus transport mechanisms in relation to the effect of high frequency chest compression (HFCC) on mucus clearance. Pediatr Pulmonol 1994; 17(2): 113–118.
93. Scherer TA, Barandun J, Martinez E, et al. Effect of high-frequency oral airway and chest wall oscillation and conventional chest physical therapy on expectoration in patients with stable cystic fibrosis. Chest 1998; 113(4):1019–1027.
94. Darbee JC, Kanga JF, Ohtake PJ. Physiologic evidence for high-frequency chest wall oscillation and positive expiratory pressure breathing in hospitalized subjects with cystic fibrosis. Phys Ther 2005; 85(12):1278–1289.
95. Dolmage TE, De Rosie JA, Avendano MA, et al. Effect of external chest wall oscillation on gas exchange in healthy subjects. Chest 1995; 107(2):433–439.
96. Hansen LG, Warwick WJ. High-frequency chest compression system to aid in clearance of mucus from the lung. Biomed Instrum Technol 1990; 24(4):289–294.
97. Jones A, Rowe BH. Bronchopulmonary hygiene physical therapy in bronchiectasis and chronic obstructive pulmonary disease: a systematic review. Heart Lung 2000; 29(2):125–135.
98. Servera E, Sancho J, Zafra MJ, et al. Secretion management must be considered when reporting success or failure of noninvasive ventilation. Chest 2003; 123:1773.
99. Rideau Y, Gatin G, Bach J, et al. Prolongation of life in Duchenne's muscular dystrophy. Acta Neurol (Napoli) 1983; 5(2):118–124.

29
The Importance of Overnight Monitoring in the Management of Chronic Respiratory Failure

ROGER S. GOLDSTEIN
West Park Healthcare Centre, University of Toronto, Toronto, Ontario, Canada

LORI DAVIS
West Park Healthcare Centre, Toronto, Ontario, Canada

I. Introduction

When deciding whether to initiate elective mechanical ventilatory support for patients with chronic respiratory failure, the decision can be facilitated by the clinician having objective information about the patient's nocturnal ventilation and gas exchange. Some of this information may be deduced from the patient's daytime arterial blood gases (ABG), especially if hypoventilation is present, as the carbon dioxide tension (P_{CO_2}) will be elevated. However, in many patients, the daytime gases underestimate the severity of nocturnal hypoventilation (1). The recognition of respiratory changes during sleep is important as it may result in an approach that could reduce morbidity and mortality. The relationship between altered pulmonary function and disordered sleep is not a precise one. In patients with amyotrophic lateral sclerosis, neither forced vital capacity nor negative inspiratory pressure could predict sleep-disordered breathing (2). In patients with myasthenia gravis, pulmonary function was documented as an associated risk factor for abnormal breathing during sleep (3). In our experience (4), the vital capacity of 30 patients with kyphoscoliosis and respiratory failure was $27\% \pm 9\%$ predicted, their maximum inspiratory pressure was $25\% \pm 14\%$ predicted, and their maximum expiratory pressure was $73\% \pm 50\%$ predicted. As the underlying conditions progress, impaired mechanics are accompanied by altered resting awake arterial gas tensions, with P_{CO_2} levels of 56 to 61 mmHg and Pa_{O_2} levels of 37 to 70 mmHg in representative studies (5–7). Not surprisingly, the relationship between altered arterial blood gas tensions and pulmonary function is not precise. A study, designed to determine at what level of mechanical impairment respiratory failure was likely to occur, measured 53 patients with proximal myopathies. The authors reported that hypercapnia occurred when respiratory muscle strength fell below 30% predicted in uncomplicated myopathies and when the vital capacity fell below 55% predicted in those with or without parenchymal involvement (8).

It is at night when the changes in pulmonary mechanics and control of breathing, which occur in healthy individuals during sleep, are superimposed on patients whose conditions are characterized by altered pulmonary mechanics and control of breathing (9). This is especially important during rapid eye movement (REM) sleep when there is loss of intercostal muscle tone, decreased chemoresponsiveness, a rapid shallow breathing pattern,

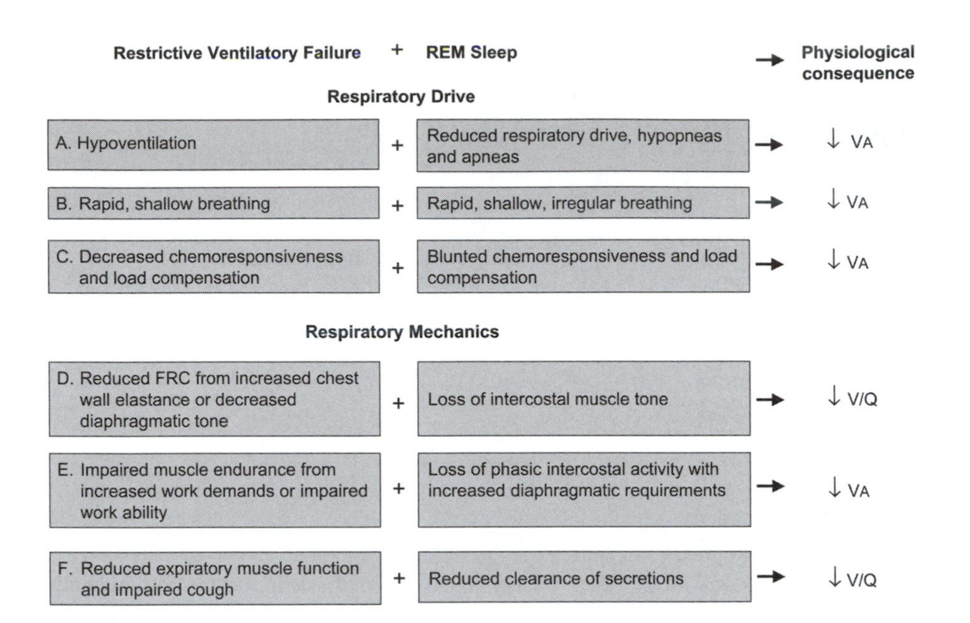

Figure 1 Schematic equation describing the changes in respiratory drive and mechanics that occur when respiratory failure is combined with REM sleep. The physiological consequences that result are shown on the right side. *Abbreviation*: REM, rapid eye movement.

increased upper airway resistance, and less vigorous secretion clearance, compared with non-REM sleep (10). Accordingly, a qualitative "equation" can be written, which in schematic terms describes the interaction between the pathophysiology of respiratory failure and the physiological elements of REM sleep (1,11). Although the relative importance of each of these interactions will vary, Figure 1 summarizes some of the important changes that occur. On the left side are the changes in respiratory drive and mechanics found in conditions associated with respiratory failure and on the right side the changes in respiratory drive and mechanics associated with REM sleep. The consequences, as shown in the equation, are reductions in alveolar ventilation and increases in ventilation/perfusion mismatching.

Therefore, although gas exchange may be altered during the day, the patient experiences the greatest elevations in Pco_2 and dips in oxygen saturation (Sao_2), at night, most noticeably during REM sleep (12). It is not surprising that for patients with respiratory failure, sleep, instead of being a period of refreshment and tranquility, presents a serious physiologic challenge. It has been suggested that these changes may influence the development of pulmonary hypertension, right ventricular dysfunction, and cor pulmonale, contributing to their premature death.

Night monitoring will help identify and characterize respiratory failure among patients with conditions, such as neuromuscular disease (NMD), thoracic restriction (TR), or chronic obstructive pulmonary disease (COPD), which may progress to respiratory failure. Night monitoring may also identify overlapping respiratory conditions, such as sleep apnea, as well as other comorbidities, such as cardiac dysfunction. In addition to their diagnostic value, studies over time are useful in monitoring trends in developing respiratory failure. By identifying a gradual progression of respiratory failure, such studies enable the patient, the family, and the health care system to benefit from planned, elective noninvasive ventilation, rather than requiring emergency intubation and ventilation in the ICU.

Patients who develop sleep-related disturbance may have a variety of signs and symptoms, such as nocturnal restlessness, frequent awakening, snoring, daytime sleepiness, fatigue, or headaches. Polysomnography is helpful in distinguishing among the different types of sleep disturbances and in assessing their severity.

The management of hypoventilation is based on the premise that preventing further reductions in alveolar ventilation during sleep will result in an improvement in nighttime and subsequently in daytime ABG, a reduction in pulmonary hypertension and cor pulmonale, and the prevention of premature death. It is important to note that to date, there have been no prospective randomized controlled trials regarding the management of respiratory failure in patients with TR disease or NMD. Nevertheless, compelling clinical evidence suggests that elective mechanical ventilatory support, preferably with a noninvasive technique, is effective in achieving the above goals.

Oxygen alone, although preventing the nocturnal desaturation, often results in unacceptably high levels of Pco_2. Diuretics and tracheostomy alone, although providing a temporary improvement, will at best delay the need for mechanical ventilatory support.

Ventilator to patient synchrony can be evaluated at night and interface leakage, whether from the mask, mouthpiece, or tracheostomy, can be readily identified. Although this does not obviate the requirement for accurate daytime monitoring of ventilation, it adds further practical information on the effectiveness of ventilatory support at night and its influence on sleep architecture, when ventilator assisted individuals are at their most vulnerable. Such measurements allow the clinician to adjust the ventilatory mode, pressures, volume, rate, and waveform, to maximize gas exchange and reduce leaks, while minimizing patient discomfort (13) and optimizing sleep quality.

Whereas some centers use full respiratory polysomnographic studies to monitor the effectiveness of ventilation in relation to sleep stages, many centers monitor Sao_2 only, or Sao_2 plus transcutaneous Pco_2, and still others use a hybrid of respiratory excursions plus gas exchange without monitoring sleep architecture. Although there are no internationally accepted guidelines as to how frequently and comprehensively to monitor respiratory failure, it is the authors' view that sleep architecture and gas exchange should be monitored immediately prior to initiating ventilation and again after ventilatory support has been established. The frequency and complexity of subsequent monitoring depends on the underlying diagnosis, the presence of comorbidities, the rate of clinical change, and the availability of monitoring facilities. Most clinicians agree that there should be regular monitoring of at least Sao_2 and Pco_2, either at home, in a community facility, or in a hospital.

In this chapter, we provide clinical case examples that illustrate some of the ways in which the management of patients who receive ventilatory support at home may be enhanced by their being studied in a fully equipped sleep laboratory. The cases also highlight some of the clinical issues specific to a respiratory failure population, many of whom are markedly impaired. We use the term "sleep study" to mean polysomnography with comprehensive respiratory monitoring, unless otherwise stated. We make no claim that a full sleep study is the only approach to patient monitoring, indeed at times we are quite comfortable with simple bedside overnight monitoring of gas exchange. However, it is our view that measuring Pco_2 noninvasively is as important to the management of patients with respiratory failure as measuring blood pressure among those treated for hypertension.

A. Scenario 1: A Patient with Kyphoscoliosis

A woman of 45 years, with idiopathic kyphoscoliosis presented for evaluation of her respiratory function. She had recently recovered from an episode of pneumonia, managed in an acute care unit, without requiring ventilatory support. At the age of four she had undergone a spinal fusion and rod insertion for scoliosis, after which she remained well for many years, despite experiencing gradually progressive dyspnea on exertion.

Her pulmonary function tests showed a vital capacity (VC) of 1.2 L (43%), a total lung capacity of 44%, and a forced expiratory volume in 1 second/forced vital capacity (FEV_1/FVC) of 90%. ABG while breathing room air showed pH 7.39, Pco_2 46 mmHg, Pao_2 78 mmHg, and Sao_2 95%. Her baseline sleep study (Fig. 2) showed a mean Sao_2 of 94% (range 73–98%) and a mean Pco_2 of 55 mmHg (range 45–64 mmHg). Gas exchange was noted to be aggravated during REM sleep.

As her peak nighttime Pco_2 was elevated, it was decided to repeat the sleep study after six months. Although there was no change in her clinical status, her subsequent study (Fig. 3) showed a mean Sao_2 of 93% (range 73–97%) and a mean Pco_2 68 mmHg (range 53–83 mmHg). Despite good sleep consolidation, the finding of progressing hypercapnia led to a decision to initiate noninvasive positive pressure ventilation (NIPPV).

She was started on bi-level positive airway pressure ventilation 20/8 cmH_2O with a rate of 15 breaths per minute (bpm). Her nocturnal gas exchange (Fig. 4) returned to within

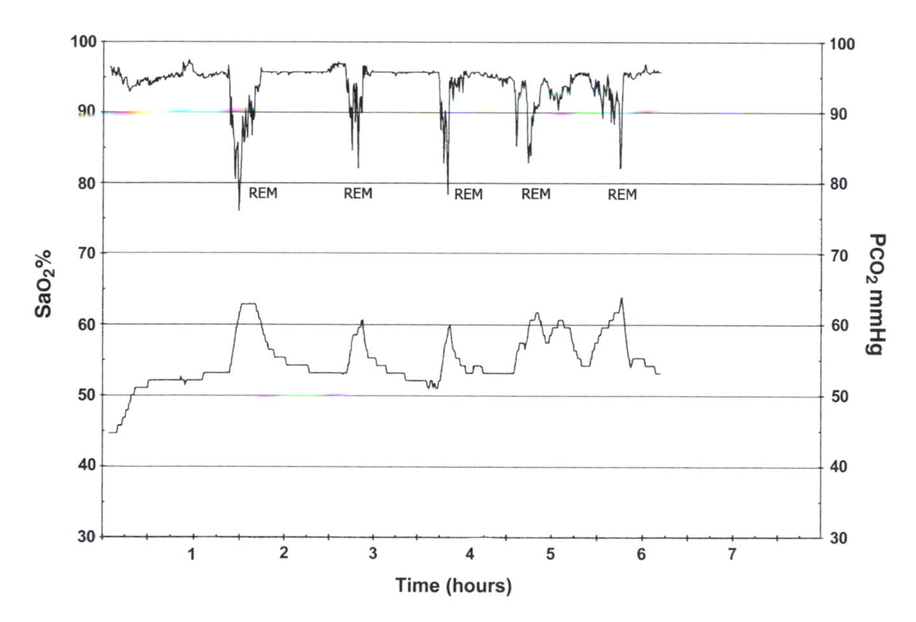

Figure 2 Recording channels for Sao_2 (*upper tracing*) and Pco_2 (*lower tracing*) from an overnight polysomnogram. A stable baseline Sao_2 of 94% and Pco_2 of 53 mmHg. Although the worst gas exchange occurs during periods of REM sleep (*marked*), on each occasion, the gases return to their baseline values during non-REM sleep. *Abbreviations*: Sao_2, saturation of oxygen in arterial blood; Pco_2, partial pressure of carbon dioxide; REM, rapid eye movement.

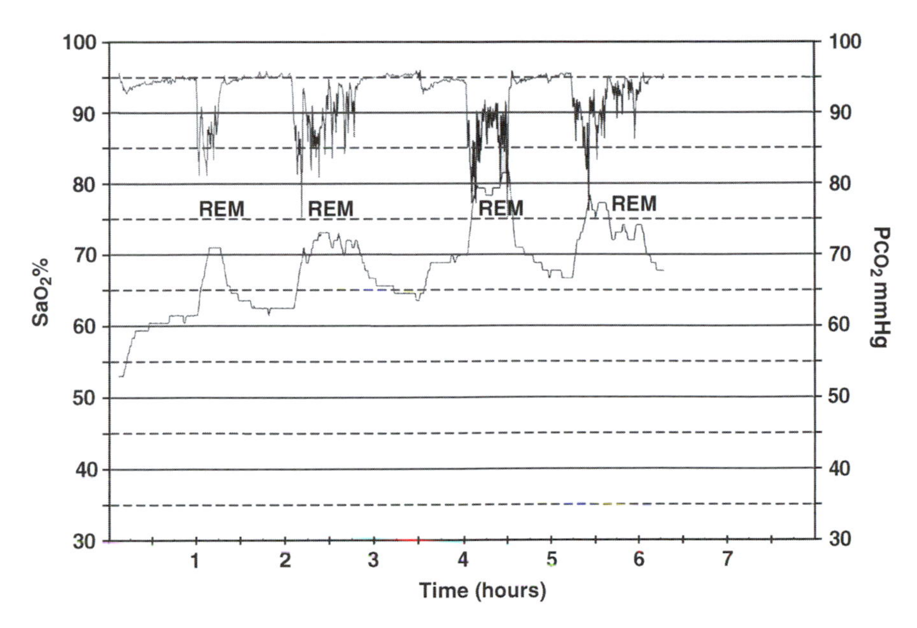

Figure 3 Recording channels for Sa_{O_2} and P_{CO_2} from an overnight polysomnogram. Note: The baseline Sa_{O_2} of 93% and P_{CO_2} of 53 mmHg. The worst gas exchange occurs during periods of REM sleep (*marked*). The Sa_{O_2} returns to baseline between REM episodes, but the P_{CO_2} gradually rises through the night. *Abbreviations*: Sa_{O_2}, saturation of oxygen in arterial blood; P_{CO_2}, partial pressure of carbon dioxide; REM, rapid eye movement.

the normal range: Sa_{O_2} 97% (92–99%) and P_2 46 mmHg (40–49 mmHg). She continued to feel well and to function well. A follow-up sleep study (Fig. 5) showed excellent synchrony between the patient and the ventilator.

This case illustrates that close to normal daytime gas exchange can occur despite hypoventilation at night. As the latter was progressive, the repeat sleep study was valuable in determining when to initiate ventilatory support.

B. Scenario 2: A Patient with Progressive Respiratory Failure

A man of 19 years had been diagnosed with Duchenne's muscular dystrophy at 6 years and became wheelchair bound by the age of 14. He had no other symptoms beyond muscle weakness and specifically denied morning headaches or dyspnea. His VC was 44% predicted and his respiratory muscle strength was reduced, with a maximal inspiratory pressure (MIP) of 28% predicted and a maximal expiratory pressure (MEP) of 13% predicted.

A baseline sleep study (Fig. 6) showed satisfactory sleep and gas exchange, with an apnea-hypopnea index within the normal range. He remained stable during annual follow-up studies for five years, during which his nighttime P_{CO_2} rose slowly to 52 mmHg. At the time of his next follow-up, he gave a history of gradually increasing fatigue and malaise. His sleep was more fragmented and his gas exchange (Fig. 7) showed a mean P_{CO_2} of

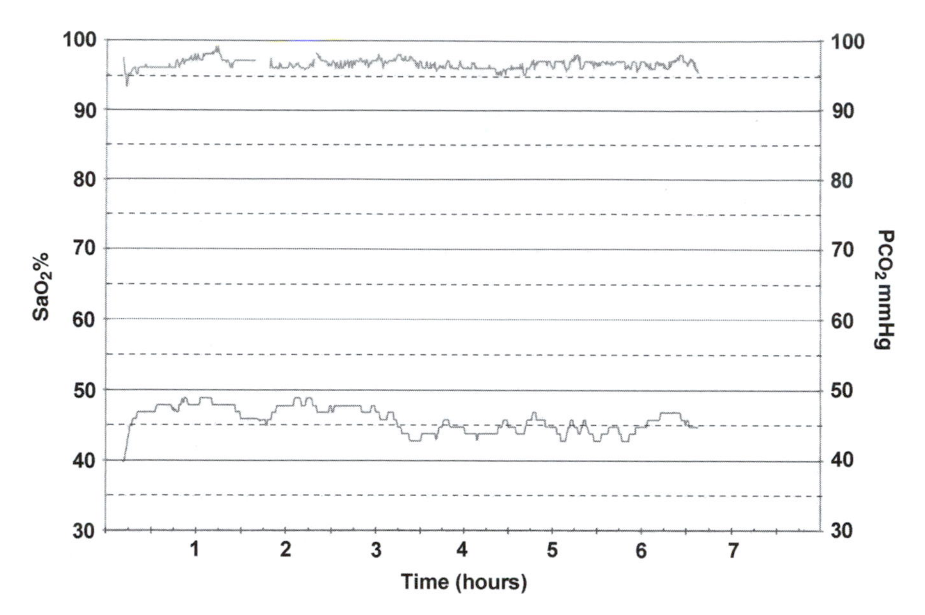

Figure 4 Recording channels for Sa_{O_2} and P_{CO_2} from an overnight polysomnogram. Patient is being ventilated with bi-level positive airway pressure using settings of 20/8 cmH_2O and a respiratory rate of 15 bpm. Note: Stable values for Sa_{O_2} and P_{CO_2}. Sleep architecture is normal and REM periods are no longer distinguishable by changes in gas exchange. *Abbreviations*: Sa_{O_2}, saturation of oxygen in arterial blood; P_{CO_2}, partial pressure of carbon dioxide; REM, rapid eye movement; bpm, breaths per minute.

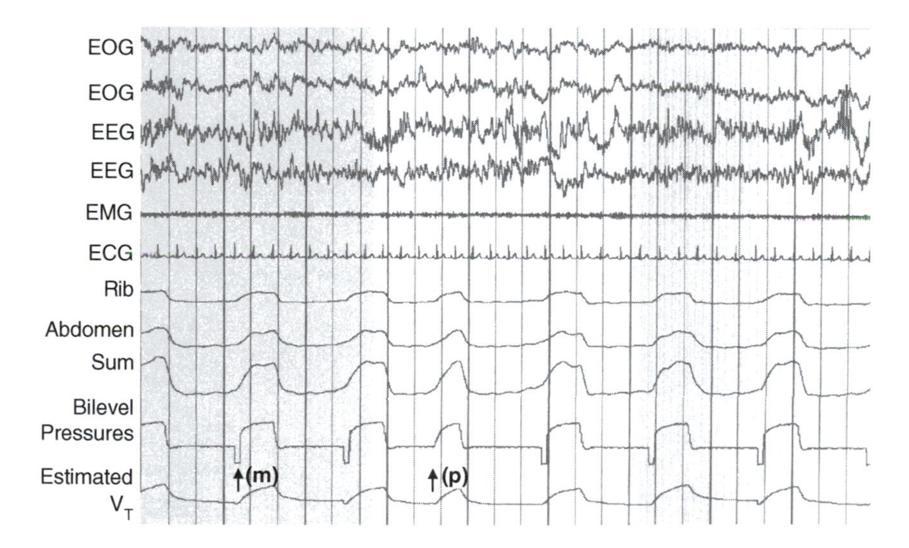

Figure 5 A representative epoch from a polysomnogram, taken during stage 2 sleep. Note: Rhythmic, synchronous respiratory movements. The channel with bi-level pressures shows both machine (m) and patient (p) initiated breaths.

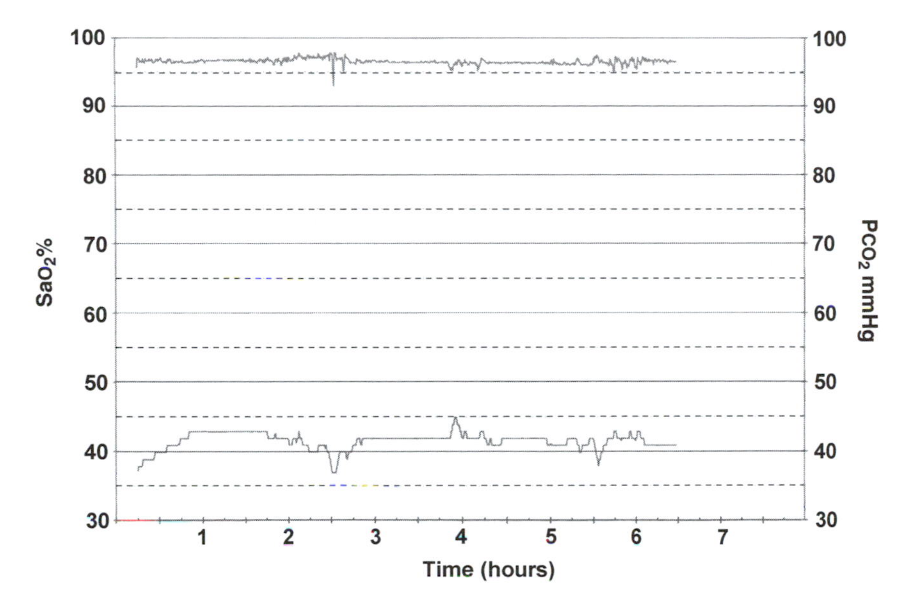

Figure 6 Recording channels for Sao_2 and Pco_2 from an overnight polysomnogram. Patient is unassisted and breathing room air. Note: Stable Sao_2 of 97% and Pco_2 of 42 mmHg. *Abbreviations*: Sao_2, saturation of oxygen in arterial blood; Pco_2, partial pressure of carbon dioxide.

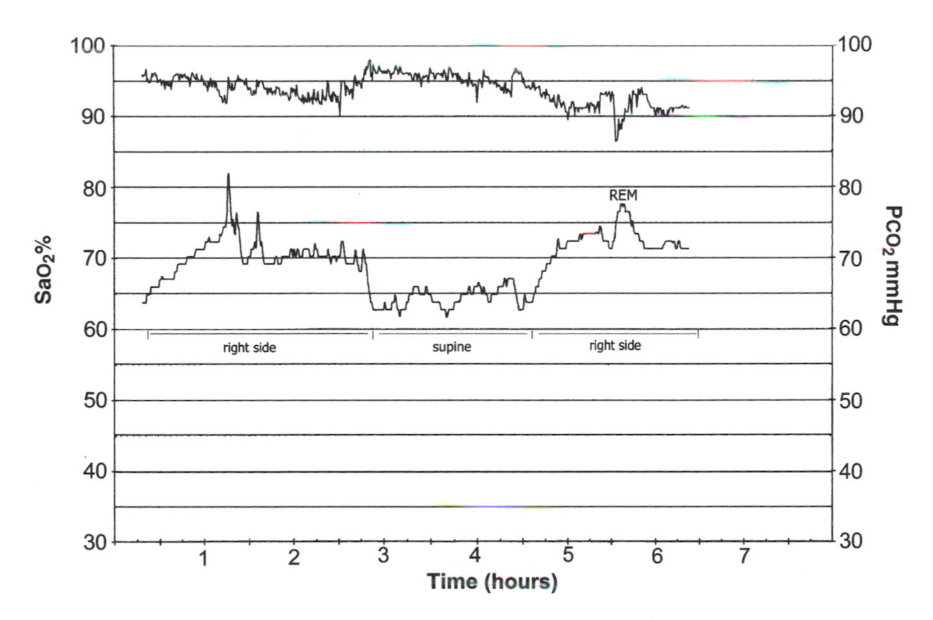

Figure 7 Recording channels for Sao_2 and Pco_2 from an overnight polysomnogram. This study is five years later than in Figure 6. Note: Mean Sao_2 of 94%. Pco_2 has risen to a mean of 69 mmHg and shows fluctuation with sleep stage and with body position. *Abbreviations*: Sao_2, saturation of oxygen in arterial blood; Pco_2, partial pressure of carbon dioxide.

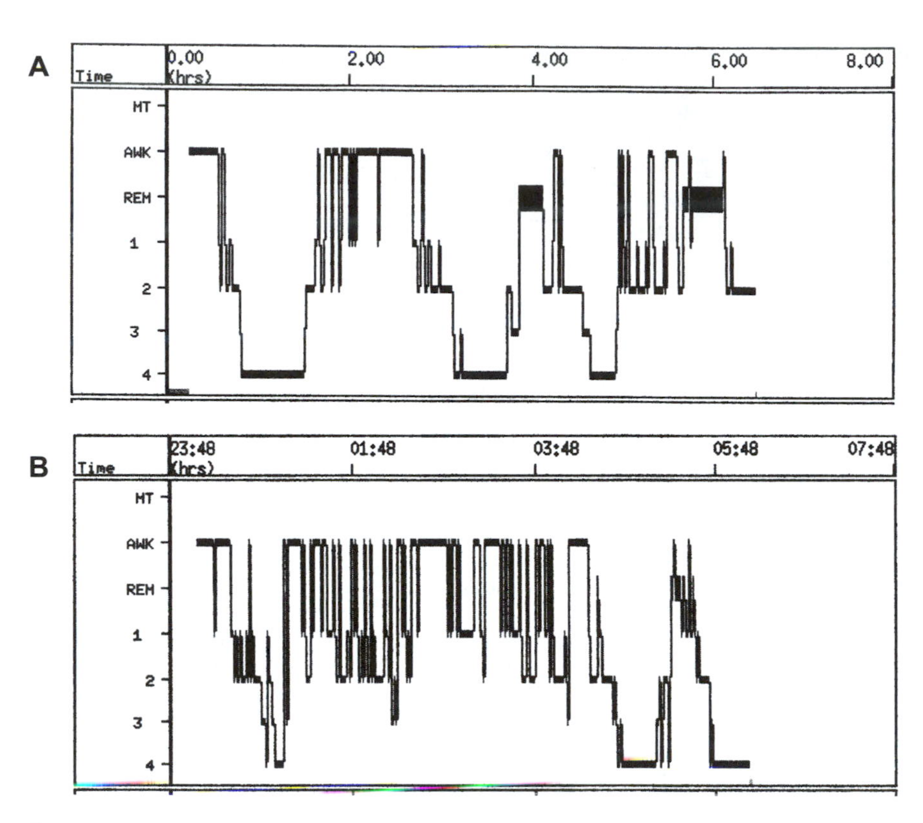

Figure 8 Overview of sleep hypnograms which illustrate changes in sleep architecture at baseline (*panel A*) and five years later (*panel B*). Note: Changes in sleep architecture correspond to clinical symptoms. The later study shows frequent awakenings with reduced slow wave sleep and REM sleep as compared to the baseline study. *Abbreviation*: REM, rapid eye movement.

69 mmHg (range 62–83 mmHg), 17 mmHg higher than his previous study. Moreover, his sleep architecture had deteriorated, with sleep fragmentation, reduced slow wave sleep, reduced REM sleep, and frequent awakenings (Fig. 8).

Despite commencing elective bi-level positive airway pressure ventilatory support, he was unable to sustain adequate gas exchange. The reduced tone of his facial muscles was addressed with the use of a chinstrap. However, an anatomical jaw malocclusion could not be remedied and he declined ventilation via a mouthpiece. He sustained marked air leakage at the mouth, such that many ventilator delivered breaths did not result in adequate ventilatory support, as seen by limited chest and abdominal excursion (Fig. 9). He was advised to consider an elective tracheostomy, but relocated and was lost to follow-up. Ultimately he agreed, at his new location, to have mouthpiece ventilation and he has remained stable.

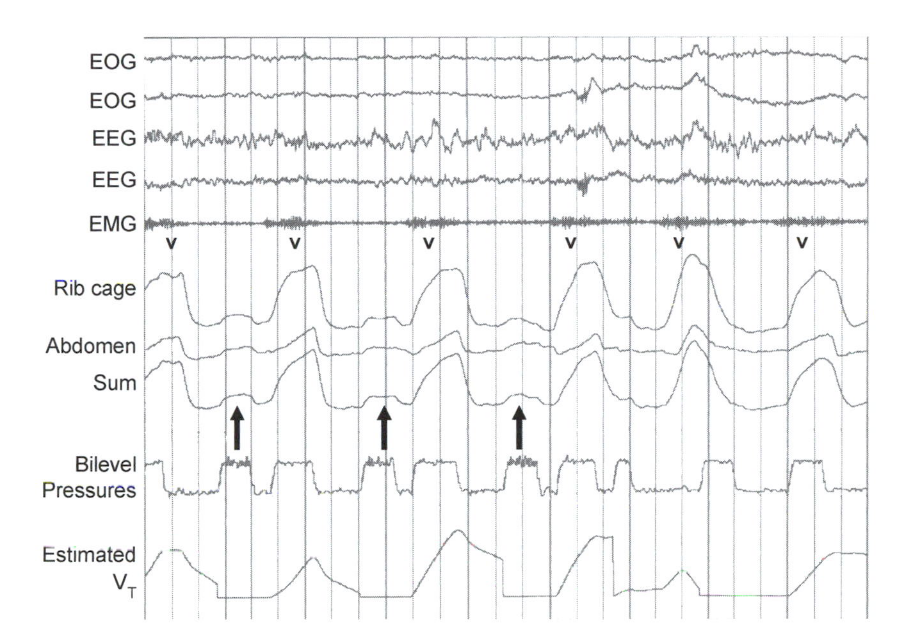

Figure 9 A representative epoch from an overnight polysomnogram. Patient is receiving bi-level pressure ventilation at 12/6 cmH_2O, respiratory rate 15 bpm. Note: Marked leakage at the mouth is reflected in the vibration (v) of the EMG channel. Some breaths (*arrows*) are associated with such severe air leakage at the mouth that they do not result in adequate respiratory excursions. *Abbreviations*: EMG, electromyography; bpm, breaths per minute.

This case illustrates the importance of serial night studies in identifying the need for ventilation, evaluating its effectiveness and providing objective evidence for the consideration of alternate options for ventilatory support.

C. Scenario 3: Respiratory Failure Requiring a Tracheostomy

A woman of 59 years, with severe post-polio kyphoscoliosis and mild asthma, was evaluated for home mechanical ventilation (HMV) following an episode of acute respiratory failure. She had required intubation and ventilation and subsequently a tracheostomy. After she was weaned her tracheostomy was closed. Her VC was 0.86 (31%), FEV_1/FVC was 81%, MIP 12% predicted, and MEP 18% predicted. ABG, while breathing ambient air, showed pH 7.39, Pco_2 53 mmHg, Pao_2 56 mmHg, and Sao_2 89%. She returned home with a prescription for nocturnal oxygen at a flow of 0.5 L/min.

A baseline sleep study on supplemental oxygen at 0.5 L/min (Fig. 10) showed an oscillating saturation profile with a mean Sao_2 of 88% (range 79–95%) and an elevated Pco_2 with a mean value of 64 mmHg (range 58–71 mmHg). She refused elective NIPPV by mask, nasal pillows, or mouthpiece and returned home with a prescription for controlled supplemental oxygen, via a venturi mask.

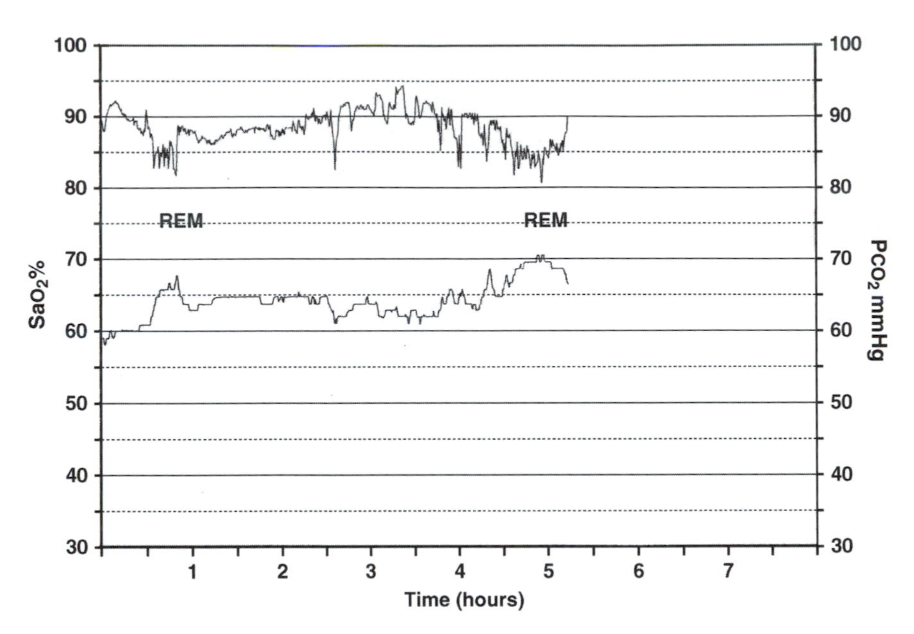

Figure 10 Recording channels for Sao_2 and Pco_2 from an overnight polysomnogram. Patient is receiving oxygen via nasal prongs at a flow rate of 0.5 L/min. Note: The oscillating Sao_2 profile at the beginning and at the end of the night, during REM sleep. The Pco_2 is elevated, with the highest value corresponding to the prolonged REM period at the end of the night. *Abbreviations*: Sao_2, saturation of oxygen in arterial blood; Pco_2, partial pressure of carbon dioxide; REM, rapid eye movement.

Two years later she presented with worsening respiratory failure. She again refused NIPPV but agreed to an elective tracheostomy, and she returned home a week later, with volume ventilation, V_T of 450cc, respiratory rate, f = 10 bpm delivered through a size 7 cuffed tracheostomy tube (Fig. 11). She was followed annually for a further 12 years, developing worsening asthma, as well as severe osteoporosis, with intermittent respiratory exacerbations, but always returning to clinical stability.

During a follow-up study she was noted to have an elevated Pco_2 associated with leakage around her tracheostomy tube. This was addressed by increasing her cuff inflation pressure by adding 1 cc of water (Fig. 12). This cuff inflation resulted in improved ventilation, as shown (Fig. 13) by increased respiratory excursions and increased exhaled volumes.

In this case, patient refusal to tolerate NIPPV eventually resulted in invasive ventilation. Serial follow-up studies confirmed clinical stability and a leak around her tracheostomy tube were addressed by increasing her cuff volume.

D. Scenario 4: Inadequate Follow-Up of Respiratory Failure

A 20-year-old woman with severe kyphoscoliosis and respiratory failure had been diagnosed as a child with NMD attributable to a congenital enzyme deficiency. She walked unaided until the age of five years, required a tracheostomy for secretion clearance at the

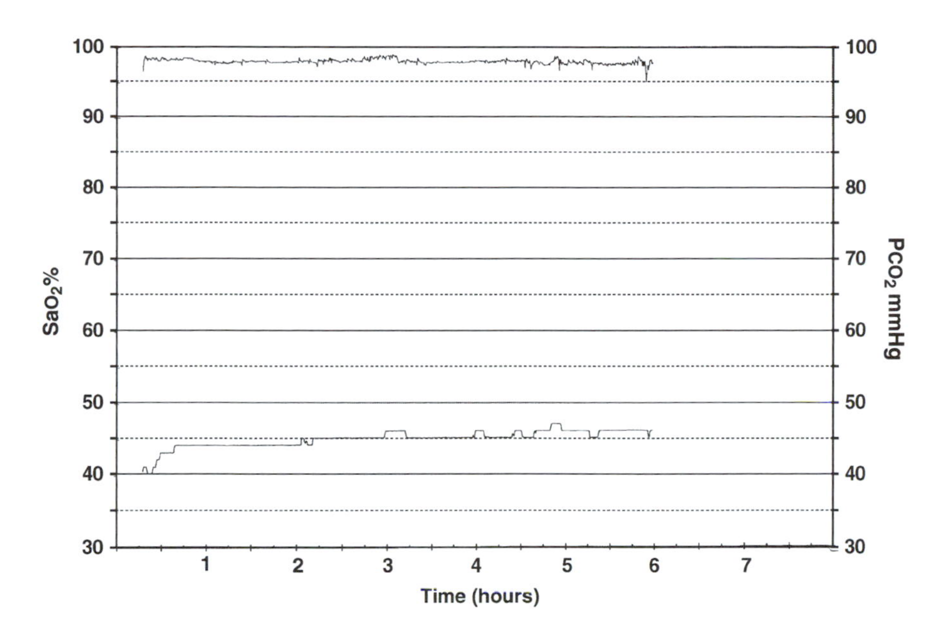

Figure 11 Recording channels for Sa_{O_2} and P_{CO_2} from an overnight polysomnogram. Patient breathing room air while receiving volume ventilation (assist control mode, VT of 500 cc with respiratory rate of 10 bpm) interfaced via a tracheostomy. Note: Stable Sa_{O_2} with a mean of 98% and stable P_{CO_2} with a mean of 45 mmHg. *Abbreviations*: V_T, volume ventilation; Sa_{O_2}, oxygen saturation; P_{CO_2}, carbon dioxide tension.

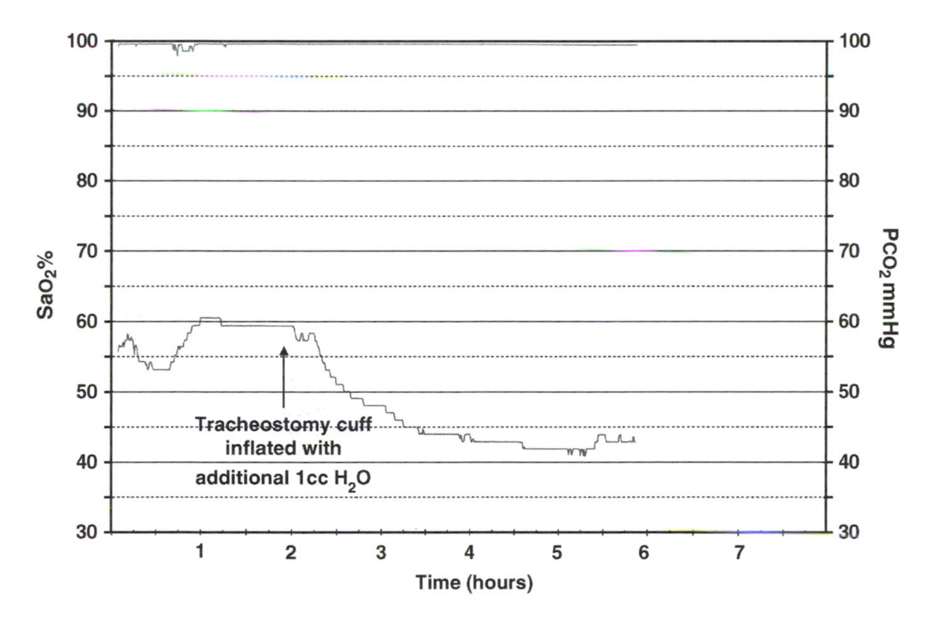

Figure 12 Recording channels and ventilatory parameters Sa_{O_2} and P_{CO_2} from an overnight polysomnogram. Note: Stable Sa_{O_2} with a mean of 99% and P_{CO_2} of 59 mmHg (14 mmHg > previous study). Cuff inflated with additional 1 ccH_2O to minimize air leakage around tracheostomy. *Abbreviations*: Sa_{O_2}, saturation of oxygen in arterial blood; P_{CO_2}, partial pressure of carbon dioxide.

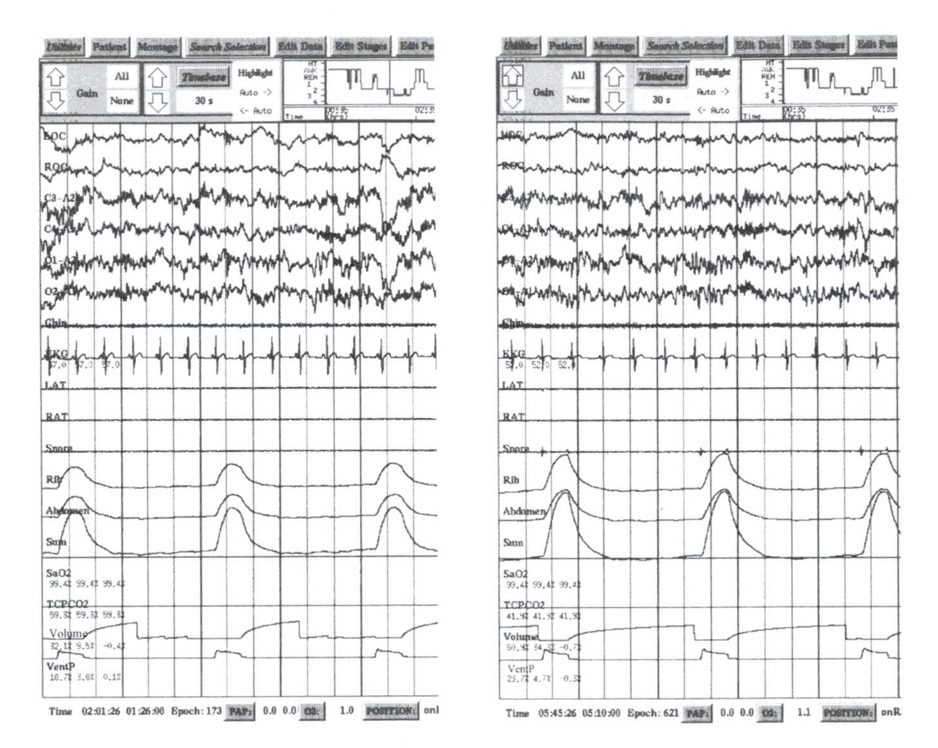

Figure 13 Representative epochs from a overnight polysomnogram, showing the effect of adequate cuff inflation on ventilation. On the left panel, respiratory excursions, ventilator pressures and exhaled volumes are reduced, associated with leakage around the tracheostomy, compared with the same measures (*right panel*), repeated after adequate tracheostomy cuff inflation.

age of 12 years, and required nocturnal ventilatory support at the age of 14 years. Although seen from time to time, she had not undergone any regular monitoring of her ventilatory support. She completed high school and was having difficulty concentrating at university when she presented for a respiratory evaluation. Her sleep study showed fragmented sleep with increased arousals and fluctuating gas exchange (Fig. 14). There were 149 arousals associated with central hypopneas, an event rate of 29/hr (normal < 10/hr). Exhaled volume was markedly reduced due to leakage around her tracheostomy tube and 50% of her time in bed was spent with a Sa_{O_2} <88%. Her P_{CO_2} also fluctuated widely with a mean of 57 mmHg (range 34–76 mmHg).

In response, her tracheostomy tube was changed from a Shiley™ #4, fenestrated uncuffed tube to a Bivona™ #6 tight to the shaft tube. Her ventilatory mode was changed from synchronized intermittent mandatory ventilation (SIMV) to assist control, so that each breath was assisted by the machine. Her V_T was reduced from 600 cc to 400 cc and her respiratory frequency from 15 to 14 bpm. With these new settings she felt more comfortable. Her Sa_{O_2} improved to 95% (range 85–99%) with zero time spent at a Sa_{O_2} <88% and her P_{CO_2} fell to a mean of 36 mmHg (range 30–46 mmHg) (Fig. 15). A further reduction in V_T was made to maintain her P_{CO_2} within the normal range.

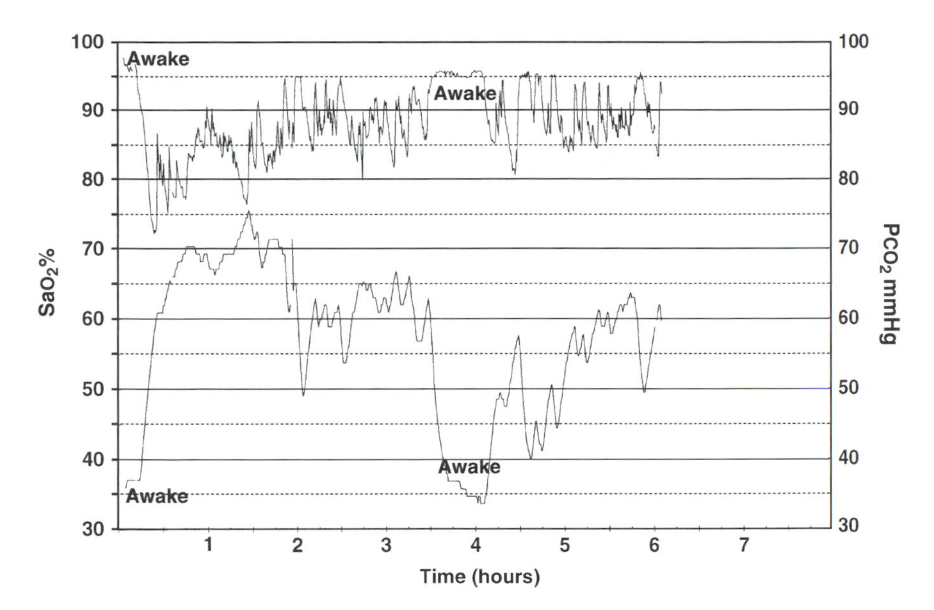

Figure 14 Recording channels for Sa_{O_2} and P_{CO_2} from an overnight polysomnogram in a patient with muscular dystrophy, volume ventilated via tracheostomy with a V_T of 600 cc in the SIMV mode. Note: The Sa_{O_2} is <88% for 50% of the study. The P_{CO_2} is markedly elevated, fluctuates widely during sleep, and returns to normal only during wake. *Abbreviations*: SIMV, synchronized intermittent mandatory ventilation; V_T, volume ventilation; Sa_{O_2}, saturation of oxygen in arterial blood; P_{CO_2}, partial pressure of carbon dioxide.

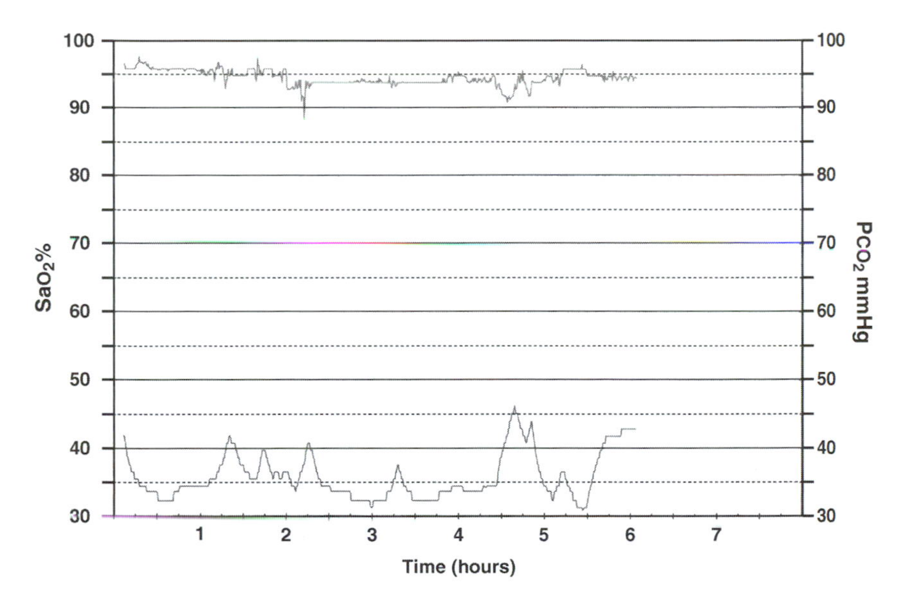

Figure 15 Recording channels for Sa_{O_2} and P_{CO_2} from an overnight polysomnogram. Note: The ventilatory mode has been changed to assist control and the tracheostomy tube from a fenestrated uncuffed tube to a "tight to the shaft" tube. There is improved synchrony between the patient and the ventilator, resulting in improved gas exchange.

This case illustrates the importance of regular follow-up of both ventilation and gas exchange especially as children transition into adulthood. It also illustrates how improved ventilation achieved by alterations to the interface and mode of ventilation will enable adequate gas exchange at a lower delivered tidal volume and breath frequency.

E. Scenario 5: Monitoring Electrophrenic Respiration

The next three examples illustrate how overnight polysomnography can be valuable in monitoring patients in whom respiratory failure is treated with electrophrenic respiration (EPR).

The first example is of a 48-year-old woman with alveolar hypoventilation consequent upon syringomyelia in whom bilateral pacers were inserted at the age of 29. Her VC was 69% predicted, FEV_1/FVC was 104% predicted, her MIP was 75% predicted, and MEP 44% predicted.

On relocation to Toronto, although she stated that she was well and despite her having normal daytime ABG; pH 7.42, Pco_2 40, Pao_2 85, Sao_2 97%, it was decided to refer her for a sleep study. As can be seen (Fig. 16), she displayed an oscillating pattern of Sao_2, consistent with obstructive sleep apnea, with a respiratory index of 34/hr. Given that she felt well, she elected to continue EPR despite our pointing out to her the increased risks associated with untreated obstructive sleep apnea. It is well established that when the diaphragm is stimulated without prior activation of the upper airway dilators and stabilizer muscles, the patient is at increased risk of partial or complete upper airway obstruction (12).

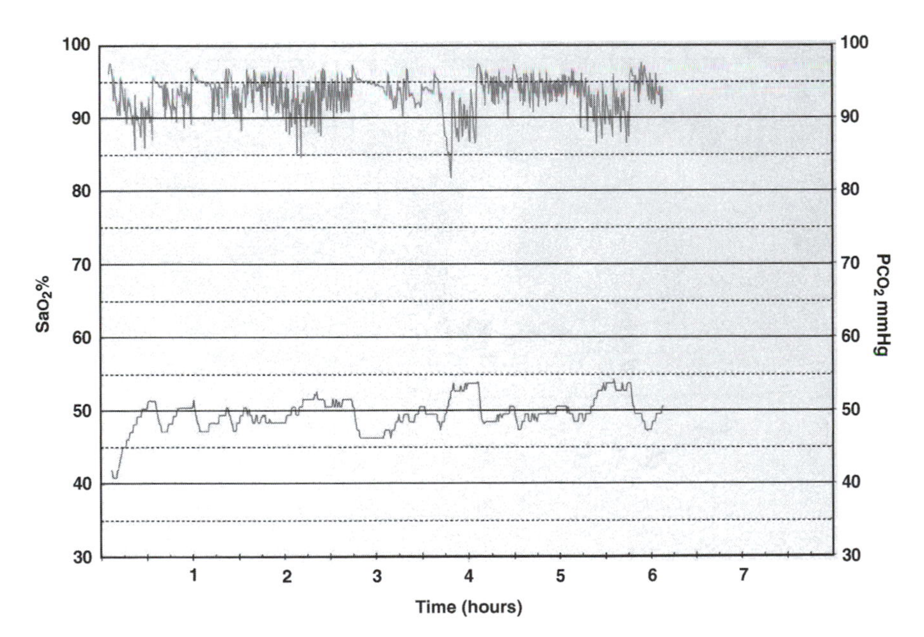

Figure 16 Recording channels for Sao_2 and Pco_2 from an overnight polysomnogram. Note: The oscillating saturation profile reflecting repeated upper airway obstruction associated with diaphragmatic pacing.

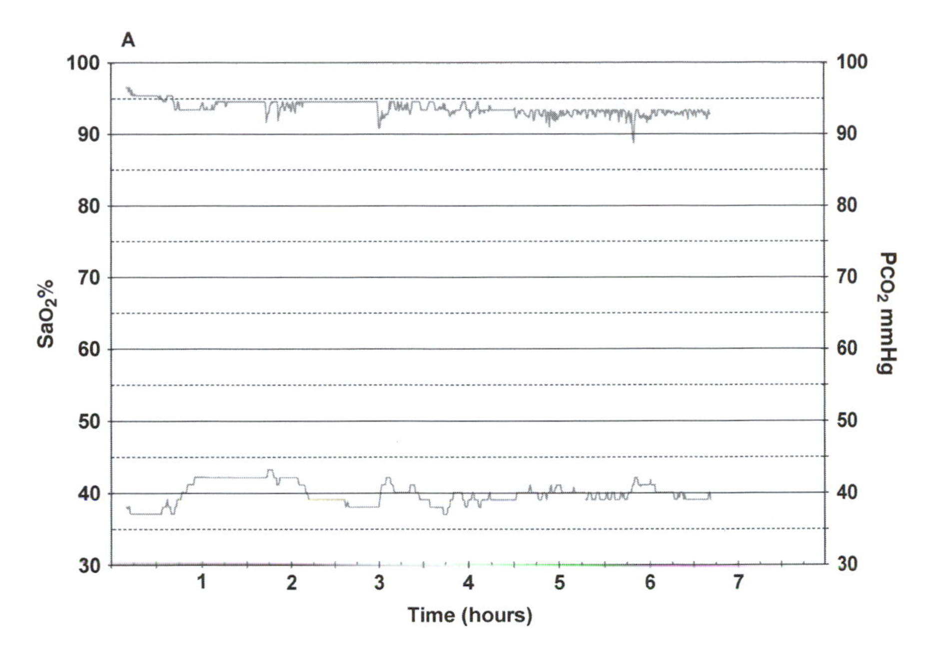

Figure 17 Recording channels for Sa_{O_2} and P_{CO_2} from an overnight polysomnogram. Note: Stable gases during bilateral diaphragmatic pacing.

The second example is of a 47-year-old woman in whom bilateral pacers were inserted at the age of 18 when she sustained a diving accident that resulted in a high spinal cord injury. Functionally quadriplegic, she lived independently, self-directing care, and maximizing her leisure activities. She insisted on her tracheostomy being closed, despite being advised of the risk of upper airway obstruction. She continued to feel very well. Her night study showed a mean Sa_{O_2} of 94% (range 88–97%) and a P_{CO_2} of 40 mmHg (range 37–43 mmHg) (Fig. 17). Although rib cage–abdominal paradox can be clearly identified, there was no evidence of upper airway obstruction (Fig. 18).

The third example is of a 48-year-old woman in whom bilateral pacers were inserted at the age of 16 because of primary alveolar hypoventilation. She remained very stable and was employed on a full-time basis. Her VC was 106% predicted, FEV_1/FVC was 88%, MIP 87% predicted, and MEP 66% predicted. Regular follow-up showed excellent gas exchange, although on assessing her pacemakers, the right side had failed to function for some years.

She presented at an unscheduled visit, with tiredness and morning headaches. ABG showed pH 7.39, P_{CO_2} 60 mmHg, Pa_{O_2} 68 mmHg, and Sa_{O_2} 93%. Her sleep study showed marked hypoventilation (Fig. 19A) with a Sa_{O_2} of 74% (range 62–94%) and a P_{CO_2} of 86 mmHg (range 62–95 mmHg). It was decided that her left side pacemaker had also failed and in the absence of either side providing ventilatory support, volume ventilation was initiated in the sleep laboratory. She responded well (Fig. 19B) with a Sa_{O_2} of 96% (range 93–97%) and a P_{CO_2} of 38 mmHg (range 35–59 mmHg). She was volume ventilated until her pacemaker receivers could be replaced.

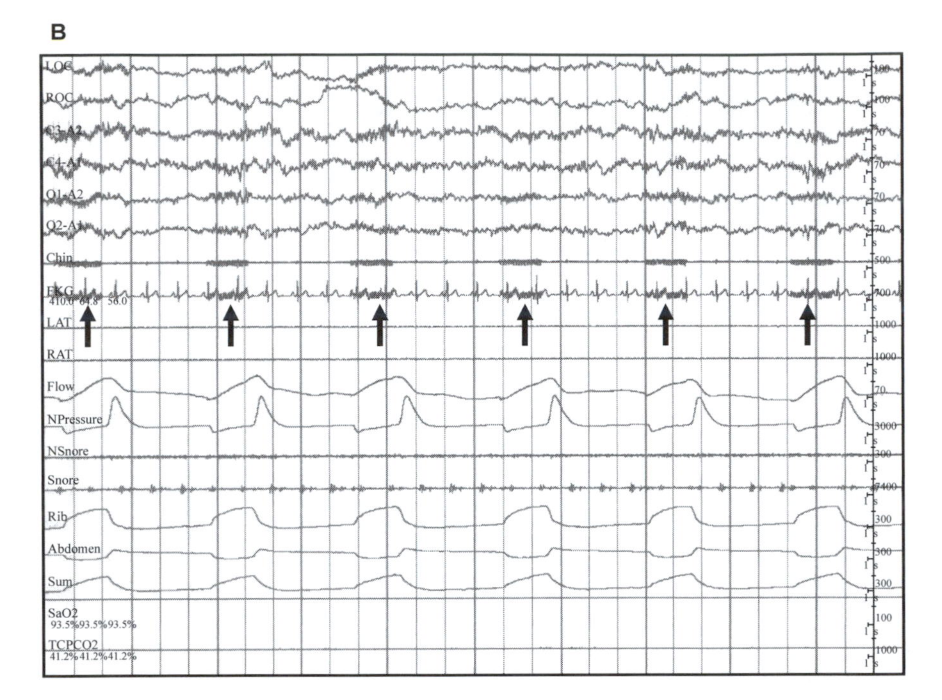

Figure 18 A complete polysomnographic montage. Note: Rib cage and abdominal paradox with no evidence of upper airway obstruction. Artifact from diaphragmatic pacing impulses is seen throughout the epoch (*arrow*).

These three cases illustrate the importance of sleep studies in respiratory failure patients receiving EPR. Such studies are able to detect pacemaker failure as well as upper airway obstruction. Patients with idiopathic primary hypoventilation may still maintain adequate gas exchange during wakefulness, even with dysfunctional pacers, but at night in the absence of cues to breathing, a sleep study will show a very different picture.

II. Comment

Although the precise mechanisms by which respiratory failure patients improve remain to be defined, clinical reports have consistently observed improvements in nocturnal gas exchange and daytime arterial gas values, with adequate ventilatory support (14,15). These changes are associated with reductions in hemoglobin and pulmonary hypertension as well as improvements in the sense of well-being (13). Patients who require only nocturnal ventilation often return to full-time activities. However, should ventilation fail, there is a prompt return to abnormal gas exchange, even after a prolonged period of stability. Therefore, ongoing follow-up of ventilated patients with respiratory failure should include a regular assessment of gas exchange.

However, there is little published information to guide the type, frequency, and location of respiratory monitoring in patients receiving long-term mechanical ventilation

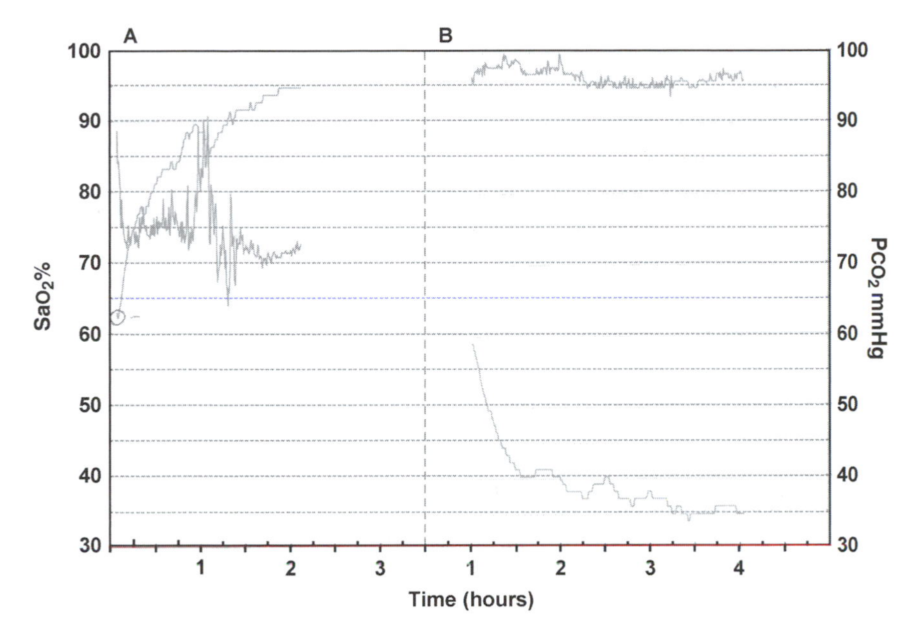

Figure 19 Recording channels for Sao_2 and Pco_2 from an overnight polysomnogram. Left panel (A) reflects failed bilateral pacemakers. The Sao_2 falls from 88% to 65%. On awakening, it returns to 88%, falling again during sleep. In parallel, the Pco_2 is seen to rise progressively from 62 mmHg to 95 mmHg. The right panel (B) illustrates the effect of volume ventilation initiated in the sleep laboratory. Note: The saturation trace is now stable. The Pco_2 falls progressively to 35 mmHg. *Abbreviations*: Sao_2, saturation of oxygen in arterial blood; Pco_2, partial pressure of carbon dioxide.

(LTMV) (16). A recent report of a U.S. consensus conference hosted by an internationally recognized physician advocacy organization, noted for its commitment to excellence in respiratory care for patients requiring LTMV, was silent on the issue of follow-up monitoring (17) as was an important European survey which included detailed questionnaires sent to 483 centers, treating 27,118 users of HMV, which did not comment on issues associated with follow-up monitoring (18,19). A multicenter French study of long-term follow-up of 259 patients with COPD receiving LTMV was able to report serial ABGs but provided no guidance as to the frequency of monitoring or the use of noninvasive measurements (20). The clinical practice guidelines on LTMV at home, authored through the American Association of Respiratory Care, mentions that the frequency of monitoring should be determined by the ongoing individualized care plan and be based on the patient's medical condition, adding that monitoring should occur after initiation of ventilation and with each change to the ventilator settings (21). However, these guidelines provide only minimal recommendations as to the nature and frequency of follow-up monitoring and do not address studies at night. The above cases exemplify the benefits of accurate night studies. Given the growing importance of home ventilation among adults and children (22), we anticipate that in the near future international guidelines that include the indications and complexity of nighttime monitoring will help guide clinicians in their management of patients with respiratory failure.

References

1. Goldstein RS, Brooks D, Davis L. Sleep in patients with neuromuscular and chest wall disorders. In: McNicholas WT, Phillipson EA eds. Breathing Disorders in Sleep. London: WB Saunders, 2002:310–322.
2. David WS, Bundlie SR, Madhavi Z. Polysomnographic studies in amyotrophic lateral sclerosis. J Neurol Sci 1997; 152:S29–S35.
3. Quera-Salva MA, Guilleminault C, Chevret S, et al. Breathing disorders during sleep in myasthenia gravis. Ann Neurol 1992; 31:86–92.
4. Goldstein RS, Molotiu N, Skrastins R, et al. Reversal of sleep induced hypoventilation and chronic respiratory failure by nocturnal negative pressure ventilation in patients with restrictive ventilatory impairment. Am Rev Respir Dis 1987; 135:1049–1055.
5. Ellis ER, Grunstein RR, Chan S, et al. Non invasive ventilatory support during sleep improves respiratory failure in kyphoscoliosis. Chest 1988; 94(4):811–815.
6. Hoeppner VH, Cockroft DW, Dosman JA, et al. Nighttime ventilation improves respiratory failure in secondary kyphoscoliosis. Am Rev Respir Dis 1984; 129:240–243.
7. Kirby GR, Mayer LS, Pingleton SK. Nocturnal positive pressure ventilation via nasal mask. Am Rev Respir Dis 1987; 135:738–740.
8. Braun NM, Aurora NS, Rochester DR. Respiratory muscle and pulmonary function in polymyositis and other proximal myopathies. Thorax 1983; 38:316–323.
9. Stradling JR, Chadwick GA, Frew AJ. Changes in ventilation and its components in normal subjects during sleep. Thorax 1985; 43:364–370.
10. Tabachnik E, Muller NL, Brian AC, et al. Changes in ventilation and chest wall mechanics during sleep in normal adolescence. J Appl Physiol 1981; 51:557–564.
11. Phillipson EA. Control of breathing during sleep. Am Rev Respir Dis 1978; 118:909–939.
12. Oren J. Control of the upper airways during sleep and the hypersomnia-sleep apnea syndrome. In: Oren J, Barnes CD, eds. Physiology in Sleep. New York: Academic Press, 1980:273–313.
13. Bach JR, Tilton MC. Life satisfaction and well being measures in ventilator assisted individuals with traumatic tetraplegia. Arch Phys Med Rehab 1994; 75:626–632.
14. Garray SM, Turino GM, Goldring RM. Sustained reversal of chronic hypercapnia in patients with alveolar hypoventilation syndromes. Long term maintenance with non-invasive nocturnal mechanical ventilation. Am J Med 1981; 70:269–274.
15. Splaingard ML, Frates RC, Harrison GM, et al. Home positive pressure ventilation: twenty years' experience. Chest 1983; 84(4):376–382.
16. O'Donohue WJ, Giovannoni RM, Golberg AI, et al. Long term mechanical ventilation. Guidelines for management in the home and at alternate community sites. Report of the Ad Hoc Committee, Respiratory Care Section, American College of Chest Physicians. Chest 1986; 90:1S–37S.
17. MacIntyre NR, Epstein SK, Carsons S, et al. Management of patients requiring prolonged mechanical ventilatory support: report of a NAMDRC Consensus Conference. Chest 2005; 128:3937–3954.
18. Lloyd-Owen SJ, Donaldson GC, Ambrosino N, et al. Patterns of home mechanical ventilation use in Europe. Results from a Eurovent survey. Eur Respir J 2005; 25:1025–1031.
19. Farre R, Lloyd-Owen SJ, Ambrosino N, et al. Quality control of equipment in home mechanical ventilation: a European survey. Eur Respir J 2005; 26:86–94.
20. Muir J, Girault C, Cardinaud JP, et al. Survival and long term follow-up of tracheostomized patients with COPD treated by home mechanical ventilation. A multicenter French study in 259 patients. French Cooperative Study Group. Chest 1994; 106:201–209.
21. American Association of Respiratory Care. AARC clinical practice guideline. Long term invasive mechanical ventilation in the home. Respir Care 1995; 40(12):1313–1320.
22. Jardine E, O'Toole M, Paton JY, et al. Current status of long term ventilation of children in the United Kingdom: questionnaire survey. Br Med J 1999; 318:295–299.

30
Management of Respiratory Infections

MIQUEL FERRER, MAURICIO VALENCIA, and ANTONI TORRES
Servei de Pneumologia, Institut Clínic del Tòrax, Hospital Clínic, Institut d'Investigacions Biomèdiques August Pi I Sunyer (IDIBAPS), CibeRes (CB06/06/0028), University of Barcelona, Barcelona, Spain

I. Introduction

Pneumonia is the most relevant respiratory infection in mechanically ventilated patients. It is defined as the presence of microorganisms in the pulmonary parenchyma leading to the development of an inflammatory response by the host, which may be localized to the lung or may extend systemically. Nosocomial pneumonia (NP) is an infectious process that develops within 48 hours after admission to hospital and was not incubating at the time of hospitalization. Ventilator-associated pneumonia (VAP) is considered a subgroup of NP and is an infectious pulmonary process that develops 48 hours after the presence of an artificial airway and mechanical ventilation (MV). Since a large proportion of the patients who develop NP are intubated and receive MV, most epidemiological and clinical studies on NP have been focused on critically ill patients and those receiving MV. From a clinical point of view, NP is of great importance, both because of its consequences in terms of morbidity and mortality and because of the high costs associated with this condition.

II. Epidemiology

Despite the large amount of data on the epidemiology of VAP, results vary widely. This may be due to the lack of a standardized diagnostic approach and variability in the populations studied. Moreover, although VAP has been well defined, disagreement as to the final diagnosis may be attributed to (1) focal areas of the lobe that may be missed, (2) negative microbiological studies despite the presence of inflammation in the lung, and (3) disagreement among pathologists as to their findings. The point of time at which VAP develops has important implications in the etiology, treatment, and diagnosis of this disease. VAP has classically been determined as early-onset pneumonia, which occurs within the first four days after hospital admission, and late-onset pneumonia, which develops five or more days after admission (1).

NP is the second most common hospital-acquired infection and is the leading cause of death in this category. The incidence of NP ranges from 4 to 50 cases per 1000 admission in community hospitals and general medical wards, and 120–220 cases per 1000 admission in intensive care units (ICUs) or among patients requiring MV. The EPIC study (2), a large one-day point prevalence study of infections, involved 1417 ICUs and included 10,038 patients. The prevalence of ICU-acquired infections was of 21%, with half of these patients having pneumonia. This was of nosocomial origin in 10%. In a large, prospective cohort study of 1014 patients receiving MV, 177 (18%) developed VAP (3). The incidence of this disease was 24% (78/322) in a Spanish study on risk factors for VAP (4). In a recently published study, the mean incidence of hospital-acquired pneumonia in non-ICU patients was 3 $\pm$ 1.4 cases/1000 hospital admissions (5). Most patients (64%) were in medical wards, had severe underlying diseases, and stayed at hospital for more than 5 days.

The overall incidence of VAP varies from 8% to 28%. A prospective Italian study on VAP including 724 critically ill patients who had received prolonged mechanical ventilation reported an incidence of 23%. This rate varied from 5% in patients receiving MV for one day to 69% in those receiving MV for more than 30 days. In a study including 567 ventilated patients, VAP evaluated with invasive procedures was 9%. In this latter study, the cumulative risk of pneumonia was estimated to be 7% at 10 days and 19% at 20 days after initiation of MV, thereby showing the classical incremental risk of pneumonia of 1% per day (6). However, in a large series of 1014 patients receiving MV, Cook et al. described a rate of VAP of 18%, and although the cumulative risk for developing VAP increased over time, the daily hazard rate decreased after day 5. The risk per day was determined to be 3% on day 5, 2% on day 10, and 1% on day 15.

Several studies have reported the rate of mortality in VAP to range from 24% to 76% (4,6,7). Ventilated ICU patients with VAP have from 2- to 10-fold greater risk of death than patients without this complication. In a study of 78 episodes of NP detected in 322 consecutive patients with MV, the overall mortality rate was 23% (4). Similarly, the Neumos 2000 study group reported a mortality of 26% (pneumonia-attributed 13.9%) in 186 non-ICU patients with hospital-acquired pneumonia (5). The mortality of patients with NP was higher (33%) when compared with rates of patients without NP (19%, $p < 0.01$). On step-forward logistic regression variables independently associated with a worse prognosis included: high-risk microorganisms (*Pseudomonas aeruginosa*, Enterobacteriaceae, and other gram-negative bacilli, *Enterococcus faecalis, Staphylococcus aureus, Candida* spp., *Aspergillus* spp., and episodes of polymicrobial pneumonia), bilateral involvement on chest X ray, the presence of respiratory failure, inappropriate antibiotic therapy, age >60 years, or an ultimately or rapidly fatal underlying condition. The increased risk ratios of mortality in patients with VAP vary from 1.7 to 4.4 (8). Although several studies have shown that VAP is a severe disease, the controversy as to attributing mortality to NP continues. However, several studies have shown NP to be an independent prognostic factor. Patients in whom the attributable mortality is increased include patients undergoing cardiac surgery, acute lung injury, and those who are immunosuppressed (9). In contrast, in patients with life-threatening medical conditions such as cardiac arrest in young patients with no underlying disease and those admitted due to trauma, NP does not seem to significantly increase the mortality [10].

III. Pathogenesis

To develop pneumonia, virulent microorganisms must invade the lung parenchyma, either as the result of a defect in defense mechanisms of the host or by an overwhelming inoculum. The normal human respiratory tract has a variety of defense mechanisms such as anatomic barriers, cough reflex, cell and humoral-mediated immunity, and a dual phagocytic system involving both alveolar macrophages and neutrophils. Virulent microorganisms can reach the alveolar space by colonization of the upper airway with potentially pathogenic microorganisms and by posterior microaspiration, macroaspiration of gastric contents, contaminated respiratory care equipment, fiberoptic bronchoscopes, tracheal suctioning catheters, nebulizers, the hematogenous route, and direct dissemination from contiguous sites such as the pleura, the pericardium, or the abdomen.

Oropharyngeal and tracheal colonization play a central role in the pathogenesis of VAP. Colonization within the first 24 hours of MV has been described in patients who are intubated and in those with MV, varying from 80% to 89% (11). One study demonstrated that 45% of 213 patients admitted to a medical ICU became colonized with aerobic gram-negative bacilli after one week. Among the 95 colonized patients, 23% developed NP while only four out of the 118 non-colonized patients developed pneumonia. Among the microorganisms colonizing trachea, *Pseudomonas* spp. has an increased affinity to ciliated tracheal epithelial cells, and these microorganisms are not usually present in the oropharynx. Adherence of *Pseudomonas* increases in desquamated epithelium following influenza virus infection, tracheostomy, or repeated tracheal suctions in intubated patients. In a study including 86 patients receiving MV, oropharyngeal colonization—which was detected either on admission or from subsequent samples—was a predominant factor of NP compared with gastric colonization. Oropharyngeal colonization with *Acinetobacter baumannii* yielded an estimated 7.45-fold increased risk of pneumonia compared with patients who had not yet, or who were not identically colonized ($p = 0.0004$). DNA genomic analysis demonstrated that an identical strain was isolated from oropharyngeal or gastric samples and bronchial samples in all but three cases of pneumonia due to *S. aureus* (12).

IV. Risk Factors

There is a great deal of data concerning risk factors for VAP. These factors are important since they may contribute to the development of effective prevention programs by indicating which patients may be most likely to benefit from prophylaxis against pneumonia. We herewith discuss the most relevant risk factors for endogenous infection in VAP, although data on many of these factors continue to be controversial. These risk factors are listed in Table 1.

A. Antimicrobial Agents

The distribution of microorganisms, especially potentially resistant bacteria, differs with prior antibiotic therapy. Likewise, previous antibiotic administration may influence the development of VAP in two different ways: its use may be associated with a protective effect against early-onset pneumonia, or it may be associated with an increased risk of late-onset

Table 1 Risk Factors for Nosocomial Pneumonia

Reintubation	Supine position
Decrease in pressure of the tracheal tube cuff	Coma and head trauma
Stress-ulcers prophylaxys (anti-H_2)	Nasogastric tube and gastric distension
Tracheostomy	Patient transport

pneumonia. To determine the baseline and time-dependent risk factors for VAP, Cook et al. evaluated 1014 patients. On multivariate analysis independent predictors of VAP were a primary diagnosis on admission of burns [relative risk (RR) 5.09], trauma (RR 5.00), central nervous system disease (RR 3.40), respiratory disease, cardiac disease (RR 2.72), MV within the previous 24 hours (RR 2.28), witnessed aspiration (RR 3.25), and paralytic agents. Exposure to antibiotics conferred protection (risk ratio 0.37), but this effect attenuated over time. Rello et al. evaluated the risk factors for VAP within the first eight days of MV in 83 consecutive intubated patients undergoing continuous aspiration of subglottic secretions (CASS). Multivariate analysis showed the protective effect of antibiotic use (RR 0.10) whereas failure of the CASS technique (RR 5.29) was associated with a greater risk of pneumonia. In addition, Sirvent et al. (13) evaluated the use of systemic prophylaxis with Cefuroxime before intubation on the incidence of VAP in 100 patients with coma, 50 of whom received one dose of 1.5 g of cefuroxime intravenously at the time of intubation and a second dose 12 hours later. The global incidence of early-onset VAP was 37% ($n = 37$): 12 (24%) in the cefuroxime groups and 25 (50%) in the control group ($p = 0.007$). All these studies demonstrate the protective effect of antibiotic therapy in early VAP caused by endogenous flora. In a prospective study in 277 patients with MV, Kollef et al. (8) determined the following four factors to be associated with VAP: index of systemic organ failure ≥ 3 [odds ratio (OR) 10.2], age ≥ 60 years (OR 5.1), previous antibiotics (OR 3.1), and supine head position within the first 24 hours of MV (OR 2.9). In addition to the importance of antibiotic therapy as a risk factor for VAP, the influence of antibiotics on the etiology of this disease is also relevant. In a prospective study, Rello et al. (14) studied 129 consecutive episodes of VAP to evaluate the influence of prior antibiotic administration on the etiology and mortality of VAP. The rate of VAP caused by gram-positive cocci or *Haemophilus influenzae* was statistically lower ($p < 0.05$) in patients who had received antibiotics previously, while the rate of VAP caused by *P. aeruginosa* was statistically higher ($p < 0.01$). Step-forward logistic regression analysis only determined previous antibiotic use (OR 9.2) to significantly influence the risk of death in VAP. Likewise, Trouillet et al. (15) demonstrated that three variables remained significantly associated with potentially resistant microorganisms as a causative etiology in VAP: duration of MV for7 days or more (OR 6.0), prior antibiotic use (OR 13.5), and prior use of broad-spectrum drugs (third-generation cephalosporin, fluoroquinolones, and/or imipenem) (OR 4.1). All of these studies have demonstrated that antimicrobial therapy has a bimodal effect on the development of VAP. Antibiotics protect against early-onset pneumonia, especially pneumonia caused by endogenous flora, but they are also responsible for the selection of resistant microorganisms causing late-onset pneumonia such as *P. aeruginosa* and methicillin-resistant *S. aureus* (MRSA).

B. Body Position

It has been demonstrated that up to 50% of healthy adults aspirate at night. However, in these subjects it is not clinically significant since lung defense mechanisms remain intact. Torres and coworkers demonstrated the importance of body position in gastroesophageal reflux and tracheal aspiration. These authors instilled a colloid with technetium via nasogastric tube, and by placing patients in a semi-recumbent position they found a significant reduction in the radioactivity of tracheal secretions compared with patients in the supine position. Moreover, in another randomized study (16) this group studied the impact of body position on the development of VAP. Patients were placed in a semirecumbent (45°) or supine (0°) body position. Microbiologically-confirmed pneumonia developed in 5% of the patients in the semi-recumbent position and in 23% of those in the supine ($p = 0.018$).

C. Gastric Colonization and Stress-Ulcer Prophylaxis

Low gastric pH prevents against bacterial growth in the gastric chamber and bacterial migration from the small bowel. The relationship between gastric pH and gastric colonization has been well established in several studies. The use of prophylactic agents for stress-ulcer which alter the gastric pH may increase gastric colonization and the rates of VAP, although this remains to be demonstrated. In a 1991 meta-analysis, Tryba found (17) that antacids and H_2-antagonists were significantly more effective in preventing stress bleeding in treated versus untreated patients. Sucralfate was superior to H_2-antagonists. Patients treated with antacids or H_2-antagonists showed a significantly higher risk for the development of NP. In a latter study, Cook et al. demonstrated a trend toward lower clinically important bleeding with H_2-antagonists and antacids than sucralfate. They found a trend toward an increased risk of pneumonia associated with H_2-antagonists compared with no prophylaxis and a significantly higher risk compared with sucralfate. Finally, another meta-analysis (18) concluded that ranitidine is not effective in the prevention of gastrointestinal bleeding and may increase the risk of pneumonia. Studies on sucralfate do not provide conclusive results. Currently, there are not enough data so as to give a concluding recommendation.

V. Diagnosis

The first problem in the diagnosis of NP and VAP is the lack of a gold standard for comparing the different techniques used to confirm the diagnosis. Despite the use of histology from pulmonary biopsy and cultures of pulmonary tissue in the immediate postmortem period, the most accurate techniques remain unclear. Suspicion of NP depends on the finding of new and persistent infiltrates on chest X ray in association with some clinical signs and symptoms (fever or hypothermia, purulent respiratory secretions, and leukocytosis or leukopenia). Based on histology and microbiological cultures of postmortem pulmonary biopsies, one study demonstrated that the presence of radiological findings plus two or more clinical criteria showed a sensitivity and specificity of 69% and 75%, respectively (19).

In recent years, the clinical pulmonary infection score (CPIS), validated by Pugin and coworkers, has been widely used. This score combines different clinical, radiological, physiological, laboratory, and microbiological parameters (Table 2) in order to increase the specificity of the clinical diagnostic approach. A score >6 demonstrates a good correlation with the presence of pneumonia. The results of different studies on the diagnostic performance of this score are contradictory with values of sensitivity and specificity of around 77% and 42%, respectively (19). Some studies have been aimed at increasing the diagnostic yield of this score with the addition of gram staining of secretions of the lower respiratory tract (20).

The diagnostic tests performed on suspicion of VAP have two objectives. The first is to determine whether the patient really has an infectious pulmonary process as indicated by the signs and symptoms leading to the use of these tests. The second is the isolation of the causative microorganisms of the disease.

Table 2 The Clinical Pulmonary Infection Score

Criterion	0	1	2
Tracheal secretions	Absent	Nonpurulent	Purulent
Pulmonary radiology	No	Diffuse	Localized
Temperature (°C)	≥ 36.5 and ≤ 38.4	≥ 38.5 or ≤ 38.9	≥ 39 or ≤ 36
Blood leukocytes	$\geq 4000 \leq 11000$	<4000 or >11000	= + bands >500%
Pao_2/Fio_2	>240 or ARDS		≤ 240 no ARDS
Microbiology[a]	Negative		Positive

[a]Cultures delay evaluation at least 24 hours.
Abbreviations: Pao_2, oxygen arterial pressure; Fio_2, inspired fraction of oxygen; ARDS, acute respiratory distress syndrome.

For many years the diagnostic performance of the different techniques used to confirm suspicion of VAP has been under debate. At present, the profitability of noninvasive tests such as tracheobronchial aspirate (TBAS), and invasive bronchoscopic tests such as bronchoalveolar lavage (BAL), and the protected specimen brush (PSB) as well as the advantages and disadvantages of each has been well established (21). As a general rule, the TBAS has a very good sensitivity with a specificity a little lower than the invasive tests when using a quantitative culture of the respiratory secretions obtained by this method (22). In different studies, the sensitivity of this test varies from 38% to 100% with a specificity of 14% to 100% (23). A negative TBAS culture in a patient who has not received antibiotic treatment has a high negative predictive value for the presence of VAP. In one study on the diagnostic value of this technique, the negative predictive value was 72% in 102 patients evaluated with this technique and with invasive methods. The sensitivity of PSB and BAL are 33–100% and 42–93%, respectively; and the specificity is 50–100% and 45–100% (6). On the other hand, the current controversy lies in the role invasive and noninvasive methods have in the prognosis and use of antibiotics in these patients.

On analyzing only the randomized studies, we found that in a pilot study with 51 patients, Sánchez-Nieto and coworkers observed that bronchoscopic methods led to a greater change in initial antibiotic treatment (42% vs. 16%, $p < 0.05$) with no significant differences as regards to either global or attributable mortality or morbidity. This study was limited by its small sample size and the lack of a standard treatment protocol in the invasive group. The study by Solè Violan and coworkers demonstrated a greater number of antibiotic changes with invasive techniques with no clear influence on mortality, length of ICU stay, and number of days on MV. Ruiz and coworkers (24) compared 76 patients with suspicion of VAP (39 noninvasive and 37 invasive) and concluded that the diagnostic performance of both techniques in VAP is similar, as was mortality at 30 days, number of days on MV, and length of ICU stay. The costs of invasive studies were clearly greater. One study by Fagon and coworkers (25) reported positive results with respect to a decrease in mortality on day 14 with the Sequential Organ Failure Assessment (SOFA) score on days 3 and 7, a reduction in the use of antibiotics, and the number of antibiotic-free days with the invasive technique. Nonetheless, the study was limited by the use of qualitative cultures of the tracheal aspirates which thereby limited comparison with the remaining studies.

In summary, we suggest the following diagnostic and management approach of NP (Fig. 1). First, clinical suspicion of pneumonia should be based on classical clinical criteria or a CPIS >6. Respiratory secretions should be collected at this time by TBAS or bronchoscopy for obtaining quantitative cultures. Reevaluation should be made at 48 to 72 hours and the decision as to whether to continue antimicrobial treatment should be based on the probability of pneumonia, the results of the cultures, and the presence of an alternative diagnosis (26).

VI. Treatment

When deciding to treat a suspected episode of ICU-acquired pneumonia, several aspects should be taken into account. The importance of early initiation of an adequate antimicrobial therapy for the treatment of VAP has been emphasized in recent years in several studies. Alvarez-Lerma evaluated 430 patients with VAP and found a higher attributable mortality (24.7% vs. 16.3%, $p = 0.039$) and a higher incidence of septic shock and gastrointestinal bleeding among patients receiving inadequate initial treatment. Similar results were also reported by Luna and coworkers and Rello and cols. With mini-BAL fluid cultures, Kollef and Ward reported that inappropriate antibiotic therapy was associated with an OR for death of 3.28.

Empirical antimicrobial therapy may be inadequate as a consequence of the presence of unexpected pathogens not covered by the initial antibiotic schedule, but this may be mainly due to unanticipated resistance. In most of the previously mentioned studies, a large proportion of the episodes of inadequate antimicrobial treatment were attributed to potentially resistant gram-negative bacteria (especially *P. aeruginosa, Acinetobacter* spp., and *Enterobacter* spp.) or MRSA.

Another important aspect to be taken into account is whether modification of the initial therapy based on microbiological results improves the outcome of the patient. Studies addressing this issue did not find any improvement in mortality with this strategy. Luna and coworkers showed that therapeutic changes made after bronchoscopy led to more patients ($n = 42$) receiving adequate therapy. Nonetheless, the mortality in this group was comparable to the mortality reported among patients who continued to receive inadequate therapy ($n = 23$). In the study by Rello and coworkers, bronchoscopic results led to a change in antibiotic treatment in 27 cases (24%) considered to receive inadequate initial treatment. Despite clinical resolution in 17 of these cases (63%), the mortality was higher compared with patients with initial adequate therapy. Kollef and Ward found a high prevalence (73%) of inadequate initial antibiotic therapy in a study of 130 patients with VAP. In this study the mortality of patients in whom the antibiotic therapy had been started or changed based on the results of mini-BAL culture was significantly higher compared with patients with unchanged or discontinued treatment (60.8% vs. 33.3% and 14.3%, respectively).

The results of these studies demonstrate the need for early initiation of broad-spectrum empirical antimicrobial therapy on suspicion of VAP. The American Thoracic Society (ATS) published its first guidelines for the management of hospital-acquired pneumonia in 1995. In 1998, Trouillet et al. (15) suggested a different classification for the prediction of pathogens and the selection of antibiotic treatment based on the use or not of previous antibiotic use and the duration of MV. These classifications provide different rationale for the prediction of

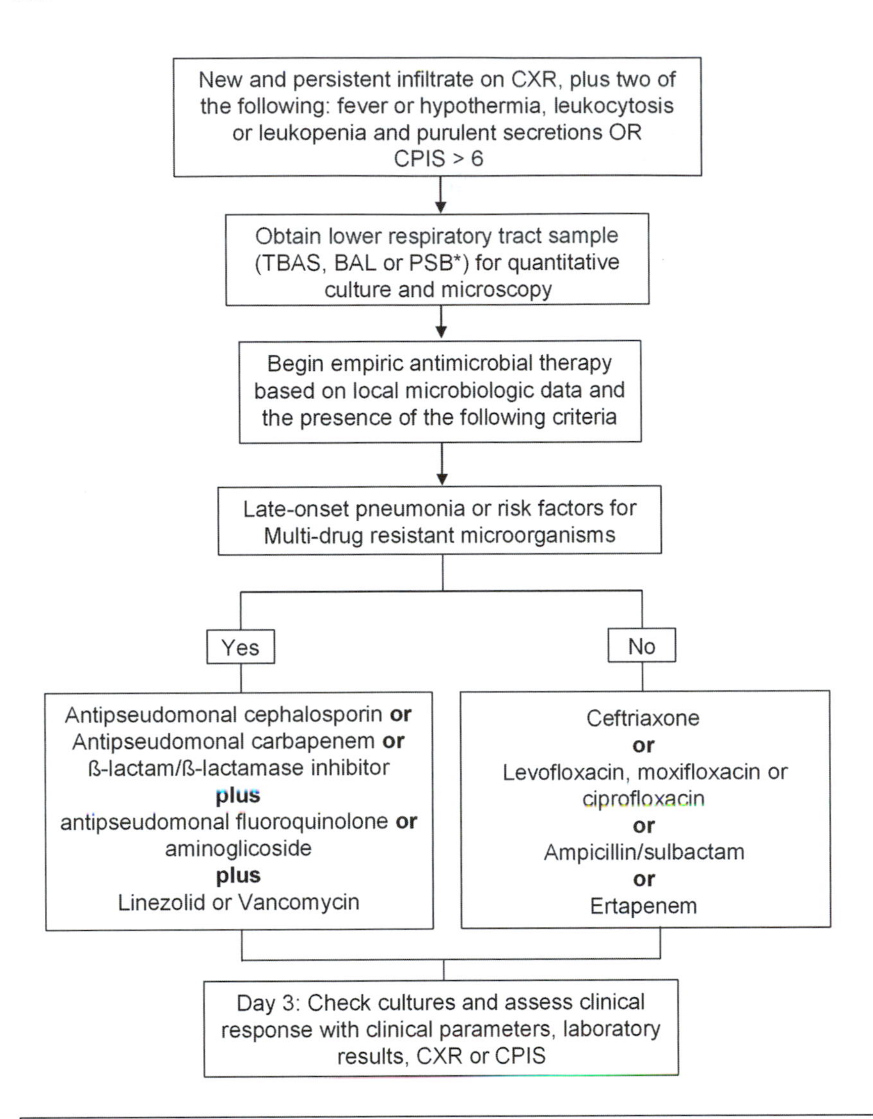

Figure 1 Algorithm for the management of patients with nosocomial pneumonia. *Abbreviations*: CXR, chest X ray; CPIS, clinical pulmonary infection score; TBAS, tracheobronchial aspirate; BAL, bronchoalveolar lavage; PSB, protected specimen brush; PaO_2, oxygen arterial pressure; FiO_2, inspired fraction of oxygen; MODS, multiple organ dysfunction syndrome.

microbial etiology with the aim of aiding clinicians in prescribing the appropriate initial empirical therapy.

In a prospective study, we recently evaluated the level of bacterial coverage and validated the adequacy of the antibiotic strategy proposed by the 1996 ATS guidelines and the Trouillet framework (27). Both classifications were found to be effective in predicting the pathogen involved (91% and 83%, respectively). However, taking the in vitro sensitivity of the pathogens isolated into account, the adequacy of the antibiotic treatment proposed by these classifications was found to be rather low (79% for ATS and 80% for Trouillet). The microorganisms involved in treatment inadequacy were multiresistant *P. aeruginosa, A. baumannii, S. maltophilia*, and MRSA. These findings underline the importance of considering additional parameters such as local microbial epidemiology and more accurate models of prediction of resistance to improve the level of coverage and the appropriateness of antibiotic treatment.

The ATS recently published the new guidelines for the management of adults with hospital-acquired pneumonia (28) and, contrary to the previous guidelines, the severity of pneumonia does not play an important role in the decision making as to the initial empirical treatment to be implemented (Fig. 1). Regardless of the severity of pneumonia, patients with risk factors for infection with multidrug resistant microorganisms or with hospital admission greater than five days should receive empirical broad-spectrum antibiotic therapy that adequately covers infection by *P. aeruginosa* (Table 3). The different schedules recommended for this group include: a cefalosporin with antipseudomonal activity, a carbapenem or piperacillin/tazobactam associated with an aminoglycoside, or a fluoroquinolone with antipseudomonal activity. Linezolide or vancomycin should be associated in cases with suspicion of MRSA infection or hospitals with a high rate of incidence. Patients who do not fulfill the previously mentioned characteristics should receive empirical treatment with schedules that cover the "core" microorganisms such as *S. pneumoniae, H. influenzae*, methicillin-sensitive *S. aureus*, and antibiotic-sensitive aerobic gram-negative bacilli. The drugs of choice include: ceftriaxone or a fluoroquinolone or β-lactam/β-lactamase inhibitor or ertapenem (28).

To date, the use of combined antibiotic therapy is still recommended in the treatment of VAP on suspicion of *P. aeruginosa* or other potentially resistant pathogens. Previous

Table 3 Etiologic Pathogens Likely to Cause Nosocomial Pneumonia

Patients with no risk factors for MDR pathogens, early onset, and any severity.	Patients with late-onset pneumonia or risk factors for MDR pathogens and any severity
Streptococcus pneumoniae	The same as the previous group plus
Haemophilus influenzae	
MSSA	
Enteric gram-negative bacilli	
Escherichia coli	*Pseudomonas aeruginosa*
Klebsiella pneumoniae	*Klebsiella pneumoniae* (ESBL)
Enterobacter spp.	*Acinetobacter* spp.
Proteus spp.	MRSA
Serratia marcescens	*Legionella pneumophila*

Abbreviations: MDR, multidrug resistant; ESBL, extended spectrum β-lactamases; MSSA, methicillin-sensitive *Staphylococcus aureus*; MRSA, methicillin-resistant *Staphylococcus aureus*.

studies on bacteremic infections caused by *P. aeruginosa* and *Klebsiella* spp. demonstrated a higher mortality associated with the use of initial empirical monotherapy compared with combined therapy. However, these studies are limited in that they were performed when less active β-lactams were used. Further trials are needed to clarify this issue. For now, the use of monotherapy should be limited to the treatment of severe NP in patients without risk factors for potentially resistant pathogens.

The length of antimicrobial treatment is also under debate. In the ATS guidelines the experts recommend that the length of treatment be shortened from the traditional 14 to 21 days to shorter periods, from seven to 10 days. The latter shorter treatment is recommended in the treatment of *S. aureus* and *H. influenzae* pneumonia. However, in specific situations such as multilobar involvement, malnutrition, cavitation, gram-negative necrotizing pneumonia, and/or isolation of *P. aeruginosa* or *Acinetobacter* spp. 14- to 21-day therapy should be initiated. Nonetheless, recent evidence has suggested that short treatment is as effective as longer treatment in VAP. Chastre and coworkers (29) evaluated 401 patients with VAP, 197 were randomized to receive short (eight-day) treatment and 204 a long (15-day) course of antibiotic treatment. No differences were observed in the mortality rate (18.8% vs.17.2%) or in the recurrence of pulmonary infection (28.9% vs. 26%) on comparing the two groups of patients. However, those treated with a short course of antibiotics had significantly more antibiotic-free days (13 ± 7.4 vs. 8.7 ± 5.2 days, $p < 0.001$). The possibility of providing adequate treatment with shorter courses of antibiotics will not only reduce health care costs but will also have favorable consequences on microbial ecology by reducing the selection pressure for resistance.

VII. Conclusion

NP is the leading cause of death among hospital-acquired infections. Its incidence ranges from 4 to 50 cases per 1000 admissions in community hospitals and general medical wards. Aspiration of colonized pharyngeal secretions is considered the most important pathogenic mechanism of NP. Risk factors to develop NP include previous use of antibiotics, supine body position, prophylaxis of stress-ulcer, and duration of hospital admission. Diagnostic approaches should start with the criteria of clinical suspicion based on the above and followed by quantitative cultures of respiratory secretions obtained through TBAS or bronchoscopic samples. The initial empirical antimicrobial therapy is based on the previous duration of hospital admission and the presence of risks factor for multidrug resistant microorganisms.

References

1. Langer M, Cigada M, Mandelli M, et al. Early-onset pneumonia: a multicenter study in intensive care units. Intensive Care Med 1987; 13:342–346.
2. Vincent JL, Bihari DJ, Suter PM, et al. The prevalence of nosocomial infection in intensive care units in Europe. Results of the European Prevalence of Infection in Intensive Care (EPIC) Study. JAMA 1995; 274(8):639–644.
3. Prod'hom G, Leuenberger P, Koerfer J, et al. Nosocomial pneumonia in mechanically ventilated patients receiving antacid, ranitidine, or sucralfate as prophylaxis for stress ulcer. Ann Intern Med 1994; 120:653–662.

4. Torres A, Aznar R, Gatell JM, et al. Incidence, risk, and prognosis factors of nosocomial pneumonia in mechanically ventilated patients. Am Rev Respir Dis 1990; 142:523–528.
5. Sopena N, Sabriá M, and the Neumos Study Group. Multicenter study of hospital-acquired pneumonia in non-ICU patients. Chest 2005; 127:213–219.
6. Fagon JY, Chastre J, Domart Y, et al. Nosocomial pneumonia in patients receiving continuous mechanical ventilation. Prospective analysis of 52 episodes with use of a protected specimen brush and quantitative culture techniques. Am Rev Respir Dis 1989; 139:877–884.
7. Craven DE, Kunches LM, Kilinsky V, et al. Risk factors for pneumonia and fatality in patients receiving mechanical ventilation. Am Rev Respir Dis 1986; 133:792–796.
8. Kollef MH. Ventilator-associated pneumonia: a multivariate analysis. JAMA 1993; 270: 1965–1970.
9. Lossos IS, Breuer R, Or R, et al. Bacterial pneumonia in recipients of bone marrow transplantation. A five-year prospective study. Transplantation 1995; 60:672–678.
10. Antonelli M, Moro ML, Capelli O, et al. Risk factors for early-onset pneumonia in trauma patients. Chest 1994; 105:224–228.
11. Cardeñosa Cendrero JA, Sole-Violan J, Bordes Benitez A, et al. Role of different routes of tracheal colonization in the development of pneumonia in patients receiving mechanical ventilation. Chest 1999; 116:462–470.
12. Garrouste-Orgeas M, Chevret S, Arlet G, et al. Oropharyngeal or gastric colonization and nosocomial pneumonia in adult intensive care unit patients. A prospective study based on genomic DNA analysis. Am J Respir Crit Care Med 1997; 156:1647–1655.
13. Sirvent JM, Torres A, El-Ebiary M, et al. Protective effect of intravenously administered cefuroxime against nosocomial pneumonia in patients with structural coma. Am J Respir Crit Care Med 1997; 155(5):1729–1734.
14. Rello J, Ausina V, Ricart M, et al. Impact of previous antimicrobial therapy on the etiology and outcome of ventilator-associated pneumonia. Chest 1993; 104:1230–1235.
15. Trouillet JL, Chastre J, Vuagnat A, et al. Ventilator-associated pneumonia caused by potentially drug-resistant bacteria. Am Rev Respir Dis 1998; 157(2):531–539.
16. Drakulovic MB, Torres A, Bauer TT, et al. Supine body position as a risk factor for nosocomial pneumonia in mechanically ventilated patients: a randomised trial. Lancet 1999; 354 (9193):1851–1858.
17. Tryba M. Risk of acute stress bleeding and nosocomial pneumonia in ventilated intensive care patients: sucralfate versus antacids. Am J Med 1987; 83:117–124.
18. Messori A, Tripoli S, Vaiani M, et al. Bleeding and pneumonia in intensive care patients given ranitidine and sucralfate for prevention of stress ulcer: meta-analysis of randomised controlled trials. BMJ 2003; 32:1103–1106.
19. Fabregas N, Ewig S, Torres A, et al. Clinical diagnosis of ventilator associated pneumonia revisited: comparative validation using immediate post-mortem lung biopsies. Thorax 1999; 54:867–873.
20. Fartoukh M, Maitre B, Honore S, et al. Diagnosing pneumonia during mechanical ventilation: the clinical pulmonary infection score revisited. Am J Respir Crit Care Med 2003; 168:173–179.
21. Ioanas M, Ferrer M, Angrill J, et al. Microbial investigation on vetilator-associated pneumonia. Eur Respir J 2001; 17:791–801.
22. Valencia M, Torres A, Insausti J, et al. Valor diagnòstico del cultivo cuantitativo del aspirado endotraqueal en la neumonía adquirida durante la ventilaciòn mecánica. Estudio multicèntrico. Arch Bronconeumol 2003; 39:394–399.
23. Torres A, Puig de la Bellacasa J, Xaubet A, et al. Diagnostic value of quantitative cultures of bronchoalveolar lavage and telescoping plugged catheters in mechanically ventilated patients with bacterial pneumonia. Am Rev Respir Dis 1989; 140:306–310.
24. Ruiz M, Torres A, Ewig S, et al. Noninvasive versus invasive microbial investigation in ventilator-associated pneumonia. Am J Respir Crit Care Med 2000; 162:119–125.

25. Fagon JY, Chastre J, Wolff M, et al. Invasive and noninvasive strategies for management of suspected ventilator-associated pneumonia. Ann Intern Med 2000; 132:621–630.
26. Torres A, Ewig S. Diagnosing ventilator-associated pneumonia. N Engl J Med 2004; 350:433–435.
27. Ioanas M, Cavalcanti M, Ferrer M, et al. Hospital-acquired pneumonia: coverage and treatment adequacy of current guidelines. Eur Respir J 2003; 22:876–882.
28. Niederman M, Craven D. Guidelines for the management of adults with hospital-acquired pneumonia, ventilator-associated pneumonia, and healthcare-associated pneumonia. Am J Respir Crit Care Med 2005; 171:388–416.
29. Chastre J, Wolff M, Fagon JY, et al. Comparison of 8 vs 15 days of antibiotic therapy for ventilator-associated pneumonia in adults: a randomized trial. JAMA 2003; 290:2588–2598.

31
Nutrition in ICU

ENRICO M. CLINI and LUDOVICO TRIANNI
University of Modena, Modena, and Ospedale Villa Pineta, Pavullo (MO), Italy

NICOLINO AMBROSINO
Pulmonary and Respiratory Intensive Care Unit-University Hospital Pisa, Italy and Pulmonary Rehabilitation and Weaning Center, Auxilium Vitae, Volterra (PI), Italy

I. Introduction

Malnutrition is a common problem among hospitalized patients and illness is frequently associated with a negative energy balance, resulting in a further deterioration in the nutritional status. One survey of admissions to a general hospital reported a prevalence of malnutrition ranging from 27% to 46% across diagnostic categories (1).

Nutritional depletion is especially common in patients with chronic obstructive pulmonary disease (COPD), when a combination of low-energy intake and high-energy requirements (2) leads to muscle wasting and dysfunction (3). Compromised nutrition has been associated with a poor prognosis in stable COPD patients, with and without respiratory failure (4–6). In a study by Sivasothy (7), chronically ventilated hypercapnic, COPD patients with a body mass index (BMI) <20 had poor survival. In a study of nutritional status in 744 patients receiving long-term respiratory treatments such as supplemental oxygen or mechanical ventilation (8), the authors noted that fat-free mass (FFM), BMI < 20, and low serum albumin were the most sensitive parameters of malnutrition. A BMI < 25 has been associated with more severe respiratory disease (9).

Therefore, nutritional assessment and management is an important therapeutic option among patients with chronic respiratory diseases (10), especially those requiring prolonged mechanical ventilation (PMV) in ICU (11). Table 1 emphasizes the effects of malnutrition on the respiratory function in patients in ICU. However, specific nutritional deficiencies such as hypophosphatemia (12) have been associated with respiratory failure and impaired lipid synthesis (13) and may cause an abnormal increase in the fat mass.

II. Approaching the Malnourished Patient

Nutritional assessment that involves screening and therapy is an essential component of pulmonary rehabilitation in COPD patients, in whom weight loss, muscle wasting, and altered muscle metabolism are typical findings that are observed as the disease progresses (14). The association between low body weight and increased mortality has been well documented in several retrospective studies (15–17). Therefore, it is essential to address

Table 1 Adverse Effects of Malnutrition on Respiratory Functions

Altered ventilatory drive
Reduction in the ventilatory response to hypoxia
Decreased mass, force, contractility, and endurance of the diaphragm
Decreased respiratory muscle strength
Hypercapnia
Reduced synthesis of alveolar surfactant
Altered humoral and cellular immunity
Increased bacterial adhesion in the lower respiratory tract

Source: From Ref. 8.

nutritional status among ICU patients. Malnutrition is defined as an unintentional weight loss >10% and serum albumin level <3.2 g/dL. It has been noted that up to 50% of hospitalized patients are malnourished (18–20). Hospital malnutrition can contribute to high rates of infection, impaired wound healing, less than optimal surgical outcome, postoperative complications, longer hospital stays, and a higher risk of death.

III. Assessment

This process includes dietary, anthropometric, and biochemical aspects. Nutritional assessment begins with a detailed nutritional history that includes clinical, dietary, socioeconomic, and family issues. Areas of interest include present and past illnesses, family illness history, food allergies or intolerance, medications, nutritional supplements, over-the-counter medications, alcohol use, work environment, and education level. A useful standardized protocol is the Prognostic Nutritional Index (PNI), which incorporates serum albumin, serum transferrin, delayed skin hypersensitivity, and triceps skinfold thickness (20,21). The PNI has been shown to correlate with postoperative complications and mortality (22). Whole body functional assessment by examining overall activity, exercise tolerance, grip strength, respiratory function, wound healing, and plasma albumin concentration can also be useful.

Anthropometric measures of body composition are based on the measurement of two compartments of the body: fat and fat-free mass (water, protein, minerals of the skeletal and nonskeletal muscle, soft lean tissues, skeleton). The proportion of fat varies and in women comprises a higher percentage of total body weight (averaging 27%) than in men (averaging 15%). Body fat is commonly assessed by skinfold thickness, an estimated measure of subcutaneous fat. This measure is taken with an instrument called caliper that squeezes the skinfold with a pressure of 10 g/mm^2 and an area of 20 to 40 g/mm^2. Experts often recommend measuring skinfolds from the triceps, subscapular, suprailiac, and abdomen. The waist-to-hip circumference ratio is a measure of the distribution of subcutaneous and intra-abdominal fat. The ratio tends to increase with age and excess weight. Mid-upper-arm circumference is indicative of muscle mass and subcutaneous fat. Changes in arm circumference are relatively easy to detect. The measure is taken using a flexible tape at the midpoint of the upper arm between the acromion process and the tip of the olecranon process. The measure of the mid-upper-arm muscle circumference is a measure used to assess protein-energy malnutrition. Mid-upper-arm muscle area is a two-dimensional measure of muscle mass and provides more accurate information.

Laboratory measures of albumin, transferrin, and prealbumin are sensitive and cost-effective methods of assessing malnutrition in patients who are critically ill or have a chronic disease. Prealbumin levels are accurate predictors of patient recovery (23,24).

Although body fat can be assessed by hydrostatic weighing, this measure would be quite impractical for patients requiring PMV. However, isotope dilution allows the estimation of body fat from the proportion of water in the fat-free mass. A dose of isotope such as deuterium or tritium labeled water is administered and the concentration of isotope in the body is measured after equilibrium. Malnourished individuals have more water per unit of fat-free mass. Dual-energy X-ray absorptiometry (DEXA) is a popular technique to measure bone density in which X rays are used to measure the composition of bone and soft tissue. DEXA provides measurements of bone mineral, fat mass, lean soft tissue mass, and percentage of body fat. Finally, the bioelectrical impedance is a simple-to-apply method based on the electrical conductivity of fat and fat-free mass. The impedance instrument measures the impedance of an electrical current passed through the body when electrodes are placed on the wrist and ankle. This method allows for the calculation of body volume. Combining this measurement with body weight, a patient's density and percentage of body fat can be determined.

The energy expenditure (EE) is the amount of energy used, i.e., required for health, growth, and a level of activity. EE can be calculated either with an equation or by direct measurement. The basal metabolic rate (BMR) is measured in calories and is primarily accounted for by the activity of the brain, heart, liver, and kidneys. The Harris-Benedict equations (following below) are commonly used for calculation of the BMR in adults.

$$\text{BMR for men (kcal)} = 66 + 13.7(\text{weight in kg}) + 5(\text{height in cm}) - 6.8(\text{age in years})$$
$$\text{BMR for women (kcal)} = 655 + 9.6(\text{weight in kg}) + 1.85(\text{height in cm}) - 4.7(\text{age in years})$$

EE can be measured by direct calorimetry (heat production of an individual, in calories, when placed in an insulated chamber where the heat is transferred to the surrounding water) or indirect calorimetry (respiratory gas exchange). Additional methods include the consumption of doubly labeled water as a marker of heat production and heart rate monitoring, as there is a close relationship between heart rate and oxygen consumption during activity.

IV. Screening

Nutritional screening will identify patients with chronic respiratory conditions who may be malnourished, or may be at a higher risk of malnutrition. The screening process is relatively simple and is summarized in Table 2. Nutritional screening may be especially important among respiratory failure patients in environments where they receive PMV.

V. Intervention Strategy

Treatment of weight loss may be achieved by increasing the dietary intake or preventing weight loss by means of protein synthesis stimulation. Muscle wasting results from an impaired balance between protein synthesis (anabolism) and protein breakdown (catabolism). However, other factors such as physical inactivity, typical of ICU patients, alterations

Table 2 Assessment for Nutritional Screening

Evaluation of food, nutrient, and fluid intake
Measurement of height (annually, in those aged 65 years and older)
Calculation of BMI at each office visit
Assessment of handgrip strength
Evaluation of exercise tolerance
Evaluation of basic and instrumental activities of daily living
Evaluation of serum albumin
Periodic spirometry testing
Evaluation of current medications use and dietary supplements
Assessment of immunization status

Abbreviation: BMI, body mass index.

in the neuroendocrine responses, and systemic inflammation contribute to a negative protein balance.

Overall, nutrition therapy is a component of medical treatment that includes oral, enteral, and parenteral nutrition (PN). However, a meta-analysis provided no evidence that nutritional support has a significant effect on anthropometric measures, lung function, or exercise capacity in patients with stable COPD (25,26). By contrast, repeated administration of ghrelin, a novel growth hormone–releasing peptide that is reduced in COPD (27), may improve body composition, muscle wasting, and functional capacity in cachectic patients with COPD, thus possibly reversing some of the systemic aspects of COPD (28).

Nutrition therapy includes oral, enteral, and PN. There are limitations to the caloric amount of supplements that can be given orally. Portion size and timing of supplements are also important (29). Ventilation is closely linked with dyspnea (30). A carbohydrate-rich energy overload (970 kcal) (31), but not a normal energy load (500 kcal) (32), may increase the carbon dioxide production. A fat-rich supplement intake, but not a carbohydrate-rich supplement, increases dyspnea (29). Leucine enhances the activity and synthesis of proteins in skeletal muscle (33).

Anabolic agents have been reported to increase muscle mass (34) in COPD, but long-term trials are needed to establish whether they have a lasting effect on protein synthesis.

Cachexia is a complex interaction between inflammatory mediators, oxidative stress and growth factors that govern skeletal muscle fiber degeneration, apoptosis, and regeneration (35). Current interest is on fatty acid modulation, since fatty acid composition of inflammatory and immune cells is sensitive to change according to the fatty acid diet intake. Fish oil (containing *n*-3-polyunsaturated fatty acids) supplementation has beneficial effects on the systemic inflammatory responses (36). The role of such supplements in the ventilated patient with chronic respiratory failure remains to be clarified.

VI. Food Intake in ICU Patients

Patients requiring PMV often have swallowing dysfunction. Although sometimes associated with neuromuscular disorders (NMD), factors such as acute illness, medications (steroids, neuromuscular blocking agents, general sedatives), prolonged inactivity of swallowing muscles, and injury from intubation or tracheostomy may all contribute to this dysfunction.

Tracheostomies limit swallowing either by compressing the oesophagus or by decreasing laryngeal elevation and anterior displacement (37). The inflated cuff anchors the strap muscles in the neck, hampering laryngeal elevation and neck rotation. This procedure results in reduced glottic closure and increased laryngeal penetration, thus increasing the chances of aspiration (38). Recent studies both in acute and chronic settings (39–41) have suggested that swallowing dysfunction and pulmonary aspiration occur in patients receiving ventilatory support through a cuffed tracheostomy tube. The actual incidence of aspiration is difficult to determine, since investigators define it with a variety of different criteria (37,39). Swallowing dysfunction may well help to avoid pulmonary related complications such as pneumonia and atelectasis (42). In a recent study (43) of patients receiving intermittent positive pressure ventilation for >15 days, bedside examination identified swallowing dysfunction in 34% of cases irrespective of the presence of underlying neuromuscular disease. In 83% of these patients, video-fluoroscopy was found to be abnormal and was frequently confirmed by direct laryngoscopy. These approaches can result in corrective actions (such as selected food, right head postures, and coached cough) to prevent respiratory complications (41).

Aspiration has been found in 16% of patients and is documented by a variety of methods, such as cough, distress after swallowing, suctioning of nutrients, or postprandial scintigrapy after 99mTc-labeled meal. On clinical assessment, 6.5% of patients negative for scintigraphy were found to have swallowing dysfunction. On the other hand, scintigraphy was positive in 6.5% of patients with a negative clinical assessment. Swallowing dysfunction was identified in 29% of patients receiving PMV. The consequence of dysphagia associated nutritional deficiencies can influence locomotion and respiratory function, especially in NMD (40).

Dysphagia for individuals with PMV is best tackled by a multidisciplinary team (neurologist, nutritionist, gastroenterologist) for prompt corrective actions such as use of higher consistency food, specific head postures, or enteral nutrition (EN) to occur. Since weight loss is associated with swallowing impairment, body weight almost invariably increases once adequate ventilatory assistance and dietary intake are provided. Noninvasive alternatives to tracheostomy are effective unless severe bulbar muscle dysfunction results in ongoing aspiration of food and saliva. If aspiration causes an arterial oxygen desaturation <95% despite assisted ventilation and secretion clearance techniques, then there is a greater risk of the development of pneumonia (44–46).

VII. Artificial Nutrition

Adequate nutritional support in the ICU is very important and guidelines for these nutritional interventions have been published (47,48). The interdisciplinary team formulates the nutritional care plan to include monitoring, the most appropriate route of administration, the method of nutritional access, the duration of therapy, and educational objectives. Figure 1 shows the algorithm for the decision to initiate specialized nutritional support. A variety of delivery routes and nutritional formulation components are available.

1. Oral feeding
2. Enteral nutrition

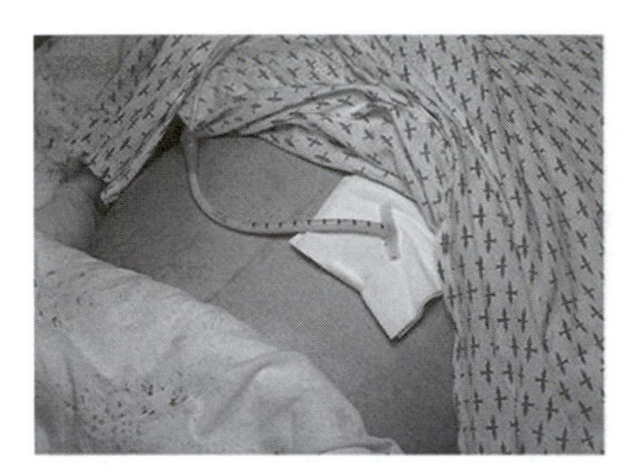
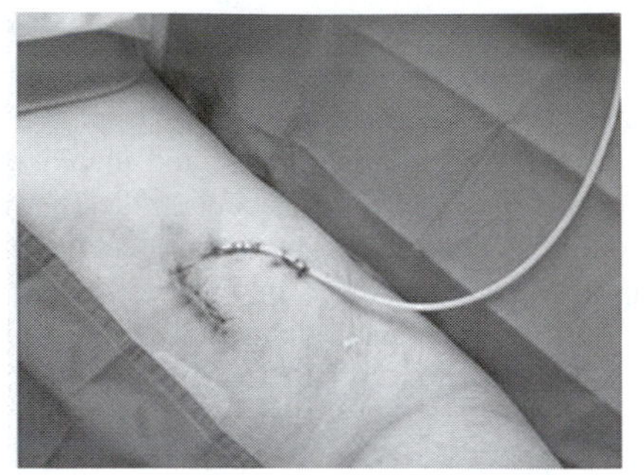

Figure 1 Algorithm for applying artificial nutrition in ICU.

- Long-term nutrition: Percutaneous endoscopic gastrostomy (PEG)
- Percutaneous endoscopic jejunostomy (PEJ)
- Short-term nutrition: nasogastric feeding (NGF)
- Nasoduodenal feeding
- Nasojejunal feeding

3. Parenteral nutrition
    - Peripheral PN (PPN)
    - Total PN (TPN)

A. Oral Feeding

Nutritional supplementation may benefit those subjects who are malnourished (BMI $<$ 18.5–20 kg/m^2 or BMI $<$ 20 kg/m^2 in surgical patients), with unintentional weight loss $>$5% within the previous three to six months, or even at risk of malnutrition (eaten very little for $>$5 days) (49).

Nutritional interventions should contain a balance of protein, energy, vitamins, and minerals. One of the goals is to correct malnutrition without increasing the respiratory quotient (50,51). A severely impaired energy balance in COPD patients during the first days of an acute exacerbation may be associated with a decreased energy and protein intake (52).

B. Enteral Nutrition

Nutritional supplements are not yet used systematically as part of comprehensive care (53). Oral supplementation during hospitalization for an acute exacerbation of chronic pulmonary disease (AECOPD) should supplement rather than replace normal dietary intake. The cost-effectiveness of nutritional supplementation among various patient groups remains to be established (54,55).

Glutamine deficiency occurs in critically ill patients, especially burn patients, as a result of increased protein turnover in the hypercatabolic state (56,57). Low levels of Glutamine on admission are associated with shock and increased hospital mortality and are more common in older persons (58). Glutamine supplementation in ICU patients was reviewed by the Italian Society of Enteral and Parenteral Nutrition (SINPE) (59), which noted that increased plasma glutamine levels were associated with improved outcomes in ICU patients. Other antioxidants such as parenteral selenium are also of interest in ICU patients (60).

These important nutrients are more easily implemented with EN than with oral feeding, although the delivery of EN is often inadequate (61). It has been recommended that EN be used in preference to PN among mechanically ventilated critically ill adult patients (62), as early use of EN has been associated with reduced ICU and hospital mortality (63) at a lower cost than PN (64). Prior to initiating EN, a detailed assessment, with subjective and objective measures, as described, should be undertaken. Most individuals require a range of 20 to 35 kcal/kg of body weight/day, with protein requirements of 1 to 1.5 g/kg of -body weight/day as well as modifications (seldom >1.5 g/kg body weight/day) to account for increased needs associated with healing wounds, and acute or chronic disease. If a patient is malnourished, then nutrient needs are greater in order to restore nutritional status. Adequacy of wound healing and improved physical strength are useful indicators of restored protein. Most "standard" 1 kcal/mL enteral formulas contain 80% water, so a patient receiving 1500 kcals will receive 1200 mL of water from the formula. Failure to account for fluid needs can lead to volume depletion and rehospitalization (65,66). Enteral formulas contain 100% of all vitamins and minerals required, if at least 1000 kcals are taken each day. Fiber containing formulas are useful in patients requiring bowel management. High calorie or calorically dense formulas provide 1.5 to 2 kcal/mL and are used for patients who have elevated calorie needs (25–35 kcal/kg) or require fluid restriction. These formulas usually contain 20–25% of the calories from protein as compared to 14–16% of calories from protein in standard formulas. Fiber can help manage diarrhea by absorbing excess water and can help manage constipation by providing bulk to the stool.

EN may be delivered to the stomach or small intestine, although EN by postpyloric feeding provides no additional advantages over gastric feeding, provided that gastric emptying is not impaired (67). Duodenal or jejunal feeding allows patients with impaired gastric emptying to be fed safely. Since the risk of aspiration is higher for patients with impaired gag reflex, altered level of consciousness, prior history of aspiration, or known gastroesophageal reflux, duodenal feedings may be preferred.

The stomach may be accessed by oro-gastric or NGF tubes and transpyloric feeding can follow the spontaneous passage of a weighted tube, endoscopic placement, or a surgical jejunostomy. Tube placement must be confirmed radiographically before feeding is initiated. Continuous gastric formula infusion is usually better tolerated than bolus methods, especially if gastric emptying is abnormal. Prokinetic agents, such as metoclopramide or cisapride, may be used to promote tube transit through the gastrointestinal tract. If four or more weeks of tube feeding are anticipated, then gastrostomy, jejunostomy, or combination gastrostomy-jejunostomy tubes should be considered.

Intermittent feeding—including a fasting period of at least eight hours—is reserved for gastric feeding. It is important to periodically check residuals depending on the bolus volume and the patient. Continuous infusion with a feeding pump will maintain a constant infusion rate, which is especially important if the distal catheter tip is in the jejunum (the area of most risk for dumping syndrome). Intermittent administration is more physiological, and transition from continuous feeds should be done over several days (68).

EN can be associated with important complications, such as nausea and vomiting (20%), gastroesophageal reflux, diarrhea (2–63%), malabsorption, aspiration (1–4%), and tube malposition. Associated causes include duodenal ulcer, pyloric channel ulcer, ileus, anticholinergic medications, opiates, central nervous system disturbances, metabolic derangements, and severe protein deficiency. Treatment with a small intestine feeding tube—nasoduodenal or jejunostomy—may overcome the problem. Medications should be in liquid form, avoiding crushed tablets. Aluminium-containing antacids or sucralfate may interact with some nutritional formulas to produce plugs or bezoars. Metabolic complications, such as hypernatremia or hyponatremia, dehydration, and hyperkalemia or hypokalemia, occur during EN, although less frequently than with PN.

Refeeding of severely malnourished patients may result in the "refeeding syndrome" in which there are acute decreases in potassium, magnesium, and phosphate, which may predispose the ventilated patient in the ICU to cardiac arrhythmias, heart failure, acute respiratory failure, coma, paralysis, nephropathy, and liver dysfunction. Refeeding syndrome occurs when the body shifts from stored body fat to carbohydrate as the primary fuel source. Serum insulin levels rise, causing intracellular movement of electrolytes for use in metabolism. Recommendations to reduce the risk of refeeding syndrome include recognizing the patient at risk (e.g., chronic condition, anorexia, prolonged hydration, alcoholism), correcting electrolyte abnormalities, administering volume and energy gradually, providing vitamin supplementation, and avoiding overfeeding.

Percutaneous Endoscopic Gastrostomy and Jejunostomy

These are measures of EN (69,70) that have gained wide acceptance and are the preferred methods (PEG in particular) for providing EN in long-term settings. The enteral tubes rest in the stomach or in the jejunum and exit through the skin of the abdomen (Fig. 2).

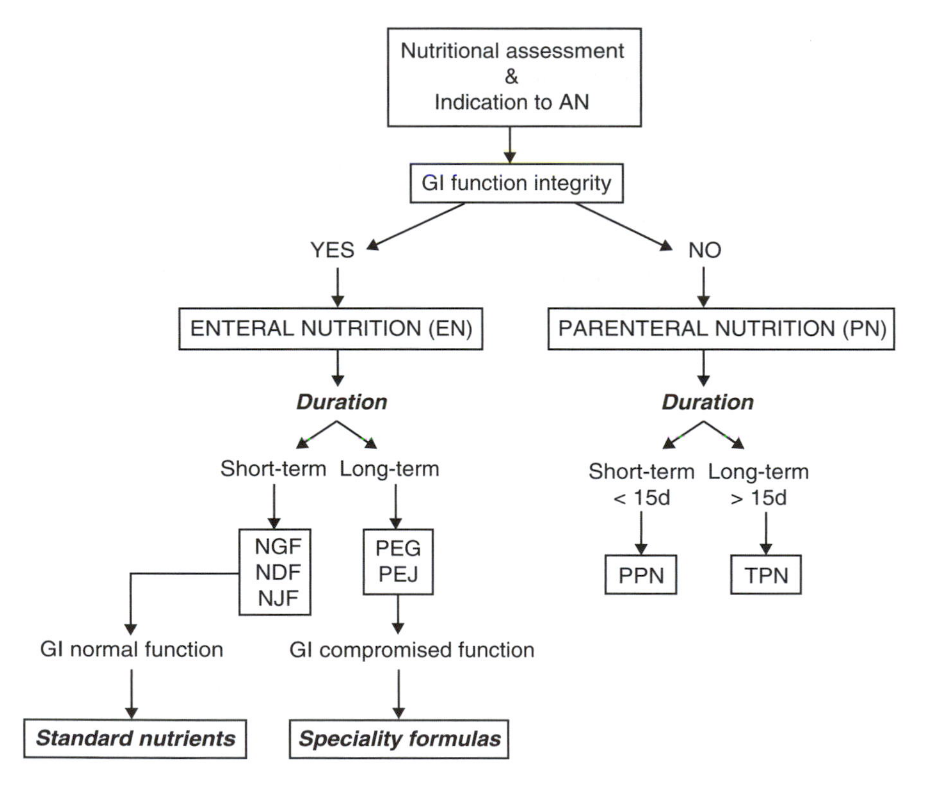

Figure 2 Percutaneous gastrostomy (*left*) and jejunostomy (*right*) tubes positioned in ICU patients.

Short-term studies have demonstrated the advantages of a PEG as compared to nasogastric tube feeding in patients with dysphagia due to NMD (71,72). PEG insertion is a quick, well-tolerated procedure with a low complication rate (73–75). It is useful in patients discharged from the ICU and can easily be removed at a later date. In patients needing PMV, a PEG is a safe and effective way of providing food, liquids, and medication. The jejunostomy tube is more frequently used to provide access in long-term situations.

C. Parenteral Nutrition

PN is the provision of nutrients intravenously for patients who cannot meet their nutritional goals by the oral or enteral routes. PN is also used for long-term nutrition support in the home setting. The principal forms of PN are total (TPN) and peripheral (PPN). In TPN, concentrated formula is delivered into a central vein. PPN has similar nutrient components as TPN, but in a lower concentration (lower osmolality) and, therefore, it may be delivered by peripheral vein. PN requires patients to be hemodynamically stable and able to tolerate fluid volume, protein, carbohydrate, and lipids included in the nutrients. Components are individualized and carefully monitored. Providing nonprotein calories as a glucose-lipid mixture has many advantages over glucose alone (76) in decreasing protein breakdown, glucose oxidation, and CO_2 production (77). Dextrose, for energy, is the mainstay of PN, and lipid emulsions are used as an energy source in a balanced nutritional regimen (78). In ventilated adult patients with acute respiratory distress syndrome, infusion of 500 mL of 10% lipid emulsion did not alter arterial oxygenation as the beneficial effect of a high cardiac output offsets the detrimental effect of increased O_2 consumption (79). Glutamine-supplemented TPN has been demonstrated to prevent and reverse intestinal atrophy associated with standard TPN use in animal models (80). It was also associated with increased nitrogen balance, fewer infections, and decreased length of stay as compared with standard amino-acid solutions (81).

Recognized complications of PN are pneumothorax, subcutaneous emphysema, arrythmias, massive hematoma during an attempt to place a central line in the subclavian vein, right atrial thrombosis, and embolism (82). Hepatic complications are seen in about 15% of patients depending on the duration and mode of application of PN (83), and metabolic bone disease may also occur (84,85).

In a systematic review, Naylor et al. (86) demonstrated that complications are reduced in patients managed by the TPN team, although it was unclear if there was a reduction in catheter-related sepsis and metabolic or electrolyte complications. Limited evidence also suggests financial benefits from the introduction of a multidisciplinary TPN team in the hospital setting (87). PN is considerably more expensive than EN (88), although accurate costing data are hard to come by. Therefore, where there are no specific data demonstrating improved outcomes with PN, EN is preferable on a cost basis (89).

VIII. Conclusions

Malnutrition is still an underestimated problem in the ICU among patients with chronic respiratory failure, and, therefore, a nutritional assessment is an important part of the management of patients requiring ventilation (90). Appropriate nutrition makes a valuable contribution to outcomes in the ICU; and whether feeding is oral, enteral, or parenteral, it should be organized to provide the best caloric and metabolic daily intake.

References

1. McWhirter JP, Pennington CR. Incidence and recognition of malnutrition in hospital. BMJ 1994; 308:945–949.
2. Debigarè R, Cote CH, Maltais F. Peripheral muscle wasting in chronic obstructive pulmonary disease. Am J Respir Crit Care Med 2001; 164:1712–1717.
3. Wouters EFM. Chronic obstructive pulmonary disease. Systemic effects of COPD. Thorax 2002; 57:1067–1070.
4. Anthonisen NR, Wright EC, Hodgkin JE. Prognosis in chronic obstructive pulmonary disease. Am Rev Respir Dis 1986; 133:14–20.
5. Jee SH, Sull JW, Park J, et al. JM body-mass index and mortality in Korean men and women. N Engl J Med 2006; 355:779–787.
6. Schols AM, Slangen J, Volovics L, et al. Weight loss is a reversible factor in the prognosis of chronic obstructive pulmonary disease. Am J Respir Crit Care Med 1998; 157;1791–1797.
7. Sivasothy P, Smith IE, Shneerson JM. Mask intermittent positive pressure ventilation in chronic hypercapnic respiratory failure due to chronic obstructive pulmonary disease. Eur Respir J 1998; 11:34–40.
8. Cano NJ, Roth H, Court-Ortune I, et al. Clinical Research Group of the Societe Francophone de Nutrition Enterale et Parenterale. On behalf of the Clinical Research Group of the SFNEP. Nutritional depletion in patients on long-term oxygen therapy and/or home mechanical ventilation. Eur Respir J 2002; 20:30–37.
9. Ambrosino N, Clini E. Long-term mechanical ventilation and nutrition. Respir Med 2004; 98:413–420.
10. Pingleton SK. Enteral nutrition in patients with respiratory disease. Eur Respir J 1996; 9:364–370.
11. Hill NS. Failure to wean. In: Fishman AP, ed. Pulm Rehabil. New York: Marcel-Dekker, Inc.1996:577–617.
12. Aubier M, Murciano D, Lecocguic Y. Effect of hypophosphatemia on diaphragmatic contractility in patients with acute respiratory failure. N Engl J Med 1985; 313:420–424.
13. Ellis DA. Intermediate metabolism of muscle in Duchenne muscular dystrophy. Br Med Bull 1980; 36:165–171.
14. ATS/ERS Task Force, Standards for the diagnosis and treatment of patients with COPD: a summary of the ATS/ERS position paper. Eur Respir J 2004; 23:932–946.
15. Schols AM, Soeters PB, Mostert R, et al. Physiologic effects of nutritional support and anabolic steroids in patients with chronic obstructive pulmonary disease: a randomised controlled trial. Am J Respir Crit Care Med 1995; 152:1248–1274.
16. Prescott E, Almdal T, Mikkelsen KL, et al. Prognostic value of weight change in chronic obstructive pulmonary disease: results from the Copenhagen City heart study. Eur Respir J 2002; 20:539–544.
17. Schols AM, Broekhuizen R, Weling-Scheepers CA, et al. Body composition and mortality in chronic obstructive pulmonary disease. Am J Clin Nutr 2005; 82:53–59.
18. Naber TH, Schermer T, de Bree A, et al. Prevalence of malnutrition in nonsurgical hospitalized patients and its association with disease complications. Am J Clin Nutr 1997; 66:1232–1239.
19. Kruizenga HM, Wierdsma NJ, Van Bokhorst MA, et al. Screening of nutritional status in the Netherlands. Clin Nutr 2003; 22:147–152.
20. Kagansky N, Berner Y, Koren-Morag N, et al. Poor nutritional habits are predictors of poor outcome in very old hospitalized patients. Am J Clin Nutr 2005; 82:784–791.
21. Asensio A, Ramos A, Nunez S. Prognostic factors for mortality related to nutritional status in the hospitalized elderly. Med Clin 2004; 123:370–373.
22. Parekh NR, Steiger E. Percentage of weight loss as a predictor of surgical risk: from the time of Hiram Studley to today. Ohio Nutr Clin Pract 2004; 19:471–476.

23. Beck FK, Rosenthal TC. Prealbumin: a marker for nutritional evaluation. Am Fam Physician 2002; 65:1575–1578.
24. Sullivan DH, Bopp MM, Roberson PK. Protein-energy undernutrition and life-threatening complications among the hospitalized elderly. J Gen Intern Med 2002; 17:923–932.
25. Ferreira IM, Brooks D, Lacasse Y, et al. Nutritional supplementation for stable chronic obstructive pulmonary disease. Cochrane Database Syst Rev 2005; 2:CD000998.
26. Mallampalli A. Nutritional management of the patient with chronic obstructive pulmonary disease. Nutr Clin Pract 2004; 19:550–556.
27. Luo FM, Liu XJ, Li SQ, et al. Circulating ghrelin in patients with chronic obstructive pulmonary disease. Nutrition 2005; 21:793–798.
28. Nagaya N, Itoh T, Murakami S, et al. Treatment of cachexia with ghrelin in patients with COPD. Chest 2005; 128:1187–1193.
29. Goris AH, Vermeeren MA, Wouters EF, et al. Energy balance in depleted ambulatory patients with chronic obstructive pulmonary disease: the effect of physical activity and oral nutritional supplementation. Br J Nutr 2003; 89:725–729.
30. Vitacca M, Callegari G, Sarvà M, et al. Physiological effects of meals in difficult-to-wean tracheostomised patients with chronic obstructive pulmonary disease. Intensive Care Med 2005; 31:236–242.
31. Pauwels RA, Buist AS, Calverley PM, et al. GOLD Scientific Committee. Global strategy for the diagnosis, management, and prevention of chronic obstructive pulmonary disease. NHLBI/WHO global initiative for chronic obstructive lung disease (GOLD) workshop summary. Am J Respir Crit Care Med 2001; 163:1256–1276.
32. Creutzberg EC, Wouters EF, Mostert R, et al. Efficacy of nutritional supplementation therapy in depleted patients with chronic obstructive pulmonary disease. Nutrition 2003; 19:120–127.
33. Morrison WL, Gibson JN, Scrimgeour C, et al. Muscle wasting in emphysema. Clin Sci (Lond) 1988; 75:415–420.
34. Schiffelers SL, Blaak EE, Baarends EM, et al. Beta-adrenoceptor-mediated thermogenesis and lipolysis in patients with chronic obstructive pulmonary disease. Am J Physiol Endocrinol Metab 2001; 280:E357–E364.
35. Borsheim E, Tipton KD, Wolf SE, et al. Essential amino acids and muscle protein recovery from resistance exercise. Am J Physiol Endocrinol Metab 2002; 283:E648–E657.
36. Yoneda T, Yoshikawa M, Fu A, et al. Plasma levels of amino acids and hypermetabolism in patients with chronic obstructive pulmonary disease. Nutrition 2001; 17:95–99.
37. Devita MA, Spierer-Rundback MS. Swallowing disorders in patients with prolonged intubation or tracheostomy tubes. Crit Care Med 1990; 18:1328–1332.
38. Bonanno PC. Swallowing dysfunction after tracheostomy. Ann Surg 1971; 174:29–33.
39. Elpern EH, Scott MG, Petro L, et al. Pulmonary aspiration in mechanically ventilated patients with tracheostomies. Chest 1994; 105:563–566.
40. Schonhofer B, Barchfeld T, Haidl P, et al. Scintigraphy for evaluating early aspiration after oral feeding in patients receiving prolonged ventilation via tracheostomy. Intensive Care Med 1999; 25:311–314.
41. Tolep K, Getch CL, Criner GJ. Swallowing dysfunction in patients receiving prolonged mechanical ventilation. Chest 1996; 109:167–172.
42. Spray SB, Zuidema GD, Cameron JL. Aspiration pneumonia: incidence of aspiration with endotracheal tubes. Am J Surg 1976; 131:701–703.
43. Coster ST, Schwartz WF. Rheology and the swallow-safe bolus. Dysphagia 1987; 1:113–118.
44. Bucholz DW, Bosma JF, Donner MW. Adaptation, compensation and decompensation of the pharyngeal swallow. Gastrointest Radiol 1985; 10:235–239.
45. Willig TN, Giladeau C, Kazandjian MS. Dysphagia and nutrition in neuromuscular disorders. In: Bach JR, ed. Pulmonary Rehabilitation. The Obstructive and Paralytic Conditions. Philadelphia: Hanley & Belfus, Inc. 1996:353–369.

46. Bach JR. Pulmonary rehabilitation in musculoskeletal disorders. In: Fishman AP, ed. Pulmonary Rehabilitation. New York: Marcel-Dekker, Inc.1996:701–723.
47. ASPEN Board of Directors and the Clinical Guidelines Task Force. Guidelines for the use of parenteral and enteral nutrition in adult and pediatric patients. JPEN J Parenter Enteral Nutr 2002; 26:1SA–6SA.
48. ASPEN Board of Directors and the Clinical Guidelines Task Force, Nutrition care process. Guideline status. JPEN J Parenter Enteral Nutr 2002; 26:7SA–8SA.
49. National Institute for Health and Clinical Excellence. Clinical Guideline 32. Nutrition support in adults: oral nutrition support, enteral tube feeding and parenteral nutrition. 2006.
50. Steiner MC, Barton RL, Singh SJ, et al. Nutritional enhancement of exercise performance in chronic obstructive pulmonary disease: a randomized controlled trial. Thorax 2003; 58:745–751.
51. Cai B. Effect of supplementing a high-fat, low-carbohydrate enteral formula in COPD patients. Nutrition 2003; 19:229–232.
52. Broekhuizen R. Optimizing oral nutritional drink supplementation in patients with chronic obstructive pulmonary disease. Br J Nutr 2005; 93:965–971.
53. Planas M. Nutritional support and quality of life in stable chronic obstructive pulmonary disease (COPD) patients. Clin Nutr 2005; 24:433–441.
54. Pritchard C, Duffy S, Edington J, et al. Enteral nutrition and oral nutrition supplements: a review of the economics literature. JPEN J Parenter Enteral Nutr 2006; 30:52–59.
55. Heys SD, Walker LG, Smith I. Enteral nutrition supplementation with key nutrients in patients with critical illness and cancer. A meta-analysis of randomized controlled clinical trials. Ann Surg 1999; 229:467–477.
56. Jackson NC, Carroll V, Russell-Jones DL, et al. The metabolic consequences of critical illness: acute effects on glutamine and protein metabolism. Am J Physiol Endocrinol Metab 1999; 276:163–170.
57. Biolo G, Fleming RY, Maggi SP, et al. Inhibition of muscle glutamine formation in hypercatabolic patients. Clin Sci (Lond) 2000; 99:189–194.
58. Oudemans-Van Straaten HM, Bosman RJ, Treskes M, et al. Plasma glutamine depletion and patient outcome in acute ICU admissions. Intensive Care Med 2001; 27:84–90.
59. SINPE Consensus Paper. Glutamitaly 2003. Riv It Nutriz Parenter Enter 2004; 22: 115–133.
60. Heyland DK, Dhaliwal R, Suchner U, et al. Antioxidant nutrients: a systematic review of trace elements and vitamins in the critically ill patient. Intensive Care Med 2005; 31:327–237.
61. Mackenzie SL. Implementation of a nutrition support protocol increases the proportion of mechanically ventilated patients reaching enteral nutrition targets in the adult intensive care unit. JPEN J Parenter Enteral Nutr 2005; 29:74–80.
62. Heyland DK, Dhaliwal R, Drover JW, et al. Canadian clinical practice guidelines for nutrition support in mechanically ventilated critically ill adult patients. JPEN J Parenter Enteral Nutr 2003; 27:355–373.
63. Artinian V, Krayern H, Di Giovine B. Effects of early enteral feeling on the outcome of critically ill mechanically ventilated medical patients. Chest 2006; 129:960–967.
64. Trujillo EB, Young LS, Chertow GM, et al. Metabolic and monetary costs of avoidable parenteral nutrition use. JPEN J Parenter Enteral Nutr 1999; 23:109–113.
65. Smith AA, Carusone SB, Willison K, et al. Hospitalization and emergency department visits among seniors receiving homecare: a pilot study. BMC Geriatr 2005; 5:9–14.
66. Daly JM, Weintraub FN, Shou J, et al. Enteral nutrition during multimodality therapy in upper gastrointestinal cancer patients. Ann Surg 1995; 221:327–338.
67. Ho KM, Dobb GJ, Webb SAR. A comparison of early gastric and post-pyloric feeding in critically ill patients: a meta-analysis. Intensive Care Med 2006; 32:639–649.
68. Baumgartner TG, Cerda JJ, Somogyi L, et al. Enteral nutrition in clinical practice. Clin Med J 1999; 40:515–527.

69. Larson DE, Burton DD, Schroeder KW, et al. Percutaneous endoscopic gastrostomy. Gastroenterology 1987; 93:4852–4861.
70. Ponsky JL, Gauderer MW, Stellato TA, et al. Percutaneous approaches to enteral alimentation. Am J Surg 1985; 149:102–115.
71. Mitchell SL, Tetroe JM. Survival after percutaneous endoscopic gastrostomy placement in older persons. J Gerontol (A) 2000; 55:735–739.
72. Norton B, Homer-Ward M, Donnelly MT, et al. A randomized prospective comparison of percutaneous endoscopic gastrostomy and nasogastric tube feeding after acute dysphagic stroke. BMJ 1996; 312:13–16.
73. Erdil A, Saka M, Ates Y, et al. Enteral nutrition via percutaneous endoscopic gastrostomy and nutritional status of patients: five-year prospective study. J Gastroenterol Hepatol 2005; 20:1002–1007.
74. Skelly RH, Kupfer RM, Metcalfe ME, et al. Percutaneous endoscopic gastrostomy (PEG): change in practice since 1988. Clin Nutr 2002; 21:389–394.
75. Hull MA, Rawlings J, Murray FE, et al. Audit of outcome of long-term enteral nutrition by percutaneous endoscopic gastrostomy. Lancet 1993; 341:869–872.
76. Askanazi J, Weissman C, Rosenbaum SH, et al. Nutrition and the respiratory system. Crit Care Med 1982; 10:163–172.
77. Bresson JL, Bader B, Rocchicciolí F, et al. Protein-metabolism kinetics and energy-substrate utilization in infants fed parenteral solutions with different glucose-fat ratios. Am J Clin Nutr 1991; 54:370–376.
78. Richelle M, Rubin M, Kulapongse S, et al. Plasma lipoprotein pattern during long-term home parenteral nutrition with two lipid emulsions. JPEN J Parenter Enteral Nutr 1993; 17:432–437.
79. Masclans JR, Iglesia R, Bermejo B, et al. Gas exchange and pulmonary haemodynamic responses to fat emulsions in acute respiratory distress syndrome. Intensive Care Med 1998; 24:918–923.
80. Kreymann KG, Berger MM, Deutz NE, et al. ESPEN guidelines on enteral nutrition: intensive care. Clin Nutr 2006; 25(2): 210–223.
81. Atkinson M, Worthley LI. Nutrition in the critically ill patient: part II. Parenteral nutrition. Crit Care Resusc 2003; 5:121–136.
82. Wengler A, Micklewright A, Heburturne Y, et al. ESPEN-home artificial nutrition working group. Monitoring of patients on home parenteral nutrition (HPN) in Europe: a questionnaire based study on monitoring practice in 42 centers. Clin Nutr 2006; 25(4): 693–700.
83. Muller MJ. Hepatic complications in parenteral nutrition. Z Gastroenterol 1996; 34:36–40.
84. Pironi L, Labate AM, Pertkiewicz M, et al. Prevalence of bone disease in patients on home parenteral nutrition. Clin Nutr 2002; 21:289–296.
85. Cohen-Solal M, Baudoin C, Joly F, et al. Osteoporosis in patients on long-term home parenteral nutrition: a longitudinal study. J Bone Miner Res 2003; 18:1989–2010.
86. Naylor CJ, Griffiths RD, Fernandez RS. Does a multidisciplinary total parenteral nutrition team improve patient outcomes? A systematic review. JPEN J Parenter Enteral Nutr 2004; 28:251–258.
87. Magnuson BL, Clifford TM, Hoskins LA, et al. Enteral nutrition and drug administration, interactions, and complications. Nutr Clin Pract 2005; 20:618–624.
88. Montero Hernandez M, Martinez Vazquez MJ, Martinez Olmos M, et al. Economic assessment of the implementation of a parenteral nutrition protocol for patients undergoing intestinal resection by a multidisciplinary team. Farm Hosp 2006; 30:20–28.
89. Kruizenga HM, Van Tulder MW, Seidell JC, et al. Effectiveness and cost-effectiveness of early screening and treatment of malnourished patients. Am J Clin Nutr 2005; 82:1082–1089.
90. Schols AMWJ, Wouters EFM. Nutrition and metabolic therapy. In: Donner CF, Ambrosino N, Goldstein RS, eds. Pulm Rehabil. London: Hodder Arnold, 2005: 229–235.

32
Skin Integrity, Bowel and Bladder Care

RITA F. BONCZEK
Hospital for Special Care, New Britain, Connecticut, U.S.A.

I. Bowel Program

Patients requiring intensive care often experience extended periods of immobility because of their primary diagnosis and, frequently, because of the presence of multiple comorbidities. It is not infrequent for them to experience dysfunction of the gastrointestinal and urological tract during their prolonged stay, either as part of their original diagnosis or as a complication during their recuperative phase. This dysfunction is aggravated by periods of inadequate fluid intake, by reduced nutritional support, or by any changes to the intestinal flora, all of which may influence the patient's ability to regulate bowel and bladder function. The situation is further complicated by polypharmacy, including medications that may adversely influence bowel and bladder motility (1).

The combination of weakened perineal muscles, urinary tract as well as other infections, and interruptions in peristalsis (whether neurogenic or medication induced) all contribute to a common problem among ventilator-dependent individuals—stool and urine incontinence—with its attending consequence of skin breakdown. Reduced ambulation, the inability to transfer to a toilet for evacuation, and general cognitive impairment often impair resolution of these issues. The resulting low self-esteem becomes a further barrier.

However, the development of an individualized, regulated program of healthy elimination can be achieved. This requires consistency and patience on the part of the patient, family and caregivers, in cooperation with the rehabilitation physician, nurse, respiratory therapist, and physical therapist. The goal of the program is for the patient to achieve continence, without breakthrough, using assistive devices and medications, with the concomitant result of having no skin breakdown (2). This continence is critical in the prevention and healing of skin breakdown, which ranges from dermatitis to infected decubitus ulcers.

A. Bowel Incontinence

Bowel incontinence is manifested by a variety of patterns of stool consistency—from soft, loose, or hard stool to no bowel movement at all but constant oozing. All of these patterns will have a negative impact on the rehabilitation process, resulting in patient frustration, fatigue, and interruption in therapy. A regulated program with timely bowel evacuations and consistent output will be part of a meaningful wellness program. The program begins at the time of admission and may be modified as the patient's health improves.

B. Pathophysiology

Central to the development of a program is a good understanding of the mixing and peristaltic functions of the gastrointestinal tract. Peristalsis is initiated by the distention of the small bowel by the passage of chyme. After meals, peristalsis is greatly increased by the distention and stimulation of gastrocolic reflex. It takes 3–10 hours for chyme to travel through the small bowel after which it is pushed into the large bowel through the ileocecal sphincter, where water is absorbed. Mass movements to the rectum occur only few times a day, most frequently after breakfast. When the mass of fecal material is in the rectum, an urge to defecate occurs. Bowel irritation from inflammation, fever, or infection can increase colonic transit time, leading to more frequent rectal evacuation.

Defecation starts with stimulation of the sensory nerve fibers of the rectum, leading to an involuntary spinal reflex that causes contraction of the rectum and the opening of the internal and external sphincters. The voluntary, somatic system completes the evacuation, after which the brain sends signals to the external sphincter to close and inhibit further elimination. Any damage to the CNS, such as a cerebrovascular accident, brain tumor, multiple sclerosis, or motor neuron diseases, can impair the bowel's voluntary and involuntary responses. These CNS changes may result in inaccurate, involuntary responses of the bowel, such as flaccidity of the rectum, expulsion of contents, or sphincter and rectal hyperactivity (3).

C. Bowel Program

Many ventilated patients are debilitated and immobile, especially after a prolonged ICU stay. They cannot sit upright on a commode for 30 minutes, and therefore, the team must start the program with a daily oral and rectal medication to begin bowel regulation. This condition is true for all types of bowel incontinence. The patient is monitored for the first seven days, during which time the program should remain constant and at the same time of the day, each day, to develop a predictable response. The ingestion of food and fluids should occur 30 minutes prior to bowel care (2).

This phase can be the most frustrating for the patient because of breakthrough stool, rectal discomfort, embarrassment, and the sensation of an unnatural process. Patients frequently decide to stop the program at this time because of their feelings, but they must be gently reeducated on the outcomes that can be achieved, including improved health, uninterrupted therapy sessions, and improved quality of life. Needless to say, this is a very challenging time, especially for the nursing team, as the patient and family may be so unhappy that they may convince the physician to alter the program, causing incontinence to return. This will interrupt the rehabilitation program and cause time loss, but it does help to demonstrate the value of a daily program to the patient. To develop the confidence to continue with the program, patients require daily emotional support from the team, together with privacy and personal hygiene. Continence can be achieved in 14 days if the program is followed.

After this period, the program can be modified every other day. If the patient does not have a bowel movement, then it may be necessary to change the routine every third day or three times a week. A spontaneous bowel movement that occurs close to the rectal stimulant is a sign that the reflex response and muscle control are improving. In this situation, the rectal medication should be held to see if the patient would continue to have spontaneous movements. It is recommended not to go more than three days without a bowel movement; therefore, rectal medication should be administered on the fourth day. During a second 14-day evaluation, if the patient develops signs of abdominal pain, loose or hard consistency stools, or rectal pain, then the oral and rectal medications should be changed.

The following bowel guidelines (Figs. 1 and 2) enable a program to be built, taking into consideration the multiple changes a patient will undergo during recovery and weaning from a ventilator. The guidelines help identify the best starting program for the assessment pattern. The rule is to start with one type of medication for the oral and rectal stimulant, and then modify on the basis of results. If the patient is not evacuating well, then change one step at a time by increasing the oral stimulant gradually until the maximum dose of the drug is achieved (4). The rectal stimulant is then modified until the goal is achieved. It is very important to pay close attention to the transit time of the medication and the time at which the bowel movement occurred. This monitoring should be done because in ventilated patients the drug response may be slower because of their chronic condition, or because of neurological dysfunction, which delays the bowel movement after the rectal medication has been administered. Under these circumstances, the medication transit time can be calculated and the oral medication administered earlier to match up with the rectal response.

Another cause of a poor rectal response is nonabsorption of rectal medication due to a bolus of stool blocking the rectal vault. This blockage must be removed before the rectal medication is administered. Blockages are a common problem and require nursing as well as patient education. Disimpaction of the rectal vault needs to be built into the program as the first step in rectal management. Unfortunately, rectal tissue often becomes red and painful with this technique. The care team needs to be aware of this issue, and administer an anti-inflammatory or anesthetic topical product in conjunction with a rectal stimulant—manual or suppository. The nurse can often anticipate potential problems and can help the patient to be comfortable during the program.

Topical preparations for the skin and rectal tissue can decrease hemorrhoids, ulcerations, fissures, and dermatitis, thus preventing secondary incontinence. In time, if the patient becomes more mobile and can tolerate being up, then the program should be conducted using a commode, a toilet, or a combination of both.

D. Skin Care with Bowel Incontinence

In reality, some patients will continue to have loose breakthrough bowel movements even with the best program. Figure 2 describes how, after ruling out infections and any additional medical diagnoses, the team can give medications to help solidify the consistency of the stool. The skin is best protected by a barrier wipe and cleanser with physiological pH of 5.5. Dimethicone, glycerin, and chlorhexidrine gluconate, followed by the application of a moisture barrier cream of the same components, are applied with petroleum on a routine basis. If dermatitis becomes open and bleeding, then the cream must be changed to a product with zinc oxide as 5% of the components (5).

Loose bowels may need to be collected in a fecal incontinence pouch, which can be challenging to keep on the patient. Rectal tube products that divert into a drainage bag are often needed for a week to give the skin the ability to heal. The rectal tube can be irrigated every two to four hours to prevent debris from clogging it, and to provide a stimulant to empty the sigmoid and rectum. This process is important because when the tube is removed, the bowel has received a daily program and responds to the rectal medication in the same

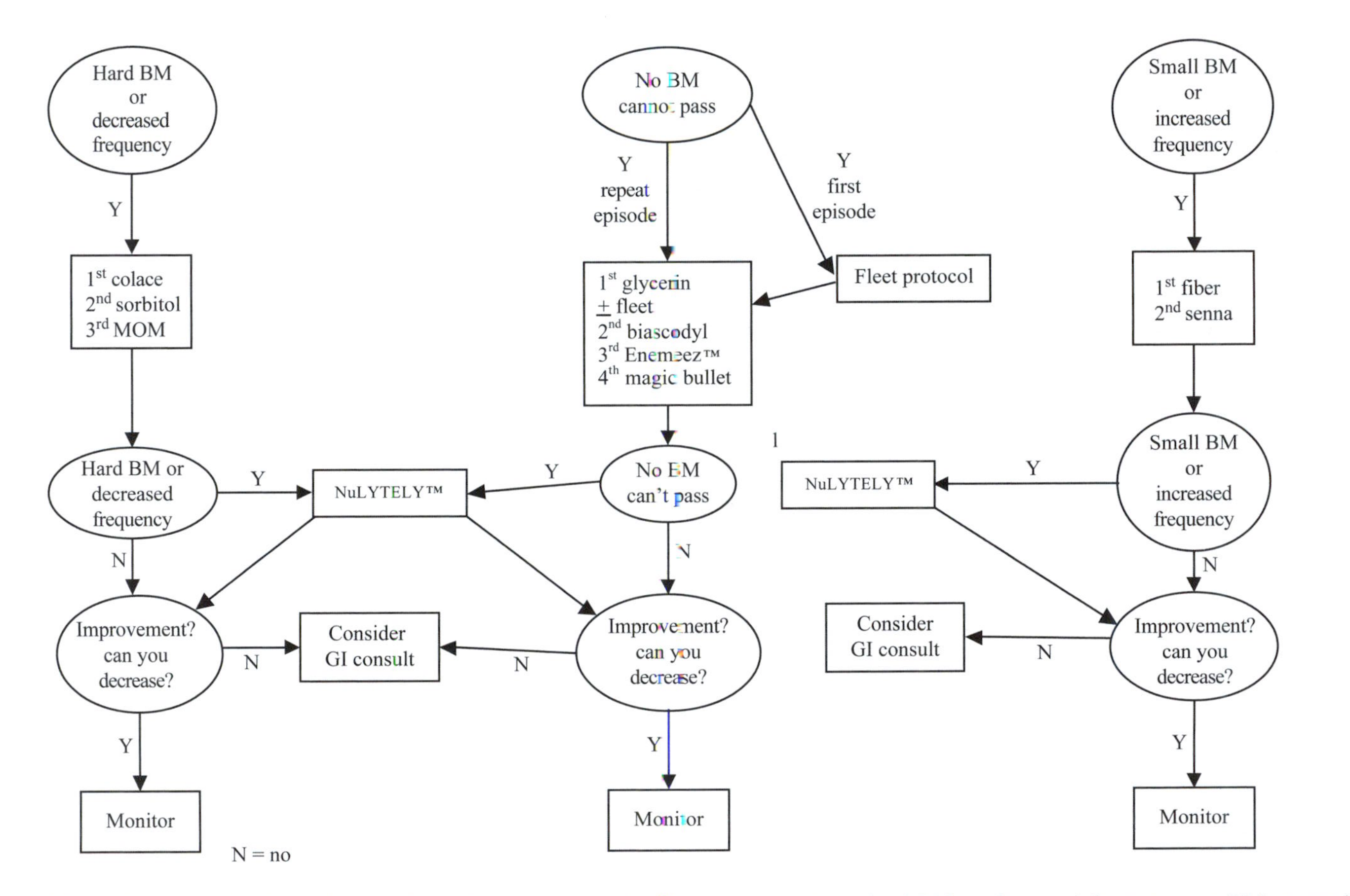

Figure 1 Bowel algorithm showing the pathways associated with each circumstance-hard BM or decreased frequency, no BM, or small BM. *Abbreviations*: BM, bowel movement; MOM, milk of magnesia; Y, yes; N, no. *Source*: From Ref. 4.

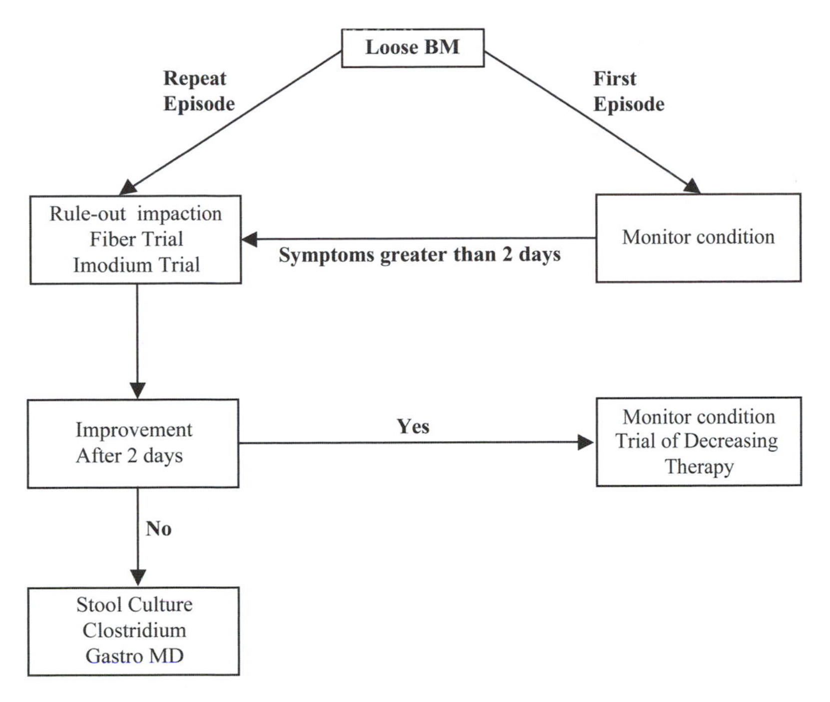

Figure 2 Bowel algorithm showing the directions for the first and repeated episodes of loose BM. *Abbreviations*: BM, bowel movement; R/O, rule out; GI, gastrointestinal.

manner as before, such that no time is lost in the bowel training. Rectal tube products may be used early to prevent superficial ulcers from developing into deep muscle ulcers. The rectal tube is a great support when the consistency is loose, but cannot be used when consistency is soft or formed.

A bowel program is essential as nothing is more disappointing for the patient than an unwelcome bowel movement after washing, dressing, and being placed in an electric wheelchair. One untimely accident can waste an entire day of rehabilitation. Bowel programs prevent skin breakdown, decrease medical complications, and improve the time spent in rehabilitation activities.

II. Bladder Program

A. Urinary Continence

Urinary continence is more difficult to establish in the ventilator patient because of the variety of medications and fluid requirements. Many patients have comorbid coronary artery disease for which they require diuretics. Maintaining a good fluid balance is a challenge for the patient with a weak bladder, due to disuse or a long-term indwelling catheter.

Reestablishing a voiding plan without breakthrough wetness requires that all the team members follow the established plan. The first step is to obtain the history of previous voiding patterns, to determine other diagnoses, such as overflow incontinence, frequency, stress incontinence, or prostatic hypertrophy (6). A clear picture of premorbid urination patterns can help the team develop a care plan.

B. Pathophysiology of the Bladder

The bladder functions as a low-pressure reservoir, filling at the rate of 2 mL/min until approximately 360–400 mL is reached, and the intravesical pressure increases. This pressure activates proprioceptive receptors in the bladder wall to signal the sacral spinal cord, thus triggering detrusor contraction. Sensory stimulation occurs at the micturation center in the brainstem that coordinates urethral sphincter relaxation as the detrusor muscle contracts. Higher controls in the frontal lobe can block this sensory message until conscious direction permits a voluntary void. Medical insults to the spinal column, peripheral sensory nerves, and cerebral cortex will cause malfunction in the voiding pattern (7).

C. Urology Guidelines

The indwelling catheter should be removed when the patient can recognize the signal to void or can tolerate wetness on the skin. The team should toilet the patient every two hours using a female or male urinal. The commode should be introduced slowly, at least once a day, to help the patient to adjust to sitting up. Initially, limited commode use helps to prevent fatigue and to build endurance. After the voiding trial is started, a postvoid volume should be determined on at least three occasions. Residual volumes >200 mL should be removed by retry of a void or an intermittent catheterization. If consistent postvoid urinary retention occurs, the plan should include toileting upright and on a "time void while awake schedule" regardless of the sensation to go. Diuretics should be administered early in the day, limiting fluids after 7 PM to 150 mL and monitoring fluid intake so as not to exceed body requirements. If retention continues, then urodynamics should be requested to evaluate the detrusor and external sphincter responses.

Patients with urinary frequency and urinary retention do benefit from urodynamical evaluation to determine the voiding pressures, the volume that triggers the void, the effect of abdominal pressure, and the volume of void. A urology nurse or a physician can prescribe appropriate medications to address the above issues. Urodynamics may be performed at the bedside by a trained nurse and can provide prompt information to assist with a plan to address incontinence. This examination will prevent unnecessary wetness and improve the continence outcomes.

Patients with specific neurological diseases, or spinal cord injuries with neurogenic bladders require closer evaluation. These injuries can cause hyperactivity or flaccidity. Urological guidelines (Fig. 3) outline the treatments that help provide continence in neurological diseases. A key objective is to remove the indwelling catheter. The voiding pattern must be followed closely; if there is no void after six hours or if the patient has symptoms of pressure or autonomic dysreflexia, then catheterization is required. If a patient cannot consistently void, or if the volumes are greater than 300 mL, then an intermittent catheterization program should be used. The program begins every four hours and is then decreased by an hour, if the catherization volumes are less than 200 mL for over 48 hours. After a week of intermittent catheterization, urodynamics, urinalysis, and a urology consult are indicated. On the basis of these results, cholinergic, anticholinergic, or adrenergic antagonist medications may be prescribed to facilitate a spontaneous or reflex void.

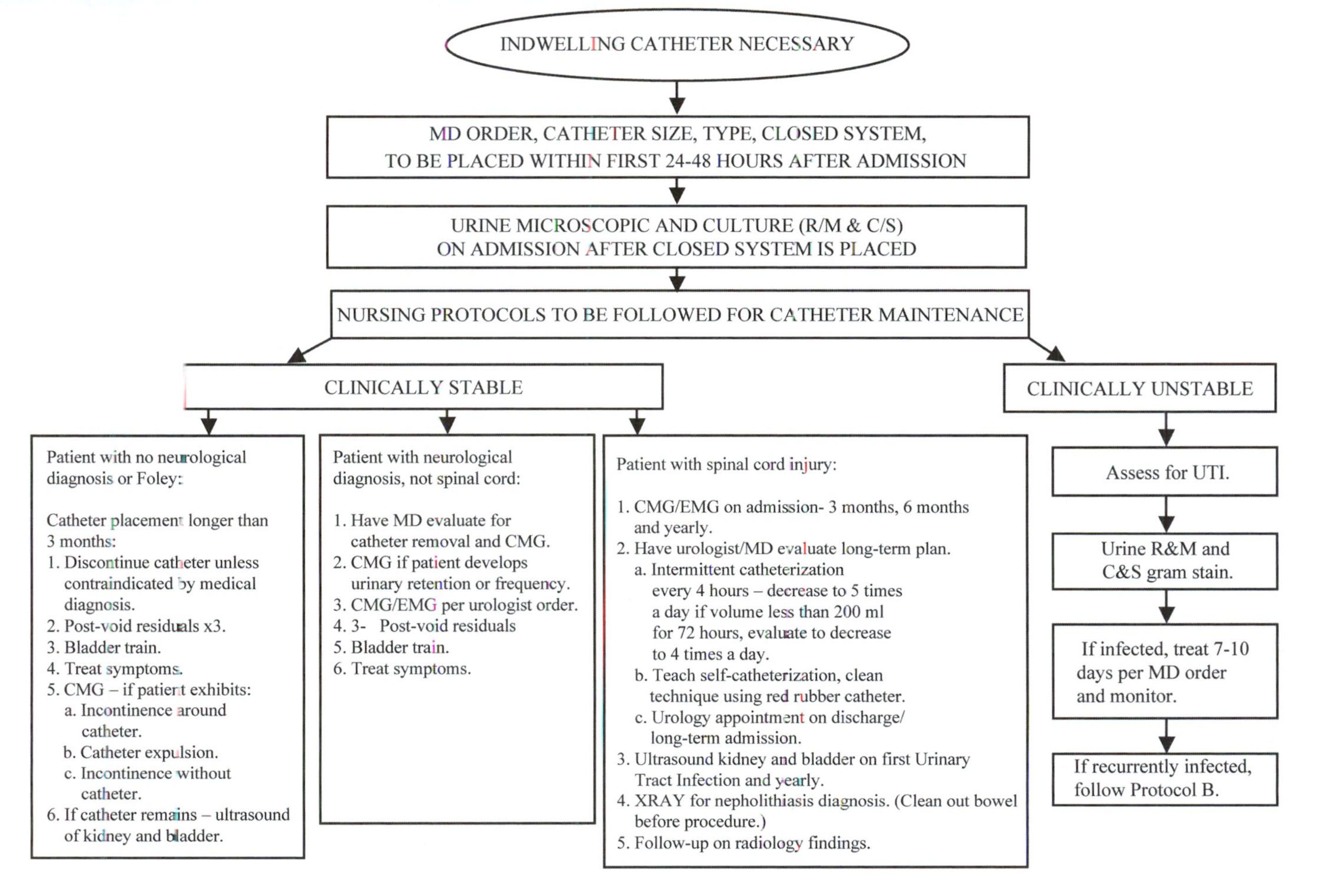

Figure 3 Urology guidelines for indwelling catheter in a patient clinically stable with the diagnoses nonneurologic, neurologic, spinal cord, and also in a patient who is clinically unstable. *Abbreviations*: UTI, urinary tract infection; CMG, cystometrogram; EMG, electromyogram; MD, doctor.

D. Skin Care with Urinary Incontinence

To prevent skin breakdown when incontinence occurs in men, an external appliance is important. These appliances come in a variety of models. If the penis is inverted, an incontinence pouch can be used. Incontinence pouches are also available for women, but are not comfortable to apply or wear. For the female who is wet and cannot achieve a continence program, a urologist may suggest an indwelling catheter or a collagen implantation to the urethra along with application of estrogen cream intravaginally to restore urethral integrity and decrease incontinent episodes. A suprapubic catheter may be considered in men and women, as it facilitates management and is comfortable when sitting and during sexual activity. Indwelling urethral catheters should be restricted to the acutely ill person who is being monitored for fluid balance, severely impaired with pain, or has stage three to four pressure ulceration (8).

To maintain intact skin during the establishment of the program, a basic barrier wash of oleic acid, soybean oil, and potassium hydroxide followed by a moisture barrier cream of dimethicone 3% and glycerin stearate should be used. Candida dermatitis should be treated with an antifungal product and a cortisone cream for at least 14 days. Severe dermatitis or skin breakdown on the penis may require the replacement of an indwelling catheter until healed. Urethral ulceration and labia inflammation or polyps from catheter pressure can be treated with anti-inflammatory cream twice a day, for seven days, and then tapered slowly to twice a week as a maintenance program.

References

1. Sine RD. Identification and management of bowel and bladder problems. In: Sine RD, Roush R, Liss SE, et al., eds. Basic Rehabilitation Techniques—A Self-Instruction Guide. Gaithersburg, Maryland: Aspen, 1998:58–61.
2. Parsons K. Neurogenic bowel management in adults with spinal cord injury. Consortium for spinal cord medicine, paralyzed veterans of America, March 1998:1–39.
3. Fried K, Fried G, Farnan C. Elimination. In: Dorstine J, Hargrove S, eds. Comprehensive Rehabilitative Nursing. Philadelphia: WP Saunders, 2001:153–162.
4. Bonczek R, Soltis T. Bowel Algorithm Flowchart, Hospital for Special Care. Adult Bowel Guideline Protocol. New Britain, CT: 2005:1–3.
5. Chand T. Cleansing and skin care. In: Templeton S, ed. Wound Care Nursing: A Guide To Practice. Seattle: Aspen, 2005:69–87.
6. Nurse B, Collin M. Indwelling Foley Catheter Management Protocol, A Hospital For Special Care. New Britain, CT: 2005:1–4.
7. Pines M. Bladder elimination and continence. In: Hoeman S, ed. Rehabilitation Nursing Process, Application and Outcomes. 3rd ed. Philadelphia: Mosby, 2002:383–415.
8. Urinary Incontinence Guidelines Panel. Urinary Incontinence in Adults. Clinical Practice Guideline: Acute and Chronic Management. Clinical Practice Guideline No. 2. AHCPR Publication No. 96-0682. Rockville MD: Agency for Health Care Policy and Research, Public Health Service, US Department of Health and Human Services, 1996.

33
Palliative Care for the Ventilator Patient: End-of-Life Issues and Approaches

ALLISON LANE-RETICKER
University of Connecticut Health Center, Hartford, Connecticut, U.S.A.

I. Introduction and Definitions

Palliative care and ventilator therapy for patients with chronic respiratory disease are by no means mutually exclusive. Indeed, optimal treatment for these patients includes alleviating distressing symptoms and providing support to the patient and family, using an interdisciplinary team. While the focus of this chapter is palliative care for the ventilator patient, it will also discuss the broader areas of palliative care for patients with end-stage lung disease and palliation of pulmonary symptoms in patients with other life-threatening illness.

Balfour Mount coined the term palliative care in 1973. It refers to comprehensive care provided by an interdisciplinary team for patients and families living with life-threatening or terminal illness. The goal of palliative care is to help the patient achieve the best possible quality of life by relieving physical, emotional, or spiritual suffering, and by achieving maximal functional capacity. On the basis of an understanding of the patient's values, beliefs, and culture, palliative care encourages evaluation of each potential treatment in terms of the balance of benefit and burden at a specific time in a patient's life.

In its most general sense, palliative care encompasses end-of-life care but does not require that the patient abandon curative efforts. Palliative care can include surgery, radiation, chemotherapy, and other very active treatments. Ideally, palliative care begins at the time of diagnosis of life-threatening illness and proceeds in parallel with curative care until the patient chooses to focus solely on comfort care. The term also includes comfort-focused care in patients who wish to forego curative efforts, but who may have a prognosis of more than six months and under some jurisdictions may be ineligible for most hospice programs. In this sense, it may be considered comfort-focused prehospice care. And in another sense, hospice care is one form of palliative care.

Hospice is both a philosophy of care, and in the United States , an insurance benefit. Hospice seeks neither to hasten nor to prolong death, but to maximize quality of life for as long as the patient lives. Care is provided by an interdisciplinary team (nurse, physician, social worker, chaplain, and others) whose members collaborate to relieve patient and family distress and, after the patient's death, provide support to the bereaved family. Often when symptoms are relieved, patients enjoy time with family and friends preparing a legacy, finding meaning, or even traveling.

While the hospice philosophy is quite uniform, the translation of the same into an insurance benefit can be variable. In the United States, the referring physician and the

Table 1 U.S. Medicare Hospice Benefit

Criteria for pulmonary disease

General

1. Patient must be eligible for Medicare Part A and must enroll in a Medicare-approved hospice program
2. The referring physician and the hospice medical director must certify that the patient is terminally ill and has a life expectancy of six months or less, if the disease runs its usual course
3. The patient or proxy must agree that the hospice benefit will replace standard Medicare coverage for the terminal illness

Disease specific

1. Disabling dyspnea (at rest or with minimal exertion), dyspnea poorly responsive or unresponsive to bronchodilator therapy, dyspnea resulting in decreased functional activity or fatigue, FEV1 $< 30\%$
2. Progression (frequent hospitalizations, emergency department or doctor visits)
3. Cor pulmonale

   Confirmatory:

   $< 90\%$ ideal body weight or $>10\%$ loss of weight

   Resting tachycardia >100 beats/min

   $Pao_2 < 55$ mmHg or $Sao_2 < 88\%$

   Continuous oxygen therapy

Abbreviations: FEV1, forced expiratory volume in 1 second; Pao_2, partial pressure of oxygen in arterial blood; Sao_2, saturation of oxygen in arterial blood.

hospice medical director must certify that the patient is terminally ill and has a life expectancy of six months or less if the illness runs its usual course. The patient or a proxy must file a statement with the selected hospice agreeing that the hospice benefit will replace standard Medicare coverage for the terminal illness as long as the hospice benefit remains in effect. In addition to the general eligibility criteria there are disease specific criteria for patients with lung disease (Table 1).

Hospice care is available at home, in nursing homes, in hospitals, and in freestanding hospices. However, most patients are cared for at home, with a nurse making regular visits as well as being available 24 hours a day by telephone or for emergency visits. A home health aide is assigned for up to two hours a day. The hospice provides equipment, such as a hospital bed and wheelchair, and medications related to the diagnosis. The comprehensive nature of the coverage prompted one author to call hospice an "an all-embracing beneficence" (1). Many hospices cannot afford expensive therapies, such as total parenteral nutrition (TPN), radiation, or chemotherapy, which may delay the patient's moving to a hospice situation. While there is no philosophical reason for a hospice patient to abandon specific therapies, there may be financial reasons.

Pulmonologists are well acquainted with pulmonary rehabilitation (PR), which shares many goals and approaches with palliative care. PR is an interdisciplinary approach to alleviating distressing respiratory symptoms, improving functional status, and enhancing quality of life in patients with chronic lung disease. In addition to a patient-specific exercise prescription and psychosocial support, PR provides education on self-management strategies, energy conservation, nutrition, and living with chronic disease. Advance directives are usually covered in the educational sessions. The initial, formal phase of PR is time-limited,

Table 2 Components of Palliative and End-of-Life Care for Patients with Cardiopulmonary Disease

Support for patient and family
Advance care planning
Maintaining and supporting the patient's dignity, including cultural and spiritual needs
Care of the patient
Relief of distressing symptoms
Management of the dying process, including withdrawal of life-sustaining treatment
Referral to appropriate hospital and community resources
Quality palliative and end-of-life care in all treatment settings
Responsibility of the professional caregiver
Assurance of education and competence in palliative and end-of-life care
Support and counseling to address professional caregiver grieving
Development of institutional, professional, and regulatory policies to ensure quality
Palliative and end-of-life care

Source: From Ref. 3.

but graduates are often welcome to continue in the program, indefinitely. Indeed, PR is presented as an enduring change in lifestyle, encouraging increased activity levels and promoting self-management in collaboration with health professionals. Most PR programs have difficulty in reaching patients who are homebound.

Management of severe chronic respiratory disease is usually aimed at alleviation of symptoms rather than cure. However, referrals to PR are infrequent and often delayed, and many hospice referrals do not occur until the patient is actively dying. Guidelines on the care of patients with chronic respiratory disease are often silent on the issue of palliative care, especially end-of-life preferences (2,3). On the other hand, both the American College of Chest Physicians and the American Thoracic Society in conjunction with the European Respiratory Society have issued position statements endorsing palliative care, including advance care planning for patients with severe cardiopulmonary disease (4,5). The American College of Chest Physicians outlines the components of palliative care (Table 2).

Although chronic obstructive pulmonary disease (COPD) is usually progressive, with disability gradually increasing over several years, the course for a given patient is quite unpredictable. The gradual decline in function may be punctuated by exacerbations, which suddenly result in respiratory failure. With good care even patients with chronic hypoxemic and hypercarbic respiratory failure may live for months or years. The median survival for patients hospitalized with an acute exacerbation of COPD is two years, and 50% of patients are readmitted within six months (6). But which patients will die in six months? Non-pulmonary organ failure is the most significant risk factor for early death from COPD (7), but studies have failed to identify reliable predictors of six-month mortality in patients with severe lung disease. In other words, the sickest patients do not necessarily die first (8). Except for dementia, COPD is the terminal diagnosis associated with the most variable survival in patients referred for hospice care (9). This uncertainty makes it difficult for some physicians to ask patients about their preferences in end-of-life care.

Given the prognostic uncertainty, any exacerbation or consideration of a new treatment modality such as lung reduction surgery or transplantation can be an opportunity to discuss the patient's goals of care and wishes for attempted resuscitation. The pulmonologist may choose to involve a palliative care specialist in these conversations. Early involvement of palliative care allows patients and families time to establish relationships with one of the teams that may be involved with their end-of-life care.

II. Symptom Management

Patients with extra-pulmonary life-threatening illnesses often have pulmonary symptoms, and patients dying of pulmonary disease often have extra-pulmonary symptoms. Patients with end-stage pulmonary disease carry a heavy symptom burden, including dyspnea, pain, insomnia, fatigue, anxiety, depression, and immobility. Many patients fear breathlessness more than pain. Ironically, dyspnea remains a prominent symptom for many patients on ventilators. To treat dyspnea we can use four management strategies: reducing ventilatory impedance, reducing ventilatory demand, improving respiratory muscle function, and altering central perception (10). Impedance can be decreased by bronchodilators and steroids, and occasionally with bronchial stents and lung volume reduction surgery, or by eliminating pleural effusions. Ventilatory demand is decreased through energy conservation strategies as diverse as exercise training early in disease, and the use of wheelchairs later in the illness. Respiratory muscle function can be improved by proper positioning and, in some cases, with supplemental oral nutrition. The perception of dyspnea can be altered by distraction, by supplemental oxygen, by opioids, and by benzodiazepines. In opioid-naïve patients, 3–5 mg of oral morphine every three to four hours is a good starting dose, with 1–2 mg intravenous morphine every three to four hours for those who need intravenous medications. For patients already on opioids for pain, a 25% increase in dose often relieves dyspnea. All opioid use must be within the context of their respiratory suppressant effects, especially among patients who are already hypercapnic.

Pain is surprisingly common in patients with end-stage lung disease. The Study to Understand Prognoses and Preferences for Outcomes and Risks of Treatments (SUPPORT) investigators found 44% of COPD patients reporting pain, as compared to 57% of lung cancer pain patients; 40% of patients who had high levels of pain in the hospital were still having pain six months later (11). Because of the respiratory depressant action of opioids, relieving pain is often complicated for patients with lung disease, but in one study, nearly half of the patients said that they preferred treatment for pain even if it meant a shorter life (11). Treating ongoing pain requires round-the-clock dosing, generally using a sustained release opioid. Patients also require medication for breakthrough pain. Usually, 10% of the total daily opioid dose is prescribed, as needed every three to four hours. There is no ceiling dose on opioids themselves, but when using fixed combinations of opioids and medicines, such as acetaminophen or nonsteroidal anti-inflammatory medications, care must be taken to avoid toxicity. It is important to remember that opioids cause constipation, which should be treated prophylactically with a stool softener and a laxative.

Delirium is common at the end of life and is very frightening for patients and families, interfering with communication just when it is most important. Restraints should be avoided whenever possible. Insomnia is also a problem for dyspneic patients, who often fear that if they go to sleep they will not wake up. Anxiety worsens dyspnea, and dyspnea leads to anxiety. Depression and anxiety are often overlooked in patients with end-stage lung disease. Like other patients with chronic debilitating illnesses, end-stage lung patients suffer losses of independence, privacy, and a sense of wholeness. The loss of work and other accustomed roles as a parent, child, partner, nurturer, etc. may bring a sense of worthlessness or a loss of meaning or hope, which can result in clinical depression or a spiritual crisis. Psychiatrists and chaplains can be helpful members of the team in this regard.

A. Communication

The most important part of communication is listening, especially to patients and their families. This activity involves some simple mechanics: sitting down and otherwise avoiding appearing rushed, treating silence and tears as legitimate forms of communication, and being willing to witness the speaker's pain without rushing in with a solution. It helps to ask open-ended questions, to repeat or paraphrase the response, to encourage further comments with "verbal leads," such as "umm," or "ah." Sometimes the physician's response should be active, as when suggesting a possible explanation for the patient's observations or remarking on discordance between words and affect. At the conclusion of a conversation it is helpful to integrate and summarize what the patient or family member has said.

The SUPPORT study of 1832 seriously ill, hospitalized patients found that only one-fourth had discussed preferences for cardiopulmonary resuscitation with their physicians, and more than half of those who had not, did not want to do so (12). In another study, fewer than one-third of oxygen-dependent COPD patients had discussed end-of-life options with their physicians, but three-quarters reported that their doctor knew their preference (2). Clearly, someone needs to be facilitating these discussions, and palliative care physicians have experience in goals-of-care conversations.

Before having such a discussion with the patient or the family, it is important to be as sure as possible of the medical facts. This information can be challenging since many subspecialties may be involved in the patient's care, sometimes with several physicians per specialty. There may be fluctuations in the parameters each follows, which may obscure the big picture. Before sharing information with the patient, the physician should find out what the patient understands and what he or she wants to know. Some patients are reassured by having great detail; others want to know nothing and have the physician or someone else make all decisions. American culture emphasizes autonomy over other ethical principles, but in other cultures, elders or families may make decisions for the patient. Substitute decision making is especially challenging. One useful opening is "tell me about your father," followed by, "if he could take part in this discussion, what would he say?" Although physicians often feel a sense of urgency about goals-of-care discussions, it is helpful to view individual conversations as part of a series of discussions (Table 3).

In this context, the words we choose are important. Some physicians prefer "allow natural death" to "do not resuscitate." "Withholding" or "withdrawing" sounds unfeeling or undutiful, while "stopping the ventilator since it is burdensome and no longer fits our goals for your mother" sounds caring. It may be helpful for the physician to practice some phrases to use to introduce difficult topics, such as "if time were short," "hoping for the best and still preparing for what we will do if the treatment doesn't work," etc. Equally important is recognizing that there are some things we should never say, especially, "there is nothing more I can do for you." When cure is no longer possible and the patient wants to focus on quality of life, a transition to hospice may be appropriate. Janet Abrahm suggests framing hospice referral positively by noting that because of the progression of the disease, the

Table 3 Conducting a Family Meeting

Preparation
Clarify conference goals and establish agenda with key clinicians
Agree on basics of medical situation, prognosis and options
Agree on leadership of meeting, note taker
Agree on attendees—ask patient and family who they want
Invite nursing, case management, social service as appropriate
Identify place that assures privacy and comfort
Introductions
Introduce all participants, identify official proxy, leader explains role
If patient cannot attend, bring patient as a person into the room ("Tell me about ___)
Establish ground rules and ask how they like to deal with information
Explain proxy's role
Assess family's understanding of current situation
Ask everyone to speak
Ask family about changes over last weeks and months
Review patient's current medical status
Outline condition, prognosis, and treatment options
Consider making a recommendation
Ask each family member for questions
Respond empathetically to emotional reactions
Family discussion
Ask patient what decisions he or she is considering, and ask family members if they have concerns about plan.
If patient is not participating, ask each family member what he believes the patient would choose
Ask if they would want time alone to discuss options
Wrap-up
Summarize areas of consensus and disagreement
If there is no consensus, identify other resources, such as clergy, other physicians, ethicists, and schedule a follow-up meeting
If there is consensus, caution against unexpected outcomes, and identify a family spokesperson for ongoing communication
Document in chart: those present, decisions made, and follow-up plan

Source: From Ref. 13.

patient is now eligible for additional care and support (14). The patient needs to know that redirecting goals to "intensive caring" can improve symptoms and provide excellent quality of life.

Often patients and families tell us they want "death with dignity." By that they mean they want care in a context that recognizes their uniqueness as human beings, care that honors who they were and are before and in spite of their disease (15). Harvey Max Chochinov promotes "dignity-conserving care," which values the patient as an individual and emphasizes the patient as a whole person (16). It starts with simple questions, such as "is there anything we can do to make you more comfortable?" It involves allowing the patient as many choices and as much normalcy as possible. The tenor of care is important; this is as simple as focusing on the person, not the incontinence. Restraints are not part of dignity-conserving care.

It is not unusual for physicians to feel a sense of failure, as a patient gets sicker. Sometimes the palliative care physician can reframe the situation, pointing out that the attending physician has been successful in helping the patient through many challenges, but now the disease is so extensive that even the best efforts at cure will be fruitless and the primary goal should be comfort. The patients and families fear abandonment and are comforted by the presence and continued active involvement of a trusted doctor or team. Often supporting the patient and family through a comfortable death is as satisfying for the pulmonologist or intensivist as the previous phases of treatment.

B. End of life

Patients contemplating death identify five domains of quality end-of-life care: adequate pain and symptom control, avoiding inappropriate prolongation of dying, achieving a sense of control, relieving the burden on their families, and strengthening relationships with loved ones (17). Surveys of families of ICU patients show that they have parallel needs: to be assured of the patient's comfort, to be with the patient and to be able to help the patient, to be informed of changes in the patient's condition and the treatment plan, to be heard and reassured that their decisions were right, to have their own comfort addressed, and to find meaning in the death of their loved one (18).

There is a growing recognition that palliative care and intensive care are not mutually exclusive. ICUs that were once seen as sterile and inhospitable to families are now attuned to their needs. Often, it is reasonable for patients who have been cared for in the ICU to make a transition to less technologically intense care, supported by the staff they know and trust.

One of the most critical parts of palliative care is to ensure a good death, and this often means stopping treatments that are no longer appropriate to the patient's goals. These treatments may include blood transfusions, hemodialysis, vasopressors, antibiotics, TPN, tube feedings, and even ventilatory support. Before removing the patient from the ventilator support, it is important to make sure that all members of the medical team are in agreement, or at least, that all parties have been heard and that the responsible physician and the patient or representative are in agreement. Inputs should be sought from nursing, respiratory therapy, social work, and pastoral care. The organ procurement organization should be notified, if appropriate. The family should understand that the patient may not die right away and may in fact be transferred out of the ICU, and in rare cases, may even leave the hospital. They should be prepared for what they may see. It is important to have a specific plan. If the patient is on paralytic medication, it should be stopped so that any distress will be apparent and thus treated. The physician decides whether the endotracheal tube will be removed or the ventilator settings gradually decreased to zero. With extubation there may be airway problems, but the physician's intent is clear. The family is often relieved that the patient is free of the tube. Turning down the ventilator settings may be easier for the family to watch than extubation, but this may be confused with efforts at therapeutic weaning. In either case, it is important to treat respiratory distress promptly and aggressively with opioids and benzodiazepines. When the patient is extubated rather than weaned, treatment of respiratory distress should be prophylactic unless the patient is brain dead. Special attention must be paid to the family. They are likely to recall this scene for years. Where will the family be when support is withdrawn? Will they want to say a prayer with the chaplain? Will they be present for extubation or be perhaps behind the curtain or outside the door? Who will be there to support the family? Palliative care includes bereavement support, usually through notes and telephone call, but sometimes by attending the funeral.

III. Clinical Vignettes

These three cases represent common situations in pulmonary palliative care. The first is a patient who was never on a ventilator. The second was a patient who was removed from a ventilator, and the third was a patient who died at home on a ventilator after a long hospital course.

VL is an 86-year-old man with advanced COPD and severe hypertension. He attended the PR clinic until severe dyspnea precluded outpatient visits. The same pulmonologist followed him for many years, and they had repeated discussions about goals of care. The patient made it clear that he did not want intubation, or resuscitation, or even hospital admission. He became progressively more homebound and elected hospice, but used very few services. Reluctantly, he has come to accept a small dose of morphine for dyspnea once or twice a day. Although he clearly met hospice eligibility criteria for end-stage lung disease when he enrolled in hospice (disabling dyspnea, progression of pulmonary disease, and body weight $< 90\%$ ideal), he has survived 18 months and has been recertified for hospice twice. Perhaps his social isolation (he has not been outside in over a year) has protected him from respiratory infections, which might have led to a fatal exacerbation otherwise.

In this case, a series of discussions with a trusted pulmonologist clarified the patient's goals of care and prevented the patient from receiving interventions he never wanted. His survival in hospice has surprised him, his physician, and his hospice nurses. While he is able to stay at home with his wife, his quality of life is severely compromised by his dyspnea. He remains reluctant to use opioids to treat the dyspnea. This case exemplifies the difficulty in predicting which patients with severe lung disease will die within six months.

JB was a 29-year-old man with cystic fibrosis. He had undergone bilateral lung transplantation, but suffered from severe chronic rejection. He was severely ill with non-reversible airway obstruction and chronic respiratory failure, complicated by methicillin-resistant *Staphylococcus aureus* (MRSA) and Pseudomonas colonization, malnutrition, and diabetes. He could not tolerate bi-level positive airway pressure, and he and his family chose a time-limited trial of invasive ventilation. After several days there was no significant improvement, so he was extubated and started on a morphine drip with the understanding that he would not be reintubated. On the morphine drip his breathing improved and he was comfortable and able to respond to questions. He lived for approximately two weeks, dying peacefully in the hospital with his family at his bedside.

In this case, the patient and his family had initially chosen a very active level of care, including transplantation. When his respiratory condition worsened and they had to make another decision regarding the intensity of therapy in the face of apparently irreversible disease, they chose a time-limited trial of intubation. Patients often tell us they do not want to be on a long-term ventilator, but they would like a trial to see if some part of the clinic picture is reversible. Chronic rejection meant this patient's survival off the ventilator was not possible, and the patient and his family elected to prioritize comfort care. The morphine drip was begun as part of the patient's end-of-life care, and to the surprise of his family and some of his physicians and family, it relieved dyspnea without worsening respiratory failure. Apart from its central effects on the perception of dyspnea, morphine may have helped by decreasing dynamic hyperinflation via a decrease in tachypnea. Opioids allowed the patient two comfortable weeks and a peaceful death.

MC was a 69-year-old woman with a history of hypertension and depression who was admitted to the hospital with progressive weakness. She was found to have a progressive degenerative neurologic disease. She developed aspiration pneumonia and respiratory failure and was intubated. Her complicated course spanned more than eight months and included bowel ischemia, a massive intra-abdominal bleed, thromboembolic problems requiring bilateral femoral embolectomies, MRSA infection, cholecystitis, an ischemic stroke, and a GI bleed requiring many transfusions. Although she regained consciousness, she was not able to make decisions and her health care proxy refused to act. Her family members disagreed frequently among themselves, but in general insisted that "everything be done." They avoided family meetings, making it difficult to plan for her transfer to a skilled nursing facility. Eventually, they decided to take her home on a ventilator on hospice. For the first ten days or so she had round-the-clock nursing care, but, eventually, one daughter took over the bulk of her care and nurses visited several times a week. She survived at home for about seven weeks.

This case illustrates the challenges of ventilator care for patients with progressive neurologic disorders. The patient's wishes were unclear; the family was in disarray, and frequently threatened legal action. The hospitalist found the case overwhelming. Several extended care facilities (ECF) declined to accept the patient. She was marooned in the hospital until her family eventually agreed to home hospice care.

Ventilation in degenerative neurologic conditions is very challenging. Ventilation can be used to tide the patient over a complication or it can be a permanent treatment. In some cases patients and families elect a trial of ventilation. Although there may be no ethical difference between not starting a treatment and withdrawing it, there is an emotional difference. This condition is particularly true for ventilation, both invasive and noninvasive. Most often, patients come to ventilation in the course of sudden respiratory failure. They are intubated and ventilated, and cannot be weaned. The progressive neurologic disorder means that their quality of life is diminishing. Long-term hospital care is usually not an option, and the patient and family must choose between care in an ECF and care at home. Often patients say they would die rather than go to an ECF. Care of a ventilator patient at home puts tremendous burdens on the family, and these strains are compounded by the fact that some patients, such as those with amyotrophic lateral sclerosis, may survive for years on home ventilation. Even a brief period at home is extremely stressful to the family.

IV. Summary

Palliative care is an important modality for patients with chronic respiratory disease, whether or not they receive ventilatory support. It is also important for patients with extrapulmonary disease suffering from respiratory failure. Despite uncertainty about the prognosis, the input from many specialists must be integrated; the patient and family supported and helped to articulate goals of care, all while the patient is kept as comfortable as possible.

References

1. Gore JM, Brophy CJ, Greenstone MA. How well do we care for patients with end stage chronic obstructive pulmonary disease (COPD)? A comparison of palliative care and quality of life in COPD and lung cancer. Thorax 2000; 55:1000–1006.
2. Knauft E, Nielsen EL, Engelberg RA. Barriers and facilitators to end-of-life care communication for patients with COPD. Chest 2005; 127:2188–2196.
3. Kvale PA, Simoff M, Prakash UB. Palliative Care. Chest 2003; 123:284S–311S.
4. Selecky PA, Eliasson AH, Hall RI, et al. Palliative and end-of-life care for patients with cardiopulmonary diseases—American college of chest physicians position statement. Chest 2005; 128:3599–3610.
5. Celli BR, MacNee W, and committee members. Standards for the diagnosis and treatment of patients with COPD: a summary of the ATS/ERS position paper. Eur Respir J 2004; 23:932–946.
6. Connors AF, Dawson NV, Thomas C, et al. Outcomes following acute exacerbation of severe chronic obstructive lung disease. Am J Respir Crit Care Med 1996; 154:959–967.
7. Afessa B, Marales I, Scanlon P, et al. Prognostic factors, clinical course, and hospital outcome of patients with chronic obstructive pulmonary disease admitted to an intensive care unit for acute respiratory failure. Crit Care Med 2002; 30:1610–1615.
8. Fox E, Landrum-McNiff K, Zong Z. Evaluation of prognostic criteria for determining hospice eligibility in patients with advanced lung, heart or liver disease. JAMA 1999; 282:1638–1645.
9. Christakis NA, Escarce JJ. Survival of Medicare patients after enrollment in hospice programs. N Engl J Med 1996; 335:172–178.
10. Luce JM, Luce JA. Management of dyspnea in patients with far-advanced lung disease—"Once I lose it, it's kind of hard to catch it." JAMA 2001; 285:1331–1337.
11. Desbiens Nam Wu AW. Pain and suffering in seriously ill hospitalized patients. J Am Geriatr Soc 2000; 48:S183–S186.
12. Hoffman JC, Wenger NS, Davis RB, et al. Patient preferences for communication with physicians about end-of-life decisions. Ann Intern Med 1997; 127:1–12.
13. Weisman, D. 1998 Fast Fact #16 Conducting a Family Meeting. End of Life Physician Education Resource Center www.eperc.mcw.edu
14. Abrahm JL, Hansen-Flasschen J. Hospice care for patients with advanced lung disease. Chest 2002; 121:220–229.
15. Murray SA, Kendal M, Boyd K, et al. Exploring the spiritual needs of people dying of lung cancer or heart failure: a prospective qualitative interview study of patients and their carers. Palliat Med 2004; 18:39–45.
16. Chochinov HM. Dignity-conserving care—a new model for palliative Care. JAMA 2002; 287:2253–2260.
17. Singer PA, Martin DK, Kelner M. Quality end-of-life care: patients' perspectives. JAMA 1999; 281:163–168.
18. Truog RD, Cist AFM, Brackett SE, et al. Recommendations for end-of-life care in the intensive care unit: The Ethics Committee of the Society of Critical Care Medicine. Crit Care Med 2001; 29:2332–2348.
19. Classens MT, Lynn J, Zhong Z, et al. Dying with lung cancer or chronic obstructive pulmonary disease: insights from SUPPORT. J Am Geriatr Soc 2000; 48:S146-S153.

34
Management of Chronic Respiratory Failure and Obesity

JEAN-FRANÇOIS MUIR and ANTOINE CUVELIER
Pulmonary Department and Respiratory Intensive Care Unit, Rouen University Hospital, Rouen, France

I. Introduction

Obesity is defined as an excessive accumulation of fat, with a resulting increase of body mass index (BMI) > 30 kg/m^2. A BMI > 25 (overweight) represents a health-risk factor, and obesity is the most frequently found health risk in the United States, where more than one in three adults weigh 20% over the ideal value. The prevalence of obesity is 3.5 million in the United States (26% adults of 20–75 years), reaching 31% of the male and 35% of the female population. The prevalence of extreme obesity (BMI $\geq$ 40 kg/m^2) has quadrupled and that of BMI $\geq$ 50 kg/m^2 has increased fivefold (1). Obese patients frequently present with acute on chronic respiratory failure (CRF) in the emergency ward, or are discovered in a chronic status as they are investigated for suspicion of obstructive sleep apnea syndrome (OSAS), for assessment of CRF, or for preoperative evaluation.

The majority of obese subjects with obstructive sleep apnea (OSA) have normal alveolar ventilation when awake. However, in a subgroup of subjects, hypoventilation while awake will be present. Approximately 10–15% of patients with OSAS present with daytime chronic respiratory failure with hypoxia, hypercapnia, and pulmonary hypertension (PH) (2), half of them having an overlap syndrome that associates with OSAS and chronic obstructive pulmonary disease (COPD) (3,4) and the other half presenting with obesity hypoventilation syndrome (OHS) (5).

OHS, previously called the "Pickwickian syndrome" (6), is defined as the association of obesity, sleep-disordered breathing (SDB) with daytime hypersomnolence, and hypercapnia (PaCO_2 > 45 mmHg) in the absence of any other respiratory disease (Fig. 1). SDB can present as obstructive apneas and hypopneas, obstructive hypoventilation due to increased upper airway resistance, and/or central hypoventilation (7). The prevalence of OHS is 36% in patients with BMI between 35 and 40 kg/m^2, and 48%, if BMI equals or exceeds 50 (8). Without adequate treatment, patients with OHS develop cor pulmonale and recurrent episodes of hypercapnic respiratory failure, and loss of survival (Fig. 2). OHS is one of the many etiologies of CRF and has become a growing indication to initiate long-term noninvasive ventilation (NIV) in most European countries (9,10).

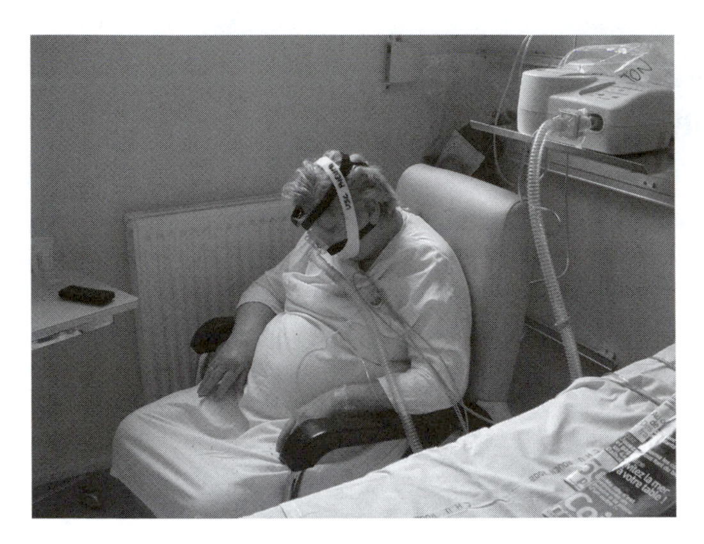

Figure 1 Patients presenting with OHS. *Abbreviation:* OHS, obesity hypoventilation syndrome.

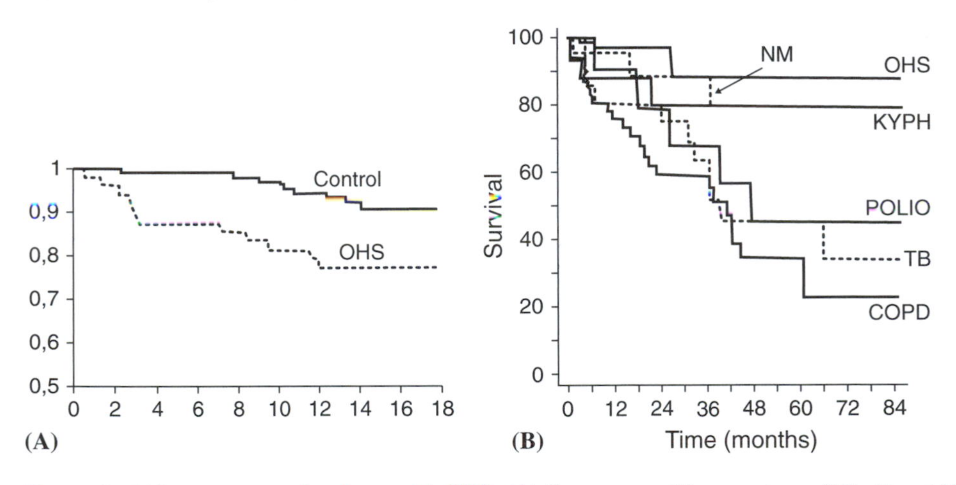

Figure 2 Life expectancy of patients with OHS. (**A**) Spontaneous life expectancy (38), N = 148 patients. (**B**) Comparison between OHS and various etiologies of CRF (9). *Abbreviations*: OHS, obesity hypoventilation syndrome; CRF, chronic respiratory failure.

II. Pathophysiology

Obesity reduces the emergency relief value and, to a lesser extent, the functional residual capacity (FRC). In more severe disease, it also reduces the vital capacity and the total lung capacity. Obesity is also associated with an increase in respiratory resistance and a reduction in thoracic cage compliance. It doubles the work of breathing and quadruples the energy cost of breathing (11). To meet these demands, ventilatory drive is doubled with a higher respiratory rate and a smaller tidal volume. When the obese patient is awake and supine, the compliance of the ribcage is decreased, and, therefore, the supine FRC is lower than the upright FRC, with a reduction in ventilation-perfusion ratio inequality and secondary hypoxemia (12).

Breathing during sleep is also modified by obesity and may present with different patterns, e.g., no hypoxemia and (heavy) snoring, with possible upper airway resistance syndrome; periodic hypoxemia with hypopneas; periodic hypoxemia and sleep apneas, and continuous hypoxemia, with or without long periods of hypoventilation (13).

The mechanisms that contribute toward the development of OHS include abnormal pulmonary mechanics with an excessive work of breathing and alteration of the central control of ventilation. Altered hypoxic and hypercapnic ventilatory responses are present, but do not explain the development of OHS, as tracheostomy or noninvasive ventilation (NIV) do not always modify these responses, even if hypoxia and hypercapnia are improved. These altered ventilatory responses seem to be partly linked to the chronic hypoxemia and poor sleep quality, upper airway obstruction, and possibly the influence of leptin (14,15). Leptin is produced in white adipose tissue and acts in the hypothalamus to inhibit appetite (16). Obese humans demonstrate very high levels of leptin that do not seem to suppress appetite, suggesting that human obesity may be a leptin-resistant state. Thus, central leptin resistance in some obese individuals may lead to depressed ventilatory drive and consequent OHS (17). Conversely, serum leptin decreases in patients with OHS when treated with NIV, further suggesting a relationship between OHS pathogenesis and leptin signaling (15,18). Another factor to explain OHS is the frequent presence of an OSA pattern during sleep, which could act according to the duration of the interapneic period through a nocturnal accumulation of CO_2 (19).

OHS may present with various possible sleep respiratory patterns (obstructive apneas, hypoventilation, and sometimes, central apneas, or a combined pattern) (7) and needs polysomnographic evaluation to adapt the ventilatory treatment, which is then mandatory (Fig. 3) either as nasal continuous positive airway pressure (nCPAP) or bi-level positive airway pressure ventilation, generally with oxygen supplementation if severe desaturation is present.

Using nasal or facial interfaces, NIV alleviates respiratory failure of various origins. Its mechanisms of action include resting the respiratory muscles, increasing thoracic compliance, and resetting the respiratory centers (20). In OHS, nocturnal NIV has been shown to be clinically effective because of a rapid and sustained improvement in daytime arterial blood gas levels (9) and a net reduction of daytime sleepiness. However, mechanisms of improvement remain unclear, as well as the pathophysiology and the natural history of the disease.

Fifteen OHS patients were recently evaluated by full nocturnal polysomnography (PSG) and thereafter, stratified according to their diurnal CO_2 ventilatory responses (21). With NIV, the Epworth sleepiness scale and Osler test scores significantly improved only in patients having low CO_2 sensitivity. Sleep latencies were significantly shorter in patients having low CO_2 sensitivity. No clinical characteristics could differentiate the patients having normal or impaired CO_2 sensitivity at baseline, since they had similar BMIs, similar daytime hypoxemia and daytime hypercapnia levels, similar indices of nocturnal respiratory disturbances, and similar severity of desaturation during sleep. Domiciliary NIV would have reset the respiratory centers and therefore improved CO_2 sensitivity, but this was not the case for five of seven patients (71%). NIV improved Pa_{CO_2}, restored sleep architecture (increased stage 3–4 and rapid eye movement sleep), corrected nocturnal desaturations, and decreased the respiratory disturbance index and microarousals. The mechanisms of the improvements in sleep and daytime Pa_{CO_2}, without any significant change in CO_2 sensitivity and without concomitant weight loss, are unclear.

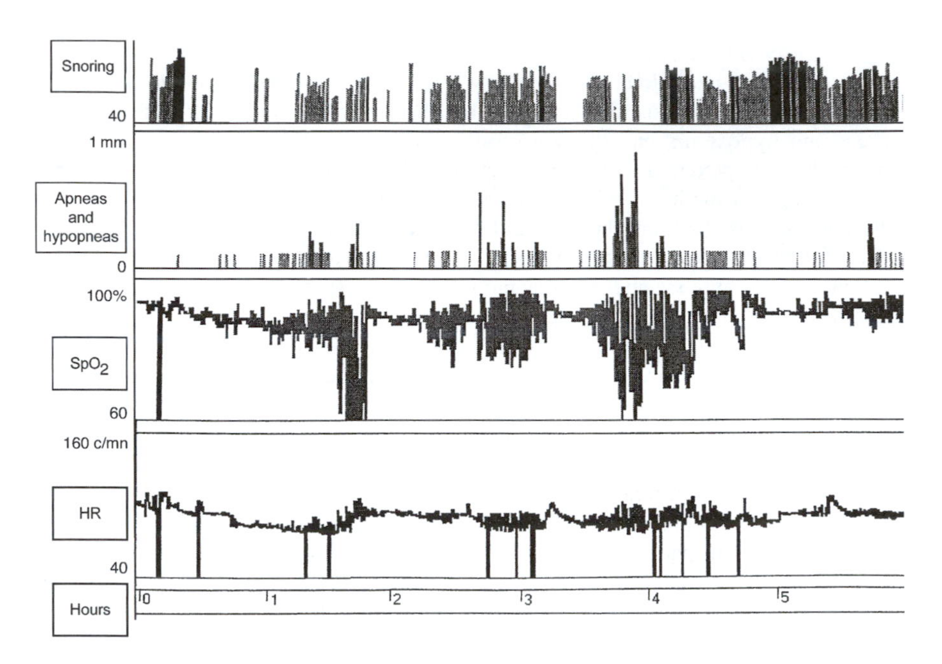

Figure 3 Ventilatory polygraphy of a patient with severe OHS. IAH = 26; Pao_2 = 9.6 kPa; $Paco_2$ = 8.5 kPa (O_2 3L/min). *Abbreviations*: OHS, obesity hypoventilation syndrome; IAH, intra-abdominal hypertension; $Paco_2$, partial pressure of carbon dioxide in arterial blood.

It may be suggested that the coexistence of OSAS in all the OHS patients could be an explanation for the observed improvement of $Paco_2$ values. OSAS occurs in approximately 70% to 90% of all OHS cases (7), but previously published studies in these patients did not analyze the response to NIV according to the nocturnal pattern (i.e., hypoventilation with or without OSAS). Perhaps the patients in the present study took advantage of bi-level NIV because the ventilatory assistance suppressed underlying obstructive apneas and hypopneas, and partly prevented CO_2 load in the same way. Because NIV regularly improves OHS patients but not always normalizes CO_2 response, the specific impact of the ventilatory assistance remains to be evaluated on each component of the OHS pathophysiology: correction of OSAS, correction of hypoventilation, unloading of respiratory muscles (22), improvement in the forced vital capacity (23), or more recent factors, such as leptin resistance, inflammation, or genetic factors (24).

III. Management of Obese Patients and CRF

A. Ventilatory Management

nCPAP Versus Bi-level NIV

Approximately 10–15% of patients with OSAS present with daytime CRF along with hypoxia, hypercapnia, and PH (2). When these patients present with a stable respiratory status, their nocturnal pattern of predominant OSA leads to a discussion on the use of nCPAP as the first step, rather than bi-level NIV. No clear answer has been given and there are no long-term studies to confirm whether this is a good initial choice, even in the presence of hypercapnia.

In a recent study (25), the impact of continuous positive airway pressure (CPAP) titration on the sleep architecture, respiratory events, and nocturnal hypoxemia was compared in 23 patients with OHS and significant daytime hypercapnia and also in 23 patients with eucapnic OSA matched for BMI, apnea-hypopnea index (AHI) with severe SDB, and lung function. Both groups were extremely obese (BMI > 50). After a full night diagnostic PSG, the two groups had a full night of CPAP titration without supplemental oxygen therapy. CPAP resolved SDB and nocturnal hypoxemia in 57% of patients with OHS. The optimal CPAP of 13.9 ± 3.1 cmH_2O was reached within one hour of sleep onset. CPAP was unable to resolve refractory hypoxemia in 43% of patients with OHS; these patients had a higher BMI, more severe nocturnal hypoxemia at baseline, and a higher residual AHI during the night of CPAP titration than those with successful titration. Overall, CPAP led to significant increase in rapid eye movement sleep and significant reduction in arousal index and AHI both in patients with eucapnic OSA and OHS. Thus, time spent with $Spo_2 < 90\%$ during sleep with nCPAP in OHS could be proposed to identify those who may not respond to nCPAP, for whom NIV is indicated.

A recent, large retrospective study (26) looked at the effect of CPAP adherence on respiratory failure in patients with OSA. This study shows that good compliance with CPAP leads to an improvement in respiratory failure with comparable improvements in those subjects receiving bi-level ventilation. There was also a reduction in the need for oxygen supplementation, with time. However, patients who continued to spend a significant percentage of their thallium stress test with $Spo_2 < 90\%$, despite the elimination of upper airway collapse, would be good candidates for NIV. Randomized prospective studies are necessary to confirm this hypothesis.

Bi-level NIV

Mechanical ventilation (MV) with bi-level NIV must be considered in the presence of nocturnal hypoventilation, especially if accompanied by cor pulmonale, nocturnal arrythmias, morning headache, impaired cognitive function, or reduced daytime vigilance. Right heart failure is also frequently present. The "obese sleepy patient" (27) with chronic hypoxia and hypercapnia is the typical presentation of OHS. To adapt to NIV, it is important to identify the nocturnal respiratory pattern of such patients.

Masa et al. (28) reported on the treatment of 22 pure OHS patients (AHI < 20) with nocturnal NIV, using either a volume-cycled ventilator or bi-level NIV; 11 patients also required supplemental oxygen. Symptoms of daytime somnolence and dyspnea improved with $Paco_2$ falling from 58 ± 10 to 45 ± 5 mmHg after four months. NIV with either volume-cycled or bi-level pressure ventilation is the mainstay of treatment (28–30). The past years have seen an increase in the use of bi-level pressure respirators for this indication. After treatment with NIV, breathlessness on exertion, quality of sleep, daytime sleepiness and fatigue, and early morning headaches improve (28). Furthermore, nocturnal and daytime arterial blood gas levels improve, often within the first few days of treatment (29–31). Recent data about a very large group of patients who had OHS treated with NIV (9) in 29%, and pressure-cycled ventilators in 90% showed a very significant decrease in the number of hospital stays for cardiac or respiratory illness for the three years after the use

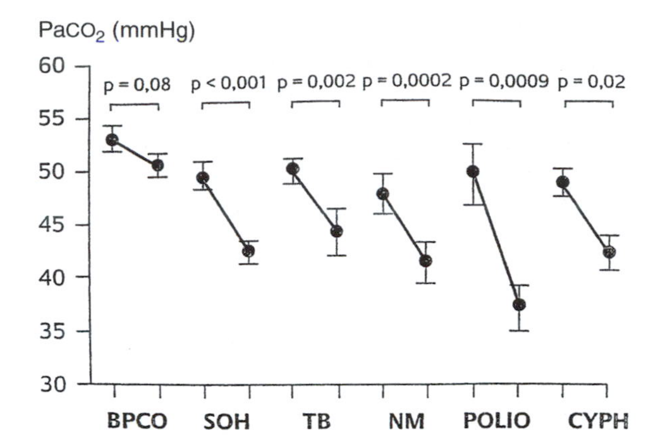

Figure 4 Improvement of ABG in different etiologies of CRF receiving long-term home ventilation. *Abbreviations*: ABG, arterial blood gas volume; CRF, chronic respiratory failure. *Source*: From Ref. 9.

of noninvasive positive pressure ventilation (NPPV) therapy, compared to the year before, as well as a marked improvement in blood gases (31) (Fig. 4).

Good compliance suggested that this treatment was cost-effective as well as improving morbidity and mortality in such patients (Fig. 2).

A previous study (14) has suggested that nocturnal NIV could be used as an interim measure in subjects with severe OSA and hypercapnia until ventilatory decompensation is reversed (possibly by alterations in ventilatory drive and ventilatory responses to hypercapnia and hypoxia) and CPAP therapy can then be used long term. Others (30) have shown that a proportion of patients may be switched over to CPAP once respiratory failure has been controlled. CPAP therapy from the start, rather than bi-level ventilation followed by CPAP, may be just as effective (particularly improving sleep architecture and arousals) and potentially more cost-effective in patients with OHS, even if blood gases are not corrected immediately.

Nocturnal hypoventilation, which persists during the day in obese patients with nocturnal apneas and hypoventilation may be associated with COPD, defining the "overlap syndrome" (3). In 264 OSAS patients (32), 30 had coexistent COPD, with hypoxemia in 57%, hypercapnia in 27%, and PH in 37% of them. In the other 234 "pure" OSAS patients, only 26% were hypoxic, 8.5% were hypercapnic, and 11 % had PH at baseline. The same schedule may be proposed for OHS, but long-term studies are also warranted to confirm the initial choice and continuation of nCPAP or bi-level NIV.

B. Technical Aspects

Short-term studies have shown that among obese patients with OSAS and hypercapnic respiratory failure there is a subgroup of patients who require NIV to correct their arterial blood gas (ABG) levels and to treat symptoms of hypercapnic respiratory failure. These patients have a higher BMI (mean $\geq$ 40 kg/m^2), a higher daytime $Paco_2$, and lower daytime Pao_2, or nocturnal Sao_2 than those who can be managed with CPAP alone (29,33–35). Long-term NIV therapy was also shown to be effective in improving arterial blood gas levels and in treating symptoms of hypercapnic respiratory failure in patients with OHS but without severe OSAS (AHI < 20) (28). Two studies (23,30) confirm improvements in respiratory failure by treatment with bi-level ventilation over a period of at least one year.

Occurrence of dyssynchrony in OHS during NIV has been recently described in 20 OHS patients in stable clinical condition treated by NIV for at least three months with a bi-level pressure support and submitted to single-night PSG under NIV including transcutaneous measurement of Pco_2 ($TcPco_2$) (36). Four types of respiratory events were defined and quantified: patient/ventilator desynchronization, periodic breathing, autotriggering, and apnea-hypopneas. Eleven patients (55%) exhibited desynchronization occurring mostly in slow-wave sleep and rapid eye movement sleep and associated with arousals but not inducing significant changes in $TcPco_2$ or oxygen saturation using Spo_2. Eight patients (40%) showed a high index of periodic breathing, mostly occurring in light sleep and associated with more severe nocturnal hypoxemia. Autotriggering was sporadic and usually limited to one or two breaths, although prolonged and asymptomatic autotriggering occurred in one patient during 10.6% of total sleep time. Thus, patient/ventilatory asynchrony and periodic breathing are respiratory patterns occurring frequently in OHS patients treated using NPPV. Nocturnal monitoring of Spo_2 and $TcPco_2$, commonly used to assess the efficacy of ventilatory support, do not adequately explore this aspect of therapy that might influence its efficacy as well as sleep quality.

Bi-level NIV may be used as a first-line treatment, with supplemental oxygen (27). Expiratory airway pressure is titrated to control hypopneas and apneas, and inspiratory airway pressure is added to control $Paco_2$. If bi-level NIV fails, nasal volume ventilation may be used (29). In many patients with OHS and predominant OSA, once hypercapnia has improved (which may take several weeks) nCPAP may be used (29). Thirteen obese patients (n = 13) with a BMI > 35, aged 28–69 years with severe OSAS and hypercapnia (8.2 ± 0.3 kPa) and failing to respond to initial CPAP therapy, were treated via a nasal nocturnal volume-cycled ventilator, which was tolerated by all patients. Significant improvements in daytime arterial blood gas levels were obtained after 7 to 18 days of nasal intermittent positive pressure ventilation (29) in 10 of the 13 patients; three months later, 12 of the 13 patients could be converted to nCPAP therapy and one patient remained on NIV. In another study (37), the same results were observed after three months of home nocturnal bi-level NIV in seven patients, three of whom had severe obesity.

Thus, the indications for a trial of bi-level NIV in obese patients with CRF are progressive respiratory failure with excessive sleepiness, with daytime hypercapnia and OHS in the setting of OSAS that has not correctly responded to nCPAP, with disorders of ventilatory control and daytime hypercapnia or sleepiness (27,38,39) (Fig. 5).

C. Medical Management

Weight loss has proven effective. A reduction of 5% to 10% of body weight can result in a significant fall in $Paco_2$ (40,41). Unfortunately, weight loss by diet alone is difficult to achieve and sustain; thus, bariatric surgery has been advocated. After weight reduction surgery in 31 patients with OHS who had initial and follow-up (1 year) arterial blood gas data, BMI fell from 56 ± 13 to 38 ± 9 kg/m^2 and $Paco_2$ from 53 ± 9 to 44 ± 8 mmHg (42). However, operative mortality (defined as occurring within 30 days) was 4% in the total of 126 OHS patients subjected to a variety of bariatric surgical techniques, compared to 0.2% in the 884 eucapnic patients (42). It is possible that laparoscopic bariatric surgery may be

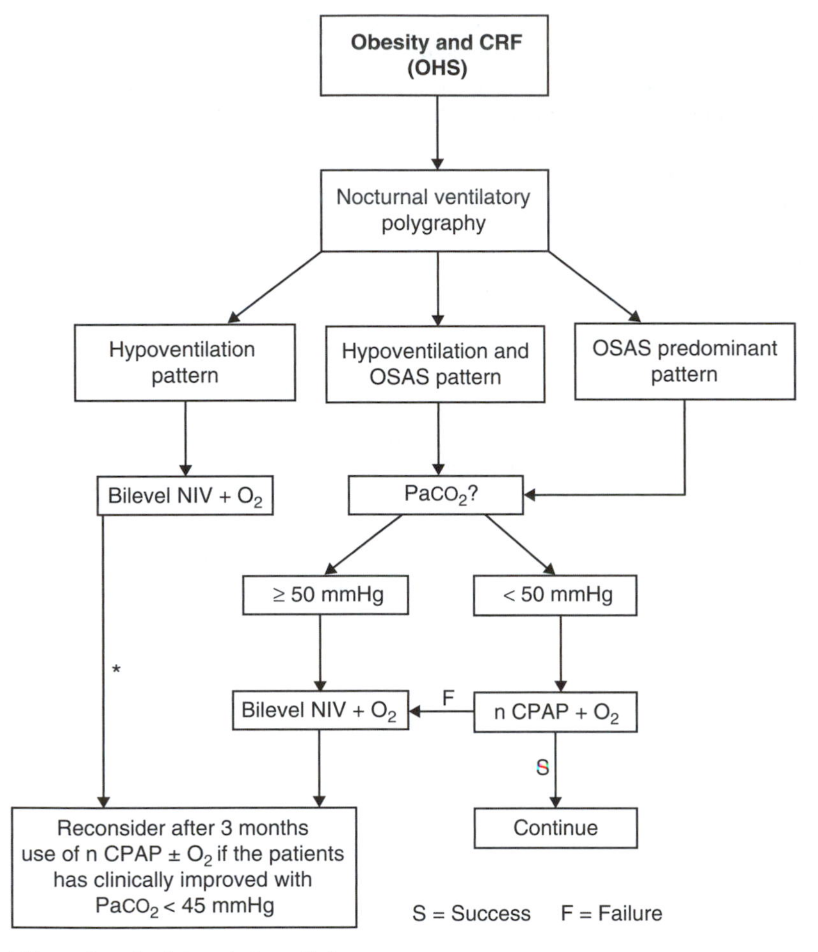

Figure 5 Ventilatory management algorithm in OHS and presenting with CRF. *Abbreviations*: OHS, obesity hypoventilation syndrome; CRF, chronic respiratory failure. *Source*: From Ref. 38.

more broadly and safely utilized in the future, even if general anesthesia always represents a risk in patients with CRF and general severe obesity (40).

IV. Acute-on-Chronic Respiratory Failure and Obese Patients

Acute respiratory failure (ARF) is nowadays a frequent reason for admission to a respiratory intensive care unit (RICU). In a recent study of 150 patients, mortality after hospitalization was 23% in 47 patients with OHS and 9% in 52 patients with isolated obesity. Morbidity for OHS patients was higher, related to a more important need for MV, with more frequent stays in RICU, and the need for subsequent care in a long-term care facility (8). NIV has largely improved the prognosis of OHS and ARF.

Six patients with morbid obesity (159 ± 19% predicted body weight) and OSAS in ARF (pH 7.23 ± 0.03; $Paco_2$ 10.6 ± 0.5 kPa) were immediately treated with nCPAP and oxygen with an improvement in clinical and respiratory status within 24 hours of MV (43). These data were confirmed in six other patients with ARF and encephalopathy (44) (BMI, 50.3 ± 4.8 kg/m^2; pH, 7.26 ± 0.06; $Paco_2$, 10.5 ± 2.5 kPa; Pao_2, 6.3 ± 0.8 kPa breathing air). Bi-level NIV was applied at a back-up respiratory frequency of 10/min, with an inspiratory positive airway pressure (IPAP) of 18 cmH_2O and an expiratory positive airway pressure (EPAP) of 6 cmH_2O at the beginning of the management. Increments of 2 cmH_2O were applied, according to the clinical status, with supplemental oxygen at 2–4 L/min. A rapid improvement was observed in clinical status and arterial blood gas levels, within 24 hours. No intubation was required and the AHI on discharge from the ICU facility was 63 ± 9.

In a population of 207 OSAS patients (45), 25 had been diagnosed as having OSAS after an ARF episode requiring endotracheal ventilation; 182 were diagnosed on PSG without any previous ARF episode. The ARF etiology was an episode of bronchial infection in 10 cases and a slow worsening of previous CRF in 12 patients. The Simplified Acute Physiology Score was 13 + 3 and the duration of MV was 12 ± 2 days. Survival in the ICU was observed in all 25 patients presenting with ARF. Three months after the ARF episode, six patients were treated at home with MV and 19 with nCPAP; three years later, three deaths secondary to new episodes of ARF were observed and four patients were lost to follow-up. Comparing the 25 OSAS with ARF and the other 182 OSAS patient without previous ARF, the two predictive factors were forced respiratory value in one second and the level of baseline hypercapnia. No differences were found between the two groups in AHI, age, BMI, and sex ratio. In another retrospective study of 20 obese patients (46), immediate success was obtained in 18 patients initially treated with NIV via a facial or nasal mask; two patients had to be intubated after initial failure with NIV. One month later, PSG recordings at steady state showed that nine patients had OSAS and 11 had OHS. Of these, 11 were secondarily discharged under NIV. In this group, the primary use of pressure support ventilators (seven patients) was associated with quicker improvements in Pao_2/Fio_2 ratio, $Paco_2$, and pH compared to the use of volume ventilators (seven patients). Because of the initial failure of volume ventilation, four patients had to be moved to pressure support ventilation with secondary success. In another report (34), 41 obese patients with ARF were treated via bi-level NIV as the first-line ventilatory treatment with 16 cmH_2O IPAP and 4 cmH_2O EPAP as primary ventilatory settings. EPAP and IPAP were secondarily adapted to stabilize Sao_2. The mean age was 63 ± 11 years, the BMI was 42 ± 9 kg/m^2, pH was 7.32 ± 0.04, Pao_2 was 9.4 ± 1.7 kPa, and $Paco_2$ was 6.0 ± 0.9 kPa. Of 41 patients, 39 were successfully treated without need for endotracheal ventilation. After seven days, $Paco_2$ was 6.7 ± 0.8 kPa. Six patients were pure OSAS, 19 had OHS, four had COPD without OSAS, and 10 had an overlap syndrome. A therapeutic algorithm has been proposed to manage such conditions, which may occur until 25% of admissions in the RICU (47) (Fig. 6).

NIV is efficient in ARF and CRF and obesity; parallel monitoring with PSG improves the assessment of the etiology of respiratory failure to decide the immediate and long-term treatment and to adjust to MV (48). Future studies are warranted to assess the long-term effects of MV, optimal choice of the best kind of respiratory assistance (barometric vs. volumetric vs. nCPAP) and of the long-term progress of patients with OHS.

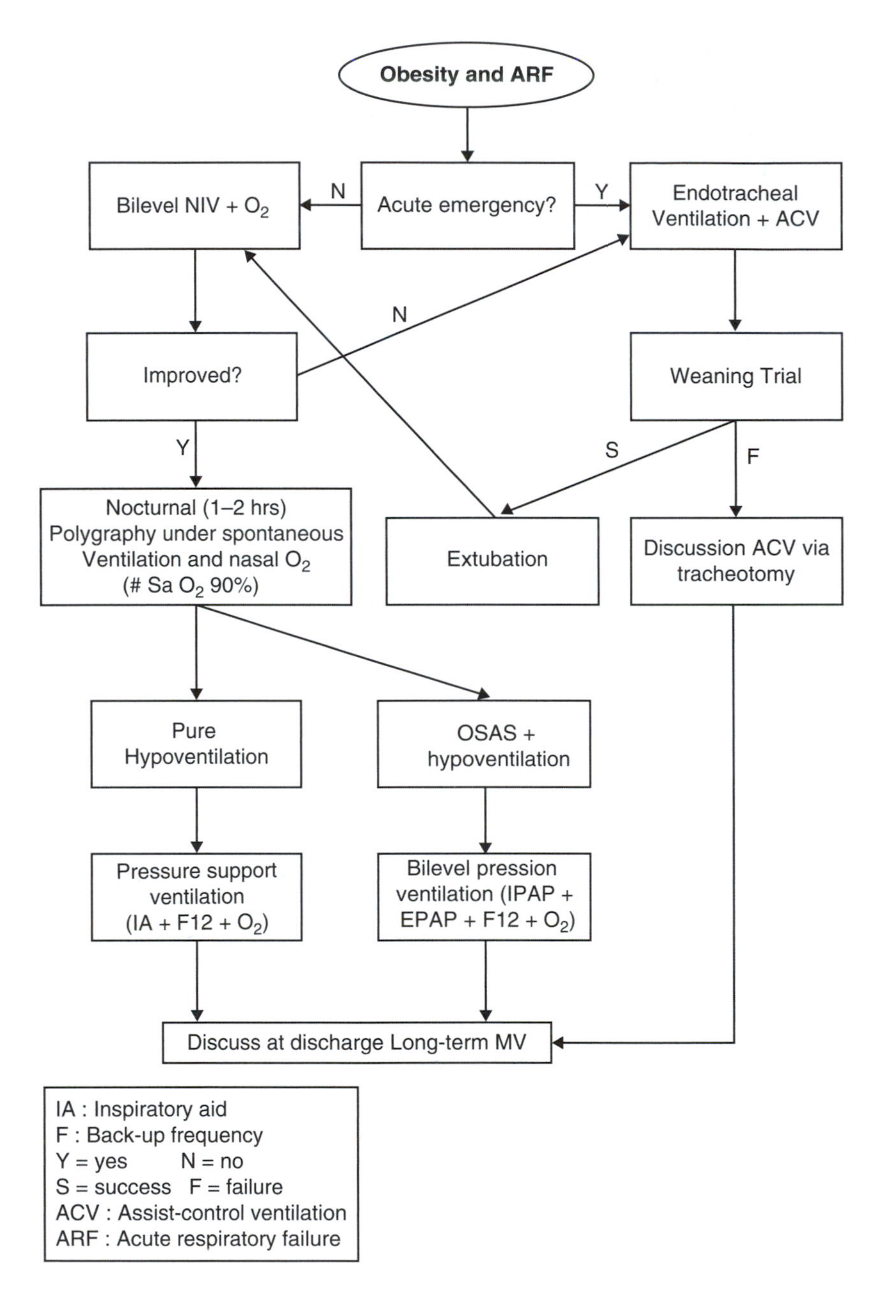

Figure 6 Ventilatory management in OHS and ARF. *Abbreviations*: OHS, obesity hypoventilation syndrome; ARF, acute respiratory failure. *Source*: From Ref. 47.

References

1. Freedman DS, Khan LK, Serdula MK. Trends and correlates of class 3 obesity in the US from 1990 through 2000. JAMA 2002; 288:1758–1761.
2. Weitzenblum E. Syndrome d'apnées du sommeil et insuffisance respiratoire. Rev Mal Respir 1994; 11:1–3.
3. Flenley DC. Sleep in chronic obstructive lung disease. Clin Chest Med 1985; 6:651–661.
4. Fletcher EC, Schaaf JM, Miller J, et al. Long-term cardiopulmonary sequelae in patients with sleep apnea and chronic lung disease. Am Rev Respir Dis 1987; 135:525–533.
5. – Association of COPD and OSAS, and Chaouat A, Weitzenblum E, Krieger J, et al. Am J Respir Crit Care Med 1995; 151:82–86.
6. Burwell CS, Robin ED, Whaley R, et al. Extreme obesity associated with alveolar hypoventilation. A Pickwickian syndrome. Am J Med 1956; 21:811–816.
7. Kessler R, Chaouat A, Schinkewitch P, et al. The obesity-hypoventilation syndrome revisited: a prospective study of 34 consecutive cases. Chest 2001; 120:369–376.
8. Nowbar-Burkart KM, Gonzales R. Obesity associated hypoventilation in hospitalized patients: prevalence, effects and outcome. Am J Med 2004; 116:1–7.
9. Janssens JP, Derivaz S, Breitenstein E, et al. Changing patterns in long-term noninvasive ventilation: a 7-year prospective study in the Geneva Lake area. Chest 2003; 123:67–79.
10. Krachman S, Criner GJ. Hypoventilation syndromes in sleep disorders. Clin Chest Med 1998; 19:139–156.
11. Ray CS, Sue DY, Bray G, et al. Effects of obesity on respiratory function. Am Rev Respir Dis 1983; 128:501–506.
12. Rochester DF. Obesity and pulmonary function. In: Alpert MA, Alexander JK, eds. The Heart and Lung in Obesity. New York: Futura Publishing Co., 1997; 109–131.
13. Koenig SM, Suran PM. Obesity and sleep disordered breathing. DF obesity and pulmonary function. In: Alpert MA, Alexander JK, eds. The Heart and Lung in Obesity. New York: Futura Publishing Co., 1997:147–198.
14. Oison AL, Zwillich C. The obesity hypoventilation syndrome. Am J Med 2005; 118:948–956.
15. Phipps PR, Starritt E, Goünszein RR, et al. Association of serum leptin with hypoventilation in human obesity. Thorax 2002; 57:75–76.
16. Klein S, Coppack SW, Mohamed-Ali V, et al. Adipose tissue leptin production and plasma leptin kinetics in humans. Diabetes 1996; 45:984–987.
17. O'Donnell CP, Schaub CD, Haines AS, et al. Leptin prevents respiratory depression in obesity. Am J Respir Crit Care Med 1999; 159:1477–1484.
18. Yee B, Cheung J, Phipps P, et al. Treatment of obesity hypoventilation syndrome and serum leptin. Respiration 2006; 73:209–212.
19. Ayappa I, Berger KL, Norman RG, et al. Hypercapnia and ventilatory periodicity in OSAS. Am J Respir Crit Care Med 2002; 166:1112–1115.
20. Hill NS. Non invasive ventilation. Does it work, for whom, and how? Am Rev Respir Dis 1993; 147:1050–1055.
21. Chouri-Pontarollo N, Borel J-C, Tamisier R, et al. Impaired objective daytime vigilance in obesity-hypoventilation syndrome: impact of non-invasive ventilation. Chest 2007; 131:148–155.
22. Pankow W, Hijjeh I, Schuttler F, et al. Influence of noninvasive positive pressure ventilation on inspiratory muscle activity in obese subjects. Eur Respir J 1997; 10:2847–2852.
23. de Lucas-Ramos P, de Miguel-Diez J, Santacruz-Siminiani A, et al. Benefits at 1 year of nocturnal intermittent positive pressure ventilation in patients with obesity-hypoventilation syndrome. Respir Med 2004; 98:961–967.
24. Jokic R, Zintel T, Sridhar G, et al. Ventilatory responses to hypercapnia and hypoxia in relatives of patients with the obesity hypoventilation syndrome. Thorax 2000; 55:940–945.

25. Bannerjee D, Yee BJ, Piper AJ, et al. Obesity hypoventilation syndrome: hypoxemia during CPAP. Chest, 2007; 131:1678–1684.
26. Mokhlesi B, Tulaimat A, Evans AT, et al. Impact of adherence with positive airway pressure therapy on hypercapnia in OSA. J Clin Sleep Med 2006; 2:57–62.
27. Claman OM, Piper A, Sanders MA, et al. Nocturnal noninvasive positive pressure ventilatory assistance. Chest 1996; 110:1581–1588.
28. Masa JF, Celli BR, Riesco JA, et al. The obesity hypoventilation syndrome can be treated with noninvasive mechanical ventilation. Chest 2001; 119:1102–1107.
29. Piper AJ, Sullivan CE. Effects of short term NIPPV in the treatment of patients with severe obstructive sleep apnea and hypercapnia. Chest 1994; 105:434–440.
30. Perez de Llano LA, Golpe R, Ortiz Piquer M, et al. Short-term and long-term effects of nasal intermittent positive pressure ventilation in patients with obesity-hypoventilation syndrome. Chest 2005; 128:587–594.
31. Laaban JP. SAOS et obésité. In: Répercussions respiratoires de l'obésité, Vol 1. Paris: Margaux Orange, ed. 2005: 63–74.
32. Kessler R, Chaouat A, Weitzenblum E, et al. Pulmonary hypertension in the obstructive sleep apnea syndrome: prevalence, causes and therapeutic consequences. Eur Respir J 1996; 9:787–794.
33. Resta O, Guido P, Picca V, et al. Prescription of nCPAP and nBiPAP in obstructive sleep apnoea syndrome: Italian experience in 105 subjects; a prospective two-center study. Respir Med 1998; 92:820–827.
34. Rabec C, Merati M, Baudouin N, et al. Management of obesity and respiratory insufficiency: the value of bi-level pressure-cycled nasal ventilation. Rev Mal Respir 1998; 15:269–278.
35. Schafer H, Ewig S, Hasper E, et al. Failure of CPAP therapy in obstructive sleep apnoea syndrome: predictive factors and treatment with bi-level positive airway pressure. Respir Med 1998; 92:208–215.
36. Guo YF, Sforza E, Janssens JP. Respiratory patterns during sleep in OHS patients support. Chest 2007; 131:1090–1099.
37. Waldhorn RE. Nocturnal nasal intermittent positive pressure ventilation with bi-level airway pressure (BIPAP) in respiratory failure. Chest 1992; 101:516–521.
38. Kessler R. Le syndrome obésité hypoventilation ou le syndrome de Picwick re-visité. In: Laaban JP, ed. SAOS et obésité, in Répercussions respiratoires de l'obésité, Vol 1. Paris: Margaux Orange, ed. 2005:49–62.
39. Muir JF, Cuvelier A, Bota S, et al. Arch Chest Dis 1998; 53:556–559.
40. Casey KR, Contillo KO, Brown LK. Sleep related hypoxemic/hypoventilation syndromes, Chest 2007; 131:1936–1948.
41. Tirlapur VG, Mir MA. Effect of low calorie intake on abnormal pulmonary physiology in patients with chronic hypercapnic respiratory failure. Am J Med 1984; 77:987–994.
42. Sugerman HJI, Fainnan RP, Sood RK, et al. Long-term effects of gastric surgery for treating respiratory insufficiency of obesity. Am J Clin Nutr 1992; 55:597S–601S.
43. Shivaram U, Cash ME, Beal A. Nasal continuous positive airway pressure in decompensated hypercapnic respiratory failure as a complication of sleep apnea. Chest 1993; 104:770–774.
44. Sturani C, Galavotti Y, Scarduelli C, et al. Acute respiratory failure due to severe obstructive sleep apnea syndrome, managed with nasal positive pressure ventilation. Monaldi Arch Chest Dis 1994; 49:558–560.
45. Ordronneau J, Chollet S, Nogues B, et al. Le syndrome d'apnées du sommeiJ en réanimation. Rev Mal Respir 1994; 11:51–55.
46. Muir JF, Bota S, Cuvelier A, et al. Acute respiratory failure and obesity. Incidence of management with noninvasive mechanical ventilation. Am J Respir Crit Care Med 1998; 157:S309.
47. Cuvelier A, Rabec C. La ventilation mécanique au cours de l'IRA hypercapnique du sujet obése, spécificités de la VNI, Réanimation 2007; 16:75–81.
48. Cuvelier A, Muir JF. Obesity hypoventilation syndrome: new insights in the Pickwick papers [editorial]. Chest 2007; 131:7–8.

35
Progressive Neuromuscular and Degenerative Diseases

JOHN R. BACH
University of Medicine and Dentistry of New Jersey–The New Jersey Medical School, Newark, New Jersey, U.S.A.

I. Introduction to Respiratory Muscle Aids

Patients with neuromuscular disorders (NMD) develop ventilatory failure because of a combination of dysfunctions of the inspiratory, expiratory, and bulbar-innervated muscles. Respiratory failure and the need for a tracheostomy are avoidable in most cases, using the approaches and interventions presented in this chapter.

Pulmonologists are more accustomed to managing impairments of gas exchange with supplemental oxygen and bronchodilators than impairments of muscle function, using respiratory muscle aids. Also, for patients with central or obstructive apneas, clinicians may prescribe continuous positive airway pressure (CPAP) or low span bi-level positive airway pressure (BiPAP) [inspiratory positive airway pressure (IPAP)-expiratory positive airway pressure (EPAP) < 10 cmH_2O]. However, for patients with weak inspiratory and expiratory muscles, CPAP is useless and low-span BiPAP provides inadequate rest for weak inspiratory muscles as well as fails to provide optimal lung volumes for coughing (1). With advancing inspiratory and expiratory muscle weakness, ventilatory failure ensues. This is often managed with invasive mechanical ventilation, even though noninvasive techniques are effective and preferable.

Oxygen therapy increases the risk of ventilatory failure compared with ventilatory assistance or with no treatment at all (2) and can obscure recognition of mucus plugging as it alleviates desaturation without attending to secretion clearance. Oxygen therapy can also prolong hypopneas and apneas during rapid eye movement (REM) sleep (3), and result in reduced muscular activity needed for effective noninvasive intermittent positive pressure ventilation (NIPPV) during sleep (4). In short, for patients with NMD, these are not substitutes for noninvasive mechanical ventilation.

Ventilatory impairment results from inspiratory muscle weakness, central hypoventilation, thoracic restriction, upper airway narrowing, extreme obesity, abdominal distension, and improperly fitting thoracolumbar orthoses. In NMD, pulmonary infiltrates and respiratory failure are precipitated by mucus plugging due to an ineffective secretion clearance, especially during acute respiratory infections (2,7).

Patients with advanced ventilatory muscle dysfunction develop a rapid, shallow breathing pattern with an inability to take deep breaths, leading to chronic microatelectasis and decreased lung and chest wall compliance (8,9). Acute respiratory tract infections with pulmonary scarring and spinal deformity cause further loss of lung compliance. Hypercapnia decreases respiratory muscle strength, and respiratory control centers reset to accommodate hypercapnia, depressing ventilatory drive (2,4).

Patients with generalized muscle dysfunction also have expiratory and oropharyngeal muscle weaknesses that decrease cough peak flows (CPF). When CPF do not exceed 2.7 L/sec, cough may be completely ineffective (10). CPF are also reduced by airway obstruction from tracheal stenosis, laryngeal incompetence, vocal cord dysfunction, hypopharyngeal collapse, or obstructive pulmonary disease. The CPF are reduced further when the vital capacity (VC) is <1.5 L (11). The lower the CPF, the more likely that airway secretions will result in pneumonia and acute respiratory failure. Smoking and the presence of invasive endotracheal tubes increase the tendency for mucus plugging, which may predispose to "ventilator-(actually, "invasive interface")-associated pneumonia" (12).

Ventilatory insufficiency occurs initially during REM sleep, later extending throughout sleep and eventually to waking hours. Normocapnic arterial hypoxemia is also common during sleep, reflecting the ventilation-perfusion mismatching associated with microatelectasis, scoliosis, and pulmonary scarring.

Malnutrition, acidosis, electrolyte disturbances, cachexia, infection, fatigue, and muscle dysfunction, all exacerbate ventilatory insufficiency. Narcotics, sedatives, and supplemental oxygen reduce ventilatory drive and exacerbate alveolar hypoventilation.

Many patients with NMD develop CO_2 narcosis with supplemental oxygen. Hypoventilation is often first recognized during a respiratory infection when bronchial mucus plugging triggers acute respiratory failure. Ventilatory failure can also develop suddenly or over a period of hours or days in patients with acute cervical myelopathies, Guillain-Barré syndrome, myasthenia gravis, acute poliomyelitis, or exacerbations of multiple sclerosis.

Whereas dysfunctional respiratory muscles may be supported to avoid respiratory failure, there are no effective noninvasive aids or substitutes for the bulbar-innervated muscles. Bulbar dysfunction leads to loss of speech and swallowing, resulting in aspiration and desaturation despite respiratory muscle aids. This is the only indication for tracheostomy among the NMD population (13).

Respiratory muscle assistance involves the manual or mechanical application of forces to the body or pressure changes to the airway to assist inspiratory or expiratory muscle function. Negative pressure applied to the airway during expiration assists the expiratory muscles for coughing, just as positive pressure applied to the airway during inhalation (noninvasive IPPV) assists inspiratory function.

A manual thrust applied to the abdomen during expiration, especially when in combination with mild chest compression, assists expiratory muscle function and increases cough flows (11). The intermittent abdominal pressure ventilator (IAPV) involves the intermittent inflation of an elastic air sac that is contained in a corset or belt worn beneath the patient's outer clothing (Fig. 1). A positive pressure ventilator inflates the sac. Bladder action against the abdominal wall moves the diaphragm upward, causing a forced exsufflation. During bladder deflation, the abdominal contents and diaphragm return to the resting position, and inspiration occurs passively. A trunk angle of 70° to 80° from the horizontal is ideal for use. The patient who has any inspiratory capacity or is capable of glossopharyngeal breathing (GPB) can gulp in volumes and thereby add to the mechanical insufflations. The IAPV generally augments tidal volumes by about 300 mL, but volumes as high as 1200 mL have been reported when there is no scoliosis or obesity (14).

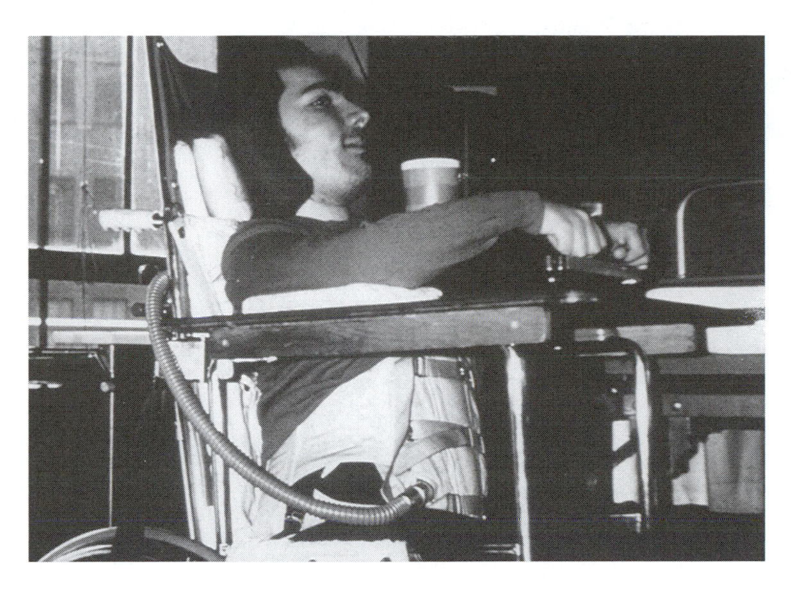

Figure 1 The girdle of the IAPV with its air sac connected to the tubing of a volume-cycled ventilator. This 45-year-old DMD patient, continuously ventilator dependent for 24 years and having no measurable vital capacity, used the IAPV for daytime ventilatory support for 15 years. *Abbreviations*: IAPV, intermittent abdominal pressure ventilator; DMD, Duchenne muscular dystrophy.

II. Clinical Goals

The goals of management are to maintain pulmonary compliance and promote chest wall and lung growth (in pediatric patients), to maintain normal alveolar ventilation, and to maximize CPF.

A. Lung and Chest Wall Mobilization

Lung and chest wall mobilization can be achieved through air stacking (18), deep insufflations, or nocturnal noninvasive ventilation for infants (16). The maximum insufflation capacity (MIC) is the largest volume of air that can be held with a closed glottis. The patient "air stacks" consecutively delivered volumes from a volume-cycled ventilator or a manual resuscitator with the expiratory valve blocked, holding these volumes with a closed glottis until no more air can be held. The air is delivered via a mouthpiece, a lipseal (Fig. 2), or a nasal interface. Air stacking is performed multiple times in three daily sessions. Most patients can also learn GPB to expand their lungs beyond their VC. The difference between the MIC and the VC correlates with glottic integrity (11). If the glottis is incompetent for air stacking, deep insufflations are passively provided via a mechanical insufflator-exsufflator at 40–70 cmH_2O three times daily.

Air stacking increases voice volume, maximizes CPF, improves pulmonary compliance, prevents atelectasis, and indicates effective use of NIPPV. Anyone who can air stack can be extubated to NIPPV. Such patients can be extubated without being ventilator

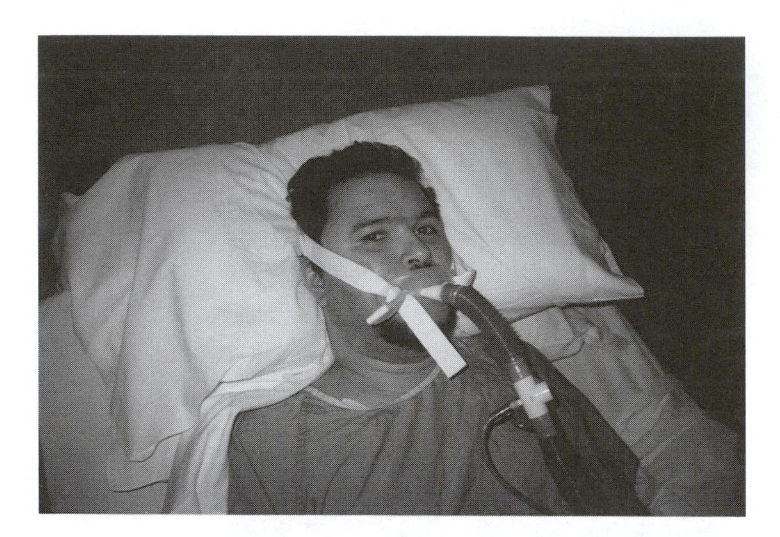

Figure 2 A 37-year-old with Duchenne muscular dystrophy, vital capacity 270 mL, continuously dependent on noninvasive ventilation seen here using lipseal ventilation for nocturnal ventilatory support.

weaned. While infants cannot air stack, nocturnal use of high span (IPAP-EPAP $>$ 10 cmH_2O) BiPAP prevents pectus excavatum and promotes lung and chest wall growth for infants with spinal muscular atrophy (SMA) (19).

B. Maintain Normal Alveolar Ventilation

Ventilatory support can be provided with NIPPV from volume-cycled ventilators via an angled mouthpiece, lipseal, nasal, or oral-nasal interface. Simple 15- or 22-mm-angled mouthpieces are most convenient for daytime ventilatory support (Fig. 3). To use mouthpiece IPPV, adequate neck rotation and oral motor function are necessary to prevent leakage from the mouth or nose. In addition, the patient must open the glottis and vocal cords, dilate the hypopharynx, and maintain airway patency to receive the air.

If the lips are too weak to grab a mouthpiece, the patient can use an IAPV (14) or nasal IPPV for daytime as well as for nocturnal support (Fig. 4). Nasal interfaces can be alternated to vary skin pressure. Inconspicuous nasal interfaces that permit the use of eyeglasses can also be used. The patients can most conveniently be trained and equipped to use NIPPV in the outpatient and home settings.

We have only found oronasal interfaces to be useful in patients with amyotrophic lateral scoliosis (ALS) who have no remaining bulbar-innervated muscle function. Most such patients will require indwelling tracheostomies.

Closed systems NIPPV are unnecessary unless ventilatory drive is blunted by oxygen therapy, sedative medications, or excessive hypercapnia, which can lead to excessive air leakage from the nose or mouth (4). If necessary, one can provide an essentially closed system of ventilatory support by using a lipseal (Respironics International Inc., Murrysville, Pennsylvania, U.S.), placing cotton pledgets in the nostrils, and sealing the nostrils with a

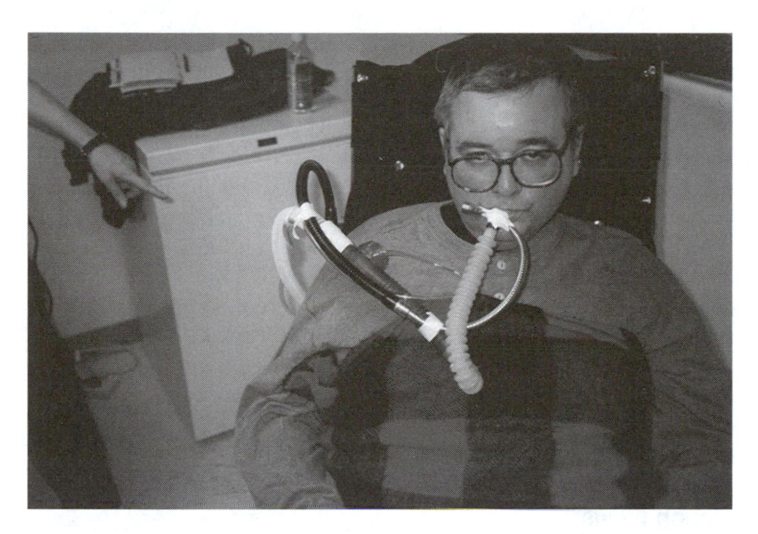

Figure 3 A 51-year-old man with ALS and no ventilator-free breathing ability using daytime mouthpiece IPPV. *Abbreviations*: ALS, amyotrophic lateral scoliosis; IPPV, intermittent positive pressure ventilation.

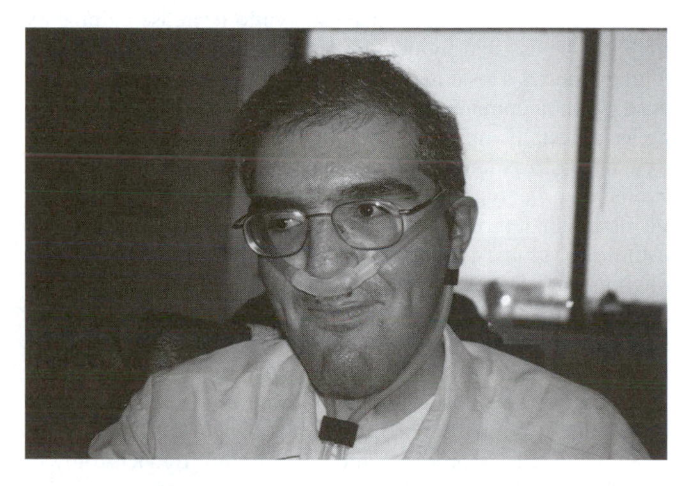

Figure 4 A 30-year-old lawyer with Duchenne muscular dystrophy, vital capacity 280 mL, continuously dependent on noninvasive ventilation, using a Nasal-Aire interface (Fisher-Paykel Inc. Irving, CA) for daytime ventilatory support.

band-aid. Orso-nasal interfaces like the Hybrid (Teleflex Medical Inc., Research Triangle Park, N.C.) can also be used. Patients with little or no measurable VC can be safely ventilated with open systems of nasal or oral ventilation.

The benefits of NIPPV include respiratory muscle rest, increasing alveolar ventilation, lung compliance, chemosensitivity, and ventilation/perfusion matching (4). To accomplish optimal rest, high volumes or pressure spans are used. Assist-control mode is set at volumes of 800 to 1500 mL for adults and IPAP to EPAP spans of 15 to 22 cmH_2O for BiPAP users with little residual glottic function. Patients vary the volume of air inhaled from the ventilator, cycle to cycle, to vary their tidal volume, speech volume, and cough flows as well as to expand their lungs. BiPAP does not enable patients to air stack, so it should not be used by adults with NMD unless glottic closure is lost.

Besides mild orthodontic deformities, other potential difficulties include allergy to the plastic lipseal or silicone interfaces (13% vs. 5% for nonsilicone interfaces), dry mouth (65%), eye irritation from air leakage (about 24%), nasal congestion (25%) and dripping (35%), sinusitis (8%), nose bleeding (4–19%), gum discomfort (20%) and gum receding from nasal interface or lip pressure, maxillary flattening in children, aerophagia (20,21), and, as for invasive ventilation, barotrauma. Occasional patients express claustrophobia. Abdominal distention tends to occur sporadically. It can be decreased by pressure limiting volume-cycled ventilators, or at times by switching from one ventilator style to another. It is relieved as the air passes as flatus once the patient sits up in the morning or by "burping" through the gastrostomy tube if present. Barotrauma is rare in NMD.

C. Maximize Cough Flows

Whereas the mucociliary elevator is the primary mechanism for clearing the peripheral 21 divisions of the airway, coughing clears the most central 6 divisions. Chest percussion and vibration can help mobilize peripheral airway secretions but they are not substitutes for coughing and, unlike for assisted coughing, have never been shown to decrease pulmonary morbidity and mortality. Cough can be assisted by manual and mechanical means.

Manually assisted coughing requires substantial lung inflation through air stacking or deep lung insufflation, followed by an abdominal thrust applied as the glottis opens. If the VC is < 1.5 L, air stacking is especially important before the abdominal thrust (11). Whereas inspiratory, expiratory, and bulbar-innervated muscles are needed for spontaneous coughing, only bulbar-innervated muscle function is required for assisted coughing as airway pressure changes and abdominal thrusts substitute for respiratory muscles; but nothing noninvasive can substitute for glottic function.

Manually assisted coughing requires a cooperative patient, good coordination between the patient and caregiver, and adequate physical effort and often-frequent application by the caregiver. When inadequate, the most effective alternative is mechanically assisted coughing (MAC). The combination of mechanical in-exsufflation (MI-E) with an abdominal thrust is MAC. MI-Es deliver deep insufflations followed immediately by deep exsufflations. The MAC cough volumes normally exceed 2 L at flows of 10 L/sec. MI-E pressures of +40 to –40 cmH_2O delivered via oronasal interface or adult tracheostomy or translaryngeal tubes with the cuff inflated are usually most effective. However, machine pressures are secondary. What is important is to fully expand and then fully and rapidly empty the lungs.

Whether via the upper airway or via indwelling airway tubes, routine airway suctioning misses the left main stem bronchus about 90% of the time. This explains high rates of left lower lobe pneumonia. MAC, on the other hand, provides the same exsufflation flows in both left and right airways without discomfort, fatigue, or airway trauma and it can be effective when suctioning is not.

Patients who benefit from MAC have weak respiratory muscles but adequate bulbar-innervated muscle function for airway patency, although insufficient for air stacking to assist CPF to over 5 L/sec. MAC is not usually necessary for patients with intact bulbar-innervated muscle function who can air stack sufficiently for CPF to exceed 6 L/sec, with an abdominal thrust. MAC will not avert a tracheostomy if bulbar-innervation is inadequate, as in advanced bulbar ALS.

III. The Oximetry Feedback: Respiratory Aid Protocol

Oximetry feedback can be used for monitoring alveolar ventilation and, especially, for maintaining clear airways. Respiratory aids will maintain saturation of oxygen in arterial blood (Sa_{O_2}) >94% without supplemental oxygen. Oximetry feedback is most important during respiratory tract infections and when extubating patients with little or no ventilatory capacity. NIPPV and MAC with oximetry feedback have averted hundreds of hospitalizations for patients with Duchenne muscular dystrophy (DMD) (15), SMA (16), ALS (13), and other NMDs (22). Tracheostomy is indicated if aspiration causes the Sa_{O_2} to remain <95% despite optimal use of NIPPV and MAC, which generally only occurs in advanced bulbar ALS. Without tracheostomy, most patients with ALS whose Sa_{O_2} has decreased to <95% despite using respiratory aids will be deceased within two months (13–15).

A. Glossopharyngeal Breathing

Both inspiratory and, indirectly, expiratory muscle activity can be assisted by GPB. This technique involves the glottis capturing air and propelling it into the lungs. One breath usually consists of six to nine gulps of 60 to 100 mL each. GPB can provide an individual with no inspiratory muscle function with normal ventilation throughout daytime hours without using a ventilator, and safety in the event of ventilator failure during sleep (17). The safety and versatility afforded by GPB are key to avoiding tracheostomy or removing one in favor of using noninvasive aids for neuromuscular ventilatory failure. About 65% of patients with functional bulbar-innervated musculature have been reported to be able to use GPB to increase tidal volumes (17,27).

B. Extubation and Decannulation

Intubation is often avoidable by using NIPPV and assisted coughing. It is the ability to successfully extubate ventilator-dependent patients to NIPPV that enables tracheostomy to be avoided in most patients with NMD (15,17).

Once intubated, the same ventilator-weaning parameters used for patients with lung disease are typically used to guide extubation in NMD, i.e., resting minute ventilation, maximum voluntary ventilation, tidal volume, VC, maximum inspiratory pressure, arterial–alveolar oxygen gradient on 100% oxygen, and ratio of dead space to tidal volume. The large number of parameters signals their lack of efficacy, as most of them relate to inspiratory rather than expiratory airway clearance ability.

Patients with NMD can be extubated to NIPPV despite little or no autonomous ventilatory capacity. Postextubation CPF is a good predictor of successful extubation as it reflects bulbar-innervated muscle integrity, and therefore, the ability to eliminate airway secretions (10,11). Preextubation peak expiratory flows have also been shown to predict success in extubating patients with primarily respiratory impairment (28).

Table 1 Extubation Protocol for Patients with Ventilatory Impairment

1. Oxygen administration limited to achieve Spo_2 no higher than 95%.
2. Mechanically assisted coughing used via the invasive tube up to every few minutes as needed to fully expand and quickly empty the lungs to reverse oxyhemoglobin desaturation due to airway mucus accumulation when baseline Spo_2 decreases, when there is auscultatory evidence of secretion accumulation, and on patient demand. Tube and upper airway are suctioned following use of expiratory aids.
3. Ventilator weaning attempted without permitting hypercapnia.
4. Extubation whether or not the patient is ventilator weaned when meeting the following criteria:
   - afebrile and normal white blood cell count
   - no supplemental oxygen required to maintain Spo_2 >94% for greater than 24 hr
   - chest radiograph abnormalities cleared or clearing
   - respiratory depressants discontinued with no residual effects from them
   - airway secretions normal and suctioning required less than 1–2×/8 hr
   - coryza diminished sufficiently to permit use of nasal ventilation
5. Extubation to continuous high span bi-level positive airway pressure or, preferably, to NIPPV via mouth/nasal interface, no supplemental oxygen.
6. Oximetry feedback used to guide the use of MAC, postural drainage, and chest physical therapy to reverse desaturations below 95% due to airway mucus.
7. With CO_2 retention or ventilator synchronization difficulties, nasal interface leaks are eliminated. For small children with rapid breathing rates who are using high span BiPAP, the inspiratory ramp may need to be shortened or the IPAP decreased. Back-up rates may need to be set at one-half the child's breathing rate to capture every other breath. Synchrony may also improve by switching to using a more trigger-sensitive volume cycle ventilator. Persistent oxyhemoglobin desaturation, despite eucapnia and aggressive MAC, can indicate impending severe respiratory distress and need to reintubate.
8. Following reintubation the protocol is used for a second trial of extubation to nasal IPPV or high span nasal BiPAP. Once extubation is successful and $Spo_2 > 94\%$ in ambient air, the patient weans himself or herself to the preintubation regime of ventilator use by taking fewer and fewer mouth piece IPPVs as tolerated and as presented in Figure 3.

Abbreviations: Spo_2, saturation of oxygen in arterial blood; NIPPV, noninvasive intermittent positive pressure ventilation; MAC, mechanically assisted cough; CO_2, carbon dioxide; IPAP, inspiratory positive airway pressure; BiPAP, bi-level positive airway pressure.

In patients with NMD, hypercapnia correlates with pulmonary complications and death (2). Weaning schedules cause anxiety as the patient is not ready to breathe autonomously or the schedule may be too conservative, delaying respiratory muscle reconditioning. An Sao_2 <95% suggests hypoventilation, airway mucus, or residual lung disease. Patients are often extubated to CPAP or, inappropriately, to low-span BiPAP, and cough aids are not used. When extubation fails, the clinician feels justified in recommending tracheostomy. A more appropriate approach for patients with primarily ventilatory impairment is presented in Table 1, which often enables tracheostomy to be averted indefinitely in NMD.

C. Preparation for Surgical Anesthesia

In NMD, the correction of spinal deformities, insertion of gastrostomy tubes, or other are sometimes avoided because of fear of respiratory complications. However, such complications are preventable if patients are trained in NIPPV and MAC before undergoing general anesthesia, and are extubated to these interventions postoperatively as in Table 1 (29).

D. Noninvasive Vs. Tracheostomy Ventilation Outcomes

SMA is the most common NMD in the floppy newborn. Infants with typical SMA type 1 have 70% mortality by 6 months and 90% by 12 months of age. In a recent study of 80 typical SMA 1 patients, all of whom developed respiratory failure at <24 months of age, the extubation (Table 1) success rate was 87% compared with 6% by conventional extubation approaches. Hospitalization rates for the noninvasively managed patients fell from 1.6 per year up to age three to 0.04 per year after age five. Eight such patients are, currently, over 10 years of age, using nasal ventilation up to 24 hours a day. Only 5 of 80 underwent tracheostomy because of severe bradycardias in two, bronchomalacia in two, and persistent desaturations due to saliva aspiration in one. SMA type 1 patients who undergo tracheostomy can also have long-term survival (16), but this is at the cost of lifetime continuous invasive ventilatory dependence and the failure of speech development. About 80% of SMA type 1 patients who are managed noninvasively develop the ability to speak and few require continuous noninvasive ventilation with no ventilator-free breathing ability.

In a study of 91 ventilator users with DMD, 51 went on to require continuous NIPPV for 6.3 $\pm$ 4.6 (range to 25) years. None of the 34 full-time NIPPV users who had access to MAC died from respiratory complications, whereas three died from severe cardiomyopathy. Five patients with no breathing capacity were extubated or decannulated to continuous NIPPV and five became continuously dependent on NIPPV for one year or more without ever being hospitalized (15). It has previously been reported that DMD patients undergoing tracheostomy tend to have a prolongation of survival of about seven years but also have a tendency to die from complications related to invasive mechanical ventilation (IMV) (24).

Although both NIPPV and tracheostomy IPPV prolong survival, NIPPV is overwhelmingly preferred by patients over tracheostomy for speech, sleep, swallowing, comfort, appearance, security, use of GPB, and overall (25). One study also demonstrated 200% cost savings by using NIPPV for patients with no ventilator-free breathing ability, by facilitating community placement with personal care attendants rather than nursing care or long-term institutionalization (26). Despite the benefits of noninvasive interventions, few clinicians are aware that they can be used instead of tracheostomy IPPV and even fewer are familiar with all of the techniques available (1). As previously noted, however, when bulbar-innervated musculature is completely dysfunctional, tracheostomy can offer further prolongation of survival.

In a recent study, 25 patients with ALS became dependent on NIPPV, including 13 who became continuously dependent for 19.7 $\pm$ 16.9 months without developing acute respiratory distress or oxyhemoglobin desaturation. For another 76 patients, the daytime Sao_2 baseline persistently decreased to <95%, 78 times because of some combination of alveolar hypoventilation and airway congestion. For 41 patients, the baseline was corrected by some combination of NIPPV and MAC for 11.1 $\pm$ 8.7 months before desaturation recurred in 27. Of the latter, 11 underwent tracheostomy, 14 died in less than two months, and two were again corrected by the addition of MAC to NIPPV. Thirty-three of the 35 patients for whom the Sao_2 could not be normalized required tracheostomy or died within two months. The difference between the patients who could be spared respiratory failure from those who could not was that the latter had significantly poorer glottic function with no ability to air stack or generate measurable assisted CPF (13). We have decannulated ALS patients with no ability to breathe unaided who have survived up to 10 years using continuous NIPPV before requiring tracheostomy. Once bulbar ALS patients undergo tracheostomy for ventilatory support, survival has been reported to be about five years before most patients die from complications related to their tracheostomies (23).

IV. Conclusion

Few, if any, patients with NMD should be left to develop unexpected ventilatory failure as appropriate assessment, self-management education, and follow-up will identify disease progression and risk of respiratory complications. When ventilatory failure occurs, tracheostomy tubes can be avoided, for the most part, irrespective of the degree of ventilator dependence, with the exception of those with insufficient bulbar-innervated musculature for speech, deglutition, and airway protection. Those with indwelling tracheostomy tubes should be offered decannulation as part of their rehabilitation, irrespective of the extent of their respiratory muscle failure. The only exceptions to this therapy are patients with advanced bulbar ALS or those with rare facioscapulohumeral muscular dystrophy, who lose all bulbar-innervated muscle function and aspirate saliva to the extent of Sao_2 remaining below 95% (13).

References

1. Bach JR, Chaudhry SS. Management approaches in muscular dystrophy association clinics. Am J Phys Med Rehabil 2000; 79:193–196.
2. Bach JR, Rajaraman R, Ballanger F, et al. Neuromuscular ventilatory insufficiency: the effect of home mechanical ventilator use vs. oxygen therapy on pneumonia and hospitalization rates. Am J Phys Med Rehabil 1998; 77:8–19.
3. Smith PEM, Edwards RHT, Calverley PMA. Oxygen treatment of sleep hypoxemia in Duchenne muscular dystrophy. Thorax 1989; 44:997–1001.
4. Bach JR. Physiology and pathophysiology of hypoventilation: ventilatory vs. oxygenation impairment. In: Bach JR, ed. Noninvasive Mechanical Ventilation. Philadelphia: Hanley & Belfus, 2002:25.
5. Neudert C, Oliver D, Wasner M, et al. The course of the terminal phase in patients with amyotrophic lateral sclerosis. J Neurol 2001; 248:612–616.
6. Polkey MI, Lyall RA, Davidson AC, et al. Ethical and clinical issues in the use of home noninvasive mechanical ventilation for the palliation of breathlessness in motor neurone disease. Thorax 1999; 54:367–371.
7. Mier-Jedrzejowicz A, Brophy C, Green M. Respiratory muscle weakness during upper respiratory tract infections. Am Rev Respir Dis 1988; 138:5–7.
8. Sinha R, Bergofsky EG. Prolonged alteration of lung mechanics in kyphoscoliosis by positive hyperinflation. Am Rev Respir Dis 1972; 106:47–57.
9. Bach JR, Kang SW. Disorders of ventilation: weakness, stiffness, and mobilization. Chest 2000; 117:301–303.
10. Bach JR, Saporito LR. Criteria for extubation and tracheostomy tube removal for patients with ventilatory failure: a different approach to weaning. Chest 1996; 110:1566–1571.
11. Kang SW, Bach JR. Maximum insufflation capacity: the relationships with vital capacity and cough flows for patients with neuromuscular disease. Am J Phys Med Rehabil 2000; 79:222–227.

12. Baram D, Hulse G, Palmer LB. Stable patients receiving prolonged mechanical ventilation (PMV) have a high alveolar burden of bacteria. Chest 2005; 127:1353–1357.
13. Bach JR, Bianchi C, Aufiero E. Oximetry and prognosis in amyotrophic lateral sclerosis. Chest 2004; 126:1502–1507.
14. Bach JR, Alba AS. Intermittent abdominal pressure ventilator in a regimen of noninvasive ventilatory support. Chest 1991; 99:630–636.
15. Gomez-Merino E, Bach JR. Duchenne muscular dystrophy: prolongation of life by noninvasive respiratory muscle aids. Am J Phys Med Rehabil 2002; 81:411–415.
16. Bach JR, Baird JS, Plosky D, et al. Spinal muscular atrophy type 1: management and outcomes. Pediatr Pulmonol 2002; 34:16–22.
17. Bach JR. Respiratory muscle aids: patient evaluation, respiratory aid protocol, and outcomes. In: Bach JR, ed. The Management of Patients with Neuromuscular Disease. Philadelphia: Hanley & Belfus, 2004:271–308.
18. Kang SW, Bach JR. Maximum insufflation capacity. Chest 2000; 118:61–65.
19. Bach JR. Prevention of pectus excavatum for children with spinal muscular atrophy type 1. Am J Phys Med Rehabil 2003; 82:815–819.
20. Leger SS, Leger P. The art of interface: tools for administering noninvasive ventilation. Med Klin 1999; 94:35–39.
21. Pepin JL, Leger P, Veale D, et al. Side effects of nasal continuous positive airway pressure in sleep apnea syndrome: study of 193 patients in two French sleep centers. Chest 1995; 107:375–381.
22. Bach JR. Home mechanical ventilation for neuromuscular ventilatory failure: conventional approaches and their outcomes. In: Bach JR, ed. Noninvasive Mechanical Ventilation. Philadelphia: Hanley & Belfus, 2002:103.
23. Bach JR. Amyotrophic lateral sclerosis: communication status and survival with ventilatory support. Am J Phys Med Rehabil 1993; 72:343–349.
24. Bach JR. Pulmonary rehabilitation considerations for Duchenne muscular dystrophy: the prolongation of life by respiratory muscle aids. Crit Rev Phys Rehabil Med 1992; 3:239–269.
25. Bach JR. A comparison of long-term ventilatory support alternatives from the perspective of the patient and care giver. Chest 1993; 104:1702–1706.
26. Bach JR, Intintola P, Alba AS, et al. The ventilator individual: cost analysis of institutionalization versus rehabilitation and in-home management. Chest 1992; 101:26–30.
27. Bach JR, Alba AS. Noninvasive options for ventilatory support of the traumatic high level quadriplegic. Chest 1990; 98:613–619.
28. Smina M, Salam A, Khamiees M, et al. Cough peak flows and extubation outcomes. Chest 2003; 124:262–268.
29. Bach JR, Sabharwal S. High pulmonary risk scoliosis surgery: role of noninvasive ventilation and related techniques. J Spinal Disord Tech 2005; 18:527–530.

36
Chronic Ventilatory Support in Obstructive Lung Disease

PETER J. WIJKSTRA
University Medical Centre Groningen, Groningen, The Netherlands

MARK W. ELLIOTT
St. James's University Hospital, Leeds, U.K.

I. Introduction

Chronic ventilatory support is currently a well-accepted therapy in patients with chronic respiratory failure due to thoracic cage abnormalities or in patients with neuromuscular disease. In contrast, the evidence to use chronic ventilatory support in patients with obstructive lung disease is less clear. Most of studies in this area have been in patients with chronic obstructive pulmonary disease (COPD) and only a few in patients with cystic fibrosis (CF) and bronchiectasis. In this chapter, we will focus primarily on COPD, discussing first the rationale of noninvasive positive pressure ventilation (NIPPV) in these patients and second all randomized controlled studies. Thereafter, we will elaborate on different issues that might be important in making NIPPV more effective in patients with COPD. Finally, we will discuss the effects of chronic ventilatory support in patients with CF and bronchiectasis.

II. Rationale for NIPPV in Patients with COPD

Several theories exist as to why chronic NIPPV might be effective in COPD: (1) resting dysfunctional respiratory muscles, thereby increasing their daytime strength and endurance and improving peripheral muscle function by improving the operating milieu (pH, Pa_{O_2}, Pa_{CO_2}); (2) preventing repeated nocturnal arousals, thereby improving the quality of sleep; (3) resetting the central chemosensitivity to carbon dioxide; and (4) reducing the load against which the respiratory muscle pump has to function.

A. Improving Respiratory Muscle Function

The respiratory muscles are in an unfavorable position in patients with severe COPD due to hyperinflation. Therefore, the diaphragm is thought to be susceptible to fatigue. Bellemare and Grassino introduced the so-called tension time index (TTI) comprising two elements: respiratory load and the respiratory duty cycle—$TTI = P_{di}/P_{di,max} \times T_i/T_{tot}$ (1). The respiratory load is represented by the pressure generated by the diaphragm P_{di} as a proportion of the maximal inspiratory pressure $P_{di,max}$. The duty cycle is represented by the inspiratory time (T_i) as a proportion of the duration of one inspiratory and expiratory cycle (T_{tot}). A value >0.15 has been associated with diaphragmatic fatigue.

It has been hypothesized that NIPVV might increase $P_{di,max}$ and reduce P_{di}, thereby decreasing the TTI and reducing the likelihood of fatigue. There was some evidence in favor of this hypothesis from a number of small short-term uncontrolled studies using negative pressure ventilators, which showed an improvement in various measures of respiratory muscle strength in association with improved blood gas tensions (2–5). An uncontrolled study of positive pressure ventilation showed a significant decrease in $Paco_2$ in association with a decrease of the pressure time product of the diaphragm. A subgroup of responders had a significantly increased transdiaphragmatic pressure and were better able to clear CO_2 (6).

In an attempt to provide a definitive answer as to whether assisted ventilation worked by resting respiratory muscles, Shapiro et al. randomized 184 patients with severe COPD to active or sham ventilation with a poncho wrap negative pressure ventilator (7). No significant changes in respiratory muscle strength were found, but a dose-response relationship was found between the amount of time that the ventilator was used per day and the six-minute walking distance (6-MWD). The most striking finding was that while patients were encouraged to use the ventilator for at least five hours each day, the average duration of use was closer to three hours. Negative pressure ventilation is rarely used for chronic domiciliary ventilation of patients with COPD, although there is some evidence of benefit in acute exacerbations (8). One consistent finding from the negative pressure studies was that when benefits were seen, it was predominantly among patients with hypercapnia. The question of whether chronic respiratory muscle fatigue exists remains controversial. It is probably unlikely as Laghi et al. failed to show any evidence of low frequency fatigue, even in COPD patients about to fail a weaning trial (9).

B. Improving Sleep Quality

Another possible explanation for the positive effects of NIPPV is improved sleep efficiency. Elliott et al. showed a significant decrease in diurnal $Paco_2$ and improved sleep efficiency after 12 months of NIPPV in 12 COPD patients (10). In a controlled trial, Meecham Jones showed that nocturnal NIPPV significantly improved sleep efficiency compared with oxygen treatment only (11). Criner also found a positive effect of NIPPV in a short-term trial in which gas exchange and sleep efficiency were measured in patients with COPD (12). They compared low-level CPAP with bi-level positive airway pressure (BiPAP) on two consecutive nights in COPD patients with a mean $Paco_2$ of 58($\pm$4) mmHg. No significant changes were found in $Paco_2$, while there was a significant improvement in sleep efficiency and total sleep time in the group treated by BiPAP.

C. Improving Central Drive

Restoration of central chemosensitivity—by the effective control of nocturnal hypoventilation—has been shown in patients with severe obstructive sleep apnea (13), neuromuscular disease (14), and chest wall deformity as well as patients with COPD (15,16).

D. Reducing the Load Against Which the Respiratory Muscle Pump Has to Function

Elliot et al. showed significant effects of nocturnal NIPPV on gas exchange in eight patients with severe COPD [mean forced expiratory volume in one second (FEV_1) = 0.53 L] and hypercapnia (mean $Paco_2$ = 8 kPa) (15). The decrease in $Paco_2$ was significantly correlated with the decrease in residual volume (RV), the decrease in gas trapping, and the increase in ventilation. The improvements in gas exchange were not related to changes in respiratory muscle strength. Budweiser et al. also showed, in a retrospective study, that NIPPV decreased the ratio of RV to total lung capacity (TLC) (17). In addition, in the patients with the most severe hyperinflation (RV/TLC > 75%) there was a significant correlation between inspiratory positive airway pressure (IPAP) and the reduction in $Paco_2$ ($r = 0.56, p < 0.05$). Diaz et al. in a sham controlled study of NIPPV used during the daytime for only three hours for five days a week (18) showed a change in the pattern of breathing to a slower and deeper pattern and an increase in the 6-MWD. In an earlier study they did not show any effect on respiratory muscle strength, but did show a reduction in hyperinflation with a significant relationship between a decrease in $Paco_2$ and a lower positive end expiratory intrinsic pressure (PEEPi) (19).

In conclusion, although several theories exist, there are currently no studies on negative predictive value (NPV) or NIPPV that have provided definitive evidence that the benefits in gas exchange were related to improvements in respiratory muscle function or in sleep efficiency. The relationship between improved gas exchange and hyperinflation needs further investigation. The restoration of the central drive to breathe is the most consistent finding. It is therefore important in any evaluation of NIPPV to be confident that nocturnal hypoventilation has been reduced.

III. Uncontrolled Trials

A number of uncontrolled trials of NIPPV have shown encouraging results in outcomes of immediate importance to patients. Perrin et al. showed that quality of life improved significantly after six months of NIPPV. In this study 14 patients with a mean $Paco_2$ of 7.8 kPa received volume ventilation during the night (20). In addition to an improved quality of life they also reported a significant improvement in arterial blood gas tensions. Similar positive results were seen in a study by Sivasothy et al. (21). Twenty-six patients with severe COPD (mean FEV_1 = 0.7 L) and hypercapnia ($Paco_2$ = 8.6 kPa) were ventilated at night using a volume ventilator. After 18 months (range 4–74) both gas exchange and quality of life improved significantly. Another long-term study by Jones et al. showed that after 24 months of pressure ventilation there were significant improvements in arterial blood gas tensions, and a reduction in hospital admissions and general practitioner visits (22). In summary, these uncontrolled studies showed that in a selected group of patients, with hypercapnia, NIPPV can control nocturnal hypoventilation and improve quality of life as well as arterial blood gas tensions during spontaneous breathing.

A. Short-Term Randomized Controlled Trials of NIPPV in COPD

There have been six randomized controlled trials(RCTs) of NIPPV for up to three months that have been published as full papers (11,18,23–26). Details of these studies are presented in Table 1. Strumpf et al. found no significant changes in any of the measured variables

Table 1 Randomized Controlled Trials of Short-Term NIPPV

Trial	Number of patients (treatment/controls)	FEV_1 mean (range)	$Paco_2$ mean (range)	Length (months)	IPAP/ EPAP	Outcome measures	Effects
Strumpf et al. (23)	Cross-over trial Enrolled: 19 Completed: 7	0.54 (0.46–0.88)	49 (35–67)	3	15/2	ABG, RM, walking test, dyspnea, PFT, sleep study, NP function	Significant effects for NP function
Gay et al. (24)	Parallel-group trial Randomized: 7/6 Completed: 4/6	0.68 (0.5–1.1)	55 (45–89)	3	10/2	ABG, 6-MWD, dyspnea, PFT, sleep study	No significant effects
Meecham Jones et al. (11)	Cross-over trial Enrolled: 18 Completed: 14	0.86 (0.33–1.7)	56 (52–65)	3	18/2	ABG, 6-MWT, HRQL, PFT, sleep study	Significant effects for ABG, sleep efficiency, HRQL
Lin (25)	Cross-over trial Enrolled: 12 Completed: 12	33% predicted	51 (±4)	2 weeks	12/2	ABG, PFT, RVEL, LVEF, sleep study	Significant effects of NIPPV and O_2 on nocturnal oxygenation
Renston (26)	Parallel-group trial Randomized: 9/8 Completed: 9/8	0.75 (0.45–1.05)	???	5 days for 2 hours	15–20/2	ABG, EMG, RM, 6-MWD, dyspnea	Significant effects for dyspnoea and 6-MWD
Diaz (19)	Parallel-group trial Randomized: 18/18 Completed: 18/18	32% predicted	56 (±6)	3 hr/day 5 day/week 3 weeks	18/2	ABG, RM, TTI, 6-MWD, dyspnea	Significant effects for BGA, dyspnoea, 6-MWD, RM, TTI

Abbreviations: IPAP/EPAP, ratio of inspiratory positive airway pressure and expiratory positive airway pressure; NP; ABG, arterial blood gas; 6-MWD, six-minute walking distance; 6-MWT, six-minute walk test; HRQL, health-related quality of life; RVEL, right ventricular ejection fraction; LVEF, left ventricular ejection fraction; NIPPV, noninvasive positive pressure ventilation; O_2, oxygen; TTI, tension time index.

apart from the neuropsychological function (23). Only seven of their 19 patients completed the study, and most patients were not hypercapnic. Gay et al. assessed the effects of NIPPV in hypercapnic patients and showed that NIPPV did not lead to an improvement in clinical parameters compared with sham ventilation (24). Again, only a small number of patients completed the study. The study of Meecham Jones et al. was the only one that showed clear evidence of clinical benefits for nocturnal NIPPV in patients with COPD (11). After three months, the combination of NIPPV and oxygen was better than oxygen alone for gas exchange, sleep efficiency, and health status. Lin et al. determined the effects of NIPPV after two weeks and found a positive effect of the combination of NIPPV and oxygen on nighttime oxygenation (25).

The reason for these negative results might be that some patients need more than two weeks of acclimatization before they are comfortable and confident with ventilator use at night. Renston et al. investigated the effects of daytime NIPPV (two hours a day for five consecutive days) (26). Despite the fact that no significant changes were found in gas exchange, patients in the BiPAP group showed both a significant decrease in level of dyspnea and an improvement in 6-MWD. However, it was not clear from the paper if BiPAP was significantly better than sham treatment. Another recent paper investigated the effects of NIPPV during the daytime for three hours, five days a week for three weeks(18). The authors found significant improvements in gas exchange, dyspnea, and walking distance.

As conflicting results exist, a meta-analysis of individual data from RCTs was carried out, comparing NIPPV with the conventional management of patients with COPD in stable respiratory failure (27). Only studies investigating NIPPV applied via a nasal or face mask for at least five hours each day for three weeks were included. Four RCTs were found that fulfilled the above-mentioned criteria (11,23,24,28) (Table 2), including the three-month data of the study of Casanova as well (28). Table 2 shows that three months of NIPPV in patients with stable COPD did not improve lung function, gas exchange, sleep efficiency, or 6-MWD. The limited number of patients in this meta-analysis precludes a clear clinical direction regarding the short-term effects of NIPPV in COPD.

Table 2 Primary Results of a Meta-Analysis on Nocturnal NIPPV

Outcomes	Contributing trials (references)	Sample size (NIPPV/control)	Treatment effect	
			Mean	95% CI
FEV_1	11, 23, 24, 28	33/33	0.02 L	−0.04, 0.09
FVC	11, 23, 24, 28	33/33	−0.01 L	−0.14, 0.13
$P_{i,max}$	23, 24, 28	24/24	6.2 cmH_2O	0.2, 12.2
$P_{e,max}$	23, 24, 28	24/24	18.4 cmH_2O	−11.8, 48.6
Pao_2	11, 23, 24, 28	33/33	0.0 mmHg	−3.8, 3.9
$Paco_2$	11, 23, 24, 28	33/33	−1.5 mmHg	−4.5, 1.5
Six-minute walk test	11, 24	12/11	27.5 m	−26.8, 81.8
Sleep efficiency	11, 23, 24	13/11	−4.0%	−14.7, 6.7

Abbreviations: NIPPV, noninvasive positive pressure ventilation; CI, cardiac index; FEV_1, forced respiratory value in 1 second; FVC, forced vital capacity; Pao_2, partial pressure of oxygen in arterial blood; $Paco_2$, partial pressure of carbon dioxide in arterial blood.
Source: From Refs. 11, 23, 24, and 28.

B. Long-Term RCTs of NIPPV in COPD

Casanova et al. reported the first long-term trial with a duration of one year (28). Fifty-two patients were randomized either to NIPPV and standard care or to standard care alone. The level of BiPAP used was only modest (IPAP 12–14 cmH_2O) and its effect was not confirmed during the night. However, this study did show some positive effects. The number of hospital admissions at three months was reduced (5% vs. 15%), but not the number after six months. There were modest improvements in dyspnea and neuropsychological function, but no changes in arterial blood gases or respiratory muscle strength at 12 months.

Another long-term randomized controlled study, by Clini et al., compared the combination of NIPPV and long-term oxygen therapy (LTOT) with LTOT alone for a period of two years (29). Only patients with a $Paco_2$ >6.6 kPa were included. One hundred and twenty patients were considered, 90 were randomized, and 47 completed the study. The level of NIPPV was again modest (IPAP of 14 ± 3 cmH_2O), although the ventilator was used for 9 ± 2 hours. Compared with the one-year period before the study, trends that did not reach between group statistical significance suggested an increase in hospital admissions and in ICU admissions in the LTOT group and a decrease in both in the NIPPV group. After two years, dyspnea decreased and health-related quality of life improved in the NIPPV compared with the LTOT group. Finally, in a study that has only been published in abstract form, Muir compared 60 patients with severe COPD who received LTOT and NIPPV with 62 patients who received LTOT alone (30). After a median follow-up of 4.7 years there were no significant differences in survival between the groups, with the exception of patients older than 65 years in whom survival was better in the NIPPV and LTOT group.

Clearly, we do not have enough evidence that NIPPV should be provided routinely to stable COPD patients with respiratory failure. Some of the inconsistencies among studies may be explained by methodological differences.

Patient Selection

Patients who are more hypercapnic seem to benefit more from NIPPV (11,29), especially when the $Paco_2$ >6.6 kPa. Meecham Jones noted that these patients had the greatest daytime decrease in $Paco_2$ after starting NIPPV. Trials that obtained negative results included normocapnic or only mildy hypercapnic patients (23–25).

Type and Adequacy of Ventilation

Whereas all RCTs used BiPAP, the uncontrolled studies used mainly volume-cycled ventilation. Assist-control ventilation is frequently selected to enhance synchrony between the patient and the ventilator (23). More importantly, the study by Meecham Jones et al. (11) is the only one to have confirmed the effectiveness of ventilation using transcutaneous $Paco_2$. Strumpf et al. monitored Pco_2 with end-tidal measurements, acknowledged to be unreliable in COPD. Therefore, a possible effect of NIPPV cannot be excluded. Meecham Jones et al. confirmed the effectiveness of NIPPV during sleep at a mean inspiratory pressures of 18 cmH_2O, and noted positive effects on most outcomes (11). In a recent retrospective report, a mean inspiratory pressure of 28 cmH_2O resulted in a fall in $Paco_2$ during spontaneous breathing from 55 to 46 mmHg (31).

Number of Hours on NIPPV

The optimal duration of ventilatory support is unknown. Two randomized controlled studies treated patients with COPD for short periods of ventilatory support during the day (18,26). In one study, the patients received BiPAP for two hours daily for five days a week, while in the other BiPAP was given for three hours daily, five days a week for three consecutive weeks. These short periods were reported to produce significant benefits in clinical parameters and changes in Pao_2 and $Paco_2$. Perhaps patients adjusted to daytime ventilation more readily than at night. In contrast, in a long-term trial of Clini (29), BiPAP was used for 9 ± 2 hours, and in the study by Meecham Jones it was used for 6.9 hours (range 4.2–10.8) (11).

Duration of Ventilation

The duration of treatment can also influence the outcome. Most studies were for three months, and two followed patients for longer periods (29,30). Clini et al. noted an improved quality of life after two years and improved dyspnea after one year, with a trend to a reduction in hospital and ICU admissions over the subsequent year. Days in hospital due to respiratory exacerbations also showed a nonsignificant trend in favor of NIPPV (12.6 ± 7.9 vs. 16.9 ± 10.3). Clinical benefits were seen after three months in the Meecham Jones study (11).

IV. Cystic Fibrosis and Bronchiectasis

There are far fewer publications about the use of NIPPV in patients with bronchiectasis and CF. However, as these conditions are characterized by airflow obstruction and hyperinflation, it is likely that many of the principles relating to NIPPV in COPD also apply to these patients. However, an important difference is the greatly increased volume of secretions and, in the case of CF, the fact that the condition is usually more rapidly progressive. This may raise practical issues with regard to palliative care in the terminal phases of the disease.

Uncontrolled studies have shown that in patients with CF, NIPPV will unload respiratory muscles, increase alveolar ventilation, and improve oxygenation during wakefulness, sleep, and an acute exacerbation. Inspiratory and expiratory muscle strengths improve following NIPPV, which may be important in facilitating secretion clearance (32). NIPPV also improves tolerance of physiotherapy (33,34).

However, there is little information regarding the impact of NIPPV on quality of life or survival. The use of NIPPV as a bridge to transplantation is well described (35,36) and while, in the absence of a transplant, patients become increasingly dependent on assisted ventilation there is no evidence that the institution of NIPPV compromises effective palliative care. The outcome for transplantation is said to be better if patients have received ventilatory support noninvasively pretransplant compared with invasive ventilation (35). Although Sood et al. described 100% one-year survival in eight patients who had been transplanted while being ventilated invasively (37), invasive ventilation for more than two weeks is usually associated with a poor prognosis (37). Therefore, noninvasive ventilation should be the mode of choice unless organs are known to be available imminently. Long-term NIPPV has also been described in patients with bronchiectasis of other causes leading to improved arterial blood gas tensions and reduced need for hospitalization (38).

V. Summary

There is insufficient evidence for NIPPV among stable patients with COPD or bronchiectasis, including those with CF. For hypercapnic patients with COPD, in whom the effectiveness of NIPPV in improving gas exchange at night has been confirmed, there might be some clinical benefit, although well-designed prospective trials of this approach are required. NIPPV is effective in the management of acute respiratory failure prior to invasive ventilation, or in patients deteriorating while awaiting transplantation. NIPPV may have an adjunctive role, together with physiotherapy in selected patients with high volumes of sputum, but its precise application needs further definition.

References

1. Bellemare F, Grassino A. Effect of pressure and timing of contraction on human diaphragm fatigue. J Appl Physiol 1982; 53(5):1190–1195.
2. Scano G, Gigliotti F, Duranti R, et al. Changes in ventilatory muscle function with negative pressure ventilation in patients with severe COPD. Chest 1990; 97(2):322–327.
3. Cropp A, DiMarco AF. Effects of intermittent negative pressure ventilation on respiratory muscle function in patients with severe chronic obstructive pulmonary disease. Am Rev Respir Dis 1987; 135(5):1056–1061.
4. Zibrak JD, Hill NS, Federman EC, et al. Evaluation of intermittent long-term negative-pressure ventilation in patients with severe chronic obstructive pulmonary disease. Am Rev Respir Dis 1988; 138(6):1515–1518.
5. Celli B, Lee H, Criner G, et al. Controlled trial of external negative pressure ventilation in patients with severe chronic airflow obstruction. Am Rev Respir Dis 1989; 140(5):1251–1256.
6. Nava S, Fanfulla F, Frigerio P, et al. Physiologic evaluation of 4 weeks of nocturnal nasal positive pressure ventilation in stable hypercapnic patients with chronic obstructive pulmonary disease. Respiration 2001; 68(6):573–583.
7. Shapiro SH, Ernst P, Gray-Donald K, et al. Effect of negative pressure ventilation in severe chronic obstructive pulmonary disease. Lancet 1992; 340(8833):1425–1429.
8. Corrado A, Ginanni R, Villella G, et al. Iron lung versus conventional mechanical ventilation in acute exacerbation of COPD. Eur Respir J 2004; 23(3):419–424.
9. Laghi F, Cattapan SE, Jubran A, et al. Is weaning failure caused by low-frequency fatigue of the diaphragm? Am J Respir Crit Care Med 2003; 167(2):120–127.
10. Elliott MW, Simonds AK, Carroll MP, et al. Domiciliary nocturnal nasal intermittent positive pressure ventilation in hypercapnic respiratory failure due to chronic obstructive lung disease: effects on sleep and quality of life. Thorax 1992; 47(5):342–348.
11. Meecham Jones DJ, Paul EA, Jones PW, et al. Nasal pressure support ventilation plus oxygen compared with oxygen therapy alone in hypercapnic COPD. Am J Respir Crit Care Med 1995; 152(2):538–544.
12. Criner GJ, Brennan K, Travaline JM, et al. Efficacy and compliance with noninvasive positive pressure ventilation in patients with chronic respiratory failure. Chest 1999; 116(3):667–675.
13. Berthon-Jones M, Sullivan CE. Time course of change in ventilatory response to CO_2 with long-term CPAP therapy for obstructive sleep apnea. Am Rev Respir Dis 1987; 135(1):144–147.
14. Annane D, Quera-Salva MA, Lofaso F, et al. Mechanisms underlying effects of nocturnal ventilation on daytime blood gases in neuromuscular diseases. Eur Respir J 1999; 13(1): 157–162.
15. Elliott MW, Mulvey DA, Moxham J, et al. Domiciliary nocturnal nasal intermittent positive pressure ventilation in COPD: mechanisms underlying changes in arterial blood gas tensions. Eur Respir J 1991; 4(9):1044–1052.

16. Nickol AH, Hart N, Hopkinson NS, et al. Mechanisms of improvement of respiratory failure in patients with restrictive thoracic disease treated with non-invasive ventilation. Thorax 2005; 60(9): 754–760.
17. Budweiser S, Heinemann F, Fischer W, et al. Long-term reduction of hyperinflation in stable COPD by non-invasive nocturnal home ventilation. Respir Med 2005; 99(8):976–984.
18. Diaz O, Begin P, Andresen M, et al. Physiological and clinical effects of diurnal noninvasive ventilation in hypercapnic COPD. Eur Respir J 2005; 26(6):1016–1023.
19. Diaz O, Begin P, Torrealba B, et al. Effects of noninvasive ventilation on lung hyperinflation in stable hypercapnic COPD. Eur Respir J 2002; 20(6):1490–1498.
20. Perrin C, El Far Y, Vandenbos F, et al. Domiciliary nasal intermittent positive pressure ventilation in severe COPD: effects on lung function and quality of life. Eur Respir J 1997; 10(12): 2835–2839.
21. Sivasothy P, Smith IE, Shneerson JM. Mask intermittent positive pressure ventilation in chronic hypercapnic respiratory failure due to chronic obstructive pulmonary disease. Eur Respir J 1998; 11(1):34–40.
22. Jones SE, Packham S, Hebden M, et al. Domiciliary nocturnal intermittent positive pressure ventilation in patients with respiratory failure due to severe COPD: long-term follow up and effect on survival. Thorax 1998; 53(6):495–498.
23. Strumpf DA, Millman RP, Carlisle CC, et al. Nocturnal positive-pressure ventilation via nasal mask in patients with severe chronic obstructive pulmonary disease. Am Rev Respir Dis 1991; 144(6):1234–1239.
24. Gay PC, Hubmayr RD, Stroetz RW. Efficacy of nocturnal nasal ventilation in stable, severe chronic obstructive pulmonary disease during a 3-month controlled trial. Mayo Clin Proc 1996; 71(6):533–542.
25. Lin CC. Comparison between nocturnal nasal positive pressure ventilation combined with oxygen therapy and oxygen monotherapy in patients with severe COPD. Am J Respir Crit Care Med 1996; 154(2 pt 1):353–358.
26. Renston JP, DiMarco AF, Supinski GS. Respiratory muscle rest using nasal BiPAP ventilation in patients with stable severe COPD. Chest 1994; 105(4):1053–1060.
27. Wijkstra PJ, Lacasse Y, Guyatt GH, et al. Nocturnal non-invasive positive pressure ventilation for stable chronic obstructive pulmonary disease. Cochrane Database Syst Rev 2002; (3): CD002878.
28. Casanova C, Celli BR, Tost L, et al. Long-term controlled trial of nocturnal nasal positive pressure ventilation in patients with severe COPD. Chest 2000; 118(6):1582–1590.
29. Clini E, Sturani C, Rossi A, et al. The Italian multicentre study on noninvasive ventilation in chronic obstructive pulmonary disease patients. Eur Respir J 2002; 20(3):529–538.
30. Muir JF, de la Salmoniere P, Cuvelier A CSTB. Survival of severe hypercapnic COPD under long-term home mechanical ventilation with NIPPV + oxygen versus oxygen therapy alone. Preliminary results of a European multicentre study. Am J Respir Crit Care Med 1999; 159:A295.
31. Windisch W, Kostic S, Dreher M, et al. Outcome of patients with stable COPD receiving controlled noninvasive positive pressure ventilation aimed at a maximal reduction of Pa(CO2). Chest 2005; 128(2):657–662.
32. Piper AJ, Parker S, Torzillo PJ, et al. Nocturnal nasal IPPV stabilizes patients with cystic fibrosis and hypercapnic respiratory failure. Chest 1992; 102(3):846–850.
33. Fauroux B, Boule M, Lofaso F, et al. Chest physiotherapy in cystic fibrosis: improved tolerance with nasal pressure support ventilation. Pediatrics 1999; 103(3):E32.
34. Holland AE, Denehy L, Ntoumenopoulos G, et al. Non-invasive ventilation assists chest physiotherapy in adults with acute exacerbations of cystic fibrosis. Thorax 2003; 58(10):880–884.
35. Madden BP, Kariyawasam H, Siddiqi AJ, et al. Noninvasive ventilation in cystic fibrosis patients with acute or chronic respiratory failure. Eur Respir J 2002; 19(2):310–313.

36. Caronia CG, Silver P, Nimkoff L, et al. Use of bilevel positive airway pressure (BIPAP) in end-stage patients with cystic fibrosis awaiting lung transplantation. Clin Pediatr (Phila) 1998; 37(9): 555–559.
37. Sood N, Paradowski LJ, Yankaskas JR. Outcomes of intensive care unit care in adults with cystic fibrosis. Am J Respir Crit Care Med 2001; 163(2):335–338.
38. Benhamou D, Muir JF, Raspaud C, et al. Long-term efficiency of home nasal mask ventilation in patients with diffuse bronchiectasis and severe chronic respiratory failure: a case-control study. Chest 1997; 112(5):1259–1266.

37
Ventilation Among the Pediatric Population

BRIGITTE FAUROUX
Pediatric Pulmonary and INSERM UMR S719 AP-HP, Hopital Armand Trousseau and Université Pierre et Marie Curie, Paris, France

FRÉDÉRIC LOFASO
Physiology Department and INSERM 841 AP-HP, Hopital Raymond Poincaré and Université Versailles Saint-Quentin en Yvelines, Garches, France

I. Introduction

Long-term ventilatory support may be indicated in a significant number of diseases encountered in the pediatric population (1,2). Indeed, respiratory center inefficiency and disorders characterized by an imbalance between the load imposed on the respiratory system and the capacity of the respiratory muscles may lead to the development of alveolar hypoventilation, which may be corrected or improved with ventilatory assistance. As such, lung diseases characterized by an impairment of the diffusion of gases, such as interstitial lung diseases, do not respond to ventilatory support and will require long-term oxygen therapy. Neuromuscular disorders, abnormalities of the upper airways (such as laryngomalacia or Pierre Robin syndrome) and of the chest wall and/or the lungs (such as cystic fibrosis, CF), and disorders of ventilatory control (such as Ondine's curse) represent the main causes of chronic alveolar hypoventilation in childhood (1,2).

In the pediatric population, long-term ventilatory support will be preferentially delivered noninvasively by means of a nasal interface. The advantages of noninvasive positive pressure ventilation (NPPV) are that it preserves the patient's airways and that it can be applied on demand, and preferentially at night, causing much less morbidity, discomfort, and disruption to social and family life than a tracheostomy. But NPPV is not applicable to all children. Noninvasive forms of mechanical ventilation are technically difficult to apply in infants and young children. Usually, NPPV is applied during the night, and during the daytime nap in young children. A minimal respiratory autonomy is thus a prerequisite for NPPV, even if the beneficial effects of NPPV can extend, after a certain period, during periods of spontaneous breathing. When alveolar hypoventilation progresses or when it persists during the day, additional ventilatory support, such as mouthpiece ventilation, may be necessary. Invasive ventilation by means of a tracheostomy remains the last option, but this invasive form of ventilatory support needs to integrate the prognosis of the underlying disease as well as the psychological and practical acceptance by the patient and his family.

NPPV is mostly used on an empirical basis in children, with a considerable gap between the expanding use and the lack of precise knowledge on physiological benefits.

This makes it difficult to establish both the appropriate timing of initiation of NPPV and the most pertinent therapeutic goals.

This chapter focuses on long-term ventilatory support in infants and children. Because of the preferential use of NPPV, we will focus on this technique. The place of a tracheostomy will be discussed in the chapter, dealing with the limits and side effects of NPPV.

II. Which Patients May Benefit from NPPV?

A. Disorders Justifying NPPV

Infants and children may require long-term ventilatory support due to three categories of diseases that may impair the ventilatory balance: increased respiratory load (due to intrinsic cardiopulmonary disorders, upper airway abnormalities, or skeletal deformities), ventilatory muscle weakness [due to neuromuscular diseases (NMD) or spinal cord injury], or failure of neurological control of ventilation (with central hypoventilation syndrome being the most common presentation) (Fig. 1).

Increase in Respiratory Load

Obstruction of the upper or lower airways may cause an increase in respiratory load. Obstructive sleep apnea (OSA) is less common in children than in adults. In this age group, enlarged tonsils and adenoids play a predominant role (3). Noninvasive continuous positive airway pressure (CPAP) ventilation has proved its efficacy and is proposed as a first therapeutic option if tonsillectomy and adenoidectomy are not able to relieve upper airway obstruction (4,5). Congenital abnormalities of the upper airways, such as laryngomalacia, tracheomalacia, or Pierre Robin syndrome, may also cause severe upper airway obstruction (6). Even in young infants, noninvasive CPAP may correct the alveolar hypoventilation (7).

Children with achondroplasia often have sleep-related respiratory disturbances, primarily hypoxemia (8). A substantial minority of them have obstructive or central apnea,

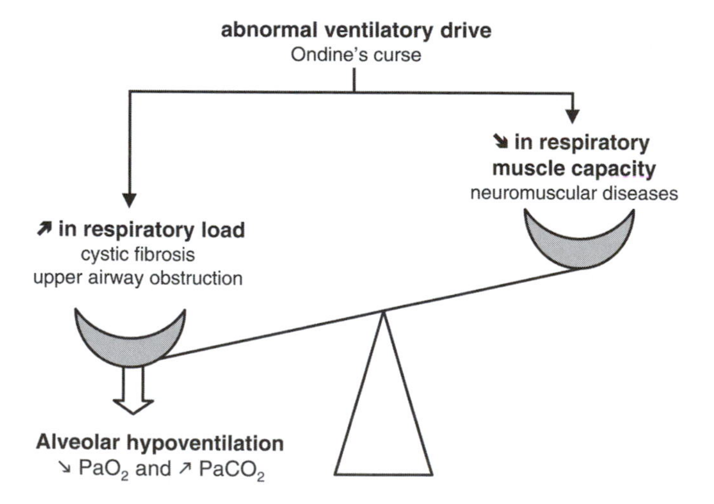

Figure 1 Causes of ventilatory imbalance in childhood.

which has been linked to brain stem compression (9). These symptoms may be adequately relieved by NPPV.

Respiratory insufficiency in CF is also characterized by the development of alveolar hypoventilation. In children and young adults with advanced pulmonary CF disease, as lung disease progresses, with a progressive fall in the forced expiratory volume in one second (FEV1), there is an increase in the respiratory muscle load (10). Indeed, in a group of children with CF, having a forced expiratory volume in one second (FEV1) between 30% and 50% of predicted value, the respiratory muscle output, assessed by the esophageal and diaphragmatic pressure time products, was increased three- to fivefold. As a result, the patients develop a compensatory mechanism of rapid shallow breathing pattern in an attempt to reduce the increase in load. Although this breathing strategy maintains the level of ventilation, partial arterial carbon dioxide pressure ($Paco_2$) rises. NPPV is able to unload the respiratory muscles and improve alveolar hypoventilation (11–13).

Chest wall abnormalities such as severe scoliosis, kyphosis, or thoracic dystrophy may cause restrictive diseases severe enough to require long-term NPPV.

Ventilatory Muscle Weakness

Ventilatory muscle weakness, dysfunction, or paralysis can occur because of NMD, or as a result of spinal cord injury. The respiratory muscles are rarely spared in children with NMD (14). Ventilatory muscle weakness is associated, in a variable degree, with inspiratory muscle weakness, which results in inability to inspire fully, resulting in atelectasis, as well as expiratory muscle weakness, causing inability to cough, predisposing these patients to pulmonary infection. The consequent hypoventilation may translate in inadequate gas exchange. The most common NMD requiring NPPV during childhood are Duchenne muscular dystrophy and spinal muscular atrophy (SMA). Duchenne muscular dystrophy is a progressive disorder and ventilatory failure is inevitable in the course of the disease, although the time course of progression varies between individuals. Home NPPV counteracts the hypoventilation and can improve survival (15–17). Respiratory failure is also common in children with SMA. The SMAs are inherited as autosomal recessive disorders. Severity is inversely proportional to the amount of survival motoneuron protein in the anterior horn cell. SMAs range from essentially total paralysis and need for ventilatory support from birth, to the relatively mild muscle weakness presenting in the young adult. Diaphragmatic strength is generally preserved and respiratory muscle weakness predominates on the other inspiratory and expiratory muscles (14). Respiratory failure is less frequent in other muscular dystrophies, such as Becker, limb-girdle, and facioscapulohumeral dystrophies. Congenital myopathies are often static (14). However, the conditions of children may deteriorate functionally with growth because weakened muscles are unable to cope with increasing body mass.

The importance of respiratory failure associated with spinal cord injury depends on the level of the injury. High spinal cord injury, above C-3, causes diaphragm paralysis. This virtually always causes respiratory failure in infants and young children. NPPV can be tried in older children who have a sufficient respiratory autonomy for at least 8 to 10 hr/day. In patients with lower cervical cord injury, expiratory muscle function is severely compromised and thus cough is defective, and the clearance of bronchial secretions is greatly impaired. As a result, retention of secretions leading to atelectasis and bronchopneumonia frequently occurs in such patients and may require short periods of NPPV during episodes of acute respiratory failure.

Failure of the Neurological Control of Ventilation

Disorders of neurological control of breathing that are severe enough to cause chronic respiratory failure are uncommon to rare. Congenital central hypoventilation syndrome (Ondine's curse) is the most common presentation in childhood and is characterized by the failure of autonomic control of breathing (18). Hypoxia and hypercapnia worsen during sleep. Infants generally require invasive ventilation by means of a tracheostomy, but NPPV may be successful in older children who are able to sustain adequate ventilation during wakefulness but require ventilatory assistance only during sleep (19,20).

B. Medical and Technical Requisites for NPPV

Medical Requisites for NPPV

The medical requisites for NPPV are summarized in Table 1. The selection of patients for home care is the most crucial point; the severity of the medical condition and the age of the patient are two major factors that must always be considered.

NPPV can only be proposed if the patient's condition may be efficiently improved by it. Polysomnographic evaluations are recommended before the initiation of NPPV, before discharge with the ventilator, and during an overnight hospital admission during the follow-up. Careful extrapolation should be made from polysomnogram evaluations performed during daytime naps because they do not always reflect what happens during the night. Discharge may be allowed when the patient's condition is perfectly stabilized in the hospital with the home ventilator for a few days and with a perfect tolerance of the mask and the ventilator. Diurnal blood gases should return within the normal limits. A minimal respiratory autonomy (of at least six hours) is preferable even if some highly skilled teams have reported a successful experience with NPPV in 24-hour-dependent children (21,22).

All caregivers and especially the parents should complete competency training in the hospital before discharge. Caregivers need to be taught how to manage the patient and all minor technical problems with the ventilator equipment. They must know the clinical symptoms that require urgent medical attention. All these points have to be checked before discharge. Written competency agreements and guides for the caregivers are strongly

Table 1 Medical and Technical Requisites for NPPV in Children

Medical requisites	Technical requisites
• The patient's condition may be corrected or improved by NPPV	• Tolerance of the interface
• Minimal respiratory autonomy	• Adaptation to the ventilatory mode and settings
• Stable condition	• Appropriate alarms (pressure and tidal volume)
• Normal gas exchange during night and day	• Education of parents and caregivers
• Adequate growth	• Adequate home environment
• Normal neurocognitive development	• Home care organization skilled in pediatric home ventilation

Abbreviation: NPPV, noninvasive positive pressure ventilation.

recommended. Proficiency should be checked by the medical team and the nurse in the hospital and by the technician of the home care organization on a regular basis.

Technical Requisites for Home NPPV

The technical requisites are summarized in Table 1. The tolerance of the interface and the perfect adaptation to the ventilatory mode and settings are the most important technical requisites. Few ventilators have been designed specifically for children. Even if bench studies and practice in the adult population have provided reassuring results, the efficacy and absence of problems with the settings, triggers, and alarms have to be checked in the hospital before discharge.

Home should be suitable for the ventilator-dependent child. No home care can be allowed if the minimal safety requirements are not fulfilled. An important role of the home care organization or social worker is to check the appropriateness of the home environment. A visit to the home is recommended before discharge. Smoking by the parents or others should be prohibited in home.

Optimal home care should be completely organized before discharge. Financial aspects have to be discussed and resolved before discharge. This organization may differ according to the country and the health care system. Assistance to the family, which may be provided by nurses, non–health care professionals, or extended family members, has to be organized.

It is possible to organize holidays sufficiently in advance with most of the home care organizations. A local referee, both concerning the home care (nurse and technician) and the medical hospital care, should be informed and made available for the patient.

III. When to Start NPPV?

A. Indications for NPPV

Evidence-based recommendations are not available to guide the decision and timing of NPPV in children. Indeed, no prospective controlled studies have evaluated the optimal timing and criteria to start NPPV according to the underlying disease. Presently, the indications for NPPV are based on recommendations of experts or scientific societies.

The most accepted indication for NPPV is diurnal hypercapnia in a stable state because it is the signature of overt ventilatory failure. Most recommendations concern patients with NMD and, in particular, patients with Duchenne muscular dystrophy in whom ventilatory support should be considered when daytime $Paco_2$ exceeds 6 kPa (45 mmHg) (23–27). No guidelines or recommendations are available for the other causes of hypoventilation such as OSA or CF, but it seems reasonable to also consider diurnal hypercapnia as a criterion to propose NPPV in these patients.

NPPV is also indicated when acute exacerbations caused by bronchitis or pneumonia precipitate the patient in acute respiratory failure. But ideally, NPPV should be initiated before an acute exacerbation, which does not represent an optimal physiological and psychological situation to start such a treatment.

These two classical criteria are preceded by a variable period of nocturnal hypoventilation during which treatable symptoms, such as frequent arousals, severe orthopnea, daytime fatigue, and alterations in cognitive function, may deteriorate the daily life of the patient. There is also a wide agreement that clinical symptoms attributable to nocturnal hypoventilation such as sleep disruption, daytime hypersomnolence, excessive fatigue, and morning headache are most important for the decision of NPPV (28). This observation underlines the importance of a polysomnographic sleep study that represents the only way to document nocturnal hypoventilation. Recently, Ward and coworkers evaluated the benefit of NPPV in a group of adults and children with congenital neuromuscular or chest wall disease having normal daytime $Paco_2$, but a peak transcutaneous Pco_2 ($Ptcco_2$) >6.5 kPa (29). Ten patients were randomized to NPPV and 10 to control, without NPPV. NPPV was associated with a decrease in the percentage of nighttime spent with a $Ptcco_2$ >6.5 kPa and an increase in mean nocturnal pulse oximetry (Sao_2). Most importantly, 9 of the 10 controls failed nonintervention by fulfilling criteria to initiate NPPV after a mean of 8.3 ± 7.3 months. In this small and heterogeneous group of patients, NPPV was associated with a significant gain in the SF-36 general health score by 18 months. Indeed, when NPPV is decided, its effect on growth and neuropsychological development such as improvements in alertness, attention/concentration, and behavior/temperament are crucial factors in children that merit further investigation (28).

It is essential that the child, if his or her age permits, and the parents should have the opportunity to discuss the NPPV therapy in advance. Discussion should start long before the anticipated need to allow the child and the family to evaluate options thoroughly and to discuss their feelings. NPPV has here an essential first place as a noninvasive therapy, but still represents an objective element reflecting a further step in the severity of a disease. It is crucial to determine short-term and intermediate-term goals of NPPV with the child and the family to explain the principles of NPPV and to underline the fact that NPPV will adapt to the child and not the opposite. A wide range of ventilators and masks are available and great care will be taken to choose the most appropriate equipment and settings. The final objective is that NPPV should translate into well-being, a better quality of life, with a total adherence of the child and his family.

B. When NPPV Is Inadequate

The general point of view is that NPPV is preferred over invasive mechanical ventilation as the first therapy of chronic respiratory failure. However, NPPV is inadequate in some circumstances, which are listed in Table 2. The inability to correct the alveolar hypoventilation

Table 2 Inadequacy of NPPV

Relative inadequacy

- Severe swallowing impairment
- Need for full-time ventilatory assistance
- Inadequate family or caregiver support

Absolute inadequacy

- Ineffectiveness of NPPV due to upper airway dysfunction
- Uncontrollable secretion retention
- Inability to cooperate
- Inadequate cough, even with assistance
- Inability to fit the mask

Abbreviation: NPPV, noninvasive positive pressure ventilation.

is the most frequent demonstration of NPPV failure. This failure of NPPV will be discussed in the last paragraph of the chapter.

It is preferable to postpone NPPV in case of a pneumothorax, which can occur in patients with advanced CF lung disease. In patients with CF, nasal polyps are common and should be treated before the initiation of NPPV.

IV. Long-Term Follow-Up

A. The Hospital and Home Care Network

Follow-up at an expert multidisciplinary pediatric center for mechanical ventilation is strongly recommended. The team comprises a pediatrician with expertise in NPPV, a coordinating nurse, a physiotherapist, a dietician along with others in specialty areas, such as a pediatric gastroenterologist, a psychologist, a social worker, a cardiologist, and an orthopedic surgeon. Follow-up by a pediatric maxillofacial surgeon is recommended for the follow-up of the interface (30).

This hospital-based team should work in close collaboration with the home team, which comprises a general practitioner or general pediatrician, a physiotherapist, and a nurse. Caregivers should have a hotline number to contact in the event of a medical problem, and emergency admission should be possible at any time. Periodic admissions aid the transition from hospital to home (Table 3). A second ventilator is necessary for any patient who is unable to breathe spontaneously for more than a few hours. This spare ventilator can be fixed on the patient's wheelchair and be available if the other device breaks down. A backup ventilator with a backup generator unit is also recommended for patients in remote rural regions.

The home care system consists of at least one nurse and a technician, both of whom should be able to recognize respiratory compromise in children of various ages. Ideally, the home care team should be present on the day of discharge to check the installation and settings of the equipment in the home and to ensure that the caregivers understand the management plan. The frequency of the home visits depends on the medical condition of the patient, but visits should be at least twice a week at the start and then every week thereafter until the patient and caregivers are reasonably independent in the home setting, at which time the frequency of visits can be reduced, depending on the medical and social situation.

Table 3 Example of Follow-up of a Child Receiving Home NPPV

	Before NPPV	Before discharge	Every 2–3 mo	Annually
Clinical examination	Yes	Yes	Yes	Yes
Arterial blood gases	Yes	Yes	±	Yes
Nighttime $Ptco_2$ and $Ptcco_2$ monitoring	Yes	Yes	±	Yes
Polysomnography	Yes	Yes		Yes
Lung function tests	Yes			Yes
Echocardiography	Yes			Yes
Other specialists[a]	Yes		Yes	Yes

[a]According to the underlying disease.

Abbreviations: $Ptco_2$, transcutaneous oxygen pressure; $Ptcco_2$, transcutaneous carbon dioxide pressure.

A second ventilatory circuit, with mask, head gear, and chin strap, as well as a preventative maintenance schedule for changing filters and checking alarms are required. Nearly all ventilators need an electrical power source and although models with built-in battery supplies are preferred, the need for a backup battery should be discussed on an individual basis. Systematic pulse oximetry monitoring is not usually necessary, but may be required initially for highly ventilator-dependent patients, and subsequently, if there are issues with secretion clearance or frequent infectious exacerbations.

Following home visits, medical and equipment information should be shared with the pediatrician, family physician, and hospital team. If there is an urgent medical problem or any immediate difficulties with the ventilator, all parties, including the equipment supplier, should be notified.

As the child grows, ventilator settings must be reevaluated to ensure adequate gas exchange. Although the optimal frequency for these evaluations has not been determined, they should be performed more frequently in infants and small children who are growing rapidly.

V. Benefits of NPPV

The potential benefits of NPPV vary according to the underlying disease. The increasing implementation of long-term NPPV in children contrasts with the scarcity of proven benefits in this age group.

A. Improvement in Survival

The major benefit of NPPV is the improvement in survival, although this has only been demonstrated in patients with NMD (16). In Denmark, the benefit of NPPV on survival of patients with Duchenne muscular dystrophy was evaluated between 1977 and 2001 (17). While overall incidence remained stable at 2 per 10^5 persons, prevalence rose from 3.1 to 5.5 per 10^5, mortality fell from 4.7 to 2.6 per 100 years at risk, and the prevalence of ventilator users rose from 0.9 to 43.4 per 100. Ventilator use is probably the main reason for this dramatic increase in survival. An increase in survival has not been demonstrated in CF patients.

B. Improvement of Nocturnal Hypoventilation and Gas Exchange

During sleep, certain key alterations in respiratory and upper airway function and ventilatory responses lead to a degree of nocturnal hypoventilation even in normal subjects, causing a rise in Pa_{CO_2} of approximately 3 mmHg (0.4 kPa) in adults. This may explain why patients with chronic respiratory failure are more vulnerable during sleep. In children with NMD, NPPV increases minute ventilation (31–33) and stabilizes the oropharyngeal airway (34). We have noted that NPPV was associated with a significant improvement in nocturnal gas exchange in 12 children with laryngomalacia (6). The benefits of NPPV in patients with CF have been shown in three short-term studies, comparing consecutive nights with and without NPPV (35–37).

These improvements in nocturnal alveolar hypoventilation translate into a decrease in diurnal hypercapnia among patients with OSA and NMD (38,39). This benefit may be due to the combined effects of several interrelated processes. Reduced cerebrospinal fluid bicarbonate concentration resets the ventilatory response to CO_2 and increases respiratory drive. Improved sleep quality influences the ventilatory response to CO_2 and improved respiratory muscle endurance is of benefit to the ventilatory system (40). NPPV may be responsible for a persistent decrease in the work of breathing during spontaneous ventilation as a result of an improvement in chest wall and lung mechanics (41).

Because sleep is an at-risk period in patients with chronic respiratory insufficiency and also for practical reasons, NPPV is preferentially performed during the night. However, daytime mechanical ventilation in awake adult patients has been reported to be equally effective in reversing chronic hypercapnia (42).

C. Improvement in Lung Function and Respiratory Muscle Performance

There is only limited evidence in support of NPPV stabilizing the decline in lung function in patients with NMD or CF, although data from the French Cystic Fibrosis Observatory have suggested that NPPV might be associated with improved lung function. In our personal unpublished experience, when 44 patients receiving NPPV were compared with matched (gender, cystic fibrosis transmembrane conductance regulator genotype, age, weight, and lung function) controls, one year before the initiation of NPPV, during the year of NPPV, and after one year of NPPV, the decline in vital capacity and FEV1 was similar between the two groups. Although Piper and coworkers reported an increase in maximal expiratory and inspiratory pressures in four adults with CF after one month of NPPV (43), this improvement may have been due to a learning effect. To date, the beneficial effect of NPPV on the respiratory muscles has not been clearly demonstrated.

D. Preservation of Normal Pulmonary Mechanics and Lung Growth

The physiological changes in the compliance of the lungs and the chest wall play a crucial role in the normal development of the lung. In infancy, the chest wall is nearly three times as compliant as the lung. By the end of the second year of life, chest wall stiffness increases to the point that the chest wall and lung are nearly equally compliant, as in adulthood. Stiffening of the chest wall plays a major role in developmental changes in respiratory system function, such as the ability to passively maintain resting lung volume and improved ventilatory efficiency afforded by reduced rib cage distortion. It would be important to know if long-term NPPV in infants and young children can preserve a near to normal chest wall compliance, both in children with too stiff chest due to thoracic deformity such as scoliosis or in those with NMD exposed to ankylosis in the costosternal and costovertebral joints and to gradual stiffening of the rib cage.

A major concern in the pediatric population is the effect of chronic hypoventilation on lung growth and whether NPPV helps promote physiological lung and chest wall growth in the developing child. Animal studies have demonstrated that efficient respiratory movements are mandatory for normal lung growth and differentiation (44,45). To our knowledge, this has not been studied in children.

E. Effect of NPPV on Quality of Life

Few studies have evaluated the effect of NPPV on quality of life in children (33,46). NPPV might influence both sleep and cognitive function, thereby influencing health-related quality of life. Early initiation of ventilatory support might improve school performance, even in the absence of permanent daytime hypercapnia (28).

VI. Limits and Side Effects of NPPV

NPPV may fail for medical or technical reasons. It may be less effective than invasive ventilation in reversing respiratory failure because of the persistence of dead space. Air leakage may encourage hypercapnia in both invasively and noninvasively ventilated NMD patients. A study of 325 ventilated NMD patients noted persistent hypercapnia in >20% of the study population (47). In these patients, simple practical measures, such as changing the mask, using a chin strap, increasing minute ventilation, and changing the type of the ventilator, were able to reduce the volume of air leaks and improve the efficacy of ventilation (48). As NPPV is difficult to use round the clock, mouthpiece ventilation is a useful adjunct to nocturnal NPPV and may delay the need for a tracheostomy (49). Technical limitations are more commonly attributable to the interface than to the ventilator. Patients with copious secretions or severe swallowing dysfunction may respond poorly to NPPV and a tracheostomy then becomes necessary. Therefore, close monitoring of the patient's physiological status and disease progression together with clear information of the family are essential.

A. Place of Tracheostomy

Most children are managed with NPPV (1,50). However, some require invasive ventilation through a tracheostomy. The main indications for a tracheostomy in children are airway abnormalities such as tracheobronchomalacia or tracheal stenosis, chronic disease of prematurity, and NMD (1,51,52). The indications for a tracheostomy are comparable to those of the adult population. They include the persistence of hypercapnia despite NPPV and additional measures such as daytime mouthpiece ventilation, aspiration, and bulbar dysfunction (53). In children, NPPV is more difficult to perform in those who might be 24-hour dependent, than in adults. Infants with primary alveolar hypoventilation (Ondine's curse) are preferentially ventilated by means of a tracheostomy (18). Tracheostomy ventilation favors airway inflammation (54) and may affect speech and language development (55). In children with progressive NMD, the decision of a tracheostomy has to be discussed on an individual basis, taking into account the familial environment and the parent's and child's perspective (52,56). In any case, sending children home with invasive ventilation is more difficult than when noninvasive ventilation is used (52).

In conclusion, NPPV is increasingly used in children and infants. This expanding use contrasts with the limited proven benefits. Pediatricians, physiologists, nurses, physiotherapists, and technicians should combine their efforts to determine more accurately the physiological effects of NPPV, especially on the respiratory muscles, respiratory compliance and growth, central drive and psychoneurological development, so that it may be introduced at a time least likely to be harmful and most likely to be of benefit in improving respiratory function and health-related quality of life.

References

1. Fauroux B, Sardet A, Foret D. Home treatment for chronic respiratory failure in children: a prospective study. Eur Resp J 1995; 8:2062–2066.
2. Fauroux B, Boffa C, Desguerre I, et al. Long-term noninvasive mechanical ventilation for children at home: a national survey. Pediatr Pulmonol 2003; 35:119–125.

3. Croft CB, Brockbank MJ, Wright A, et al. Obstructive sleep apnea in children undergoing routine tonsillectomy and adenoidectomy. Clin Otolaryngol 1990; 15:307–314.
4. Guilleminault C, Pelayo R, Clerk A, et al. Home nasal continuous positive airway pressure in infants with sleep-disordered breathing. J Pediatr 1995; 127:905–912.
5. Waters WA, Everett FM, Bruderer JW, et al. Obstructive sleep apnea: the use of nasal CPAP in 80 children. Am J Respir Crit Care Med 1995; 152:780–785.
6. Fauroux B, Pigeot J, Polkey MI, et al. Chronic stridor caused by laryngomalacia in children. Work of breathing and effects of noninvasive ventilatory assistance. Am J Respir Crit Care Med 2001; 164:1874–1878.
7. Essouri S, Nicot F, Clement A, et al. Noninvasive positive pressure ventilation in infants with upper airway obstruction: comparison of continuous and bilevel positive pressure. Intensive Care Med 2005; 31:574–580.
8. Mogayzel PJ, Carroll JL, Loughlin GM, et al. Sleep-disordered breathing in children with achondroplasia. J Pediatr 1998; 131:667–671.
9. Waters KA, Everett F, Sillence DO, et al. Treatment of obstructive sleep apnea in achondroplasia: evaluation of sleep, breathing, and somatosensory-evoked potentials. Am J Med Genet 1995; 59:460–466.
10. Hart N, Polkey MI, Clément A, et al. Changes in pulmonary mechanics with increasing disease severity in children and young adults with cystic fibrosis. Am J Respir Crit Care Med 2002; 166:61–66.
11. Fauroux B, Pigeot J, Isabey D, et al. In vivo physiological comparison of two ventilators used for domiciliary ventilation in children with cystic fibrosis. Crit Care Med 2001; 29:2097–2105.
12. Fauroux B, Louis B, Hart N, et al. The effect of back-up rate during non-invasive ventilation in young patients with cystic fibrosis. Intensive Care Med 2004; 30:673–681.
13. Fauroux B, Nicot F, Essouri S, et al. Setting of pressure support in young patients with cystic fibrosis. Eur Resp J 2004; 24:624–630.
14. Nicot F, Hart N, Forin V, et al. Respiratory muscle testing: a valuable tool for children with neuromuscular disorders. Am J Respir Crit Care Med 2006; 174:67–74.
15. Vianello A, Bevilacqua M, Salvador V, et al. Long-term nasal intermittent positive pressure ventilation in advanced Duchenne's muscular dystrophy. Chest 1994; 105:445–448.
16. Simonds A, Muntoni F, Heather S, et al. Impact of nasal ventilation on survival in hypercapnic Duchenne muscular dystrophy. Thorax 1998; 53:949–952.
17. Jeppesen J, Green A, Steffensen BF, et al. The Duchenne muscular dystrophy population in Denmark, 1977–2001: prevalence, incidence and survival in relation to the introduction of ventilator use. Neuromuscul Disord 2003; 13:804–812.
18. Gozal D. Congenital central hypoventilation syndrome: an update. Pediatr Pulmonol 1998; 26:273–282.
19. Zaccaria S, Braghiroli A, Sacco C, et al. Central hypoventilation in a seven year old boy. Long-term treatment by nasal mask ventilation. Monaldi Arch Chest Dis 1993; 48:37–38.
20. Nielson DW, Black PG. Mask ventilation in congenital central alveolar hypoventilation syndrome. Pediatr Pulmonol 1990; 9:44–45.
21. Bach JR, Niranjan V. Spinal muscular atrophy type I: a noninvasive respiratory management approach. Chest 2000; 117:1100–1105.
22. Bach JR, Baird JS, Plosky D, et al. Spinal muscular atrophy type 1: management and outcomes. Pediatr Pulmonol 2002; 34:16–22.
23. Sleep-related breathing disorders in adults: recommendations for syndrome definition and measurement techniques in clinical research. The Report of an American Academy of Sleep Medicine Task Force. Sleep 1999; 22:667–689.
24. Clinical indications for noninvasive positive pressure ventilation in chronic respiratory failure due to restrictive lung disease, COPD, and nocturnal hypoventilation—a consensus conference report. Chest 1999; 116:521–534.

25. Robert D, Willig TN, Paulus J. Long-term nasal ventilation in neuromuscular disorders: report of a consensus conference. Eur Respir J 1993; 6:599–606.
26. Rutgers M, Lucassen H, Kesteren RV, et al. Respiratory insufficiency and ventilatory support. 39th European Neuromuscular Centre International Workshop. Neuromuscul Disord 1996; 6:431–435.
27. Respiratory care of the patient with Duchenne muscular dystrophy. ATS Consensus Conference. Am J Respir Crit Care Med 2004; 170:456–465.
28. Fauroux B, Lofaso F. Non-invasive mechanical ventilation: when to start for what benefit? Thorax 2005; 60:979–980.
29. Ward S, Chatwin M, Heather S, et al. Randomised controlled trial of non-invasive ventilation (NIV) for nocturnal hypoventilation in neuromuscular and chest wall disease patients with daytime normocapnia. Thorax 2005; 60:1019–1024.
30. Fauroux B, Lavis JF, Nicot F, et al. Facial side effects during noninvasive positive pressure ventilation in children. Intensive Care Med 2005; 31:965–969.
31. Simonds AK, Ward S, Heather S, et al. Outcome of paediatric domiciliary mask ventilation in neuromuscular and skeletal disease. Eur Respir J 2000; 16:476–481.
32. Heckmatt JZ, Loh L, Dubowitz V. Night-time nasal ventilation in neuromuscular disease. Lancet 1990; 335:579–582.
33. Mellies U, Ragette R, Dohna Schwake C, et al. Long-term noninvasive ventilation in children and adolescents with neuromuscular disorders. Eur Respir J 2003; 22:631–636.
34. Ellis ER, Bye PTP, Bruderer JW, et al. Treatment of respiratory failure during sleep in patients with neuromuscular disease. Positive-pressure ventilation through a nasal mask. Am Rev Respir Dis 1987; 135:148–152.
35. Gozal D. Nocturnal ventilatory support in patients with cystic fibrosis: comparison with supplemental oxygen. Eur Resp J 1997; 10:1999–2003.
36. Regnis JA, Piper AJ, Henke KG, et al. Benefits of nocturnal nasal CPAP in patients with cystic fibrosis. Chest 1994; 106:1717–1724.
37. Milross MA, Piper AJ, Norman M, et al. Low-flow oxygen and bilevel ventilatory support. Effects on ventilation during sleep in cystic fibrosis. Am J Respir Crit Care Med 2001; 163:129–134.
38. Berthon-Jones M, Sullivan CE. Time course of change in ventilatory response to CO_2 with long-term CPAP therapy for obstructive sleep apnea. Am Rev Resp Dis 1987; 135:144–147.
39. Nickol AH, Hart N, Hopkinson NS, et al. Mechanisms of improvement of respiratory failure in patients with restrictive thoracic disease treated with non-invasive ventilation. Thorax 2005; 60:754–760.
40. White D, Douglas N, Pickett C, et al. Sleep deprivation and the control of ventilation. Am Rev Respir Dis 1983; 128:984–986.
41. Bergofsky EH. Respiratory failure in disorders of the thoracic cage. Am Rev Respir Dis 1979; 119:643–669.
42. Schönhofer B, Geibel M, Sonneborn M, et al. Daytime mechanical ventilation in chronic respiratory insufficiency. Eur Resp J 1997; 10:2840–2846.
43. Piper AJ, Parker S, Torzillo PJ, et al. Nocturnal nasal IPPV stabilizes patients with cystic fibrosis and hypercapnic respiratory failure. Chest 1992; 102:846–850.
44. Inanlou MR, Kablar B. Abnormal development of the diaphragm in *mdx:Myo -/-*^{9th} embryos leads to pulmonary hypoplasia. Int J Dev Biol 2003; 47:363–371.
45. Inanlou MR, Kablar B. Abnormal development of the intercostal muscles and the rib cage in *Myf5/* embryos leads to pulmonary hypoplasia. Dev Dyn 2005; 232:43–54.
46. Simonds A, Ward S, Heather S, et al. Outcome of domiciliary nocturnal non-invasive mask ventilation in paediatric neuromuscular-skeletal disease. Thorax 1998; 53:A10.

47. Sharshar T, Chevret S, Fitting JW, et al. Ventilation à domicile (VAD) dans les pathologies neuromusculaires: une étude prospective et multicentrique de cohorte. Rea Soins Intens Med Urg 2000; 9:88.
48. Gonzalez J, Sharshar T, Hart N, et al. Air leaks during mechanical ventilation as a cause of persistent hypercapnia in neuromuscular disorders. Intensive Care Med 2003; 29:596–602.
49. Toussaint M, Steens M, Wasteels G, et al. Diurnal ventilation via mouthpiece: survival in end-stage Duchenne patients. Eur Resp J 2006; 28:549–555.
50. Edwards EA, Hsiao K, Nixon GM. Paediatric home ventilatory support: the Auckland experience. J Paediatr Child Health 2005; 41:652–658.
51. Hadfield PJ, Lloyd-Faulconbridge RV, Almeyda J, et al. The changing indications for paediatric tracheostomy. Int J Pediatr Otorhinolaryngol 2003; 67:7–10.
52. Edwards EA, O'Toole M, Wallis C. Sending children home on tracheostomy dependent ventilation: pitfalls and outcomes. Arch Dis Child 2004; 89:251–255.
53. Baydur A, Layne E, Aral H, et al. Long term non-invasive ventilation in the community for patients with musculoskeletal disorders: 46 year experience and review. Thorax 2000; 55:4–11.
54. Griese M, Felber J, Reiter K, et al. Airway inflammation in children with tracheostomy. Pediatr Pulmonol 2004; 37:356–361.
55. Jiang D, Morrison GA. The influence of long-term tracheostomy on speech and language development in children. Int J Pediatr Otorhinolaryngol 2003; 67(suppl 1):S217–S220.
56. Carnevale FA, Alexander E, Davis M, et al. Daily living with distress and enrichment: the moral experience of families with ventilator-assisted children at home. Pediatrics 2006; 117:e48–e60.

38
The Perspective of Patients

DINA BROOKS, BARBARA GIBSON, and ROGER S. GOLDSTEIN
West Park Healthcare Centre, University of Toronto, Toronto, Ontario, Canada

I. Introduction and Definitions

Home mechanical ventilation (HMV) has been defined as "the longer-term application of ventilatory support to patients who are no longer in acute respiratory failure and do not need the sophistication of an intensive care setting" (1). A task force of the American College of Chest Physicians identified the goals of long-term mechanical ventilation as increasing longevity, decreasing morbidity, enhancing quality of life, and maximizing cost-effectiveness (2).

The move of health care provision into the community has important economic implications (3–5), as well as impact on families and caregivers (6) who take up the burden and responsibilities for providing care on a long-term basis (7–10). Ventilator users may live in private homes with community care services and family support, in long-term care facilities with formally trained care providers, or in supportive housing units with on-site services. In addition to professional health care providers, such as nurses, physiotherapists, physicians, and social workers, other paraprofessionals, such as personnel support workers and homemakers are involved in providing personal, day-to-day care and household maintenance. Personnel support workers assist with activities of daily living (11). Services may be available through a variety of funding models including private hire, insured services, and publicly funded programs and delivered by not-for-profit or for-profit agencies.

II. Quality of Life and Experiences of Ventilator Users

There remains a widespread public perception that life for a ventilator user is of poor quality, despite reports that ventilator users adapt well to ongoing mechanical ventilation, recognize its positive impact, and would choose ventilation again if the opportunity arose (12–14). While ventilator dependency does not preclude the pursuit of a satisfying existence, ventilator users encounter numerous social and material barriers that isolate and exclude them from participation in community life.

Miller and colleagues (15) surveyed 17 of the first adult ventilator users in the United States with neuromuscular conditions regarding their health, education, work, recreation, resources, and life satisfaction pre- and post-ventilation. The majority (11 of 17) indicated that their quality of life had declined over time and listed decreased mobility, increased dependence, decreased community access, and decreased activity as factors. Progression of the disease was more frequently cited than the ventilator as negatively influencing quality of life. Before commencing ventilation, about half of the respondents were satisfied with their educational activities, while only four of the 17 were satisfied after ventilation. Only three of the respondents had completed any postsecondary education. None of the respondents were employed and 11 had never been employed. The majority said that their respiratory status had an effect on their recreational activities, both pre- and post-ventilation. Fifteen of 17 men listed what the investigators termed "passive" primary recreational activities (listening to music, watching television). Ten men stated they did not see friends as much as they would like. This study did not include an in-depth exploration of the men's perceptions of these issues.

Locker and Kaufert (16) used qualitative interviews to explore the experiences of 10 ventilator users in Manitoba, Canada, with postpolio syndrome. They described a "trading off" process whereby ventilator users psychologically reorient themselves to the world after commencing ventilation. While all participants reported that tracheal ventilation increased their energy and sense of well-being, they experienced a dramatic shift in their rhythms and routines of daily life. Managing the practical aspects of the ventilator and accommodating to an even greater dependence on others led them to reassess and reorder their priorities.

More recent research has focused on socio-material barriers encountered in daily life. Ventilator users across diagnostic categories have reported experiencing challenges related to transportation, education, recreational activities, and employment (12–14). In a survey of 98 adult ventilator users (across diagnostic groups) in Ontario, Canada, Goldstein and colleagues (12) found that 81% of respondents were unemployed. Other research shows that some ventilator users do not go out alone because of the need to be suctioned or the risk of ventilator disconnection (14,17). Additional "barriers to daily living" include increased care requirements, increased personal attendant requirements, difficulty navigating health and service bureaucracies, inadequate public transportation, restrictive income assistance, and limited housing options (14). In interviews with 26 Canadian ventilator users, Brooks and colleagues (14) found that ventilator users experience negative attitudes toward their disabilities, which are amplified with the visible use of ventilation in public. Similarly, a Dutch study reported that ventilator users are concerned over the "lack of understanding on the part of those around them" (13).

Although ventilator users and their families experience frustration with the myriad of barriers encountered in daily life, they also report a number of "sources of life satisfaction" including advocacy, successful health management, and supportive relationships with family, friends, and volunteers (14). In Brooks' study, a large majority of the ventilator users report that ventilation had a positive effect on their lives, resulting in improved sleep and concentration (13,14), as indicated by one participant:

> My energy was back, I was renewed, It was wonderful . . . it was noisy because the air had to escape . . . but that didn't bother me because I was so glad to have this wonderful thing that was making me breathe (1).

Goldstein and colleagues (12) showed that ventilator users adapted well to ongoing ventilatory support, recognized the positive impact on their lives, and would choose ventilation again, if they were asked. Brooks and colleagues (14) reported that ventilator users maintained productive activities and expressed a high regard for the contribution of ventilatory support in making these activities possible. Most study participants (25 out of 26) rated their quality of life as very high and were generally proud of their involvement with family and friends, social activities, homemaking, volunteerism, advocacy, education, and employment. Notwithstanding numerous bureaucratic frustrations, they recognized the contribution of public support programs, such as supportive housing, personal attendants, assistive technology, transportation, income security, and supportive health care in making community living a viable option.

Studies that have used standardized measures of quality of life have contributed greatly to discussions of the ethics of HMV (15,18–20). These studies demonstrated that health care professionals were underestimating their patients' views of personal quality of life and were using these judgments to formulate treatment recommendations. Quality-of-life measures continue to be employed in research comparing home versus institutional care (21,22), different ventilation modalities (23), and different diagnostic groups of ventilator users (24). They report that a high percentage of ventilator users have "good" quality of life. Standardized tools are limited however because they assume a particular understanding of "quality" and "life satisfaction" according to a number of domains, that may not necessarily coincide with the understanding of the individuals being assessed. Hammell (25) argues that standardized measures rarely include components that have been identified as important to those living with serious impairment, such as the importance of "being" (e.g., reflective appreciation of nature, "small things," or being with others) and "doing" (engagement in activity that does not need to be purposeful to have personal meaning). Despite these limitations, studies using standardized measures have been valuable in challenging health professionals' assumptions and have improved disclosure practices regarding ventilation (17,26).

Socio-interpretative approaches have also been used to investigate quality of life among ventilator users. Using qualitative methods, Lindahl and colleagues (27) explored relationships between body, time, place, persons, and technologies. This approach identified some unique themes related to life as a ventilator user, not captured with other approaches. The investigators described how using a ventilator means having an ambivalent relationship with one's body, which is seen as both resilient and frail. The ventilator is experienced as incorporated into the body, but is also reflected on as both burden and relief. Life focuses on the present and the rhythms of daily routines rather than on an insecure or unimaginable future. Communion with others contributes to balancing independence and dependence. Their analysis reinterpreted "ventilator-dependency" as a "way of being" where "striving for a good life at home on a ventilator is connected with maintaining persistence and autonomy in communion with the ventilator and other people in the present time and being able to rise above yourself and your personal boundaries." Gibson (28) used critical social theory and the work of Pierre Bourdieu to examine the daily lives and identities of 10 male ventilator users with Duchenne's muscular dystrophy. She found that participants were materially, socially, and symbolically marginalized and excluded through the inaccessibility of the built environment, through social arrangements that limited their abilities to engage in community life, and through the multiple ways that their bodies and technologies were stigmatized. Furthermore, she found that marginalization was embodied by participants through processes of socialization and internalization of subordinate social positionings. The embodied marginalization of study participants was manifested through their expressions of resignation and low expectations. Whereas men created personal spaces for recognition and success through various acts of resistance and distinction, what they could hope to achieve was so severely circumscribed that it suggested a need for profound changes in health and social services.

III. Relationship Between Personal Support Workers and Ventilator Users

Personal support workers (PSW) play an important role in the lives of ventilator users, as unmet personal care needs are associated with poor health, especially in individuals with severe disability (29). Although the role of family carers, particularly among women, has received some attention (30,31), less attention has been focused on the work of paid caregivers.

A. Perspectives of PSW

Aronson and Neysmith (10) focused on the experiences of PSW who assist elderly people in their homes and explored divergence between the understandings of the home care labor process of the PSW and those of the funders and government. They interviewed 30 PSW in two nonprofit home agencies in urban southern Ontario, Canada, and conducted a focus group with their supervisors. They noted that PSW experienced a lack of clear formal work expectations and a blurring of boundaries between formal and informal relations, practical and emotional labor, and paid and unpaid work. Although clients, families, and workers may appreciate the "informal" services provided, the authors concluded that they represent "uncompensated and exploited labor unrecognized by health care policies." They further noted that PSW had low status and poor recognition in society that may be related to gender, class, and race characteristics. Immigrant women or visible minorities with "few marketable skills and occupational choices" were highly represented among the PSW. Their role in caring for elderly and disabled people who themselves have low social regard may also contribute to their devaluation (32).

A recent report by Church and colleagues (33) provides a comprehensive profile of PSW in Canada. Their research was based on the literature, government reports, training materials, consultations (using informal interviews), and site visits. The researchers noted the absence of consistent terminology, certification, or a united voice for the PSW, despite the large array of organizations that have a stake in their work. PSW are mostly women, often foreign born, with a large variation in their training and being among the lowest paid workers in Canada. The authors noted the need for research to explore the relationship between disabled persons and their support workers.

B. Perspectives of Ventilator Users

The importance of holistic care and respect beyond maintenance of the body is highlighted in two studies of people with disabilities. Marquis and Jackson (34) interviewed 50 adults with physical and cognitive disabilities who were receiving services from agencies. They described service arrangements ranging from "relationship-like care" to "abuse". The main finding was that interpersonal qualities of PSW were more important to clients than technical skill and efficiency. Skar and Tamm (35) investigated the relationship between children/adolescents with restricted mobility and their assistants and reported comparable findings. They described five categories of relationships that emerged from the study: the replaceable assistant, the assistant as parent, the professional assistant, the assistant as a friend, and the ideal assistant. Interpersonal sharing and mutual respect characterized desirable relationships.

Noyes conducted 34 face-to-face interviews with young ventilator users and their families (36). Of the 12 subjects who were living at home, there were large differences in the services delivered by PSW, with whom their relationship was often negative. Participants' complaints included incompetence, poor communication, lack of respect for family and privacy, and lack of clear role description.

Brooks noted that ventilator users considered PSW to be among the most significant facilitators of satisfaction in daily life (14). They provided care and services and, in some cases, emotional support and friendship. Participants who lived in supported housing units valued the support provided to them, although they had less control over scheduling and the manner in which care was provided than those who hired their own staff. Participants generally felt that most PSW were flexible, caring, and responsive to their needs, although some expressed concern about English language competency and the lack of staffing to meet all their needs such as accompanying ventilator users into the community. Stability in employment of PSW was considered to be an advantage as suggested by this participant:

> My workers are well paid by me. And they deserve every penny of it because they're good, they're very willing to do what you want done and they don't complain.

Unlike other research that focuses on the client side of the PSW-client relationship, a Canadian study by Roeher Institute looked at the issues from both perspectives simultaneously (37). Interestingly, the needs of both groups were similar. Ability to make choices and having control over the kinds of tasks and variety of tasks performed was important for both groups. Using an "equality of well-being" framework, the researchers found that the equality of clients and workers was interdependent, with certain conditions fostering bilateral equality, while others improving conditions for one group at the direct expense of the other. Although this study was not exclusively with ventilator users, the identified issues were similar and the findings are thus likely to have cross-applicability.

IV. Relationship Between Health Care Professionals and Ventilator Users

Health care professionals such as nurses, physicians, and physiotherapists also have a considerable impact on life satisfaction of ventilator users. The "independent living movement," which forms the basis of much disability rights activism in North America, has for many years striven to ensure that people with disabilities have control over the services they need and are enabled to direct their own care (38). For health care professionals, this conceptualization translates to ensuring that health care needs are met and, at the same time, ensuring that personal autonomy is supported. For example, health care professionals can support ventilator users to exert choice when making decisions around medical intervention and technologies, such as type of ventilators and interfaces. However, health care professionals must be cognizant of the fact that health care and rehabilitation goals must consider not only functional limitations but also social barriers (39). Table 1 provides some examples of disabling attitudes exhibited by health care professionals and an alternative "disability rights" perspective (40,41).

Different conceptualizations of disability may play a role in influencing perceptions of quality of life. Research has shown that health care professionals may significantly

Table 1 Examples of Difference Between Disabling Attitude and Disability Rights Perspective

Disabling attitude by health care professionals	Disability rights perspective
Independence is the ability to "do it by yourself"	Independence is about having control about how help is provided
Health care professionals are the gatekeepers of medical and technological resources	Individuals with disability have choice when considering health care interventions and technologies
Clients should comply with a treatment plan	Disabled people need to maintain autonomy and self-respect

Source: From Refs. 40,41.

underestimate the quality of life of their patients (42,43) including ventilator users (44,45). These studies confirm ventilator users' perceptions that health care professionals consider their lives to be negatively characterized and of lesser value. Health care providers who recognize and incorporate the knowledge and experience of ventilator users, support choice, provide education, and advocate for their patients are highly valued by ventilator users (14). Such individuals are seen as making essential contributions to the positive quality of life of ventilator users. In contrast, practitioners who lack the required specialized knowledge do not understand or integrate overall care, are inaccessible, make erroneous assumptions or provide inappropriate care, cause frustrations, and create barriers (14). These conceptualizations are demonstrated in the following comments from a ventilator user (14):

> I learned a long, long time ago, (it) doesn't matter if you've got a nurse's uniform on. Or some white overcoat doesn't mean they understand neuromuscular disorders. Don't make that assumption. So I never make assumptions anymore about what they know and don't know. They know things I don't know but in a partnership they can teach me and show me and let me figure it out and give me some trust.

V. Conclusion

Ventilator users have unique needs for technological and personal support, often requiring 24-hour support to safeguard against mechanical failure and to meet their ventilatory needs. Ventilator users enjoy a good quality of life despite the numerous social, material, and attitudinal barriers they encounter in daily life. To provide appropriate care to this growing population, it is important to understand the experiences and perceptions of individuals and the issues that impact on their daily lives. These experiences are derived from that individual's daily successes, satisfactions, supports, barriers and frustrations. Choice regarding the services and resources on which they rely appear to be greater determinants of their quality of life than the actual impairment. As persons with physical disabilities have said, it is not the physical impairment or the need to be mechanically ventilated that is disabling. Rather, it is the services and resources on which your impairment renders you dependent. As stated by one individual,

> Treat us as human beings, individuals, people. We know what we want, what we need, ask us questions, don't impose (14).

References

1. Muir J-F. Home mechanical ventilation. In: Simond AK, Muir J-F, Person DJ, eds. Pulmonary Rehabilitation. London: BMJ Publishing Group,1996.
2. O'Donahue WJ, Giovannoni RM, Goldberg AI, et al. Long-term mechanical ventilation. Guidelines for management in the home and at alternate community sites. Report of the ad hoc committee, respiratory care section, ACCP. Chest 1986; 90(suppl):1–37.
3. Adams AB, Whitman J, Marcy T. Surveys of long-term ventilatory support in Minnesota: 1986 and 1992. Chest 1993; 103:1463–1469.
4. Litwin PD, Flegel CM, Richardson BC. An overview of home mechanical ventilation in Canada. Can J Respir Ther 1991; 28:67–73.
5. Coyte PC, McKeever P. Home care in Canada: passing the buck. Can J Nurs Res 2001; 33:11–25.
6. Williams AM. The development of Ontario's home care program: a critical geographical analysis. Soc Sci Med 1996; 42:937–948.
7. Browne G, Roberts J, Gafn, A, et al. Economic evaluations of community-based care: lessons from twelve studies in Ontario. J Eval Clin Pract 1999; 5:367–385.
8. Vrabec NJ. Literature review of social support and caregiver burden, 1980 to 1995. Image J Nurs Scholarsh 1997; 29:383–388.
9. Chenier MC. Review and analysis of caregiver burden and nursing home placement. Geriatr Nurs 1997; 18:121–126.
10. Aronson J, Neysmith SM. "You're not just in there to do the work" Depersonalizing policies and the exploitation of home care workers' labor. Gend Soc 1996; 10:59–77.
11. Toronto District Health Council (2002). Towards a system of personal support and homemaking services for Toronto. Toronto District Health Council.
12. Goldstein RS, Psek JA, Gort EH. Home mechanical ventilation: demographics and users perspectives. Chest 1995; 108:1581–1586.
13. van Kesteren RG, Velthuis B, van Leyden LW. Psychosocial problems arising from home ventilation. Am J Phys Med Rehabil 2001; 80:439–446.
14. Brooks D, King A, Tonack M, et al. User Perspectives on issues that influence the quality of daily life of ventilator-assisted individuals. Can Respir J 2004; 11:547–554.
15. Miller JR, Colbert AP, Osberg JS. Ventilator dependency: decision making, daily functioning and quality of life of patients with Duchenne muscular dystrophy. Dev Med Child Neurol 1990; 32:1078–1086.
16. Locker D, Kaufert J. The breath of life: medical technology and the careers of people with post-respiratory poliomyelitis. Sociol Health Illn 1988; 10(1):23–40.
17. Gibson BE. Long term ventilation for patients with Duchenne muscular dystrophy: an ethical analysis of physicians' beliefs and practices. Chest 2001; 119(3):940–946.
18. Pehrsson K, Olofson J, Larsson S, et al. Quality of life of patients treated by home mechanical ventilation due to restrictive ventilatory disorders. Respir Med 1994; 88:21–26.
19. Bach JR. Ventilator use by muscular dystrophy association patients. Arch Phys Med Rehabil 1992; 3(3):239–269.
20. Bach JR, Barnett V. Ethical considerations in the management of individuals with severe neuromuscular disorders. Am J Phys Med Rehabil 1994; 73(2):134–140.
21. Domenach-Clar R, Nauffal-Manzu D, Perpina-Tordera, et al. Home mechanical ventilation for restrictive thoracic diseases: effects of patient quality-of-life and hospitalizations. Respir Med 2003; 97(12):1320–1327.
22. Guber A, Morris E, Chen B, et al. First experience with the home care management system for respiratory patients in Israel. Isr Med Assoc J 2002; 4(6):418–420.

23. Markstrom A, Sundell K, Lysdahl M, et al. Quality-of-life evaluation of patients with neuromuscular and skeletal diseases treated with noninvasive and invasive home mechanical ventilation. Chest 2002; 122(5):1695–1700.
24. Narayanaswami P, Bertorini TE, Pourmand R, et al. Long-term tracheostomy ventilation in neuromuscular disease: patient acceptance and quality of life. Neurorehabil Neural Repair 2000; 14(2):135–139.
25. Hammell KW. Quality of life among people with high spinal cord injury living in the community. Spinal Cord 2004; 42:607–620.
26. American Thoracic Society. Respiratory care of the patient with Duchenne muscular dystrophy: ATS consensus statement. Am J Respir Crit Care Med 2004; 170:456–465.
27. Lindahl B, Sandman P-O, Rasmussen BH. Meanings of living at home on a ventilator. Nurs Inq 2003; 10(1):19–27.
28. Gibson BE. Men with Duchenne muscular dystrophy: a Bourdieusian interpretation of identity and social positioning. (Dissertation) University of Toronto, 2006.
29. Nosek MA, Fuhrer MJ. Independence among people with disabilities, a heuristic model. Rehabil Couns Bull 1992; 36:6–20.
30. Paolettu I. Caring for older people: a gendered practice. Discourse Soc 2002; 13:805–817.
31. Kersten P, McLellan L, George S, et al. Needs of careers of severely disabled: are they identified and met adequately. Health Soc Care Community 2001; 9:235–243.
32. Schmid H, Hasenfeld Y. Organizational dilemmas in the provision of home-care services. Soc Serv Rev 1993; 67:40–54.
33. Church K, Diamond T, Voronka J. In Profile: Personal Support Workers in Canada. Toronto: RBC Institute for Disability Studies Research and Education, Ryerson University, 2004.
34. Marquis R, Jackson R. Quality of life and quality of service relationships: experiences of people with disabilities. Disabil Soc 2000; 15:411–425.
35. Skar L, Tamm M. My assistant and I: disabled children's and adolescents' roles and relationships to their assistants. Disabil Soc 2001; 16:917–931.
36. Noyes J. Life as a young 'ventilator dependent'' person. J Soc Work Pract 1999; 13:177–190.
37. The Roeher Institute (2001). Disability Related Support Arrangements: Policy Options and Implications for Women's Equality. Ottawa: Status of Women Canada. ISBN 0-662-65323-8.
38. Litvak S, Enders A. Support systems: the interface between individuals and their environments. In: Albrecht GL, Seelman KD, Bury M, eds. Handbook of Disability Studies. Thousand Oaks, California: Sage Publications, 2001:252–266.
39. Richardson M. Addressing barriers: disabled rights and the implications for nursing of the social construct of disability. J Adv Nurs 1997; 25:1269–1275.
40. Morris J. Care or empowerment? A disability rights perspective. Soc Policy Admin 1997; 31:54–60.
41. Bricher G. Disabled people, health professionals and the social model of disability: can there be a research relationship? Disabil Soc 2000; 15(5):781–793.
42. Gerhart KA, Koziol-McLain J, Lowenstein SR, et al. Quality of life following spinal cord injury: knowledge and attitudes of emergency care providers. Ann Emerg Med 1994; 23(4):807–812.
43. Schneiderman LJ. Do physicians' own preferences for life sustaining treatment influence their perceptions of patients' preferences? J Clin Ethics 1993; 4:28–33.
44. Bach JR, Campagnola DI, Hoeman S. Life satisfaction of individuals with Duchenne muscular dystrophy using long term mechanical ventilatory support. Am J Phys Med Rehabil 1991; 70:129–135.
45. Bach JR, Tilton MC. Life satisfaction and well-being measures in ventilator assisted individuals with traumatic tetraplegia. Arch Phys Med Rehabil 1994; 75:626–632.

39
The Perspective of Family and Caregivers

PAMELA A. CAZZOLLI
The ALS/Neuromuscular Education Project, Canton, Ohio, U.S.A.

I. Introduction

Family caregivers of long-term mechanical ventilation (LTMV) users may face the greatest challenges of any group of caregivers. Their attitudes and how they cope with day-to-day problems greatly affect the well-being, quality of life, and survival of their ventilator-dependent loved ones. Family perspectives may also directly affect their loved ones' desire to live or die, and the decisions they make. Moreover, the attitudes and circumstances of ventilator users, and the quality of their relationships with their loved ones, can make a significant difference in the ability and willingness of family members, or significant others, to take on the responsibilities of long-term, round-the-clock care.

Survival beyond respiratory failure may last months or years [when mechanical ventilation (MV) is used] (1–3). When planning optimal management of care, physicians and health care providers may unintentionally overlook crucial problems regarding the needs of family caregivers who are held hostage in their homes. Those who are severely disabled and ventilator dependent rarely visit their physicians. Furthermore, health care professionals may have limited experience in observing LTMV patients in the home setting.

The focus of this chapter is on the perspectives of family caregivers of amyotrophic lateral sclerosis (ALS) patients using LTMV. ALS is a disabling neurologic disease that can strike any adult. Progressive disability and ongoing changes and losses ensue. ALS has a profound effect on the family. Survival of ALS patients using MV can vary considerably. For some patients, survival may exceed five years for users of nasal positive pressure ventilation (NPPV) (2,4), and more than 10 or 15 years when tracheostomy positive pressure ventilation (TPPV) is used (1–3). Thus, the use of LTMV in ALS may result in severe disability (2,5), a high burden of care (2), and high costs if caregivers are hired (2).

This chapter consists of the following:

1. Personal observations of family caregivers of ventilator users with ALS over a 22-year time frame
2. Common misconceptions of family caregivers, 1984–1999
3. Impact of slow communication on the burden of care
4. Impact of totally locked-in patients on families
5. Impact of immobility on the burden of care
6. Hired caregivers
7. Motivating factors for continuing LTMV

8. Need for social interaction
9. Life satisfaction of family caregivers, 1984 to the present
10. The impact of strife on family caregivers
11. Burden of care
12. Common observations of each caregiver group
13. What physicians and nurses can do to help family caregivers achieve life satisfaction and optimal outcomes

II. Background

Since 1984, my nursing practice has focused on serving as a nurse consultant and clinical care investigator to help improve standards of care and survival of ALS patients, particularly for MV users. This long-term investigation of family caregivers of ALS patients using home mechanical ventilation (HMV) was predominantly based on personal observation and interviews with patients and their families. Over the years, I have followed and consulted with several thousand ALS patients and their family caregivers to help make a significant difference in their lives. Serving in the community-based setting, I have visited hundreds of ALS families at their homes or care facilities. Because two hours was the average length of time per visit, there was ample opportunity to observe closely how LTMV users and their families lived day to day. Follow-up consultation and patient family support were provided via the phone on almost a daily basis. However, I have learned firsthand that phone or online assessment of patients and families is an inadequate substitute for actual visits to the home.

Because of the enormous number of patient families that I have closely followed for many years, along with the numerous variables involved, it was not possible to database every observation. The following text includes data from my personal observations of family caregivers whose loved ones used LTMV.

III. Common Misconceptions of Family Caregivers: 1984–1999

In my original investigation of 93 ALS patients using TPPV from 1984 to 1999, 68 (73%) of the 93 patients and their family caregivers believed MV would be a short-term treatment (6). However, 20 patients survived for 8 to 17 years after they commenced TPPV (7). They were unaware that the outcome would be severe disability, high costs, and high burden of care. Most of these patient families were referred for nursing consultation after they began TPPV. My initial visits to the majority of these cases began in the 1980s and early 1990s, an era in which the majority commenced MV during emergency hospitalizations. Many were still able to walk or talk and not ready to die, when TPPV was initiated (2). Families later shared with me their common experiences at the hospital, since I was not present when the MV decision was made. While their loved ones gasped for air, the families tended to panic at the bedside. They did not consider that the future outcome could be severe disability. At that time, 86 (93%) of the 93 commenced MV use when both the patients and the families perceived that MV was an immediate treatment for the respiratory crisis (6). Because they were told "ALS is fatal," they believed death would occur due to the progression of paralysis and that quadriplegia was the predictor of death. Family members perceived that emergency MV was only temporary treatment (6).

In comparison, 82 (87%) of 94 patients preplanned NPPV use, and 12 (13%) of 94 began NPPV during an emergency (6). Survival with NPPV ranged from 6 to 77 months in patients who were nonbulbar when they began NPPV (6). Although family caregivers believed that NPPV may help treat symptoms or improve sleep, many were oblivious to the potential of survival beyond respiratory failure with optimal use of NPPV. Family caregivers of patients who became severely disabled were surprised at the long-term outcome.

Overall, family caregivers of MV users perceived that the progression of immobility was the predictor of death, despite the use of MV. Also, hired caregivers, particularly nurses from hospices and home care agencies, have generally perceived this misconception. Often, families did not comprehend that respiratory failure is the primary cause of mortality of ALS and that MV can prevent respiratory failure and death.

Misconceptions, therefore, either resulted in unexpected outcomes of survival that families did not anticipate, or early mortality due to implementation of hospice services as disability progressed. The perspective of the home care/hospice nurses greatly influenced the views of families (observations on the perspectives of nurses, however, were not databased).

In my opinion, the prevalent misconception of the progression of immobility as the signal for end-of-life care is the reason morphine sulfate and oxygen were given as a substitute for NPPV. I observed that these two treatments were often administered by hospices in successful users of NPPV. This was based on their perspective that since "ALS is fatal," and that their protocols are the treatment of choice, rather than the optimal use of NPPV and airway clearance. In addition, some hospices consider that NPPV should be used intermittently to provide comfort only and not to extend survival. Furthermore, the use of bi-level ventilators by hospices, without backup rates, has increased for ALS patients. The hospice nurses had based their opinion on the belief that backup rates promote survival and had not understood that a backup is necessary for optimal relief of hypoventilation.

In a number of incidences, I learned of previously successful NPPV users with ALS who were given a prognosis of "24 hours to live." During these emergency hospitalizations, however, I was permitted to educate the health care professionals and patient families on the comfortable use of NPPV, the choices for survival, and that respiratory failure could be treated, if desired. As a result, by using NPPV appropriately, many patients had a dramatic reversal of symptoms and lived up to 24 months or more.

IV. Impact of Slow Communication on the Burden of Care

Severe disability was a usual outcome for ALS patients who used LTMV for two to five years or more. Although suctioning of the tracheostomy increased the burden and intensity of home care (2), most family caregivers reported that slow communication and immobility were the primary factors in the burden of care, rather than caring for the tracheostomy.

Methods of communication varied widely for patients who did not have intelligible speech. They included writing, push button devices, alphabet boards, augmentative communication systems, or computers with voice synthesizers that are activated by switches. Unless patients had the ability to write or push buttons speedily, communication devices usually require diligent effort and concentration. This process was extremely slow, despite the use of the most sophisticated communication technology. Some patients were unable to grasp a pen but had sufficient arm mobility to move their hand and some could write legibly and quickly with a writing device (8). The fastest method of communication that I have ever observed, among people who were immobile and unable to articulate, is a system using alphabet letters on a card or a board. After dividing and numerating the alphabet into five or six rows, patients can readily select, by eye blinks, the rows and letters to spell words.

Overall, family members indicated that slow communication caused the greatest frustration. During home visits, caregivers were observed demonstrating impatience and anger. When patients struggled to communicate their wishes, the process was often slow and unintelligible. Most sophisticated communication devices took a great deal of time and effort to use. When tempers flared, patients were often reduced to tears. This further hampered their communication efforts to become even slower. Immobile patients often indicated that impaired speech exacerbated their feelings of helplessness. If rapid methods of communication were not used, family caregivers, in turn, indicated that this compounded their feelings of hopelessness and depression. In contrast, family caregivers of patients who were nonbulbar and who could articulate effectively had a significantly reduced burden of care. Patients who were able to talk could express their wishes quickly. This greatly expedited the providing of care. The ability to express their feelings reduced misunderstandings and strife in patient-family relationships. The consensus of almost all patients and families is that the ability to communicate is the most essential factor. Effective communication is the primary requirement for maintaining quality of life. When communication became exceedingly difficult, the burden of care increased and the quality of life decreased.

V. Impact of Totally Locked-in Patients on Families

As immobility progressed, it was not uncommon for patients using TPPV to become totally locked in (after using TPPV for more than five years). I describe this state as having no reliable ability to move a single skeletal muscle, including the eyes. Consequently, the patient who is totally locked in has no ability to communicate or respond to any question. During my investigation from 1984 to 1999, 16 (17%) of 93 TPPV patients became totally locked in (6). Prior to losing all ability to blink or move their eyes, 8 of the 16 indicated that they also lost their vision or became blind (perhaps the inability to blink for a long term led to corneal damage and the permanent loss of vision). Hence, before becoming totally locked in, the impaired vision precluded the use of alphabet boards or communication devices because the patients could not see them. Besides the totally locked-in patients, I have observed many others who almost became locked in. They still had one reliable muscle that slightly moved in response to questions. Thus, I define this as a pre-totally locked-in state and final opportunity to communicate.

As patients became locked in, family caregivers indicated that the burden of care subsided significantly. The frustration with communication ceased because there was no longer an effort to communicate. Patients who had previously been demanding became despondent and silent forever. Family caregivers often referred to their loved ones as "living corpses." Many family members, especially children, became terrified by the physical appearance of someone they loved who had become locked in. They could no longer endure either visiting or assisting with care of their loved one.

In Ohio, the incidence of ventilator users becoming totally locked in since 2000 is significantly less than what I observed in the 1980s and 1990s. Because of increased education about life choices and advance directives, most patients are now indicating their wishes in advance and withdrawing from MV if they can no longer communicate. During visits to Japan, however, I have observed a high number of LTMV users who were severely paralyzed.

VI. Impact of Immobility on the Burden of Care

After impaired communication, immobility was the second most significant unpreventable challenge faced by family caregivers. Immobility was a leading factor for the high burden of care. If patients were quadriplegic, the constant positioning and repositioning of the limbs, trunk, and head were ongoing round-the-clock, never-ending tasks. Patients who had lost the use of their upper extremities were totally dependent on others for care. Those families reported a higher burden of care than families whose members were non-ambulatory, but still retained the use of their upper extremities.

Family members who received adequate help when it was needed had experienced significantly less burden of care than those without help. Some family caregivers reported no burden of care, despite having loved ones with severe disability, if they had the finances and benefits to receive hired help at home everyday. They either had built-in family support or were forced to hire caregivers. Life satisfaction of family caregivers also depended on whether their loved ones were satisfied. Patients who had acquired the ability to cope with the physical and emotional aspects of the disease often had peace of mind. That enhanced the family caregivers' ability to cope and still enjoy life. Despite severe disability, many families continued to respond positively to the patient.

Immobile patients using TPPV could never be left alone, unlike MV users with mobility. If a patient could execute self-care of a tracheostomy, they were occasionally left home alone.

Some patients had private duty nursing insurance benefits in which licensed nurses provided care for at least one shift per day. This had greatly minimized the burden of care for the family, and made it possible for the majority of MV patients to live at home rather than in care facilities. In the 1980s and 1990s, benefits for private duty nursing by third party payers were more widely available (2) than in the previous five years. Since 2000, the number of patients who were forced to hire caregivers without financial aid, if round-the-clock care and supervision were needed, has risen sharply. The lack of private duty nursing benefits has also caused more patients to move to skilled nursing facilities than in the previous years. Thus, the reduced healthcare benefits for caregiver assistance and the increased "out-of-pocket" expenses have resulted in higher direct costs and the depletion of life savings. The hiring of caregivers, not the purchase or rental cost of equipment and supplies, was the primary factor for the high costs of using MV (2). The significant costs and the high burden of care were the most common causes for patients with ALS to withdraw from MV.

On the basis of close observation, most family caregivers provided meticulous care, usually as good as hired nurses (2). Initially, family caregivers were trained on tracheostomy care and were supervised by a registered nurse. Most school-age children and teens assisted with care. Older children usually provided tracheostomy care (2,9), while younger children were often educated on intervening in the event of an emergency.

VII. Hired Caregivers

The number of patient families with hired caregivers varied widely, and was dependent on their health care benefits and/or their incomes. Surprisingly, many families were unaware of their specific health care benefits, both before and after commencement of LTMV. In the United States, patients with poverty status actually obtained the most health care benefits.

This usually included coverage for care by the government for either a part-time hired caregiver at home or full-time admission to a care facility.

All families who hired private duty nurses or caregivers did not like the care attendants in their homes continuously, despite the critical need for help. Some felt that the presence of care attendants in the home invaded their privacy. In addition, married couples did not often have time alone. When families lacked sufficient home care benefits and were forced to pay "out-of-pocket" for care, the majority preferred hiring nonagency nurses. Nurses from home care agencies were significantly higher in cost than nonagency nurses (6). Also, families often complained that agency nurses followed their own protocols, not always the wishes of patients and families.

VIII. Motivating Factors for Continuing LTMV

A motivating factor for continuing long-term MV was the hope for a miracle. In my previous study of 84 patients using TPPV, 26 hoped to stay alive because they were waiting for a cure. Four had faith that God would heal them, while 22 patients and their family members were sustained by the hope that a cure for ALS would be found. On the basis of "time for a cure" campaigns and news on ALS research, they all believed if a cure for ALS was discovered, their paralysis would be reversed. They believed this could happen "almost anytime."

IX. Need for Social Interaction

Despite their immobility, MV patients who maintained a method of communication and experienced regular social interaction could achieve life satisfaction (6,7). Patients and caregivers were satisfied with their quality of life on LTMV as long as social interaction continued, and resources were available. Social interaction included regular contact with people and participation in activities with family, friends, church groups, or caregivers. With the use of portable ventilators, powered wheelchairs, accessible vans, ramps, and laptop computers for communication, these ventilator users were able to go outdoors. They could travel, attend church, school activities, sporting events, and the theater. Others who were homebound enjoyed frequent interaction with their hired caregivers. They could enjoy social or church meetings at their homes every week and also interact with online support groups. This communication greatly minimized the feelings of social isolation, abandonment, and helplessness.

X. Life Satisfaction of Family Caregivers: 1984 to the Present

Studies have shown that the majority of MV patients were "glad to be alive" and that both patients and family caregivers "would choose MV again if given the choice" (2,9,10). The majority of family caregivers indicated that despite the heavy burden, they often continued to be willing caregivers to keep their loved ones alive (2). Use of MV (survival beyond respiratory failure) ranged from one to more than ten years. This included both TPPV and NPPV users and their families (2,10). In the investigation by Moss et al. (10), I visited 31 patient families, or majority of the study subjects. One consideration of this study (10) was that the patient/family visits occurred only once at any given moment of time. Months or years later, during a follow-up investigation, I learned that perspectives of many caregivers changed as circumstances and conditions of their loved ones using MV progressed. Thus, perspectives of family caregivers may change if disability increases significantly, burden of care becomes significantly higher, life savings become depleted, health status of family caregivers markedly deteriorates, and survival of those who become severely disabled exceeds five years.

Over the years, I have found that those patients who rated their quality of life as high and were glad to be alive had happier family caregivers. In contrast, the patients with severe disability, who suffered extreme depression and no longer desired to live, had family caregivers who shared their depression.

Family caregivers have often indicated that the most stressing period for using MV was from the time of commencement of TPPV through the following six months after their loved one became ventilator dependent. Thereafter, as family caregivers mastered ventilator care procedures, the anxiety and fear subsided.

Male caregivers seemed to have been more creative in their approach to care and tended to "invent" devices that made life easier. Women tended to purchase commercial products to simplify tasks.

Learning the skills for providing care and enhancing mobility, comfort, and safety made a significant difference among family caregivers. There are helpful educational resources on the art of caregiving (11). Some communities offer volunteer services to help family caregivers. One such program is "Share the Care." (12).

The ability to anticipate and engage in pleasurable activities and to maintain an environment where family members live in harmony with one another are essential components for life satisfaction. Family caregivers and LTMV patients need to know they have a purpose for living (13), and must have a desire to live their lives to the fullest potential, despite their circumstances (14).

For many, spirituality also played a key role in life satisfaction. Family caregivers, who expressed that they had faith in God and prayer, attributed their peace of mind to God. Many believe that they "would not have been able to make it" without God's help. "Courage To Live: The Story of Charlie and Lucy Wedemeyer" (15) is an inspirational DVD about a LTMV user with ALS and his wife. They believe that through the power of faith and the love of family and friends, they have been able to face daily challenges. They believe that there is no obstacle that they cannot overcome. The DVD also gives profound words of encouragement to other LTMV user families. Faith is a predictor for caregivers achieving life satisfaction (Table 1).

XI. The Impact of Strife on Family Caregivers

Family caregivers and/or patients who are quick to anger, who are impatient and demanding, and who have a tendency to display mood swings or temper outbursts from daily situational stress frequently create an atmosphere of strife in the home. These preexisting characteristics usually become significantly worse after LTMV is initiated. Offensive communication and refusal to forgive may ultimately result in deep bitterness, hatred, and the inability to cope. Patients who are demanding, manipulative, and seldom express appreciation to their family caregivers will foster resentment.

Table 1 Predictors for Caregivers Achieving Life Satisfaction

- Availability of willing, competent caregivers
- Adequate assistance with care
- Adequate finances and healthcare benefits
- Accessible home environment, including exit and entry of home
- Accessibility of appropriate durable medical equipment and self-help devices
- Achieving and maintaining effective methods of communication
- Regular social interaction and participation in pleasurable activities
- Supportive family and friends
- Harmonious family relationships
- Faith and close relationship with God

Table 2 Predictors of Caregiver Stress

- Strife or unresolved conflict between patient, primary family caregiver and/or with relatives of the patient
- Slow or ineffective method of communication by patient, including use of augmentative communication systems
- Severe disability of loved one, particularly if upper extremities are immobile
- Insufficient help with care
- Depression, hopelessness, despair, and no desire of patient to live
- Unmanaged anxiety and fear
- No social interaction or opportunity to enjoy pleasurable activities
- Lack of sleep
- High costs for equipment/supplies, hired help and/or depletion of life savings

Family caregivers attributed strife as a major stress factor (Table 2). Unresolved conflict robs families of "peace of mind," the ability to sleep, and the attainment of joy in life. Families who harbor strife never achieve their potential life satisfaction. Women, more often than men, reported that strife was often sparked by hypercritical remarks by their in-laws. Adult children have often reported conflicts among siblings when one person takes on all the caregiving or household tasks for a parent, while the others offer little or no assistance. Becoming consumed with anger and unresolved conflict is destructive to both the physical and emotional well-being of patients and their families. It destroys the spirit of unity. Conflicts in the home compound stress, grief, and interfere with the ability to cope. Anger may also trigger respiratory failure and result in early mortality.

XII. Burden of Care

Caregivers without a supportive family or who lack finances to hire help are often held hostage in an environment with little or no opportunity for pleasurable activities. Prolonged isolation and physical or emotional fatigue will result in caregiver burnout. Prolonged inability to cope may lead some to become emotionally dysfunctional to the point of jeopardizing the safety of their ventilator-dependent loved ones. Family caregivers who lack family support may turn to alcohol or tranquilizers for relief.

XIII. Common Observations of Each Caregiver Group

A. Well Spouse Caregivers

In my experience, the majority of primary caregivers of ALS patients using LTMV at home were the patients' spouses. Men or women in their prime of life with a full-time career and/or those who are parents to dependent children living at home have significantly higher caregiver stress levels than those male or female well spouses who are retired and without children living at home. Unless well spouses who work full time have adequate family assistance and finances to hire help, it is difficult, if not impossible, to pursue the task alone when their partners are physically helpless. Slow communication compounds the burden of care. Caregivers without adequate assistance often feel the sense of pending doom. They suffer from frequent headaches and back pain. Their lack of sleep often escalates into outbursts of anger, followed by guilt and depression. These are a few signs of caregiver burnout.

The responsibility of round-the-clock care can result in caregiver breakdown. Because use of LTMV may continue for years, care facility placement may be the only solution to assure the availability of round-the-clock caregivers. In my overall experience, I have observed significantly more caregiver husbands who were less able to provide ongoing care for more than two years than caregiver wives. Feeling the burden of care on their spouses and children, more women than men withdrew from MV, anticipating death.

B. Children Caregivers

Adult children who have a disabled parent living home alone have the constant burden of coordinating daily care and household tasks. Often a parent resists moving to a care facility, despite the risk of falling or dependent use of NPPV. Unless the parent has advance directives that are clearly understood, conflicts may arise among siblings on sharing the responsibilities of care or addressing life support issues.

Teenagers with a parent at home using LTMV faced increased responsibilities. They often resented caregiving tasks, especially if the duties interfered with their social activities or studies. Watching their beloved parent wither away was also very devastating. Through the years, I observed more strife and conflict in the home when the TPPV user with ALS was the father, rather than the mother. If the father previously governed discipline and then became inarticulate and helpless, mothers with "burnout" and rebellious teens often encountered compounded stress. Poor grades, discipline problems at school, and teen pregnancies were not uncommon in such households, particularly if there was unresolved conflict. Some teens attempted suicide. Younger children adapted better than older children. Small or school-age children in the home usually assisted with minor tasks.

C. Parent Caregivers

Of all the categories of family caregivers, parents had the most difficulty in adapting to the catastrophic diagnosis and threat to their child's life, regardless of the age of the child. Some parents tended to overprotect their child and hover over hired caregivers to assure that every procedure of care was performed with perfection. In addition, some tended not to support the wishes of their child to withdraw or refuse LTMV. Occasionally, I heard, "I plan to keep my baby alive." Parents, who were elderly, sometimes could not physically or emotionally endure the caregiving tasks. Some of them kept their adult child bed bound with diapers, and kept visitors away. In general, however, parent caregivers tended to demonstrate the most tolerance in their caregiving role.

XIV. What Physicians and Nurses Can Do to Help Family Caregivers Achieve Life Satisfaction and Optimal Outcomes

1. Provide accurate, understandable, and necessary information on the patient's diagnosis and the possible survival and outcome of LTMV. Inform patient families that (*i*) immobility will progress; (*ii*) if TPPV is used, ongoing tracheal suctioning will be required and round-the-clock caregivers will be necessary; (*iii*) if dependent on NPPV, periodic interface adjustment and supervision will be required; (*iv*) survival of nonbulbar NPPV users may be long term (2); (*v*) paralysis is likely irreversible; (*vi*) quadriplegia is not a predictor of survival; (*vii*) costs for hiring caregivers are high, and may deplete life savings, if survival is long; (*viii*) heavy family burdens or nursing home placement may ensue (2); and (*ix*) the patient has the right to withdraw from MV, if desired.
2. Respect patient family wishes and regard each MV patient's life as precious. Do not perceive that quality of life is over if tracheostomy ventilation is used, nor believe that the patient must live like a "vegetable" and be held hostage to a bed. Be aware that portable, lightweight ventilators are available, as well as technology to enhance mobility. Understand that many MV users are glad to be alive and would choose MV again, if given the choice. Recognize that many patient families have financial resources to hire help or have available, willing, and competent family caregivers to assist with care.
3. Tell families not to promise their loved ones that they will never allow them to live in a care facility. This will help eliminate conflict, guilt, and stress in the event facility placement becomes necessary.
4. Help patient families obtain adequate caregiver assistance. Assess their health-care benefits and financial resources, if necessary. Identify all possible resources for help and arrange respite care services, or care facility placement, periodically, to help prevent caregiver burnout.
5. Help patient families achieve and maintain an effective and rapid method of communication. Although augmentative communication systems can be accessed by the severely disabled, most commercial systems require concentration and are slow. Encourage patients and families to memorize an audible alphabet system for fast communication if the patient has one reliable muscle to signal rows and letters of the alphabet, as the caregiver says the rows and letters out loud. Plan and post charts of lists of the patient's possible wants and needs to spare time and to help caregivers understand what the patient is expressing or requesting.
6. Help family caregivers plan a reliable and easily accessible method for the patient to signal for help, contact their families, or send an alert in the event of an emergency situation.

7. Arrange a professional assessment of the patient's home environment to obtain recommendations for making the home accessible. Obtain appropriate durable medical equipment, mobility aids, and self-help devices for enhancing mobility, comfort, and safety. Make all activities of daily living as easy as possible. Be sure to see that the home has accessible means for the patient to leave and enter the home.
8. Plan professional counseling services for households with unmanaged emotions, troubled teens, and broken marriages. Also, encourage patient families to regularly engage in pleasurable activities, leave the home, visit friends, and take trips, despite the patient's disability and use of MV. Provide education and refer to helpful resources for traveling with ease.
9. Visit or arrange for a registered nurse or social worker to visit the homebound patient using LTMV periodically, despite the appearance that all is stable. Monthly visits are ideal. I highly recommend that physicians visit their homebound patients at least once a year to assess firsthand the patient/family's well-being, wishes, and other concerns. Family circumstances may change each year.

By understanding the perspectives of your family caregivers, you can help your patient families avoid misconceptions, obtain necessary information for making best choices, and help them to achieve and maintain the best life possible. The outcomes of family caregivers and their loved ones using LTMV may depend on you.

Acknowledgments

This chapter is dedicated to the late Edward A. Oppenheimer, MD, FCCP, who has served as a special colleague, mentor, and advocate of this long-term investigation. His dedication to improving the quality of life of people with ALS and ventilator users will always be remembered. The author also gives special thanks to the many patients and families who participated in the studies, as well as their physicians, nurses, respiratory therapists, and social workers.

References

1. Oppenheimer EA. Decision-making in the respiratory care of amyotrophic lateral sclerosis: should home mechanical ventilation be used? Palliat Med 1993; 5(suppl 2):49–64.
2. Cazzolli PA, Oppenheimer EA. Home mechanical ventilation for amyotrophic lateral sclerosis: nasal compared to tracheostomy-intermittent positive pressure ventilation. J Neurol Sci 1996; 139(suppl):123–128.
3. Bach JR. Amyotrophic lateral sclerosis. Communication status and survival with ventilatory support. Am J Phys Med Rehabil 1993; 72:343–349.
4. Bach J R. Amyotrophic lateral sclerosis: prolongation of life by noninvasive respiratory aids. Chest 2002; 122:92–98.
5. Hayashi H, Kato S, Kawada A. Amyotrophic lateral sclerosis patients living beyond respiratory failure. J Neurol Sci 1991; 105:73–78.
6. Cazzolli PA, Oppenheimer EA. Use of nasal and tracheostomy positive pressure ventilation in patients with amyotrophic lateral sclerosis (ALS). Abstracts of Papers, 7th International Conference on Noninvasive Ventilation Across the Spectrum from Critical Care to Home Care, Orlando, Florida, March 14–17, 1999.

7. Cazzolli PA, Oppenheimer EA. Use of nasal and tracheostomy positive pressure ventilation in patients with ALS: changing patterns and outcomes. Neurology 1998; 50(suppl 4):A417–A418.
8. Writing Angel. Solutions for Living, PO Box 36116, Canton, Ohio, U.S.A., 44735 (888-884-5483) www.solutionsforliving.us.
9. Cazzolli PA, Oppenheimer EA. Home mechanical ventilation for motor neuron disease (MND/ALS): nasal compared to tracheostomy intermittent positive pressure ventilation (IPPV). Abstracts of Papers, 6th International Symposium on ALS/MND, Dublin, Ireland, November 17–19, 1995.
10. Moss AH, Oppenheimer EA, Casey P, et al. Patients with amyotrophic lateral sclerosis receiving long-term mechanical ventilation: advance care planning and outcomes. Chest 1996; 110:249–255.
11. Arbuckle C. A Caregiver's Journey with a Terminal Patient. Los Angeles: Milligan Books, 2004.
12. Caposella C and Warnock S. Share the Care: How to Organize a Group to Care for Someone Who is Seriously Ill. New York, NY: Simon & Schuster, 2006.
13. Warren R. The Purpose Driven Life: What on Earth Am I Here For? Grand Rapids, Michigan: Zondervan, 2002.
14. Osteen J. Your Best Life Now: 7 Steps to Living at Your Full Potential. New York, NY: Warner Books, 2004.
15. Wedemeyer C, Wedemeyer L. Courage to Live: The Story of Charlie and Lucy Wedemeyer. DVD 2006. Available at: www.couragetolive.com.

40
The Perspective of Physicians: The Intensive Care Specialist and the Pulmonary Specialist

MIGUEL DIVO and BARTOLOME R. CELLI
Caritas St. Elizabeth's Medical Center, Tufts University School of Medicine,
Boston, Massachusetts, U.S.A.

I. Introduction

Since the polio epidemic of the 1950s, mechanical ventilation (MV) has been the cornerstone of modern intensive care units (ICUs) where it has had a significant impact on the survival of patients with respiratory failure (1). Although the main purpose of initiating MV is to serve as a bridge until spontaneous breathing can be restored, in as many as 20% of ventilated patients, liberation from MV is not easily or will never be achieved (2,3). Thus, prolonged MV has become an alternative for those patients who having reached a level of stability, nevertheless, require ventilatory support. Prolonged ventilatory support has evolved substantially over the last decades mainly because of the rapid evolution of noninvasive positive pressure ventilation (NIPPV), which has facilitated MV in the home setting.

The greatest impact on quality of life and survival has been documented in those patients afflicted with neuromuscular diseases (NMD), spinal cord injury (SCI), thoracic restriction (TR), and sleep-disordered breathing (4,5). This is likely due to the nature of the disease process and the relative ease with which a ventilatory steady state is reached. In this group of diseases patients can be ventilated with simple modes and little monitoring.

However, as a consequence of the highly sophisticated modern critical care units a new breed of patients is being created: the chronically, critically, ill-debilitated difficult-to-wean patient. Due to the multifactorial nature of their respiratory failure and series of recurrent complications, this subgroup of patients poses several clinical and ethical challenges for the physicians. Caring for these patients becomes a fascinating journey into the comprehensive "rehabilitative" multidisciplinary model of care where creativity, challenge, and a solid patient–health care provider rapport become the cornerstones on which the relationship is built. The aim of this process is to improve patient-centered quality of life, interrupt the cycle of frequent medical complications, and help the patients achieve their maximal potential (Fig. 1). The best way to achieve these aims is to funnel all of the resources needed through a multidisciplinary effort led by competent professionals and the patients' families to obtain the societal support needed to be successful. For the physician, the hope is to build consensus between the patient and caregivers and set realistic expectations, while helping patients cope with their disease. When consensus is hard to reach at the crossroad of either ceasing weaning efforts or accepting chronic ventilator

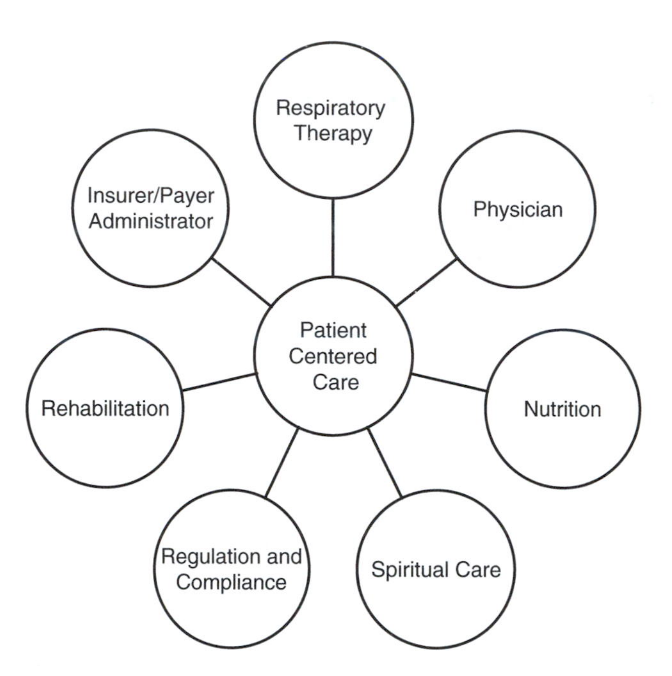

Figure 1 Elements of multidisciplinary, rehabilitative, patient-centered model of care.

dependence, the clinical and ethical dilemma is perceived by the clinician as a pendulum tilting between extending life or prolonging agony.

We often wonder to what extent our patients understand the consequences of their complex situation that often involves infections, deconditioning, limited communication, dependency for self-care, chronic institutionalization, and increased morbidity and mortality. It can be difficult to know when care is futile, especially in patients who have recovered from critical illness and are left with multiple organ damage but in a state compatible with survival at the expense of intense life support. The dilemma in such cases is further compounded by the fact that proposed models designed to predict weaning success, long-term survival, need for acute readmission, chronic institutionalization, and functional outcomes are far from accurate, lack adequate validation, and may not apply to the majority of patients faced in the acute setting (6,7) (Fig. 2).

Expert opinion has proposed a three-month period for attempting liberation from MV (8). However, relying on a strict time line to define futility is inappropriate as other factors, such as recurrent failure to progress with weaning, the lack of ventilatory reserve if weaned, or economic pressure by third-party payers, may influence the decision to abandon further weaning. Since many of the ramifications of long-term mechanical ventilation (LTMV) are difficult to discuss during an acute episode of MV, the initial discussion and counseling should be, whenever possible, proactively moved upstream by the primary care physician and directly with the patient. Although there has been improvement in this area, much work is needed to ensure that patients in the medical system learn how important it is to have advanced directives in case of a medical catastrophe.

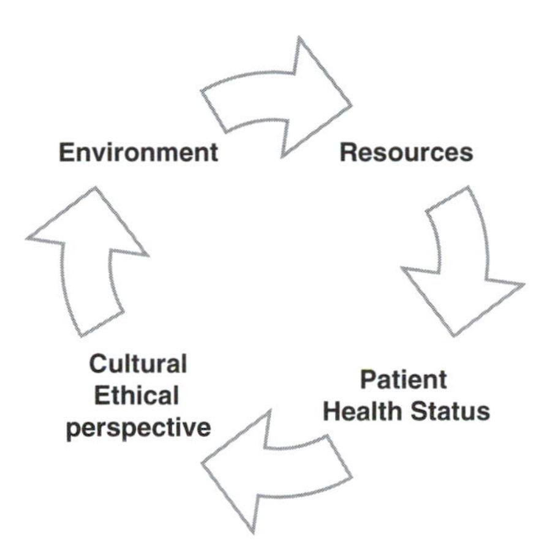

Figure 2 The prolonged mechanical ventilation care process cycle. Patient health status determines the potential for liberation of chronic ventilation dependency. However, environmental influence (reduction of infection, adverse drug reactions, etc.), available resource either professional or economic, and the cultural and ethical beliefs are also important interdependent factors for success.

II. Venues for LTMV

The venues for LTMV consist of institutionalization in chronic ventilator units or home ventilation. Although home mechanical ventilation (HMV) is the place of choice for patient and families (9–11), it also represents a burden for the caregiver and a source of direct and indirect cost to the whole family unit. Ventilator-dependent patients who can be successfully discharged to home are increasing in number (10,12–14). However, they continue to represent a highly selected group with dedicated family members willing to become trained as "uncertified respiratory therapists and nurses," who assume the hidden nonreimbursable cost (i.e., electricity to operate the ventilator 24 hours a day) and the responsibility of dealing with acute complications. HMV is more likely to be successful in industrialized countries with better-organized health care systems, more economic resources, and technology. Chronic institutionalization in an LTMV unit, though technically satisfactory, may be plagued by fractured and impersonal care.

The best environment might be an intermediate option of an LTMV unit that is more homelike and less institutional in its functioning, where family members are directly involved in care, supported by trained staff. This model would enable the ventilator user to benefit from the best of both worlds, the support of technically competent professionals and the personal loving care of families. Our challenge remains to turn this ideal model into a reality.

III. Role of the Physician

For the pulmonary and critical care physician and the generalist caring for ventilator assisted individuals (VAI), the inclusion of rotations during specialty training will provide trainees with a broader perspective on the care continuum from the acute ICU admission to weaning or home ventilation. Specific experience in LTMV for obstructive, restrictive, and neuromuscular conditions; weaning strategies, alternatives methods of ventilation, airway management, infection control, resource utilization, care processes, palliative care, and multidisciplinary rehabilitative patient-centered care will be invaluable for those who will care for patients requiring LTMV.

Most training of critical care specialists is understandably focused on management of the acutely ill patient. Economic pressures have driven ICUs to shorten the length of stay at all costs. Thus, critical care trainees are very good in saving what is salvageable but have a somewhat skewed perspective on the comprehensive care of the patient. In most institutions in the United States, patients surviving an acute illness are transferred to a distant institution under a totally different team, thus depriving the trainee of the opportunity to fully appreciate the result of the team effort and the complexity of the problems.

Given the rapidly expanding population of candidates for LTMV, it is the authors' view that funding sources should give a higher priority to clinical care, teaching, and basic and clinical research among this fascinating population (15).

References

1. Ibsen B. The anaesthetist's viewpoint on the treatment of respiratory complications in poliomyelitis during the epidemic in Copenhagen, 1952. Proc R Soc Med 1954; 47:72–74.
2. Brochard L, Rauss A, Benito S, et al. Comparison of three methods of gradual withdrawal from ventilatory support during weaning from mechanical ventilation. Am J Respir Crit Care Med 1994; 150(4):896–903.
3. Esteban A, Frutos F, Tobin MJ, et al. A comparison of four methods of weaning patients from mechanical ventilation. Spanish Lung Failure Collaborative Group. N Engl J Med 1995; 332(6): 345–350.
4. Wijkstra PJ, Avendano MA, Goldstein RS. Inpatient chronic assisted ventilatory care: a 15-year experience. Chest 2003; 124(3):850–856.
5. Markstrom A, Sundell K, Lysdahl M, et al. Quality-of-life evaluation of patients with neuromuscular and skeletal diseases treated with noninvasive and invasive home mechanical ventilation. Chest 2002; 122(5):1695–1700.
6. MacIntyre NR, Epstein SK, Carson S, et al. Management of patients requiring prolonged mechanical ventilation: report of a NAMDRC consensus conference. Chest 2005; 128(6): 3937–3954.
7. MacIntyre NR, Cook DJ, Ely EW Jr., et al. Evidence-based guidelines for weaning and discontinuing ventilatory support: a collective task force facilitated by the American College of Chest Physicians; the American Association for Respiratory Care; and the American College of Critical Care Medicine. Chest 2001; 120(6 suppl):375S–395S.
8. MacIntyre NR. Evidence-based ventilator weaning and discontinuation. Respir Care 2004; 49(7):830–836.
9. Ambrosino N, Vianello A. Where to perform long-term ventilation. Respir Care Clin N Am 2002; 8(3):463–478.
10. Goldstein RS, Psek JA, Gort EH. Home mechanical ventilation. Demographics and user perspectives. Chest 1995; 108(6):1581–1586.
11. Smith CE, Mayer LS, Parkhurst C, et al. Adaptation in families with a member requiring mechanical ventilation at home. Heart Lung 1991; 20(4):349–356.

12. Cox CE, Carson SS, Holmes GM, et al. Increase in tracheostomy for prolonged mechanical ventilation in North Carolina, 1993–2002. Crit Care Med 2004; 32(11):2219–2226.
13. Lloyd-Owen SJ, Donaldson GC, Ambrosino N, et al. Patterns of home mechanical ventilation use in Europe: results from the Eurovent survey. Eur Respir J 2005; 25(6):1025–1031.
14. Make BJ. Home care for ventilator-dependent individuals. Chest 1985; 87(3):412.
15. Darwin C. The Origin of Species. PF Collier & Son, 1909.

41
The Perspective of the Allied Health Professionals

JANE REARDON
Hartford Hospital, Hartford, Connecticut, U.S.A.

CATHY RELF
West Park Healthcare Centre, Toronto, Ontario, Canada

DEBBIE FIELD
Lane Fox Respiratory Intensive Care Unit, St. Thomas' Hospital, London, U.K.

I. Introduction

A well-motivated, experienced, and caring health care team (HCT) is key to the successful management of patients receiving long-term mechanical ventilation (LTMV). Although the LTMV population represents <10% of intensive care unit (ICU) admissions, it consumes >50% of financial resources (1). Specialized centers, within or outside the acute care hospitals, offer a more appropriate setting for patients requiring LTMV, as they provide evidence-based, cost-effective, holistic care to patients recovering from critical illness. The HCT updates care plans daily, based on the patient's physical, nutritional, psychological, emotional, and spiritual needs. The core team (Table 1), which varies among jurisdictions, collaborates with many other consulting staff (Table 2). This chapter will address the allied health professionals' perceptions of the issues, challenges, and barriers to the care of the LTMV patient population, in three different venues.

II. Venues of Care

Acutely ill patients who fail to wean are increasing in prevalence (2–4). More than half are >65 years and most have multiple comorbid conditions (5). A prolonged stay in the ICU is associated with many clinical issues (Table 3), including that of being a low priority, unpopular patient. Repeated futile weaning attempts result in frustration and poor communication between the ICU team and the patient. Usually the last to be seen in the ICU daily rounds, these patients receive little time. In addition, little effort is given by the ICU team in developing a collaborative care plan. Thus, there is a need to transfer such patients to a less acute level of care such as a step-down unit, a specialized respiratory care unit (RCU) or, in the United States, a long-term acute care center. In Canada, LTMV patients unable to return to the community may be effectively cared for in chronic assisted ventilatory care (CAVC) units. In the above settings, multidisciplinary teams and well-developed rehabilitation programs maintain good outcomes at a significant cost savings. A description of three very

Table 1 Suggested Members of Health Care Team

- Medical director or attending physician
- APRN or PA
- Nurse
- Respiratory care practitioner
- Physical therapist
- Social worker
- Case coordinator

Abbreviations: APRN, advanced practice registered nurse; PA, physician assistant.

Table 2 Collaborating HCT Partners

- Wound care specialists
- Geriatric services
- Recreational therapists
- Pastoral care personnel
- Pharmacist
- Integrative medicine therapists
- Nutritionist
- Psychiatry and psychology practitioners

Abbreviation: HCT, health care team.

Table 3 Potential Consequences of a Prolonged ICU Stay

- Skeletal and respiratory muscle weakness
- Cardiorespiratory deconditioning
- Nosocomial infections
- Malnutrition
- Decubitus wounds
- Adverse drug events
- Fatigue
- Dyspnea
- Anxiety
- Delirium
- Depression
- Sleep deprivation
- Cognitive dysfunction
- Impaired communication
- Loss of control

Abbreviation: ICU, intensive care unit.

Table 4 Criteria for Admission to a Respiratory Care Unit

- Acutely ill but in recovery phase of illness
- Hemodynamically stable (may be on low dose vasopressors)
- Intubated with tracheostomy or endotracheal tube
- Requires high level of ventilator support
- Failed weaning trials in ICU
- Potential to wean in 21 days
- Plan established for overall medical care
- Formal rehabilitation evaluation completed
- Evaluation by the RCU team before transfer
- Transferred to the service of an attending pulmonologist
- Family meeting prior to transfer to establish expectations

Abbreviations: ICU, intensive care unit; RCU, respiratory care unit.

different LTMV venues illustrates the advantages and shortcomings of each from the perspective of the allied HCT.

A. A Specialized RCU in the United States

An 8-bed RCU is housed in an 800-bed acute care hospital with distinct medical, cardiac, neurosurgical, and surgical ICUs in Hartford, Connecticut. It was developed to decrease the ICU length of stay (LOS), accepting patients who met predetermined criteria (Table 4). A major goal of this unit is to gather LTMV patients with similar respiratory needs from the ICUs. The HCT manages patients using evidence-based protocols and best practices. A pleasing, comfortable, family-friendly environment was created, with planned natural light for each cubicle and unobtrusive, state-of-the-art technology. The registered nurses (RNs) undergo a 40-hour educational core course and skills training prior to working in the unit.

Staffing

The RCU is managed collaboratively by a pulmonologist and a nurse manager. The nurse to patient ratio is 1:3 for six beds and 1:2 for two beds. A dedicated respiratory care practitioner (RCP) is assigned to the unit and 24-hour respiratory therapy (RT) coverage is available. A physical therapist (PT) provides 20 hr/wk coverage, and occupational therapy (OT) is accessed on a consulting basis. Nurse practitioners (NPs) and physician assistants (PAs) provide medical coverage in 12-hour shifts throughout the week. House-staff provide emergency coverage only when NPs or PAs are not present. A social worker is assigned for 20 hr/wk. Two patient care assistants provide bathing and other physical care.

Daily, 1-hour team bedside rounds result in a new plan of care for the next 24 hours. The previous day's goals are updated on a flow sheet and a dry erase board on the door of the patient's room. Weaning trials follow a standardized protocol for work to rest modes and duration. The care plan includes patient safety recommendations (6), prevention strategies to avoid ventilator-associated infections (7), and policies for central line and surgical site care (8). Daily clinical rounds also serve as a teaching role to discuss research questions, clinical evidence, and other patient-related issues. This aspect helps maintain high motivation and interchanges among core team members. Notwithstanding any differences of opinion, each team member is committed to supporting the final care decisions.

Table 5 RCU Team Building

- **Strengths:**
  - Patient-focused mission is important
  - Each team member is vital to a good patient outcome
  - Good interpersonal relationships—"like a big family"
  - Good communication among team, patients, and families
  - Staff willing to learn and few lines are drawn between roles
  - Commitment to excellence
  - Educational and skills support from NPs and PAs
- **Barriers to care:**
  - Sick calls
  - Nursing staff transferred to other short-staffed units
  - Lack of experienced nurses on all shifts
  - Confined work space
  - Poor management communication
  - Lack of 24-hr physician and advanced nursing coverage
- **Perceived needs:**
  - Regularly scheduled team meetings
  - Focus on problem solving
  - Honest opinions without fear of reprimand
  - Smoother transfer process from the ICU

Abbreviations: RCU, respiratory care unit; ICU, intensive care unit; NP, nurse practitioners; PA, physician assistant.

New care protocols and ideas are introduced at mandatory, yearly half-day retreats, which serve to bond the team and emphasize the unit's positive outcomes (Table 5). The retreats are also a forum for discussing any negative feelings. Labels such as "communicator" for the unit secretary, "caregiver" for the nursing aid, and "organizer" for the stocking and cleaning assistant are used to emphasize the importance of these team members.

Frustrations occur when weaning strategies vary with the attending pulmonologist, when continuity of care is compromised by 12-hour shift scheduling, and when inappropriate candidates are admitted to the unit. Patients who cannot be weaned remain on the unit for weeks because of the lack of long-term care facilities for the ventilator-assisted individual (VAI). Morbidly obese patients and those with anoxic encephalopathy present physical and ethical dilemmas that threaten staff morale. A difficult issue is the combination of LOS and reimbursement schedules, which together negatively affect the financial viability of the unit.

The team ensures that patients have at least four hours of uninterrupted sleep each night, resting in the assist control mode (9,10). Sepsis or critical illness neuromuscular abnormalities (11) delay weaning and rehabilitation for weeks and, if ICU transfer is not possible, result in the stress of providing more intensive care in an RCU. The team is aware of the many factors that might negatively influence weaning, including electrolyte imbalance (12), sepsis (13), poor glycemic control (14), corticosteroids (15), and nosocomial infections such as ventilator associated pneumonia (VAP) (16,17).

Many trauma surgeons favor early percutaneous tracheostomies to reduce the chances of VAP and to reduce days of mechanical ventilation (MV) (18). As the diversity and

Table 6 Aspiration Precautions

- Maintain cuff pressures at 20 cmH_2O to prevent leakage into the LRT
- Suction subglottic secretions before deflating tracheostomy cuff
- Empty contaminated condensation from ventilator circuits q12 hr or p.r.n.
- Head of bed >30° at all times, and 90° during and 30 min after meals
- Turn tube feedings off 30 min before bathing, turning
- Brush teeth for 5 min BID
- Mouthwash to all oral surfaces TID
- Early speech and swallow evaluation

Abbreviations: LRT, lower respiratory tract; BID, two times a day; TID, three times a day.

complexity of the many types of tracheostomy products can confuse the nursing staff (19), examples of tracheostomy equipment are displayed on teaching charts. The HCT initiated measures (Table 6) to decrease the risk of VAP. In keeping with the Berwick safety initiative (8), each HCT member is responsible for monitoring the action of all others and immediately brings any issue to the attention of the whole team.

Polypharmacy is a constant concern, as most of our patients are prescribed an average of 12 different medications. As the risk of adverse drug events is >80%, when seven or more medications are prescribed in people >65 years (20,21), the drug list is constantly reevaluated.

We use a defined set of weaning predictors (22–24) as a readiness assessment tool prior to a spontaneous breathing trial (SBT). During the SBT, a nurse or RT remains at the bedside for at least five minutes to coach the patient and monitor tolerance, recognizing that patients may require several minutes to adjust to a decrease in pressure support (25).

Psychological factors such as anxiety, delirium, and depression play an important role in daily patient management (26), with patients ventilated for >22 days having the highest level of anxiety (27). Other stress creating factors include dyspnea (28), pain (29), inability to communicate (30), thirst, and difficulty in sleeping. We try to promote nonpharmacologic strategies (Table 7) to manage these problems (31–35), although benzodiazepines, narcotics,

Table 7 Strategies to Minimize Anxiety During MV

- Alter level of ventilatory support
- Direct fans over the face
- Use communication boards or laptops
- Adjust ventilator to enable short periods of speech
- Minimize noise and excessive light
- Offer soothing music or book tapes
- Provide comfort and cleanliness
- Establish a regular sleep schedule
- Encourage family presence
- Discuss topics of interest
- Relaxation techniques
- Massage

Abbreviation: MV, mechanical ventilation.

hypnotics and sedatives are readily prescribed by some clinicians. Such drugs contribute to constipation, agitation, and the risk of aspiration, all of which delay weaning and rehabilitation (36). We use an assessment tool for delirium, the Confusion Assessment Method in the ICU (37), which has proved to be very helpful in determining the patient's level of awareness and ability to participate in the weaning process.

Rehabilitation

After a prolonged ICU stay, rehabilitation is the foremost goal. Bed rest, medications, trauma, and poor nutrition all affect the musculoskeletal and cardiorespiratory systems (38–40). The PTs play a major role in the prevention and treatment of musculoskeletal complications. The addition of exercise training to routine mobilization improves walking distance beyond that of mobilization alone (41). In practice, careful attention has to be paid to PT and nursing schedules, for this to occur. Involvement of the HCT in getting patients out of bed and where possible out of the unit has improved patient, family, and staff confidence that progress is being made. The PT also teaches the nurses and family members to provide individualized interval training, as well as an active and passive range of motion for nurses and family members.

Despite general agreement on the ethics of patient care, there is variability in the HCT approach to withholding or withdrawing care (42–45), an issue addressed elsewhere in this book. Decision making must be based on well-founded information, and consideration of the patient's and family's views (46–48). It is often the nurse or NP who first recognizes these issues and this can create interdisciplinary conflict (49). Palliative care consultation is invaluable in helping to resolve these conflicts and improve communication between clinicians and the family (50). Most medical updates to the family are done by NPs or PAs, as they are most often present during the time that the family visits.

B. CAVC: a Canadian Perspective

CAVC patients vary on a day-to-day basis and at the same time provide constancy insofar as they are always there to challenge the most dedicated health care professional. These perspectives come from the staff of a 22-bed CAVC unit set in a beautiful 27-acre park environment in Toronto, Ontario, Canada. Most patients require 24-hour ventilation.

The nursing staff ratio is lower than that of the ICU setting, from which most patients are referred, being 1:2 on days, 1:3 on evenings, and 1:4 on nights. The unit employs a balanced nursing skill mix with RNs and registered practical nurses, supported by a nursing team leader who rotates every 10 weeks. There is no in-house medical coverage out of hours or at weekends, beyond an on call duty physician who responds to a pager. However, an attending staff physician makes daily rounds during working hours, and a respiratory specialist makes rounds with the whole multidisciplinary team at least once a week.

The core nonnursing support comes from respiratory therapy with one assigned RT plus one RT technician on days, as well as hospital wide on-site coverage for nights and weekends throughout the year. Physiotherapy and occupational therapy provide care during weekday business hours, with weekend coverage on a physician's order. Recreation therapy provides individual and group programming to help enhance quality of life of the CAVC patients. In addition to group outings, individual computer and Internet access is available, with modifications to facilitate access. Other team members, including those in social work, psychology, and chaplaincy are available as required.

Perspectives

Some staff arrived by choice, some by default due to seniority, and some stayed after covering a leave of absence. Those who stay, do so because they feel they are effective in delivering excellent, patient centered care.

The work is heavy, physically and emotionally. It is essentially about routine care plans, which become more complex as the patients' underlying condition and comorbidities progress. Connecting with the patients and understanding the issues that influence their perception of quality of life are vital components of care. The team will go home satisfied if they believe that they are fulfilling the needs of the patients. Everyone wants to make a difference, if only a small one, for patients who trust their care to you.

Separating the patient from the ventilator means knowing who they were; what was their occupation; did they have hobbies, family, and friends? What are their favorite music, movies, and food? In the absence of this deeper relationship, the CAVC unit is no more than an assignment, a task, or a treatment.

Empathy with the patients' perspectives will prevent overlooking simple things that might markedly affect their mood. An understanding of their hopes and dreams, their losses and diminished control over their own bodies helps us appreciate how vulnerable they are.

The qualities our team most admires about their coworkers include caring, kindness, enthusiasm, a positive attitude, patience, humor, flexibility, tolerance, compassion, and good communication. Respect for the patient is manifest in many ways—for example, asking the patients' permission to enter the room, deliver care, or change position. These small but important issues enable patients who are medically very dependent to regain a sense of control over their environment.

Many members of the multidisciplinary team were initially aware of their lack of experience with markedly impaired patients in an environment of high technology. This was addressed by substantial on-site training from the respiratory therapists and the advanced practice nurse.

The responses to team questionnaire on two important issues are summarized below:

What makes CAVC satisfying?

- Providing the patient with opportunities to do things that we take for granted
- Increasing a patient's independence
- Knowing that the patient is safe and content
- Delivering care that a patient looks forward to
- Solving problems
- Chatting outside the therapeutic relationship
- The expression of satisfaction from the patient or family

What makes CAVC frustrating?

- Poor patient communication
- Lack of respect from a patient
- Tension within the team
- Not being able to meet the patient's needs
- Working with staff members who are just doing a job

Nurses struggle with "patient-focused care" as those patients who refuse care risk serious complications. For example, refusing a bowel routine may result in a life-threatening bowel obstruction and drinking a beer is accompanied by a risk of aspiration. The other challenge to patient-focused care is when the patient's needs are not in step with the family's needs.

The team also struggles with ethical issues such as when a patient declines to a point where quality of life is perceived, by the caregiving team, to be very poor. An understanding of how the patient regards quality of life becomes of paramount importance. Sometimes the patient's family insists on heroic measures, to preserve the life of their loved one. This becomes very delicate, especially if the patients can no longer communicate their own wishes. The toughest ethical issue is the patient's right to refuse treatment, especially when this means disconnection from the ventilator and death. Team and family conferences with the support of an ethicist and a psychologist have been of great help in tackling these difficult situations. Although the multidisciplinary team works closely in a mutually supportive environment, specific perspectives of nursing, physical therapy, respiratory therapy, and recreational therapy are summarized below.

Team Perspectives

The caseload is heavy, especially for nurses, who have unique responsibilities as they are there on evenings and weekends when other team members are off site. For the respiratory therapist, working on the CAVC unit requires a combination of respiratory therapy and psychology. There are many rewards to working in a less formal environment, with a well-defined team in which everyone knows one another. The work demands excellent care coupled with acceptance that some patients will not adopt the clinical recommendations. Many of the practical issues are not found in textbooks, but come with experience. Best practice involves evaluating new equipment, being open to change in mode of ventilation, use of positive end expiratory pressure, newer tracheostomy tubes, alternative methods of secretion clearance, and specialized dressings.

Few physiotherapists or occupational therapists have the opportunity to work with LTMV patients and, therefore, the on-call staffs are sometimes intimidated by ventilators, airway clearance issues, and communication challenges. The PT and OT work closely together, the former helping patients to maintain muscle strength and function and the latter focusing on transfers, seating, and communication. The recreational therapist enables CAVC patients to participate in many individualized activities. Specialized equipment is always in short supply and staff support is required for community outings.

All team members feel highly valued and find the work to be very satisfying, noting that even limited gains in function do enhance a patient's quality of life. Contact with others, through educational events, is an essential part of maintaining high standards.

C. Long-Term Mechanical Ventilation: a U.K. Nursing Perspective

In the United Kingdom, resources for LTMV patients (ventilated > 21 days) outside of the acute care setting are extremely limited, with few specialist chronic respiratory care centers, despite the fact that LTMV patients are increasing. The following comments describe a management strategy developed by a nurse consultant (NC), to meet the needs of LTMV patients.

LTMV in the ICU

Few guidelines exist to assist in the management of the LTMV patient in a critical care environment, despite their developing many clinical issues secondary to their prolonged ICU stay (Table 3). LTMV patients require management strategies that differ from those usually applied in the ICU. Challenges to good care include: allocation of a different nurse for each shift, seeing the patient last, very limited availability of speech language pathology and OT, and changing plans as attending clinicians rotate. Finally, specialist units and intermediate care facilities for the LTMV patients are few, and support facilities to enable patients to go home are poorly resourced.

The Experience of a Nurse Consultant Within a Critical Care Network

I was appointed as NC for a critical care network in the southeast of England, which comprised of four district general hospitals with a total of 47 critical care beds. An audit identified the most difficult patient group to manage as those requiring LTMV. My role was to develop and implement pathways for care of the LTMV patient.

A weaning pathway (Fig. 1) was developed to accommodate those who might be weaned from MV. A rehabilitation framework (Fig. 2), which focused on whole body rehabilitation, also enabled some patients to be weaned and discharged home. ICUs identified core teams of

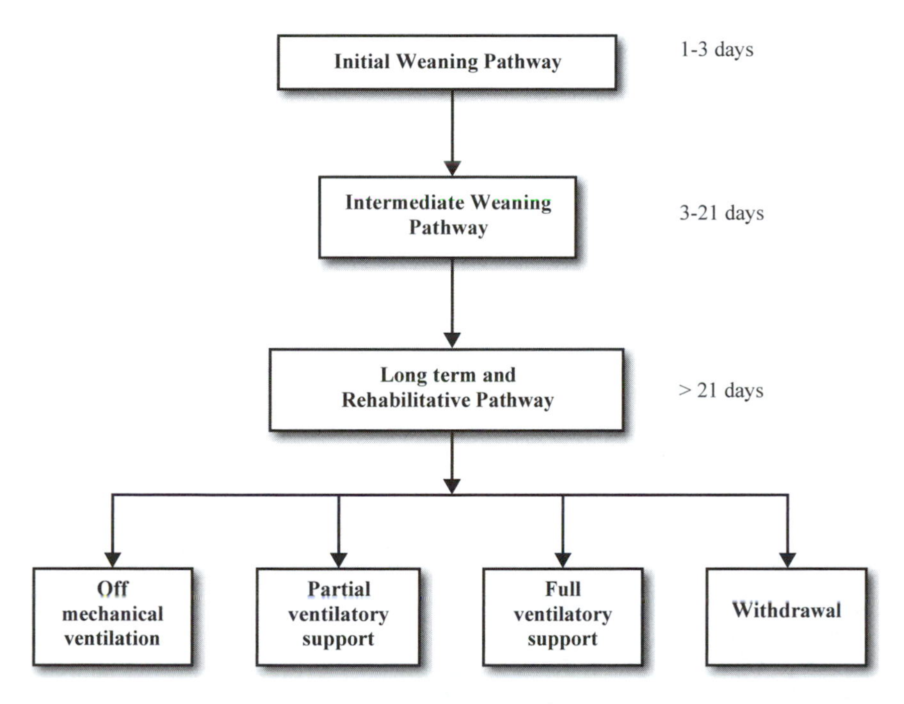

Figure 1 Three-stage weaning pathway to identify who are the LTMV patients. *Abbreviation*: LTMV, long-term mechanical ventilation.

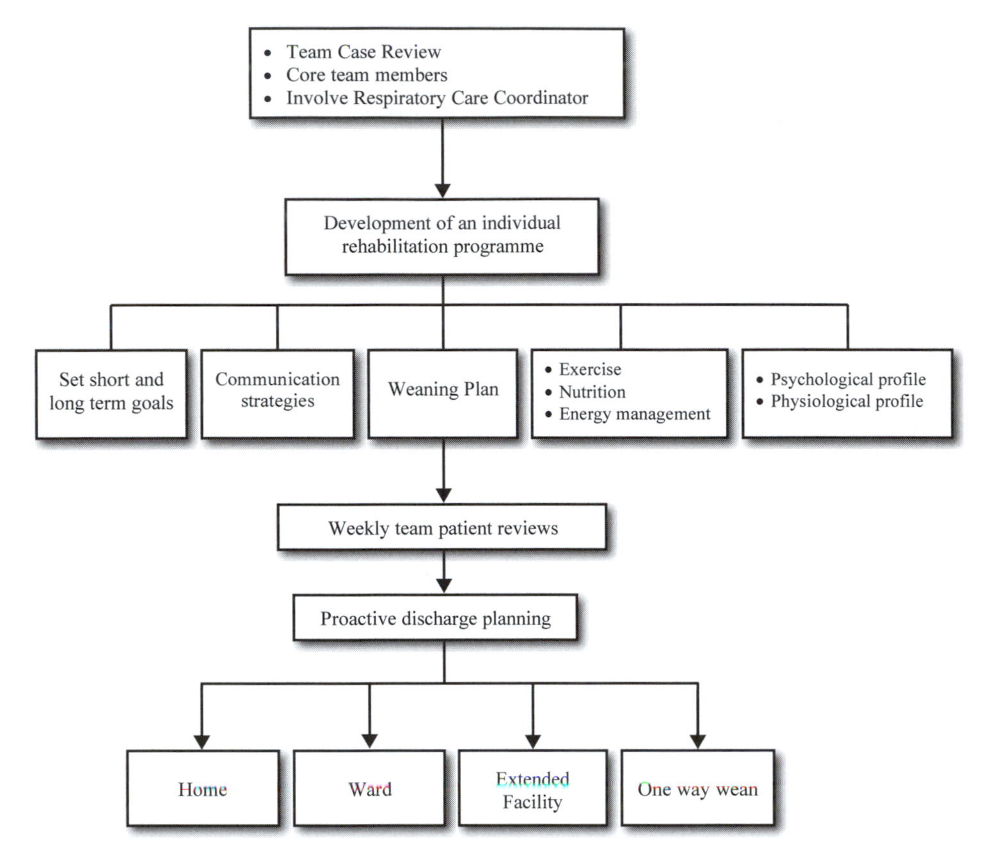

Figure 2 Long-term and rehabilitation framework for the LTMV patient. *Abbreviation*: LTMV, long-term mechanical ventilation.

staff and appointed coordinators, usually senior physiotherapists (respiratory therapists are not available in the United Kingdom) who had patient contact on a daily basis, to care for the LTMV patients.

The Process of the Rehabilitation Framework

An example of a care plan for patients in the rehabilitation framework is shown in Table 8. Distinguishing features included daily and weekly goal setting, weekly collaborative structured case reviews, and proactive discharge planning. It became clear that a structured pathway between secondary and primary care providers was needed to meet the unique needs of LTMV patients who might be transferred home or to a community facility. The model of community critical care (Fig. 3) embraced primary care trusts, general practitioners, and secondary care hospitals, with the NC as the case manager, to assist the LTMV patient in moving through the health care system. Private industry provided the domiciliary ventilators

Table 8 Rehabilitation Plan of Care

Long-term goals:

- Partial or full ventilatory support via facemask or tracheostomy.
- Discharge to long-term facility or home with a continuing care package
- PEG

Short-term goals:

- Reduce fluid overload
- Establish tolerance for cuff deflation
- Communication through PMV
- Trial of facial NIV once per day
- Inflation with three deep breaths per hour to double resting V_T.
- Daily physiotherapy
- Remove neck line and urinary catheter

Set Parameters:

- $Spo_2 > 92\%$
- $V_T >= 300$mLs during day, $V_T \geq 380$mLs when asleep
- $Paco_2 < 9.5$ kPa (70 mmHg)

Respiratory plan:

- Increase ventilator settings at night to ensure adequate V_T
- Increase respiratory endurance through respiratory muscle training
- Increase body strength and endurance with physiotherapy
- Tracheostomy to be corked and mask NIV for 5 min/day.

How to cork the tracheostomy tube:

- Deflate cuff, remove inner tube, cork tracheostomy with size 4.0, attach mask to ventilator tubing, and apply by hand or secure with straps. Encourage slow deep breathing while observing for signs of distress, reconnect after 5 min and reinflate cuff.
- Daily trials of cuff deflation and PMV extended if patient is coping, ensure PMV is out and cuff is inflated at night and during day rest, encourage phonation when PMV is in situ.
- Swallow test by the end of the week if patient is coping.

Abbreviations: PEG, possible percutaneous enteral gastrostomy; PMV, Passy Muir™ valve; NIV, non-invasive ventilation; Spo_2, pulse oximetry; $Paco_2$, partial pressure of carbon dioxide in arterial blood.

and technical support. The following case study demonstrates how coordinated management of a patient prone to respiratory failure will reduce costs and improve quality of life.

Case Study

A 53-year-old woman with severe chronic obstructive pulmonary disease, on home oxygen, had been admitted to the ICU on three occasions in 2003, for acute respiratory failure consequent upon an acute exacerbation, always unresponsive with a Glasgow Coma Scale 8/15 (Table 9). She received noninvasive positive pressure ventilation (NIPPV) by mask on each admission and after 24 hours had greatly improved. On each occasion, her LOS was 17 days before discharge home, representing acute care cost of £8880 (seven days ICU = £6300 plus 10 days ward = £2580, for a total of £8880 per admission).

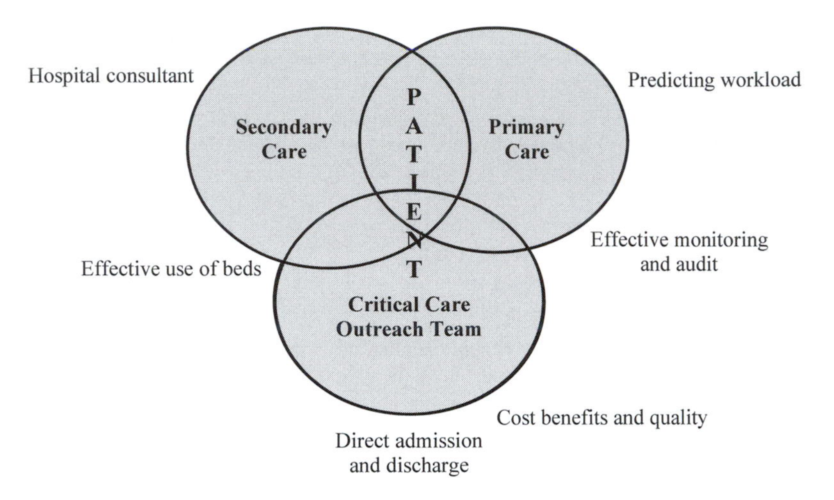

Figure 3 Conceptual model of community critical care.

Table 9 Glasgow Coma Scale

GLASGOW COMA SCALE

Patient Name: ______

Rater Name: ______

Date: ______

Activity		Score
EYE OPENING		
None	1 = Even to supra-orbital pressure	
To pain	2 = Pain from sternum/limb/supra-orbital pressure	
To speech	3 = Non-specific response, not necessarily to command	
Spontaneous	4 = Eyes open, not necessarily aware	____
MOTOR RESPONSE		
None	1 = To any pain; limbs remain flaccid	
Extension	2 = Shoulder adducted and shoulder and forearm internally rotated	
Flexor response	3 = Withdrawal response or assumption of hemiplegic posture	
Withdrawal	4 = Arm withdraws to pain, shoulder abducts	
Localizes pain	5 = Arm attempts to remove supra-orbital/chest pressure	
Obeys commands	6 = Follows simple commands	____
VERBAL RESPONSE		
None	1 = No verbalization of any type	
Incomprehensible	2 = Moans/groans, no speech	
Inappropriate	3 = Intelligible, no sustained sentences	
Confused	4 = Converses but confused, disoriented	
Oriented	5 = Converses and oriented	____
	TOTAL (3–15):	____

Source: From Ref. 51.

The patient was reviewed by the nurse consultant after her third admission. She had no experience with community specialist support and her primary caregiver was her husband who was experiencing very negative consequences to his business. The following goals were agreed upon:

- Patient to take control of her disease process
- Reduce hospital admissions
- Improve quality of life for patient and husband
- Discuss end-of-life care

The patient underwent education, pulmonary rehabilitation, and training in home NIPPV, and a continuing care package was negotiated between the primary care trust and the family. The NC called weekly and visited monthly. Continuing care costs for the following year were home ventilator service contract £700 plus disposable supplies £300, for a total of £1000. The patient was successfully managed at home, with optimized bronchodilators and exacerbation management using oral steroids and antibiotics, such that her *general practitioner* made only three home visits in 2004. As shown below (Fig. 4), her quality of life and sense of well-being improved markedly after the management plan had been implemented.

III. Conclusion

Despite considerable success with LTMV patients in the ICU, some barriers remain. These include the LTMV patient being undervalued in the ICU setting, the lack of investment in home ventilation and specialist centers, and the need for more research into the optimal

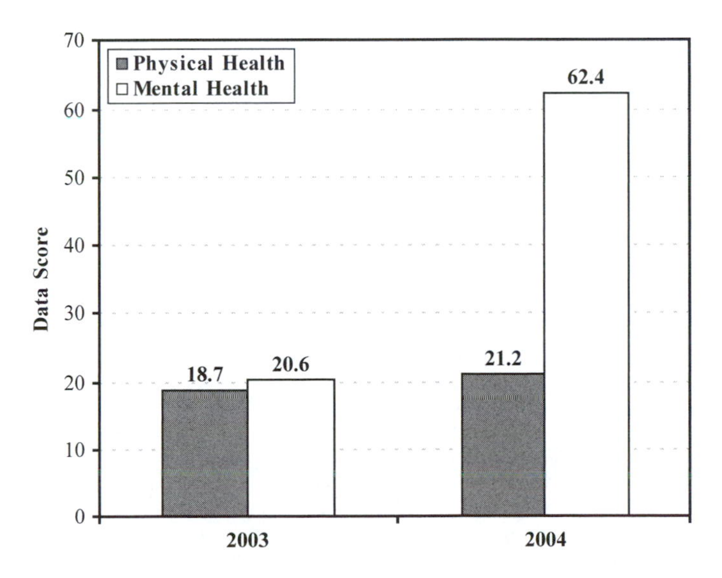

Figure 4 Quality of life after introduction of a care plan. Lynn SF-36 Summary Scores 2003 and 2004.

management of the LTMV patient. In all the three jurisdictions described, the essence of good care revolved around a coordinated multidisciplinary HCT, focused on the maintenance of high standards of care; the importance of physical, psychological, and social issues; and a cost-effective argument for investing in more facilities. The perspectives of the HCT are important in ensuring clinical success for this important group of patients.

References

1. Cohen IL, Booth FV. Cost containment and mechanical ventilation in the United States. New Horiz 1994; 2:283–290.
2. Epstein SK. Weaning from mechanical ventilation. Respir Care 2002; 47(4):454–466.
3. Cooper LM, Linde-Zwirble WT. Medicare intensive care use: analysis of incidence, cost and payment. Crit Care Med 2004; 32:2247–2253.
4. Carson SS. What are the costs of weaning problems? Abstracts of Papers, International Consensus Conference in Intensive Care Medicine: Weaning from Mechanical Ventilation, Budapest, Hungary, April 28–29, 2005. Convened by five major scientific societies.
5. Carson SS, Bach PB. The epidemiology and costs of chronically critically ill patients. Crit Care Clin 2002; 18:461–476.
6. Kress JP, Pohlman AS, O'Connor MF, et al. Daily interruption of sedative infusions in critically ill patients undergoing mechanical ventilation. N Engl J Med 2000; 342(20):1471–1477.
7. American Thoracic Society. Guidelines for the management of adults with hospital-acquired, ventilator-associated, and healthcare-associated pneumonia. Am J Respir Crit Care Med 2005; 171:388–416.
8. Berwick DM, Calkins DR, McCannon CJ, et al. The 100,000 lives campaign: setting a goal and a deadline for improving health care quality. JAMA 2006; 295(3):324–327.
9. Chen HI, Tang YR. Sleep loss impairs inspiratory muscle endurance. Am Rev Respir Dis 1989; 140(4):907–909.
10. Parthasarathy S, Tobin MJ. Effect of ventilator mode on sleep quality in critically ill patients. Am J Respir Crit Care Med 2002; 166(11):1423–1429.
11. DeJong B. Critical care neuropathy and myopathy. Abstracts of Papers, International Consensus Conference in Intensive Care Medicine: Weaning from Mechanical Ventilation, Budapest, Hungary, April 28–29, 2005. Convened by five major scientific societies.
12. Aubier M, Murciano D, Lecocguic Y, et al. Effect of hypophosphatemia on diaphragmatic contractility in patients with acute respiratory failure. N Engl J Med 1985; 3(13):420–424.
13. Hussain SN. Respiratory muscle dysfunction in sepsis. Mol Cell Biochem 1998; 179(1–2): 125–134.
14. Laghi F, Tobin MJ. Disorders of the respiratory muscles. Am J Respir Crit Care Med 2003; 168:10–48.
15. Akkoca O, Mungan D, Karabiyikoglu G, et al. Inhaled and systemic corticosteroid therapies: Do they contribute to inspiratory muscle weakness in asthma? Respiration 1999; 66(4):332–337.
16. Chastre J, Fagon JY. Ventilator-associated pneumonia. Am J Respir Crit Care Med 2002; 165:867–903.
17. Torres A. Ventilator associated pneumonia, aspiration and sepsis. Abstracts of Papers, International Consensus Conference in Intensive Care Medicine: Weaning from Mechanical Ventilation, Budapest, Hungary, April 28–29, 2005. Convened by five major scientific societies.
18. Rumbak MJ, Newton M, Truncale T, et al. A prospective, randomized study comparing early percutaneous dilational tracheostomy to prolonged translaryngeal intubation (delayed tracheotomy) in critically ill medical patients. Crit Care Med 2004; 32(8):1689–1694.
19. Littlewood KE. Evidence-based management of tracheostomies in hospitalized patients. Respir Care 2005; 50(4):516–518.

20. Prybys K, Melville K, Hanna J, et al. Polypharmacy in the elderly: clinical challenges in emergency practice. Part 1: Overview, etiology and drug interactions. Emerg Med Rep 2002; 23(11):145–153.
21. Fulton MM, Allen ER. Polypharmacy in the elderly: a literature review. J Am Acad Nurse Pract 2005; 17(4):123–132.
22. Tobin MJ. Role and interpretation of weaning predictors. Abstracts of Papers, International Consensus Conference in Intensive Care Medicine: Weaning from Mechanical Ventilation, Budapest, Hungary, April 28–29, 2005. Convened by five major scientific societies.
23. MacIntyre NR, Cook DJ, Ely EW Jr., et al. Evidence-based guidelines for weaning and discontinuing ventilatory support: a collective task force facilitated by the American College of Chest Physicians, the American Association of Respiratory Care, and the American College of Critical Care Medicine. Chest 2001; 120(6 suppl):375S–395S.
24. Meade M, Guyatt G, Cook D, et al. Predicting success in weaning from mechanical ventilation. Chest 2001; 120(6 suppl):400S–424S.
25. Brochard L, Rauss A, Benito S, et al. Comparison of three methods of gradual withdrawal from ventilatory support during weaning from mechanical ventilation. Am J Respir Crit Care Med 1994; 150:896–903.
26. Chlan LL. Description of anxiety levels by individual differences and clinical factors in patients receiving mechanical ventilatory support. Heart Lung 2003; 32(4):275–282.
27. Jubran A. Psychological factors (anxiety, post-traumatic stress). Abstracts of Papers, International Consensus Conference in Intensive Care Medicine: Weaning from Mechanical Ventilation, Budapest, Hungary, April 28–29, 2005. Convened by five major scientific societies.
28. Powers J, Bennett SJ. Measurement of dyspnea in patients treated with mechanical ventilation. Am J Crit Care 1999; 8(4):254–261.
29. Bergbom-Engberg I, Haljamae H. Assessment of patients' experience of discomfort during respirator therapy. Crit Care Med 1989; 17(10):1068–1072.
30. Rotondi AJ, Chelluri L, Sirio C, et al. Patients' recollections of stressful experiences while receiving prolonged mechanical ventilation in an intensive care unit. Crit Care Med 2002; 30(4): 746–752.
31. Schwartzstein RM, Lahive K, Pope A, et al. Cold facial stimulation reduces breathlessness induced in normal subjects. Am Rev Respir Dis 1987; 136:58–61.
32. Wong HL, Lopez-Nahas V, Molassiotis A. Effects of music therapy on anxiety in ventilator-dependent patients. Heart Lung 2001; 30(5):376–387.
33. Hoit JD, Banzett RB, Lohmeier HL, et al. Clinical ventilator adjustments that improve speech. Chest 2003; 124(4):1512–1521.
34. Knebel AR, Janson-Bjerklie SL, Malley JD, et al. Comparison of breathing comfort during weaning with two ventilatory modes. Am J Respir Crit Care Med 1994; 149(1):14–18.
35. Holliday JE, Hyers TM. The reduction of weaning time from mechanical ventilation using tidal volume and relaxation feedback. Am Rev Respir Dis 1990; 141:1214–1220.
36. Kress JP, Gehlbach JP, Lacy M, et al. The long term psychological effects of daily sedative interruption on critically ill patients. Am J Respir Crit Care Med 2003; 168(12):1457–1461.
37. Ely EW, Inouye S, Bernard G, et al. Delirium in mechanically ventilated patients: validity and reliability of the confusion assessment method for the intensive care unit (CAM-ICU). JAMA 2001; 286:2703–2710.
38. Harper CM, Lyles YM. Physiology and complications of bed rest. J Am Geriatr Soc 1988; 36:1047–1054.
39. Dittmer DK, Teasell R. Complications of immobilization and bedrest. Part 1: musculoskeletal and cardiovascular complications. Can Fam Physician 1993; 39:1428–1437.
40. Gosselink R. Rehabilitation. Abstracts of Papers, International Consensus Conference in Intensive Care Medicine: Weaning from Mechanical Ventilation, Budapest, Hungary, April 28–29, 2005. Convened by five major scientific societies.
41. Nava S, Ambrosino N. Rehabilitation in the ICU: the European phoenix. Intensive Care Med 2000; 26:841–844.

42. Angus DC, Barnato AE, Linde-Zwirble WT, et al. On behalf of the Robert Wood Johnson Foundation ICU End of Life Peer Group. Use of intensive care at the end of life in the United States: an epidemiologic study. Crit Care Med 2004; 32:638–643.
43. Cook DJ, Guyatt GH, Jaeschke R, et al. Determinants in Canadian health care workers of the decision to withdraw life support from the critically ill. JAMA 1995; 273:703–708.
44. Prendergast TJ, Claessens MT, Luce JM. A national survey of end-of- life care for critically ill patients. Am J Respir Crit Care Med 1998; 158:1163–1167.
45. Vincent JL. Forgoing life support in Western European intensive care units: results of an ethical questionnaire. Critical Care Medicine 1999; 16:1626–1633.
46. Cook D, Rocker G, Marshall J, et al. Withdrawal of mechanical ventilation in anticipation of death in the intensive care unit. N Engl J Med 2003; 349:1123–1132.
47. Curtis JR. Terminal care for the ventilator dependent patient. Abstracts of Papers, International Consensus Conference in Intensive Care Medicine: Weaning from Mechanical Ventilation, Budapest, Hungary, April 28–29, 2005. Convened by five major scientific societies.
48. McDonagh JR, Elliott TB, Engelberg RA, et al. Family satisfaction with family conferences about end-of-life care in the ICU: increased proportion of family speech is associated with increased satisfaction. Crit Care Med 2004; 32:1484–1488.
49. Meltzer LS, Huckabay LM. Critical care nurses' perceptions of futile care and its effect on burnout. Am J Crit Care 2004; 13:202–208.
50. Azoulay E, Chevret S, Leleu G, et al. Half the families of intensive care unit patients experience inadequate communication with physicians. Crit Care Med 2000; 28:3044–3049.
51. Teasdale G, Jennett B. Assessment of coma and impaired consciousness, a practical scale. Lancet 1974; 13; 2(7872):81–84.

42
Long-Term Ventilation: The North American Perspective

INDERJIT HANSRA
Tufts-New England Medical Center, Boston, Massachusetts, U.S.A.

ALEX WHITE and NICHOLAS S. HILL
Tufts-New England Medical Center, Boston and New England Sinai Hospital, Stoughton, Massachusetts, U.S.A.

I. Introduction

Long-term mechanical ventilation (LTMV) refers to a variety of techniques available to treat chronic respiratory failure. The definition is predicated on prolonged mechanical ventilation (PMV), but the requisite length of time varies. For practical purposes, this discussion considers LTMV as ventilation taking place for >21 days, for at least 6 hr/24 hr. The techniques to provide LTMV have evolved over the past century, in parallel with advancing understanding of the pathophysiology of chronic respiratory failure. The ultimate goals of LTMV are similar worldwide—to maintain adequate gas exchange and return the patient to the highest level of function, ideally at home. However, depending on the patient's care needs, the attainment of these goals can consume large amounts of resources, both human and financial. The following provides a perspective on how countries in North America—the United States, Canada, and Mexico—deal with these challenges and care for patients requiring LTMV. The focus will be on the care of adult patients, but pediatric LTMV issues overlap those of adults, and some comments will be made on them as well.

II. Historical Perspective

The polio epidemics of the 1930s through the 1950s created a large demand for ventilatory assist devices (1), starting with the prototype negative pressure ventilator, the iron lung (2). Of the many thousands who were afflicted with respiratory paralysis, many died, others weaned successfully, and some required long-term ventilatory support. The need to support ventilation long term and desire to send some patients home spawned the development of more portable and comfortable "body ventilators" such as negative pressure ventilators like the chest cuirass and jacket ventilator as well as devices that employed the force of gravity to augment diaphragm excursion like the pneumobelt (intermittent abdominal pressure ventilator) and the rocking bed (3). Complementary devices like the cough in-exsufflator were also developed at this time to assist cough in polio patients.

The 1960s witnessed the continued support of some polio patients at home, as well as the introduction of mouthpiece ventilation for long term, even continuous, support at some specialized rehabilitation hospitals (4). The 1960s also ushered in intensive care units (ICUs) that served as specialized centers to treat patients with acute respiratory failure. Sophisticated mechanical ventilators were developed to treat these patients. Some of whom failed to wean and often spent weeks or months in these units because no other facilities were available to adequately care for them.

During the 1970s, more patients with respiratory failure due to neuromuscular disorders and chest wall deformities received long-term ventilatory assistance at home, either via tracheostomy or "body ventilators," which provided effective nocturnal noninvasive ventilation (NIV) (5,6). In the 1970s, the development of home respiratory therapy companies improved support for home mechanical ventilation (HMV). Respiratory therapists could now set up ventilatory equipment, educate the patient and caregivers about using the equipment, and be available to deal with problems.

During the 1980s, nasal continuous positive airway pressure (CPAP) was developed to treat obstructive sleep apnea, and investigators in France began using nasally assisted ventilation (7). The large demand attributable to obstructive sleep apnea stimulated the creation of many different types of nasal masks, which were connected to portable positive pressure ventilators. Several case series reported consistent improvements in gas exchange and symptoms among patients with restrictive thoracic disorders treated with nocturnal nasal ventilation, starting a shift toward the use of this technology that persists today (8,9).

The bi-level positive airway pressure respiratory assist device (BiPAP™, Respironics, Inc., Murrysville, Pennsylvania, U.S.) was also introduced during the late 1980s. Although initially developed to enhance comfort in obstructive sleep apnea patients who were having difficulty tolerating high levels of CPAP (10), the bi-level device proved to be an effective, highly portable, and inexpensive positive pressure ventilator (11). Long-term acute care (LTAC) facilities also proliferated in the late 1980s and 1990s as health care facilities where patients unable to wean from ICU mechanical ventilation could be safely transferred. In the United States, this development was partly a consequence of the diagnosis-related group (DRG) reimbursement system, which paid a fixed amount for a given diagnosis. This provided a strong incentive for acute care hospitals to transfer difficult-to-wean patients as quickly as possible.

The 1990s also saw an increasing use of bi-level ventilators instead of volume-limited ventilators for NIV as well as a shift from tracheostomy to NIV. Comfortable masks designed specifically for NIV helped to facilitate its use, as did favorable reimbursement policies. More recently, changes in the epidemiology of chronic respiratory failure as well as in the reimbursement system have led to further evolution in the delivery of LTMV. More options are available for placement of patients requiring LTMV, including skilled nursing facilities (SNFs), LTAC hospitals, rehabilitation facilities, and home with the assistance of home health agencies. Advances in the technology used to provide LTMV have also helped patients live in the community or at home.

III. Epidemiologic Trends in LTMV

A. Incidence of LTMV

Reliable information on the incidence of LTMV in the United States is difficult to obtain because of the disjointed organization of the reimbursement and delivery systems. The number of patients receiving LTMV within health care institutions has not been reported. Several past surveys have extrapolated figures for the number of patients using HMV in the United States, indicating that the population of such patients has been growing rapidly. In a 1983-Massachusetts survey, Make et al. (12) estimated that there were approximately 6000 home ventilator users nationwide. A subsequent 1990-Illinois survey by Goldberg and Frownfelter (13) projected that there were 10,000 home ventilator users. According to a Minnesota survey, the extrapolated projections for the United States were 5777 users in 1986, 12,279 in 1992, and 17,824 in 1997 (14). The total number of home ventilator users in the United States is unquestionably higher now, but more recent estimates are unavailable. On the basis of the 1997 estimate, the incidence of HMV users in the United States is 5.9/100,000 population, remarkably close to the 6.6/100,000 incidence obtained in the 2001-Eurovent survey, representing the average for all European countries (15). Similar trends have been apparent in Canada (16), but specific incidences have not been reported. The trend spans both adult and pediatric populations, with most pediatric patients having congenital neuromuscular conditions (17). Published data on the incidence of LTMV are not available for Mexico.

B. Diagnoses of LTMV Patients

The Minnesota survey (14) provided information on the composition of patients receiving HMV. The largest single diagnostic category was respiratory failure due to neuromuscular disease (NMD), with muscular dystrophy and cervical trauma patients constituting equal numbers, post-polio patients slightly less, and amyotrophic lateral sclerosis (ALS) patients fewer still. As would be anticipated, since the epidemics have become increasingly remote, the post-polio population decreased between 1986 and 1997, whereas the muscular dystrophy population increased. For unexplained reasons, ALS patients decreased in number by 36% between 1992 and 1997, although this number would be expected to be substantially larger now, with the increasing use of NPPV for ALS in North America (18).

The second most common diagnostic category was chronic obstructive pulmonary disease (COPD), usually in older patients who tended to be ventilated for shorter durations at home than neuromuscular patients. Although COPD patients constitute a significant number of the patients receiving HMV, they remain a much lower proportion of patients than those with NMD or thoracic restriction. Between 1992 and 1997, NPPV became more common among pediatric patients, with 16/42 patients started on NPPV being younger than 16 years and mainly with congenital abnormalities.

Although specific numbers are unavailable, trends in NIV use at home include a decrease in the number of patients with COPD since 1999 when the Centers for Medicare and Medicaid Services (CMS) created new guidelines for reimbursement (19). A Swiss Registry found that the single diagnosis responsible for the greatest increase in home NIV use between 1992 and 2000 was obesity hypoventilation (20). In parallel with an increasing number of obese individuals as the "obesity epidemic" spreads through most Western countries, North America undoubtedly reflects this trend.

C. Trends in LTAC Facilities

As noted above, an important trend in the management of LTMV patients has been the proliferation of so-called LTAC facilities that receive most of their patients from acute care hospitals, often with tracheotomies, many of whom are undergoing weaning. LTAC facilities accept patients recovering slowly from acute respiratory failure, especially from COPD exacerbations or the acute respiratory distress syndrome (ARDS), reflecting the increasing survival related to use of NIV (6) and low tidal volume ventilation (21), respectively. In the United States, from 1993 to 2005, the number of LTACs increased from 105 to 330 and associated costs increased from $398 million to $3.1 billion (22).

LTAC hospitals improve the quality of care by weaning some patients and providing intensive rehabilitation. Most patients entering LTAC facilities have spent weeks or months in ICUs and therefore require more specialized care such as weaning, rehabilitation, round-the-clock respiratory care, dialysis, intravenous antibiotics, pain management, and—most importantly—time to recover from their acute illness. LTACs are designed to offer a post-acute care option for patients whose needs exceed those available at SNFs and for longer periods of time. Figure 1 shows the flow of patients between LTACs, acute care hospitals and home. The greatest number of facilities is available in New England and the southwest. In a report by CMS, the five states with the greatest number of LTAC beds per thousand Medicare beneficiaries account for 39% of the available beds, but only 12% of the total Medicare population (23).

A recent National Association of Long-Term Hospitals (NALTH) survey at 23-member institutions analyzed 1419 LTMV patients (24). Ninety-seven percent were transferred from acute care hospitals after an average length of stay (LOS) of 33 days. Sixty percent had medical diagnoses and 40% were postsurgical. The patients were on average 72 years old, with acute on chronic illness and 2.6 premorbid diagnoses per patient. Most had cardiovascular disease, 42% had COPD and 12% had neurological disease. In contrast to HMV population, fewer than 1% of the NALTH patients had NMD. Over a median of 15 days, 54% were weaned, 21% remained ventilator dependent, and 25% died. Patients returned home (28%), were transferred to another extended care facility (49%), or transferred to acute care (19.5%), and fewer than a third were alive after 12 months (25). Whereas these observations underline the very ill nature of the patient population, they also demonstrate that a substantial minority can return to the community.

In another report, 12-month mortality for LTMV patients in a single LTAC was 50%, with few returning to a fully functional status (26). Predictors of mortality included: age, reduced preadmission functional status, renal failure, and diabetes. In one study, it was suggested that LTMV patients treated in an LTAC were noted to have comparable mortality rates to an acute care hospital, but were treated at a lower cost (27,28).

In Canada, similar facilities are termed chronic assisted ventilatory care (CAVC) units. These are led by pulmonologists and staffed by a multidisciplinary team similar to American LTACs. In a 1995 analysis of one such unit, Wijkstra et al. (29) reported on the outcomes of 50 tracheostomized patients managed over a 15-year period. Most patients had NMD or spinal cord injury, and the minority had COPD or thoracic restriction. Although a third died, another third were discharged home or to another long-term facility in a stabilized state. The authors concluded that the CAVC units provide a safe environment for LTMV patients, at much lower cost than in an acute care center. Based on the large difference in the proportion of NMD patients, the CAVC population differs from the LTAC population in the U.S. by being less acute, the LTAC being more reflective of patients admitted directly from medical or surgical ICUs.

D. Trends in Use of Mechanical Ventilation for Long-Term Ventilatory Failure

Over the past 15 years, surveys in North America and Europe have detected a dramatic shift in LTMV from invasive to noninvasive modalities. In the Minnesota survey (14), half of the new ventilator starts between 1992 and 1997 were noninvasive, whereas virtually none were in this category prior to 1992. This trend can be attributed to the greater comfort, portability, autonomy, and fewer complications of NIV. This improved autonomy usually translates into better quality of life (30). Patients who have used both modalities prefer NIV; although in one report, invasive ventilation was rated by patients as being superior for sleep and for providing a feeling of security (31). With NIV airway suctioning is avoided and infectious complications are fewer. Demands on caregivers and associated costs are less, enabling some patients to remain at home whereas invasive ventilation would have necessitated institutionalization (31). A parallel rise in the use of NIV has occurred in the acute setting, especially for patients with acute respiratory failure due to COPD or congestive heart failure (CHF) (6), such that more physicians are familiar with this technology and willing to use it in outpatient settings.

NIV is not always preferred to tracheostomy ventilation. If patients lose their ability to protect their airway or if they develop vocal cord paralysis, invasive mechanical ventilation may be preferred, although some patients with severe impairment of speech and swallowing still respond favorably to NIV (32). Some patients feel more secure with invasive ventilation because of direct access for secretion clearance (4). Both approaches require skilled and dedicated caregivers, but many patients requiring continuous ventilatory support elect for tracheostomy ventilation unless they are closely managed by a highly skilled team, staffed and experienced in NIV for patients with no ventilator-free time.

E. Trends in Equipment for LTMV

Bi-level positive pressure ventilators are the most commonly used for NIV. Although precise numbers are difficult to ascertain, it has been estimated that more than 90% of NIV patients use these devices (N. Hill, personal observation). Compared with volume-limited positive pressure ventilators, these devices are easier to use, more comfortable and portable, quieter, and less expensive. Their major disadvantages compared with volume-limited ventilators are their lack of sophisticated alarms, lack of internal batteries, and requirement for high capacity external batteries to support their continuously functioning turbines. They are also unable to assist patients who wish to enhance secretion clearance by breath stacking, as can volume-limited ventilators (33). It is likely that the North American experience parallels that of Switzerland, where ventilators for NIV shifted from 100% volume-limited in 1992 to 85–95% bi-level or pressure support in 2000 (20).

This dramatic shift occurred partly because of the advantages of bi-level devices as listed above, but also because of technical advances. Bi-level devices are now available that weigh just a few pounds, are quieter, have built-in humidifiers, and newer, potentially more comfortable modes that lower airway pressure early during expiration (BiFlex™, Respironics, Inc., Murrysville, Pennsylvania, U.S.). Patients receiving tracheostomy ventilation are still ventilated most often using volume-limited ventilators, partly because of their more sophisticated alarm capabilities than those of bi-level devices.

Other trends in mechanical ventilation equipment such as hybrid ventilators, which provide various pressure and volume-limited modes as well as alarm systems (34) are addressed elsewhere in this text, as are developments in mask technology. Such advances include softened silicone sealing gaskets, gel seals, very compact masks, and others that minimize skin seal pressure.

F. Summary of Trends

Similar trends are occurring in the United States, Canada, and Mexico, at least for those with health insurance. Increasingly, NMD patients and those with obesity hypoventilation or CHF receive LTMV at home. The trend toward NIV is increasing. More patients requiring LTMV but who are unable to return home are being cared for in LTACs.

IV. Challenges to the Care of LTMV Patients in North America

Given the expanding population of patients with advancing age and multiple comorbidities, there will be a need for an increased number of skilled personnel to care for the growing LTMV population. Skills related to management of LTMV patients such as weaning, optimization of function, and minimization of risk are not widely taught in our current training programs for physicians or nonphysician health care professionals. There is little evidence to guide ongoing issues such as tracheostomy management. Identification of risk factors for infection such as excessive use of catheters, strict hand washing, barrier nursing, and the appropriate use of antibiotics must be rigorously implemented in LTAC facilities.

Other challenges may override the medical issues. Financial resources are limited, and in the United States, reimbursement has driven the current care process. These issues will continue to be the major force shaping the nature of care for LTMV patients. The availability of institutions for placement of chronically ventilated patients as well as the infrastructure to manage LTMV patients in the home all depend on funding. Ethical issues also influence the management of chronically ill patients. These issues are considered below.

A. Reimbursement Issues

In the United States, 70% of LTMV patients are covered by Medicare, the national insurance program for those older than 65 years, or for those who are disabled. For reimbursement, long-term care hospitals must have an average inpatient LOS >25 days. This pressures the LTACs to keep the average LOS above this limit, in contrast to acute care hospitals that are under pressure to minimize their LOS (35). Before October 2002, long-term care hospitals were paid on the basis of their average cost per discharge. Since then, a prospective payment system was developed that pays facilities based on the patient's diagnosis. Facilities that care for patients with multiple diagnoses and higher acuity levels accrue higher reimbursement from Medicare (36).

Some LTACs have created "satellite units" on the campuses of acute care hospitals, so that they receive transfers directly from the acute care setting. To discourage inappropriate transfers these units can accept no more than 50% of patients from the host hospital. Plans are to have the percentage go to 25% in 2008, which would probably lead to the closure of most of the satellite units. Medicare payments to LTACs have increased from $1.7 billion in 2001 to $3.3 billion in 2004 and are estimated to reach $5.2 billion in 2007. This increase is attributed to the aging population, and the growing need for chronic care facilities to care for them (37). Options for discharge from LTACs are limited because SNFs do not get reimbursed for chronic ventilator patients as well as LTACs (35), which makes them reluctant to accept such patients unless the patients have private insurance. SNFs also commonly lack rehabilitation services and offer less respiratory care than LTACs, so that they are suitable only for patients with no further rehabilitation potential.

Medicare does not provide for custodial services (35) so that few LTMV patients covered by Medicare are able to return home. Some private insurers are more generous, providing 8 to 12 hours of skilled nursing care per day. Even then, the family has to assume a large share of the caregiving and financial burden so that management at home is still difficult.

In the United States, respiratory care equipment vendors provide equipment in the home. Much of this is now reimbursed on a fixed rental basis, meaning that a fixed number of monthly payments are made until the device is paid for. This has substantially reduced revenues for home respiratory care equipment vendors who previously received unlimited monthly payments, forcing them to reduce staff and services as well as select patients who consume the fewest resources and making it even more difficult to send patients home from LTACs.

Those managed in the home are likely to be younger patients with NMD and have dedicated parents to manage their care. Some are helped by independent living centers that arrange for personal care attendants, and others receive aid from religious or other community organizations that provide volunteers or even financial assistance. Regardless, LTMV patients are rarely able to live independently at home without substantial family support and the ability to incur financial strain. Even with supplemental insurance to Medicare, coverage is often partial and the patient is left paying for the majority of the costs. In one survey, ALS patients receiving invasive mechanical ventilation paid more than $200,000 annually to stay at home (14).

Canada has a universal payer system, but faces many of the same issues regarding LTMV. The expense of LTMV strains provincial health budgets, as a result of which the provinces provide only partial support for the home. This is much more of an issue for very disabled patients with NMD than it is for those receiving nocturnal NIV whose needs are easily met. CAVC units serve a similar role in Canada as LTACs do in the United States, although patients enrolled in a CAVC unit tend to be more stable. Whereas it is apparent that there are too few facilities in the healthcare system, there is insufficient data to assess their impact on the Canadian system, largely because each province has its own insurance, unlinked to other provinces. The CAVC unit may also be used as a resource for patients on HMV if their medical or social circumstances change, if the caregivers require respite care, or if the patients cannot continue to live independently (29).

Mexico has separate insurance coverage systems including one for those employed by the private sector—the Mexican Institute of Social Services, another for state workers—the Institute of Security and Social Services for State Workers, a third for military, petroleum, and electric company workers, and a fourth for those uninsured by other programs. Published information on coverage of LTMV in Mexico is unavailable.

B. Ethical Issues

Patient autonomy—the right of each individual to make his or her own health care decisions—is a central tenet of medical ethics. In ICUs many patients do not have sufficient mental competence to participate in their own decisions, and in LTACs some patients are also unlikely to be mentally competent. Therefore, families may serve as proxies. This situation has not been well studied in LTACs, although older patients and those with poor functional status are less likely to survive and, clearly, patients failing to manifest weaning progress within the first few months are unlikely to wean. Discussions with the patients and families regarding continuing or discontinuing ventilatory support, require substantial

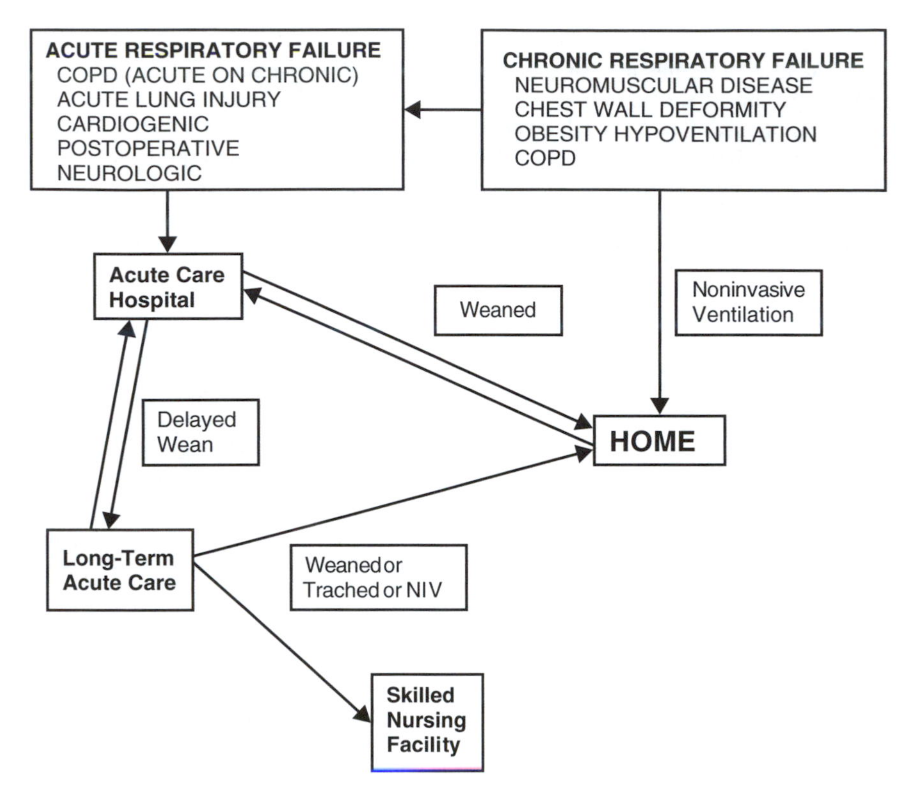

Figure 1 The management of respiratory failure in the United States. Many patients are admitted initially to an acute care hospital. If they wean promptly, they may spend time in an LTAC hospital for rehabilitation, and eventually return home. If they fail to wean, they undergo tracheostomy and are transferred to an LTAC when stable. Weaning attempts continue, and a minority of patients return home; the rest remain at the LTAC or are transferred to a SNF. Patients who deteriorate while at LTACs or at home return to the acute care hospital for stabilization. Some patients with chronic respiratory failure do not require acute care but are ventilated noninvasively and remain home. *Abbreviations*: COPD, chronic obstructive pulmonary disease; NIV, noninvasive ventilation; LTAC, long-term acute care; SNF, skilled nursing facility.

emotional investment and careful considerations of a patient's cognitive ability and capacity to understand the consequences of their decisions.

If the onset of respiratory failure is foreseeable, such as in progressive NMD, end-of-life issues should be discussed early on. One survey found that if patients had previously decided to have a tracheostomy, 88% would do so again compared with only 38% of patients who had not decided before an acute deterioration (38). This emphasizes the importance of discussing the issue of tracheostomy early with patients who have degenerative neurological conditions, so that they can be prepared for the respiratory crises and not undergo an unwanted tracheostomy or hospitalization if they would prefer to be cared for at a hospice or at home. Families should be involved in these decisions, if possible, as they bear much of the burden of care, often at the cost of their own personal lives (16).

V. Future Perspectives

The U.S. Department of Heath and Human Services Administration on Aging reports that 36.8 million Americans were older than 65 years in 2005 and that this number is expected to rise to 71.5 million by 2030 (16). As the population continues to age, there will be an increasing number of patients requiring LTMV. People are increasingly obliged to factor in the cost of long-term care in their retirement calculations. Where and how such individuals are cared for will be a major challenge. Medicare continues to reduce reimbursements for long-term care in the home. Although NIV is more commonplace in the home, home care for LTMV patients is very expensive, often depending on their monitoring and personal care needs. LTACs are currently the favored destination for LTMV patients transferred from acute care, as they allow for rehabilitation as well as the specialized nursing and respiratory care required. Returning patients to their homes or to an independent living environment remains a desirable outcome, but may not be realistic for most LTMV patients given the current reimbursement climate. It is likely that SNFs will be required to play a bigger role in the long-term care of these patients. In Canada and Mexico, similar situations are present—an aging population, with increased survival as a result of better ICU care and improved LTMV options. More CAVC type facilities will be required, as well as an enhanced linked database for national statistics and increased funding for home support of the patient receiving LTMV.

References

1. Wilson JL. Acute anterior poliomyelitis. N Engl J Med 1932; 206:887–893.
2. Drinker P, Shaw LA. An apparatus for the prolonged administration of artificial respiration: I. Design for adults and children. J Clin Invest 1929; 7:229–247.
3. Hill NS. Clinical applications of body ventilators. Chest 1986; 90:897–905.
4. Bach JR, Alba AS, Saporito LR. Intermittent positive pressure ventilation via the mouth as an alternative to tracheostomy for 257 ventilator users. Chest 1993; 103:174–182.
5. Curran FJ. Night ventilation by body respirators for patients in chronic respiratory failure due to late stage Duchenne muscular dystrophy. Arch Phys Med Rehabil 1981; 62:270–274.
6. Mehta S, Hill NS. Noninvasive ventilation-state of the art. Am J Respir Crit Care Med 2001; 163:540–577.
7. Raphael JC, Chevret S, Chastang CI, et al. Home mechanical ventilation in Duchenne's muscular dystrophy: in search of a therapeutic strategy. Eur Respir Rev 1993; 12:270–274.
8. Bach JR, Alba A, Mosher R, et al. Intermittent positive pressure ventilation via nasal access in the management of respiratory insufficiency. Chest 1987; 94:168–170.
9. Ellis ER, McCauley VB, Mellis C, et al. Treatment of alveolar hypoventilation in a six-year-old girl with intermittent positive pressure ventilation through a nose mask. Am Rev Respir Dis 1987; 136:188–191.
10. Sanders MH, Kern NB. Obstructive sleep apnea treated by independently adjusted inspiratory and expiratory positive airway pressure via nasal mask. Chest 1990; 98:317–324.
11. Strumpf DA, Carlisle CC, Millman RP, et al. An evaluation of the Respironics BiPAP bi-level CPAP device for delivery of assisted ventilation. Respir Care 1990; 35:415–422.
12. Make B, Dayno S, Gertman P. Prevalence of chronic ventilator dependency. Am Rev Respir Dis 1986; 132:A167.
13. Goldberg AI, Frownfelter D. The ventilator-assisted individuals study. Chest 1990; 98:428–433.
14. Adams AB, Shapiro R, Marini JJ. Changing prevalence of chronically ventilator-assisted individuals in Minnesota: increases, characteristics, and the use of noninvasive ventilation. Respir Care 1998, 43:643–649.

15. Lloyd-Owen SJ, Donaldson GC, Ambrosino N, et al. Patterns of home mechanical ventilator use in Europe: results from the Eurovent survey. Eur Respir J 2005; 25:1025–1031.
16. Litwin PD, Flegel CM, Richardson BC. An overview of home mechanical ventilation in Canada. Can J Respir Ther 1991; 28:67–73.
17. Schreiner MS, Donar ME, Kettrick RG. Pediatric home mechanical ventilation in children. Pediatr Clin N Am 1987; 34:47–60.
18. Borasio GD, Elinas DF, Yanagisawa N. Mechanical ventilation in amyotophic lateral sclerosis: a cross-cultural perspective. J Neurol 1998; 245 (suppl 2):S7–S12.
19. ACCP NAMDRC Consensus Group. Clinical indications for noninvasive positive pressure ventilation in chronic respiratory failure due to restrictive lung disease, COPD, and nocturnal hypoventilation—a consensus conference. Chest 1999; 116:521–534.
20. Janssens J-P, Derivas S, Breitenstein E, et al. Changing patterns in long-term noninvasive ventilation: a seven year prospective study in the Lake Geneva area. Chest 2003; 123:67–79.
21. The Acute Respiratory Distress Syndrome Network. Ventilation with lower tidal volumes as compared with traditional tidal volumes for acute lung injury and the acute respiratory distress syndrome. N Engl J Med 2000; 342:1301–1308.
22. McIntyre NR, Epstein SK, Carson S, et al. Management of patients requiring prolonged mechanical ventilation: report of a NAMDRC consensus conference. Chest 2005; 128:3937–3954.
23. Miller ME. Long-term care hospitals. Testimony before the Subcommittee on Health Committee on Ways and Means U.S. House of Representatives. Medicare Payment Advisory Commission. March 15, 2006:1–10.
24. Scheinhorn DJ, Hassenpflug MS, Votto JJ, et al. Ventilator-dependent survivors of catastrophic illness transferred to 23 long-term care hospitals for weaning from prolonged mechanical ventilation. Chest 2007; 131:76–84.
25. Scheinhorn DJ, Hassenpflug MS, Votto JJ, et al. Post-ICU mechanical ventilation at 23 long-term care hospitals: a multicenter outcomes study. Chest 2007; 131(1):85–93.
26. Carson SS, Bach PB, Brzozowski L, et al. Outcomes after long-term acute care. An analysis of 133 mechanically ventilated patients. Am J Respir Crit Care Med 1999; 160 (5 pt 1):1788–1789.
27. Seneff MG, Wagner D, Thompson D, et al. The impact of long-term acute-care facilities on the outcome and cost of care for patients undergoing prolonged mechanical ventilation. Crit Care Med 2000; 28:342–350.
28. Martin C. The emperor has no clothes: a misguided case for long-term acute-care facilities? Crit Care Med 2000; 28(2):576–577.
29. Wijkstra PJ, Avendano MA, Goldstein RS. Inpatient chronic assisted ventilatory care, a 15-year experience. Chest 2003; 124:850–856.
30. Bourke SC, Williams TL, Bullock RE, et al. Noninvasive ventilation in ALS: indications and effect on quality of life. Neurology 2003; 61:171–177.
31. Bach JR. A comparison of long-term ventilatory support alternatives from the perspective of the patient and care giver. Chest 1993; 104:1702–1706.
32. Bourke SC, Tomilinson M, Williams TL, et al. Effects of non-invasive ventilation on survival and quality of life in patients with amyotrophic lateral sclerosis: a randomized controlled trial. Lancet Neurol 2006; 5:140–147.
33. Bach JR. Update and perspective on noninvasive respiratory muscle aids. Part 2: The expiratory aids. Chest 1994; 105:1538–1544.
34. Kacmarek R, Hill NS. Ventilators for noninvasive positive pressure ventilation: technical aspects. In: Muir JR, Simonds A, Ambrosino N, eds. Noninvasive Mechanical Ventilation. European Respiratory Monograph Series. Sheffield, UK, 2001.
35. Gracey DR. Costs and reimbursement of long-term ventilation. Respir Care Clin N Am 2002; 8(3): 491–497.

36. Mantone J. Two in one. The CMS' strict admissions criteria make long term acute care hospitals consider co-locating with skilled-nursing facilities. Mod Healthc 2005; 35(45):26–28.
37. Department of Health and Human Services. Statistics on the Aging Population. Available at: http://www.aoa.gov/prof/Statistics/statistics.asp. Accessed November 11, 2006. February 22, 2007.
38. Cazzolli PA, Oppenheimer EA. Home mechanical ventilation for amyotrophic lateral sclerosis: nasal compared to tracheostomy-intermittent positive pressure ventilation. J Neurol Sci. 1996; 139 (suppl):123–128.

43
Long-Term Ventilation: The European Perspective

JAMES GOLDRING and JADWIGA WEDZICHA
Royal Free and University College Medical School, London, U.K.

I. Introduction

Chronic health care in Europe, like the rest of the developed world, is characterized by an increasingly aging population often with complex medical problems, an increase in societal expectations, and an increase in the dependence on expensive technology. Chronic respiratory failure is no different and is expected to rise in prevalence because of the aging population and possibly because of increased tobacco use. The expansion in Europe (1–3) and the United States (4) over the last three decades in the use of home mechanical ventilation (HMV) mirrors this trend. HMV is used to treat chronic hypercapnic respiratory failure in both adults and children and is usually delivered noninvasively (NIV) with the majority of patients using only nocturnal or nocturnal plus part daytime NIV. NIV has been shown to reduce mortality and morbidity (5,6) and to improve quality of life (7).

The magnitude of the rise in HMV is impressive with the number of patients receiving home ventilatory support increasing in one survey from 130 patients in 1988 to 3120 patients in 1998 (1). This expansion has been driven not just by the swelling population of individuals with chronic respiratory failure but also by the increasing recognition that NIV can be of benefit in many different causes of ventilatory failure (8). Technological advances have meant that ventilators are easier to use and that the interfaces are more comfortable. Additionally, HMV offers the individual the advantage of retaining an independent lifestyle and offers the state a health economic benefit, as it is less costly when compared to invasive mechanical ventilation (9). Along with the patient, there are the industrial manufacturers and distributors of the machines who will also be benefiting from the increasingly widespread use of HMV. It is, of course, important that the growth of HMV in Europe is on a properly planned basis and not simply driven by market considerations. However, it will be seen from this chapter that the use of HMV is not presently standardized, regulated, or consistent in Europe.

This chapter will describe and explore the wide variation in practices that occur within and between the countries of Europe with regard to HMV. Firstly, it will look at the situation in the 1990s and then again in the current decade.

II. The Situation in Europe in the 1990s

The most comprehensive early questionnaire survey of HMV to have been undertaken in Europe took place in 1992 (10). The European Working Group on Home Treatment for Chronic Respiratory Insufficiency looked at the organization of HMV, continuous positive airway pressure (CPAP), and long-term oxygen therapy (LTOT) in 13 European countries. The Group members were well aware that differences existed between the countries, and their stated aim was to characterize these variations and to allow the individual countries to benefit from the comparison of data. The Group's efforts were hampered by information that was "incomplete, erratic in detail and characterized only by its paucity in outcome modalities." Only France, with its National Association for Home Care Patients with Chronic Respiratory Insufficiency (ANTADIR), and Switzerland (Swiss Lung Association) had national registers at this time for HMV, which facilitated comprehensive data gathering. Since 1981, ANTADIR has been responsible for managing approximately 70% of patients receiving HMV in France and, since 1984, a subgroup of these patients have been surveyed annually (11). The Group was also able to obtain complete information on HMV from Denmark and Belgium via health service data and commercial supply companies. The information gathered from the remaining countries was much patchier and was generally easier to obtain for LTOT than for MV or CPAP, perhaps because, on the whole, LTOT has been established for longer in most of the countries studied.

The main findings from this survey were that HMV was being used substantively for chronic lung disease, chest wall deformities (CWD), and neuromuscular disease (NMD) in all of the countries apart from Poland, which had a negligible number of ventilated patients being treated at home. The majority of ventilators in use were positive pressure and, of these, most were volume cycled as opposed to pressure cycled. Italy and Belgium used volume-cycled machines exclusively. Both respiratory physicians and nonspecialist physicians were writing prescriptions for HMV. Prescription rules existed in only a few countries with most having no regulation of prescribing whatsoever. The ventilators were supplied through commercial companies or nationalized health services and paid for primarily by the latter. Specific details on supervision and technical support for HMV were difficult to extract from the article because the data was combined with that for LTOT.

The authors concluded that major differences occurred between the 13 European countries and that these were probably explained by the "historical origin of home care in each country, the different impact of commercial companies, and the supervision of insurance companies on doctor's prescriptions." To improve the uniformity and quality of HMV provision, they proposed the establishment of further national registries to improve data collection, a standardized Europe-wide set of guidelines to advice clinicians, and finally a system that would ensure adequate equipment performance and maintenance.

There are other notable single European country reviews of home respiratory care from the 1990s. A follow-up study between 1992 and 2000 provided longitudinal data on changes in HMV practice in Geneva (3). Janssens et al. noted that during the course of the study there was a marked increase in the proportion of patients with chronic obstructive pulmonary disease (COPD) and obesity hypoventilation syndrome (OHS) from 0% and 14%, respectively, at the outset to 25% and 39% by the end of the study. The advent of cheaper, smaller, and arguably easier to use pressure-cycled ventilators also heralded a change from the exclusive use of volume-cycled ventilators in 1992 to predominantly pressure-cycled ventilators by the end of the study. A similar longitudinal study in Sweden (2) also highlighted the rapid growth of HMV prescription for patients with OHS.

Midgren et al. (12) reported on cross-sectional data from the Swedish register of HMV, which was set up in 1996 by the Swedish Society of Chest Medicine. The salient findings here were that the prevalence of HMV use varied widely between health care regions from 1.2/100,000 inhabitants to 20/100,000 inhabitants, and only 3% of patients had COPD as the indication for HMV. The authors believed that the difference in prevalence of HMV between health care regions could be because "the indications for HMV are not well defined, which may make room for more individual decision making." Further analysis by Laub et al. (2) demonstrated that the disparity between the regions could not be explained by socioeconomic or demographic differences. The under-representation of COPD patients was put down to a lack of "enthusiasm among Swedish physicians to offer patients with these diagnoses HMV" perhaps because of the conflicting evidence of a long-term benefit for ventilation in this patient group (7,13,14). Another finding reported from the Swedish registry was that the age distribution was bimodal. The authors contrasted this discovery with Denmark whose age distribution was unimodal because of a heavy bias toward young patients with muscular dystrophy. The bias was attributed in part to the high profile Danish Muscular Dystrophy fund. Finally, with regard to the Swedish registry, there were some similarities with the Geneva study (3) in that prospective analysis of the registry data suggested that the choice of ventilator was changing from volume cycled to pressure cycled.

III. The Situation in Europe in 2002

Another pan-European questionnaire survey, funded by a European Union Concerted Action grant (the Eurovent survey), was undertaken to survey custom and practice in the different countries (15) to determine if the state of affairs had changed some 10 years after the study by Fauroux et al. (10).

This survey was more expansive with 16 countries included, which provided data on 329 centers and 21,526 HMV users. More national registers were available this time and so documentation concerning HMV from the member countries had improved over the preceding 10 years. However, the survey, like the previous one, continued to show wide variations in practice. For example, the prevalence of HMV per 100,000 inhabitants ranged from 0.6 in Greece to 17 in France. Overall prevalence of HMV in Europe was 6.6 per 100,000. Countries that started their HMV program earlier (Fig. 1) had a greater prevalence and a larger center size (Fig. 2), although this could not be the only explanation for the wide variation in prevalence. The proportion in different disease categories was also wide ranging (Fig. 3), with Denmark having proportionately more individuals with NMD being ventilated whereas patients with COPD predominated in Italy and Portugal. This discrepancy also seems to be related to the date at which the HMV program started, with the newer centers tending to focus on COPD patients. Overall, 34.4% of patients suffered from lung and airway problems, 31.2% had CWD, and 34.4% had NMD.

Other findings from the Eurovent survey were that patients were more likely to have their HMV initiated and maintained by a university hospital rather than by a nonuniversity hospital. The study also demonstrated that there was a bimodal distribution of users with older patients (>66 years) having predominantly lung and chest wall diseases and younger

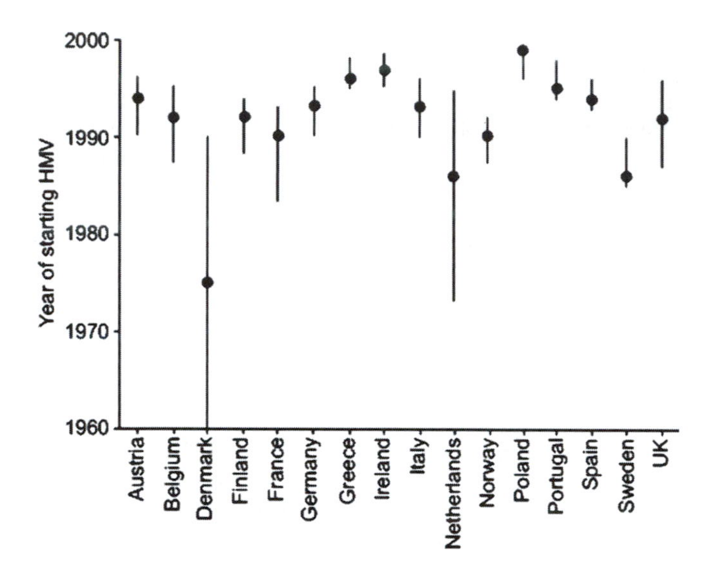

Figure 1 Median (interquartile range) year of starting HMV for each country. Denmark shows the median and full range as only two centers were included. *Abbreviation*: HMV, home mechanical ventilation. *Source*: From Ref. 15.

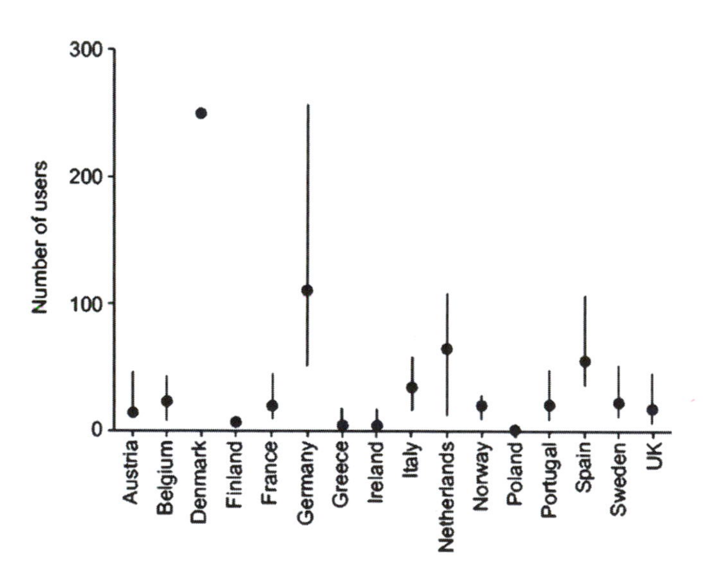

Figure 2 Median (interquartile range) center size for each country measured by number of home ventilation users. Denmark shows median only (range 250–253 for its two centers). *Source*: From Ref. 15.

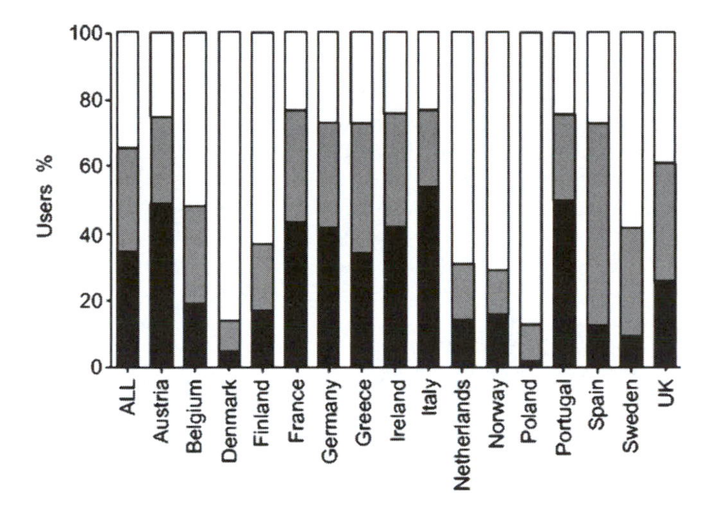

Figure 3 Percentage of users in each disease category by country. The symbol ■ represents lung/airways (COPD, cystic fibrosis, bronchiectasis, pulmonary fibrosis, and pediatric diseases); ▩, chest wall deformities (kyphoscoliosis, old TB, OHS, surgical resection); and □, neuromuscular disorders (muscular dystrophy, motor neuron disease, post-polio kyphoscoliosis, central hypoventilation, spinal cord damage, and phrenic nerve palsy). *Abbreviations*: COPD, chronic obstructive pulmonary disease; TB, tuberculosis; OHS, obesity hypoventilation syndrome. *Source*: From Ref. 15.

patients (<65years) having predominantly neuromuscular and neurological diseases. The latter group of patients were most likely to be ventilated for longer periods (>10 years), while the majority of those with intrinsic lung diseases had been on HMV for less than one year. Patients with CWD ran a more intermediate course, with most of them being ventilated between six and 10 years. The length of time that patients have spent on HMV can be explained partly by the expected survival differences between the different diagnostic categories (6), and partly by the fact that some centers had only recently begun recruiting COPD patients.

Pressure-cycled machines predominated in 2002 (70.6% of the total) and only a very small percentage of patients (0.005%) were still using forms of negative pressure ventilators. Ventilation was performed via a tracheostomy in just 13% of the overall survey population and the patients with NMD accounted for most of these. Tracheostomy ventilation was more common in France, Greece, Italy, and Belgium and probably reflects local expertise in this area (16).

IV. Quality Control of HMV Equipment in Europe

HMV is considered to be relatively safe (17), but a recent study demonstrates that there are sometimes considerable differences between the actual set and prescribed values of ventilator variables and that the alarm function when present does not always work (18).

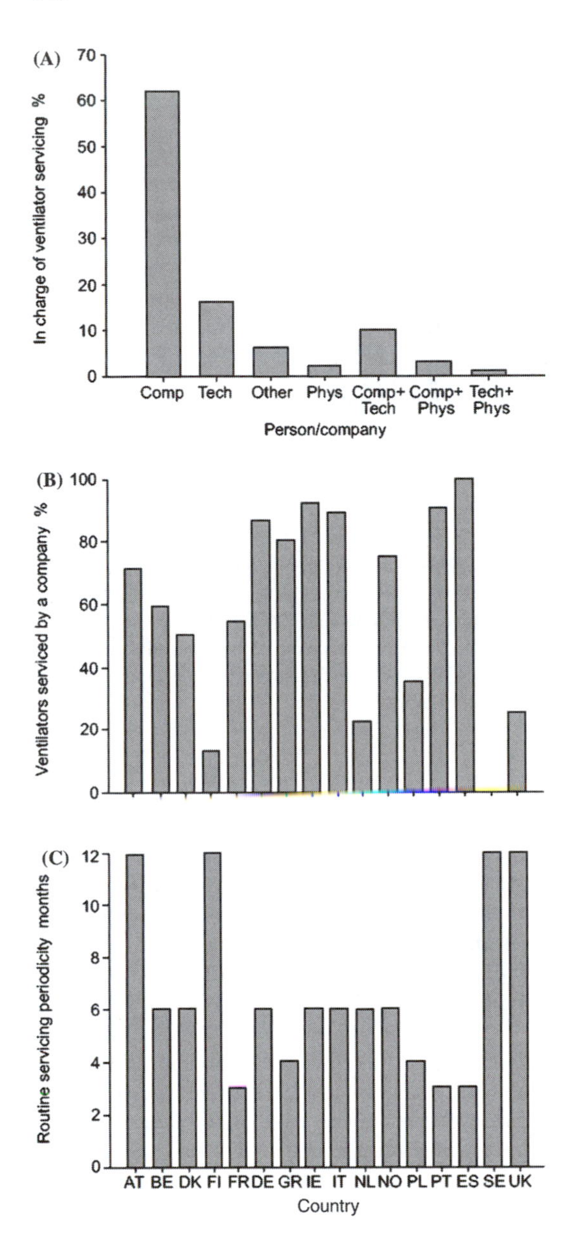

Figure 4 (**A**) Answers to the question "Who is in charge of the servicing and repair of ventilators in your center?", (**B**) centers answering that ventilator servicing was carried out by an external company, and (**C**) answers to the question "How often is your equipment routinely serviced?" by country. *Abbreviations*: Comp, ventilator company; Tech, hospital technical service; Other, other hospital department; Phys, physician in charge of patient; AT, Austria; BE, Belgium; DK, Denmark; FI, Finland; FR, France; DE, Germany; GR, Greece; IE, Ireland; IT, Italy; NL, The Netherlands; NO, Norway; PL, Poland; PT, Portugal; ES, Spain; SE, Sweden. *Source*: From Ref. 18.

As an extension of the pan-European study of 2002, Farré and colleagues (19) looked at the quality-control procedures employed at the 329 HMV centers. Predictably, wide variations existed both within and between countries. The salient findings from their study were as follows: There was a wide variation between countries as to whether the ventilator company or a hospital technician or both took a role in servicing the machine and also in the periodicity of routine servicing (Fig. 4). The timing of the servicing is unlikely to be related to technical factors so it can only be assumed that it is due to economic or administrative differences. There was also evidence of poor communication between the service provider and the clinician. An example of this is that in Sweden it was relatively common for the ventilator to be changed without the explicit agreement of the prescriber. This might be a problem for patients whose ventilatory demands are sometimes suited to a specific ventilator model. There also appeared to be some ambivalence on the part of the prescribers to involve their patients in quality control. Thus, on average, only 56% of centers assessed whether the patients or their caregivers correctly maintained the equipment and only 21% gave the patients or their caregivers written information about quality control items pertaining to their particular ventilator. This is perhaps a missed opportunity as patient self-management is now widely encouraged because of evidence of improved patient satisfaction and, more importantly, improved patient outcome (20).

V. Conclusions

The number of patients receiving HMV in Europe will continue to rise because of a combination of the background aging population, improved survival of patients with chronic respiratory disease, and a shift toward treating more people with COPD and OHS.

Other than consensus opinion on when to initiate HMV (21), there are as yet very few guidelines within Europe on how to practically implement HMV. It is probably for this reason that there is little standardization and regulation of HMV between or even within European countries. This lack of uniformity extends to quality control of the equipment itself, and this in turn impacts on patient safety as well as satisfactory patient outcomes.

References

1. National Association for Home Care Patients with Chronic Respiratory Insufficiency (ANTADIR). 1998 yearly satistics. Observatoire 1998.
2. Laub M, Berg S, Midgren B. Home mechanical ventilation-inequalities within a homogenenous health care system. Respir Med 2004; 98:38–42.
3. Janssens JP, Derivaz S, Breitenstein E, et al. Changing patterns in long-term noninvasive ventilation: a 7-year prospective study in the Geneva Lake area. Chest 2003; 123:67–79.
4. Adams AB, Shapiro R, Marinii JJ. Changing prevalence of chronically ventilator assisted individuals in Minnesota: increases, characteristics, and the use of non-invasive ventilation. Respir Care 1998; 43:635–636.
5. Leger P, Bedicam JM, Cornette A, et al. Nasal intermittent positive pressure: long term follow up in patients with severe chronic respiratory insufficiency. Chest 1994; 105:100–105.
6. Simonds AK, Elliott M. Outcome of domiciliary nasal intermittent positive pressure in restrictive and obstructive disorders. Thorax 1995; 50:604–609.

7. Meecham Jones DJ, Paul EA, Jones PW, et al. Nasal pressure support ventilation plus oxygen compared with oxygen therapy alone in hypercapnic COPD: a randomised controlled study. Am J Respir Crit Care Med 1995; 152:538–544.
8. Simonds AK. Home ventilation. Eur Respir J 2003; 47:38s–46s.
9. Bach JR, Intintola P, Alba AS, et al. The ventilator-assisted individual. Cost analysis of institutionalization vs. rehabilitation and in-home management. Chest 1992; 101:26–30.
10. Fauroux B, Howard P, Muir JF. Home treatment for chronic respiratory insufficiency: the situation in Europe in 1992. The European Working Group on Home Treatment for Chronic Respiratory Insufficiency. Eur Respir J 1994; 7:1721–1726.
11. Muir JF, Voisin C, Ludot A. Organization of home respiratory care: the experience in France with ANTADIR. Monaldi Arch Chest Dis 1993; 48:462–467.
12. Midgren B, Olofson J, Harlid R, et al. Home mechanical ventilation in Sweden with reference to Danish experiences. Respir Med 2000; 94:135–138.
13. Casanova C, Celli B, Tost L, et al. Long-term controlled trial of nocturnal nasal positive pressure ventilation in patients with severe COPD. Chest 2000; 118:1582–1590.
14. Clini E, Sturani C, Rossi A, et al. The Italian multicentre study on noninvasive ventilation in chronic obstructive pulmonary disease patients. Eur Respir J 2002; 20:529–538.
15. Lloyd-Owen SJ, Donaldson GC, Ambrosino N, et al. Patterns of home mechanical ventilation use in Europe: results from the Eurovent survey. Eur Respir J 2005; 25:1025–1031.
16. Muir JF, Girault C, Cardinaud JP, et al. Survival and long-term follow-up of tracheostomized patients with COPD treated by home mechanical ventilation. A multicenter French study in 259 patients. French Cooperative Study Group. Chest 1994; 106:201–209.
17. Srinivasan S, Doty SM, White TR, et al. Frequency, causes, and outcome of home ventilator failure. Chest 1998; 114:1363–1367.
18. Farré R, Navajas D, Prats E, et al. Performance of mechanical ventilators at the patient's home: a multicentre quality control study. Thorax 2006; 61:400–404.
19. Farré R, Lloyd-Owen SJ, Ambrosino N, et al. Quality control of equipment in home mechanical ventilation: a European survey. Eur Respir J 2005; 26:86–94.
20. Holman H, Lorig K. Patient self-management: a key to effectiveness and efficiency in care of chronic disease. Public Health Reports 2004; 119:239–243.
21. Clinical indications for noninvasive positive pressure ventilation in chronic respiratory failure due to restrictive lung disease, COPD, and nocturnal hypoventilation—a consensus conference report. Chest 1999; 116:521–534.

44
Long-Term Ventilation: The South American Perspective

EDUARDO LUIS DE VITO
Universidad de Buenos Aires, Buenos Aires, Argentina

I. Introduction

South America is the fourth largest continent. It has an area of 17,840,000 km^2 (6,890,000 mi^2), or almost 3.5% of the Earth's surface. As of 2005, its population was estimated at more than 371,000,000. This region has socioeconomic inequities, with major sectors of the population living in poverty. In many South American countries, the richest 20% may own over 60% of the nation's wealth, while the poorest 20% may own less than 5%. This wide gap can be seen in many large South American cities. In 2005, the gross domestic product (GDP) per capita (in terms of purchasing power parity) was around US $7200 (US $14,087 in Argentina; US $2817 in Bolivia). As of 2002, South America's unemployment rate was 10.8%.

Health care for the elderly is receiving increased governmental attention. Gutiérrez and Wallace (1) reported on health services for older adults in four major Latin American cities (São Paulo, Brazil; Santiago, Chile; Mexico City, Mexico; and Montevideo, Uruguay). In Argentina, Chile, Cuba, and Uruguay, over 10% of the population is ≥60 years. As in the rest of the world, health inequities in South America affect more strongly the most excluded and vulnerable sectors of the population (2).

The elimination of health inequities by using information and communication technology and the virtual health library could represent a significant advance in terms of guaranteeing the right to health for all. Coordinated by the Latin American and Caribbean Center on Health Sciences Information (BIREME), the virtual health library of the Pan-American Health Organization could democratize information and knowledge and consequently promote equity in health. The development of a network of open access journals, Scientific Electronic Library Online (SciELO) methodology, should contribute to the electronic publication of selected quality journals from developing countries. Finally, a network promotion comprising indicators of usage, quality, and impact of scientific information on health could help to overcome many difficulties (3).

This "South American Perspective" on long-term mechanical ventilation was derived from information available in publisher medline (PUBMED), BIREME, and SciELO, supplemented by abstracts presented at the Argentine National Congress of Pneumonology, its official journal Revista Argentina de Medicina Respiratoria and the digital edition of the Congress; from the Congress of Asociación Latinoamericana del Tórax (ALAT) and its official journal Archivos de Bronconeumología (Spain). Therefore, papers included here come from Brazil, Chile, and Argentina, which comprise nearly 60% of the total population in South America. These countries are among the top five with the highest GDP in the region.

Three groups of patients who require long-term ventilation (LTV) are (1) patients with neurovascular damage and cranioencephalic or cervical trauma; (2) patients with neuromuscular diseases (NMD) such as amyotrophic lateral sclerosis (ALS), Duchenne muscular dystrophy, and spinal muscular atrophy; and (3) patients who have not been weaned from invasive ventilation, but who are potentially weanable—such as those with chronic obstructive pulmonary disease (COPD), cardiac failure, and multiorgan failure.

Many of these patients remained in intensive care unit (ICU), although their needs are quite different from those of acute ICU patients. Specialized venues, management strategies, and reimbursement schemes for such patients are rapidly emerging (4). Although weaning centers provide better and more cost-effective care (5), little information has been published in South America on the outcomes of these patients.

II. Brazil

Brazil's size (>8 million km^2, or 3,287,597 mi^2), population (186 million inhabitants), inequities in access to health services, and the lack of patient associations limit epidemiologic information on NMD. In a national survey on ALS, Dietrich-Neto et al. (6) sent a requested information on ALS from 2505 Brazilian neurologists (January–September 1998). Five hundred and forty forms were returned by 168 neurologists and data on 443 patients with ALS were analyzed. Their disease characteristics were similar to those described in international studies. Although information on management was incomplete, this sample is significant, considering the disease's relatively low incidence. It is the largest cohort published to date in Brazil, and the inclusion of referral centers as well as of private clinic data reinforces the reliability of the results. De Castro-Costa (7) reported on 87 cases of motor neuron diseases at the University Hospital of Fortaleza (Northeast Brazil). These cases included a predominance of ALS patients, with a high number of cases of juvenile and early-onset adult sporadic ALS.

Nosawa et al. (8) analyzed 45 patients who between 1997 and 1999 required LTV > 10 days and had to undergo tracheostomy at the Hospital das Clínicas at the University of São Paulo. Of the 45 patients studied, 22 were weaned from mechanical ventilation within eight weeks and discharged from the ICU. Of the other 23 patients, 8 required longer-term ventilation and 15 died. The authors pointed out that patients receiving LTV consumed substantial resources.

In May 2002, Vianna et al. (9) evaluated LTV in patients with a stay $\geq$30 days, in 77 ICUs in Rio de Janeiro, noting by telephone interview that 26 were publicly funded and 51 were in the private system. There were 645 patients of whom 62 (9.6%) met the criteria for prolonged stay. The main causes were pulmonary and neurological illness. Invasive ventilation was used in 93% of public and 79% of private units. Noninvasive ventilation was not registered in public units, but used in 12% of private patients. The authors noted that noninvasive positive pressure ventilation (NIPPV) in specialized respiratory units would reduce costs as well as length of stay in the ICU. A study conducted by nurses (10) in the ventilator-dependent pediatric population improved the process of family care during their ICU stay and when at home.

Home mechanical ventilation (HMV) has been a reality in Brazil since 1994, although it is only available for people with private insurance (28% of the population). Public programs to help the low-income population receive HMV were started a few years ago. NIPPV is used for those with NMD and COPD and sometimes during weaning. The home-visiting doctor handles only a few NIPPV cases as most patients have tracheostomy intermittent positive pressure ventilation (TIPPV). Some families and caregivers prefer their ventilator user to remain in the hospital, either for social or for financial reasons (11).

The Brazilian health care system may be divided into two subsystems. The unified health system, which incorporates public providers, hospitals, and primary health centers, is associated with federal, state, and local governments. It also includes for-profit and not-for-profit providers under contract to the public system. The second system, which is the supplementary medical system, includes the private plans with voluntary affiliation as well as prepaid health plans and insurance companies.

Care for children who are dependent on technology requires consideration of societal and psychological factors. These include financial support, medicolegal discussions, ethical, social, and educational challenges, and communicating innovations in care. Some of these important issues are starting to be addressed.

III. Chile

In Chile (756,950 km^2 or 292,183 mi^2 area and 15,328,467 inhabitants), HMV in children with chronic respiratory insufficiency is increasing (12). Sánchez et al. reported on 15 children from the Pediatric Service of the Chilean Catholic University (January 1993–December 2000), aged 5 months to 15 years. Six children had NMD, four had chronic lung disease, one had thoracic restriction, and four had bronchomalacia. The decision to use HMV was made two to four months after admission and was accomplished one to four months later, taking into account the family's situation and their health insurance status. Follow-up ranged from three months to eight years. Weaning was achieved in five patients and one died from his neurological disorder.

Their experience supported the use of HMV as a therapeutic alternative. The overall monthly cost was about 2.5 to 3 times less than ICU care. Nursing studies (13) agreed that the implementation of a home program reduced hospitalization and provided continuous nursing attention from hospital to home. The program included self-care health for patients and their families. The program began in 1996 and used both the public insurance system in which people contribute with a fixed percentage of their income, and the private system in which people pay a premium based on their financial and health characteristics.

IV. Argentina

In Argentina (2,766,890 km^2 or 1,078,000 mi^2 area and 37,384,816 inhabitants), LTV occurs in designated long-term mechanical ventilation units (LTMVU) and at home. From 1990 to the present time there are six LTMVUs, all in Buenos Aires, where almost 50% of the population lives. Health coverage in Argentina is very complex and is divided into three subsystems—public, social security, and private. Home care is growing in Argentina. In the capital city of Buenos Aires and the suburbs, about 794 patients out of 1,140,000 are included, 13 of whom receive LTV. LTMVUs are a response to the need to improve the quality of life, diminish costs, and optimize weaning outside of ICU. The good results for weaning, the low incidence of complications, and the greater contact of patients with their relatives promote enthusiasm for transfer to these centers as soon as the patients are stable.

Chertcoff et al. (14) described patients from ICUs referred to LTMVUs. Between 1998 and 2002, out of 112 patients, 50 were weaned and decannulated. Their diagnoses included COPD ($n = 23$), NMD ($n = 13$), postoperative conditions ($n = 9$), and non-COPD pulmonary disease ($n = 5$). Planells et al. (15) also reported their experience with an LTMVU. Between 1997 and 2001, both NIPPV and TIPPV were established in a total of 62 patients. Their diagnoses included COPD 26%, CNS disease 35%, NMD 18%, spinal cord injury 6.6%, postoperative conditions 5%, and others 10%. Patients were enrolled for 64 days (9–150 days) after starting ventilation. Most candidates ($n = 43$) were identified in the category of weanable, some were clearly unweanable ($n = 8$) and others were using NIPPV ($n = 11$). Sixty five percent ($n = 28$) of the weanable patients were successfully weaned.

De Vito et al. described a third example of an LTMVU (16) and reported on 67 patients (aged 64 ± 19 years) admitted between 2002 and 2004. The diagnostic categories were similar to the above trials as were the results of weaning. The average time for mechanical ventilation was 50 ± 30 days. Successful weaning was defined by spontaneous breathing for seven days or a shift to NIPPV. Respiratory indices did not distinguish those who were weanable from those whose attempts were unsuccessful. The same group subsequently reported their experience with TIPPV in which cuffs were deflated or cuffless tracheostomy tubes used (leak ventilation) (17) to preserve phonation. These patients had ALS (3 bulbar onset, 3 spinal onset) and Guillain–Barré ($n = 1$). Patients had been ventilated for 18 ± 11 months and required ventilation for 19 ± 5 hrs/day. In five of the seven patients, weaning was successful. Phonation was maintained for 14 ± 10 months, lasting for 12 to 24 hours each day. Two patients with bulbar ALS failed.

Experience with HMV in Argentina is underreported both in the private (18) and the university sectors (19). In a report on 13 patients, the main features were dyspnea (100%), asthenia (100%), hypersomnia (77%), headache (69%), leg edema (46%), and memory loss (46%). All had hypoxemia and hypercapnia. Follow-up was for 2.2 years (6 months to 4 years). Within a year, all symptoms had improved and gas exchange (Pa_{O_2}/Fi_{O_2}) improved from 269 ± 65 to 337 ± 75 ($p = 0.0018$). Pa_{CO_2} improved from 71 ± 25 mmHg to 47 ± 8 mmHg ($p = 0.0013$). Ventilatory support was discontinued in five patients, two were transplanted, and eight remained stable. Long-term improvements in symptoms and arterial blood gases were obtained without significant complications.

In the case of a 62-year-old woman with bilateral carotid body paraganglioma (19) and central alveolar hypoventilation—who received mechanical ventilation in 1990 with negative pressure through a poncho wrap and subsequently NIPPV through a nasal mask—two months after treatment symptoms, signs of right ventricular failure and daytime blood gases all improved. She has successfully been ventilated for 16 years.

Finally, Minces et al. (20) analyzed, retrospectively, a cohort of seven chronically ventilator-dependent children receiving HMV. The authors concluded that in this small group of patients, respiratory support at home improved their patient's quality of life and family dynamics, while reducing the cost of their care.

V. Summary

In summary, an increasing number of patients in South America require LTMV, at least in part, because of improved ICU care. Such patients have different needs and resource consumption patterns than patients in acute ICU conditions. As LTMV is resource intense, the use of NIPPV and the creation of LTMVU outside of the ICU should be encouraged to reduce length of hospital stay, improve health-related quality of life, and optimize the weaning process. The health and medical considerations of patients who are dependent for their survival on technology must also address society's expectations and obstacles. Although financial support for adults, children, and their families is an outstanding challenge, it is also necessary to discuss medical, legal, ethical, social, educational, and financial issues, besides learning about innovations in care. South America is now undertaking some of these important matters.

Successful weaning in an LTMVU is important. Reasons to promote a quick transfer of clinically stable patients from an ICU to an LTMVU are based on the good results, the relatively low incidence of complications, a better patient-family contact, and reduced costs. HMV is an established therapeutic alternative, especially when it includes a home-visiting program. Patients and families are increasingly taught self-management of their condition.

References

1. Gutiérrez V, Wallace S. Equity of access to health care for older adults in four major Latin American cities. Rev Panam Salud Publica 2005; 17(5–6):394–409.
2. Casas-Zamora JA. Health, human development, and governance in Latin America and the Caribbean at the beginning of the 21st century. Rev Panam Salud Publica 2002; 11(5–6):397–408.
3. Filho AP. Inequities in access to information and inequities in health. Rev Panam Salud Publica 2002; 11(5–6):409–412.
4. MacIntyre NR, Epstein SK, Carson S, et al. Management of patients requiring prolonged mechanical ventilation: report of a NAMDRC consensus conference. Chest 2005; 128:3937–3954.
5. Pilcher DV, Bailey MJ, Treacher DF, et al. Outcomes, cost and long-term survival of patients referred to a regional weaning center. Thorax 2005; 60:187–192.
6. Dietrich-Nieto F, Callegaro D, Dias-Tosta E, et al. Amyotrophic lateral sclerosis in Brazil. 1998 National survey. Arq Neuropsiquiatr 2000; 58:607–615.
7. De Castro-Costa CM, Oriá RB, Do Vale OC, et al. Motor neuron diseases in the university hospital of Fortaleza (northeastern Brazil). A clinico-demographic analysis of 87 cases. Arq Neuropsiquiatr 2000; 58:986–989.
8. Nozawa E, Kobayashi E, Matsumoto ME, et al. Assessment of factors that influence weaning from long-term mechanical ventilation after cardiac surgery. Arq Bras Cardiol 2003; 80:306–310.
9. Vianna A, Zanol L, Vieira Gomez M, et al. Utilização da ventilação mecânica nos pacientes com internação prolongada nas UTI's do Município do Rio de Janeiro. Arch Bronconeumol 2004; 40:60–119.
10. Lima EC, Issi HB, Cachafeiro MEH, Hilling MG, Ribeiro NRR. Modelo de cuidado diferenciado de enfermagem à familia da criança internada na unidade de terapia intensiva pediátrica (Differentiated nursing care model to the family of child hospitalized in a pediatrics intensive care unit) Fam. Saúde Desenv., Curitiba, v.8, n.2, p. 168–177, maio/ago. 2006.
11. Ghion LG, Miranda WA. Home mechanical ventilation in Brazil revisited. Ventilator-Assisted Living 2004; 18:1. Available at: http://www.post-polio.org/IVUN/val_18-2b.html.
12. Sanchez ID, Valenzuela AS, Bertrand PN, et al. Home ventilation in children with chronic respiratory failure: a clinical trial. Rev Chil Pediatr 2002; 73(1):51–55.
13. Covarrubias VC, Farfán PI. Prolongación de la hospitalización en el domicilio. Horiz Enferm 1996; 7:23–32.
14. Plano F, Soto J, Sills N, et al. Ventilación mandatoria intermitente sincronizada y presión de soporte vs. tubo en T en el destete de la ARM prolongada. XXX Congreso de la Asociación

Argentina de Medicina Respiratoria 2002; Edición Digital de Congresos. Available at: http://www.congresosaamr.org.ar/index.htm.

15. Planells F, Delgado G, Díaz Nielsen E. Experiencia de una unidad de ARM prolongada. XXIX Congreso de la Asociación Argentina de Medicina Respiratoria 2001; Edición Digital de Congresos. Available at: http://www.congresosaamr.org.ar/index.htm.
16. Urdapilleta ME, Lebus J, Gadea G, et al. Weaning prolongado en una unidad de cuidados respiratorios crónicos. Arch Bronconeumol 2004; 40:60–119.
17. Morel Vulliez G, Lebus J, Urdapilleta M, et al. Ventilación a fuga en pacientes neuromusculares bajo ventilación mecánica prolongada. Revista Argentina de Medicina Respiratoria 2003; 2(suppl):42.
18. Casas JP, Robles AM, Pereyra MA, et al. Ventilación domiciliaria no invasiva a presión positiva en hipoventilación alveolar crónica. Medicina (B Aires) 2000; 60:545–550.
19. Montiel GC, Roncoroni AJ, Quadrelli SA, et al. Central alveolar hypoventilation with cor pulmonale: successful treatment by non-invasive intermittent positive pressure ventilation. Medicina (B Aires) 1994; 54:343–348.
20. Minces P, Schnitzler E, Perez A, et al. Asistencia respiratoria mecánica domiciliaria en la edad pediátrica. Arch Argent Pediatr 2002; 100:210–215.

45

Long-Term Ventilation: The Japanese Perspective

YUKA ISHIKAWA and KATSUNORI TATARA
National Yakumo Hospital, Yakumo, Hokkaido, Japan

HIDEKI ISHIHARA
Osaka Prefectural Medical Center for Respiratory and Allergic Diseases, Osaka, Japan

I. History of Long-Term Ventilation and Home Mechanical Ventilation

In contrast to some countries, the polio epidemics of the 1950s did not trigger the initiation of long-term ventilation (LTV) in Japan (1). The first patient to receive LTV at home was in Tokyo in 1975, when an adult with neuromuscular disease (NMD) received tracheal invasive positive pressure ventilation (TIPPV) (2). Despite the introduction of public assistance for costs associated with home mechanical ventilation (HMV), fewer than 200 patients were receiving HMV between 1990 and 1993 (Fig. 1) (2).

By 1994, fees paid by medical insurance increased to cover medical services provided by the hospital, clinic, or home care nurse as well as the costs of medical equipment, such as the ventilator rental. This led to rapid growth in the population of patients receiving HMV (2). In April 1995, of the 536 HMV cases 65% had NMD, 20% had parenchymal disease (PD), such as sequelae of tuberculosis and chronic obstructive pulmonary disease (COPD), and 15% had thoracic restriction or central hypoventilation syndrome (3,4). In June 1995, of the 1006 patients undergoing LTV for at least three months, 215 (21%) could have been discharged to a home care setting if an appropriate public assistance program had been established (3,4). By January 1997, there were 1250 patients receiving HMV of whom 461 (1.2 people/million) used noninvasive positive pressure ventilation (NIPPV) (5).

In 1998, a study of 3500 hospitals noted that there were 3400 people receiving LTV, and those with NIPPV had risen to 800, with the other 2600 receiving TIPPV (6). In the same year the rate of LTV rose to 2.6 people/million (6). By 2001, HMV was documented in 10,400 people of whom 7900 were treated with NIPPV (7). This number rose to 17,500 people (17.5 people/million) by 2004, with NIPPV being used in 15,000 (8). Most patients with TIPPV managed at home had a diagnosis of NMD. At the same time, the number of patients with LTV who resided in medical facilities increased to 13,200 of whom 7000 patients received TIPPV.

In 2004, 71% of hospitals surveyed in Japan provided home oxygen therapy for about 100,000 patients (8). Just under half of these hospitals also managed patients with NIPPV and just under a quarter performed TIPPV. Despite the increasing numbers of patients being ventilated, the medical system and especially home care support remained inadequate (8).

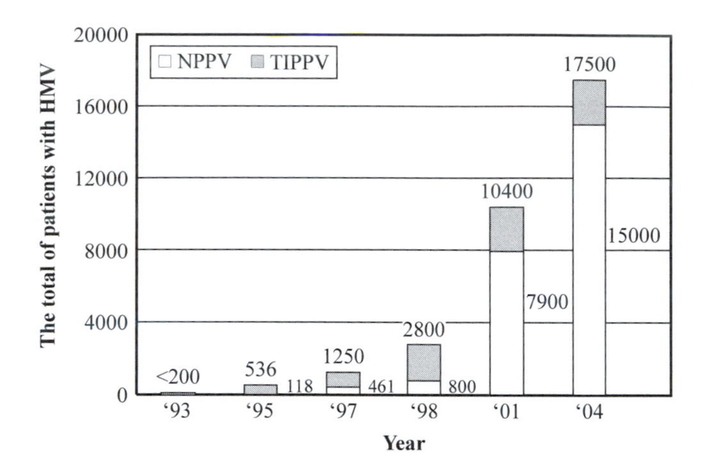

Figure 1 Transition of the number of patients with HMV. *Abbreviations*: HMV, home mechanical ventilation; NPPV, nasal positive pressure ventilation; TIPPV, tracheal invasive positive pressure ventilation.

Moreover, after requiring HMV, 35% of patients were unable to continue being employed, 21% were forced to economize to accommodate the expenses associated with HMV, and 24% felt uneasy regarding their economic outlook while receiving HMV (8). The public assistance program provided financial support for 71% of patients ventilated at home, 10% of whom were dependent on support to fully or partially cover the cost of electricity, transportation to a hospital, or a pulse oximeter (8). It was noted that some people who were eligible did not apply for assistance because of the burdensome procedures involved with the application (8). Today, the provision of public services varies among different jurisdictions and it would be useful if there was a national consensus on the level of economic assistance appropriate to support HMV.

II. LTV Outside the Home

A. Children at University Hospitals or General Hospitals

In 1993, 102 children with TIPPV could not be managed in the community, and therefore remained in pediatric wards of 52 hospitals for an average of 823 days (9). Their diagnosis included spinal muscular atrophy type 1, severe congenital myopathy, chronic lung damage after ventilatory support required by premature birth, severe mental retardation, and cerebral palsy (9).

B. LTV in a Unit for Patients with NMD and Retarded Children in the National Hospital Organization

Since 1964, expert medical care in a designated unit for children impaired by NMD has occurred in national centers under the National Hospital Organization, formerly called National Sanatoriums. The main purpose of this structure was to permit hospitalized

Table 1 IPPV and TIPPV in LTV Patients Hospitalized in Specialized Units for NMD or Other Progressive Neuromuscular Conditions Including ALS, or Mentally Retarded Children in the National Hospital Organization

		Cerebral palsy	
	Muscular dystrophy		ALS
Inpatients	2147	7154	2065
Inpatients with LTV (%)	1092 (50.9)	307 (4.3)	591 (22.7)
NIPPV (%)	61.5	3.3	4.9
TIPPV (%)	37.9	91.8	94
24-hour ventilation (%)	59.9	76	92.5

Abbreviations: TIPPV, tracheal invasive positive pressure ventilation; NIPPV, noninvasive positive pressure ventilation; ALS, amyotrophic lateral sclerosis; NMD, neuromuscular diseases; LTV, long-term ventilation.

children to attend adjacent schools for physically or mentally impaired, provide early rehabilitation, and assist the patient's family with home care.

At 27 national hospitals, 1092 (51%) of the 2147 inpatients with muscular dystrophy (MD) were receiving LTV and 61% of the patients receiving LTV were undergoing NIPPV in 2005 (Table 1) (10). NIPPV was used for 71% in Duchenne muscular dystrophy, 66% in limb-girdle dystrophy, 61% in myotonic dystrophy, 53% in Becker's MD, and 50% in Fukuyama congenital progressive MD (10). Sixty percent of the patients, on either NIPPV or TIPPV, required 24-hour ventilation.

In addition to the MD units, national hospitals care for those with severe mental retardation and cerebral palsy, and include specific units for those with amyotrophic lateral sclerosis (ALS). Of the 7154 patients with severe mental and physically impairment, 307 (4.3%) received LTV in 2005, most of whom were ventilated invasively (10). TIPPV was used for 92% of the above patients and for 94% of those with ALS—higher percentages than the 38% with MD (10). Most (76%) of the patients with LTV had no ventilator-free time (10). Similarly, of the 2605 adult inpatients with neurological conditions, 23% used LTV and 93% required 24-hour ventilation (10).

Ventilator training and follow-up occurs in regional NMD centers, designated by the National Hospital Organization. Such facilities may be directly responsible for the contract for equipment rental and will provide annual or, as required, medical follow-up in collaboration with local hospitals. They may also admit patients for rehospitalization, if required. In 2004, 906 patients and in 2005, 1039 patients were supervised by the National Hospital Organization (10).

C. Official Guidelines

The NIPPV Guidelines Development Committee of the Japanese Respiratory Society published their recommendations in June 2006 (11). There are no guidelines for HMV available in Japan, but an official subcommittee on HMV of the Japanese Society of Respiratory Care Medicine will be formulating HMV guidelines beginning in 2006.

D. Experts in Respiratory Care

Unlike the United States, a respiratory therapy–licensing system has not yet been introduced into Japan. Therefore, to be licensed as a respiratory care expert, a certification test has been used since 1996. It is the joint responsibility of the three medical societies: the Japanese Association for Thoracic Surgery, the Japanese Respiratory Society, and the Japanese Society of Anesthesiologists. Over 20,000 people including physiotherapists, nurses, and medical engineers were qualified as respiratory therapists from 1996 to 2005.

E. LTV Care System

Introduction of LTV

Specialists in pulmonology, neurology, pediatrics, or intensive care introduce LTV when it becomes clear that ongoing ventilatory support will be necessary, except for a few patients who have decided, in writing, to refuse life-sustaining procedures. Some patients cannot make the transition to home care because of insufficient family or financial support. In this case LTV is continued in hospitals, although there are insufficient facilities for this purpose.

The patient's family also participates in the decision to proceed with LTV (Fig. 2) (12), although sometimes family members are not able to support a decision to continue ventilation at home. In such cases, law does not permit discontinuation of ventilation.

Guidance on Home Care

In some hospitals, home care sections or respiratory support teams may provide guidance on home care. They include physicians, nurses, physical therapists, medical engineers, and social workers. Occupational therapists are also involved in such matters as living environment, aids, and appliances. In the absence of a specific home care transition team, discharge guidance is often provided by physicians and nurses from the wards.

Transition to home begins with the patient and family members staying together for a day in a private room of the ward—a dedicated room for home care training, if available—where medical staff members can respond at all hours. Following the above stay, if no problems arise, the patient and family members stay for a day in a lodging facility close to the hospital or return home, making the transition to a home care setting. Ward nurses prepare an individual illustrated commentary pamphlet for the family by editing digital photos that can be customized for the characteristics of the patient, family, and equipment.

When the patient returns home, the patient's physician ensures by phone or e-mail that the patient is linked to a local hospital for blood gases, vascular access, and urgent endotracheal intubation, or a clinic for home visits. Information on equipment is provided and each member of the hospital multidisciplinary team communicates with the local medical staff. The ventilator rental firm also makes contact with the local hospital to ensure the provision and servicing of the necessary respiratory equipment. Under a rental contract, equipment is rented by the hospital that in turn supplies it to the patient. The ventilator rental firm makes monthly visits to ensure that the equipment is operating correctly and in the event of failure they provide backup and repair for damaged equipment.

Home visits and rehabilitation are coordinated in the care setting to identify changes in condition and to noninvasively monitor gas exchange. Assistance with secretion clearance and support for the patients' activities are also provided at the request of the family. The family also

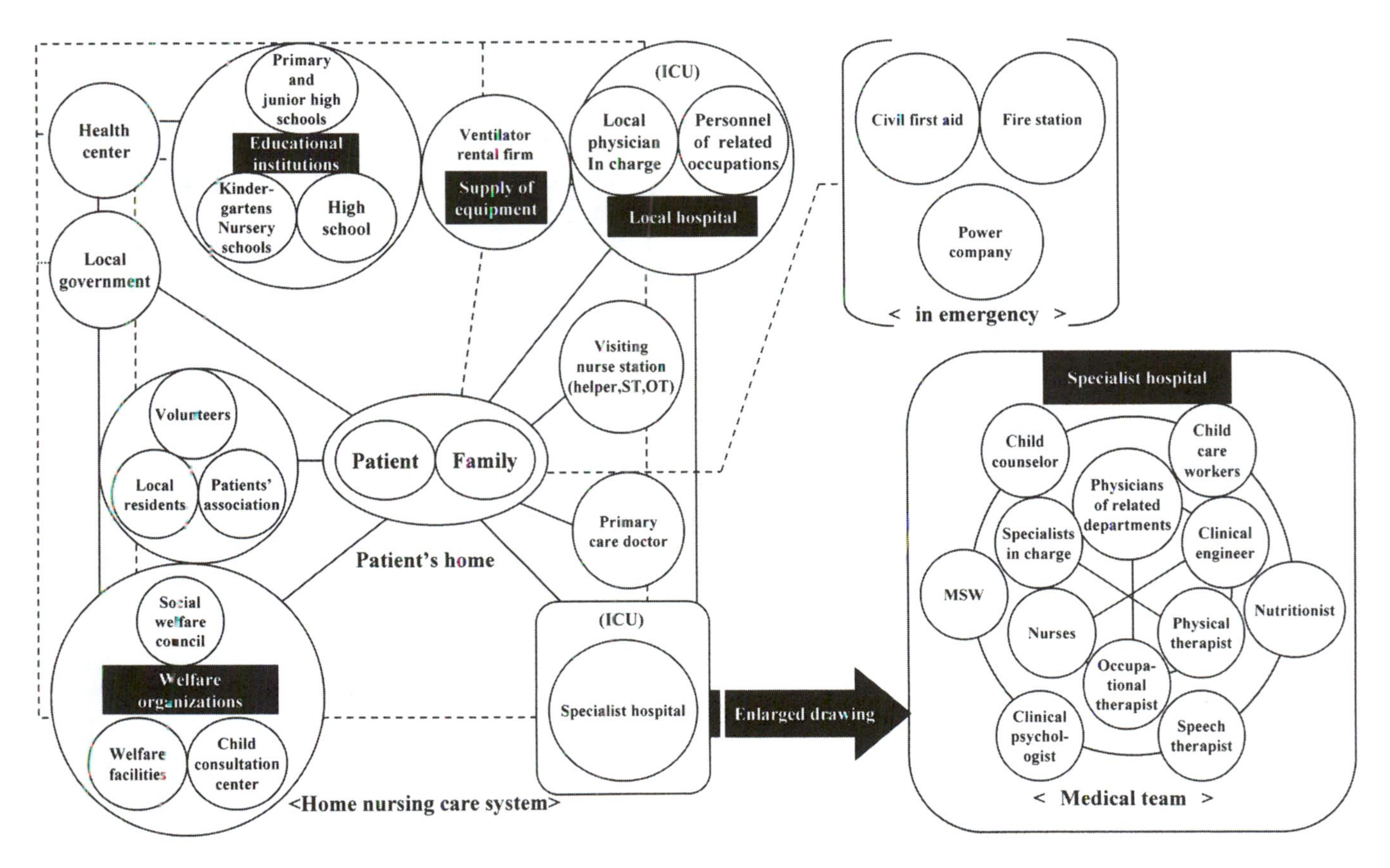

Figure 2 Home nursing care system and team medical service.

is taught when to contact the patient's primary care physician or for rehabilitation, when to access a physical therapist, occupational therapist, or assistive technology.

The municipal welfare division or health center will provide an identification booklet for the physically impaired, deliver inhalation equipment, suctioning devices, an oximeter, nursing equipment, daily necessities and a grant to pay housing conversion, medical or traveling expenses. The hospital medical social worker (MSW) may give advice as an intermediary. In many cases, the primary caregivers are the patient's family members, even at school, usually women but with men being increasingly involved. Some school nurses are able to suction through a tracheostomy.

If a family has difficulty in continuing home nursing care or in ensuring education or if child abuse is reported, the child can be admitted according to child welfare law, following the office for children's consultation, to the hospital where fundamental human rights, including the right to education are secured. With the increase of divorce and life extension through medical care, despite the trend toward a declining birthrate, the number of children requiring prolonged hospitalization continues to increase.

HMV-Related Medical Care Expenses

Medical facilities covered for HMV must have full respiratory, diagnostic, and management facilities (Tables 2 and 3). The patient is supplied with the ventilator and two sets of

Table 2 HMV-Related Medical Expenses: Medical Fees Paid to Medical Facilities

Guidance and management for HMV	¥28,000 (approx. US $255)/mo
Additions depending on the equipment	
Tracheostomy case	¥68,400 (approx. US $622)/mo
Nasal mask case	¥59,300 (approx. US $539)/mo
External negative pressure ventilation case	¥30,000 (approx. US $273)/mo
Artificial nose case	¥15,000 (approx. US $136)/mo
Inpatient ventilation case	¥7450 (approx. US $68)/day

Table 3 HMV-Related Medical Expenses: Cost to the Patient on the Health Insurance List

30% of the medical expenses as a general rule
20% of the medical expenses, if the patient is younger than three years
10% of the medical expenses or 20% according to the patient's income, if the patient is aged 70 years and older
Patients holding the physically disability certificate booklet
Outpatient individual payments vary from municipality to municipality
Specific disease patients under the specific disease care program
Payment depending on the income (except for certified severely impaired patients whose medical expenses are completely covered)

There are two medical insurance systems in Japan "Social Insurance System" for those working at a company or an office and "National Health Insurance System" for those not covered by the Social Insurance System. The hospital receives individual payments from patients and the remaining medical service fees from the medical insurance system. The fees are established for the rental rate of the equipment such as a ventilator and a humidifier. The currency has been converted using a rate of ¥110 to the US $.

accessories and is sometimes charged for the latter. The equipment used in Japan is imported from countries such as the United States, France, Germany, and Australia. The hospital pays tracheostomy costs and the municipality pays other accessories for home, such as suction equipment and nebulizers. As the patients must purchase their own resuscitator bag, many do not do so. The patient's family must purchase or rent cough assist equipment—for major items of equipment/expense (¥670,000 or US $6091) or rent (¥20,000 or US $182 per month)—with some municipalities contributing in part. Municipalities also contribute to the power required for home ventilation.

Follow-Up

Equipment Maintenance

Equipment is checked daily by a caregiver and monthly as well as annually by the supplier. In the event of equipment failure, several parties (supplier, primary care physician, home nurse station, or emergency hospital) are involved. The backup support systems are not well organized and local expertise is often scarce and poorly defined.

Medical Examination

Patients are seen monthly at the medical office or at home, with visits by home care at regular intervals, as required. Visits average twice per week for about two hours per visit. Rehabilitation staff, and most frequently, physiotherapists also visit for one hour, as required, weekly or monthly.

Follow-Up System

University and community hospitals cooperate with specialized centers and local hospitals, especially during the first month of the transition home, with open telephone consultation between the medical and nursing teams. Experienced centers also reevaluate patients regularly during the day and during sleep as well, arranging for admission to hospital if the patient's medical or social condition changes. Regular hospitalization for respite is recommended but, in practice, is difficult to organize. If a backup ventilator system has not been supplied, the patient's family is trained to perform ventilatory support with a resuscitator bag while transferring the patient to a hospital. The caregivers may also contact the rental firm to arrange a backup as well as the local HMV center for advice and assistance with increased home care.

Preparation for Disasters

Some communities have created a system under which home care patients are transferred to local hospitals in anticipation of an electric power failure or flood disaster. Local fire departments will also assist in the event of a power failure or need for evacuation. Some electric power companies will arrange power generators available for 24-hour ventilator users in case of an electrical failure.

Challenges for the Future

It is hoped that the choices available for patients receiving LTV will be broadened to include not only the home, but group homes or facilities with both amenities and medical care. Wider use of NIPPV should decrease the number of patients with TIPPV. However, as

LTV cases increase, the challenges of funding and manpower will increase. The task of improving health-related quality of life is ongoing, and there is a need for sharing information with other countries faced with similar issues around LTV to optimize care within the limits of culture and economic resources.

Acknowledgments

The authors wish to thank laboratory technician Tomoyuki Aoyagi for the drawings of the graphic charts and Rieko Watanabe and Cheryl Yamashita for the translation of the article.

References

1. Ishikawa Y. Post-polio pulmonary dysfunction [in Japanese]. Respir Circ 2003; 51(11): 1121–1127.
2. Kimura K. Home mechanical ventilation in Japan: current status and challenges for the future. In: Text for the annual leader training session about home care medical equipments [in Japanese], Tokyo Japan Association for the Advancement of Medical Equipment. 2005:2–18.
3. Sato M, Asai Y, Ando M, et al. Nationwide survey of long term ventilation and home mechanical ventilation in 1995. A 1995 annual report of the Japanese Ministry of Health, Labour and Welfare Specified Respiratory Failure Study Group [in Japanese]. 1995:106–109.
4. Ishihara H, Kimura K, Watanabe S, et al. Actual condition survey of home mechanical ventilation in 1995—summary of questionnaire responses from patients, doctors and mechanical ventilator distributors. A 1996 annual report of the Japanese Ministry of Health, Labour and Welfare Specified Respiratory Failure Study Group [in Japanese]. 1996:110–114.
5. Ishihara H, Kimura K, Watanabe T, et al. Nationwide survey of home mechanical ventilation in 1997. A 1997 annual report of the Japanese Ministry of Health, Labour and Welfare Specified Respiratory Failure Study Group [in Japanese]. 1997:93–98.
6. Ishihara H, Kimura K, Ohi M, et al. Nationwide survey of home mechanical ventilation and noninvasive intermittent positive pressure ventilation in 1998. A 1998 annual report of the Japanese Ministry of Health, Labour and Welfare Specified Respiratory Failure Study Group [in Japanese]. 1999:87–90.
7. Ishihara H, Kimura K, Ohi M, et al. Nationwide survey of home mechanical ventilation in 2001. A 2001 annual report of the Japanese Ministry of Health, Labour and Welfare Specified Respiratory Failure Study Group [in Japanese]. 2002:68–71.
8. Ishihara H, Sakatani M, Kimura K, et al. Nationwide survey of home mechanical ventilation in 2004. A 2004 annual report of the Japanese Ministry of Health, Labour and Welfare Specified Respiratory Failure Study Group [in Japanese]. 2005:31–34.
9. Sakakihara Y, Yoneyama A, Kamoshita S. Chronic ventilator-assisted children in university hospitals in Japan. Acta Pediatr Jpn 1993; 35:332–335.
10. Tatara K, Ishikawa Y, Imai T, et al. A study on effective, efficient, and safe management of long-term mechanical ventilation. A 2005 collaborative research report of the National Organization Hospital [in Japanese]. 2006 (in press).
11. Ohi M, Akashiba T, Ishikawa Y, et al. Guideline for Noninvasive Positive Pressure Ventilation (NPPV) [in Japanese]. Edited by the Noninvasive Positive Pressure Ventilation (NPPV) Guidelines Development Committee of The Japanese Respiratory Society. Tokyo, Nankodo. 2006:2–96.
12. Kishiya R. Coordinating the management of home mechanical ventilation. In: Ishikawa Y, ed. Manual for the care of patients using noninvasive ventilation. Neuromuscular Disorders. Chiba Japan Planning Center Inc., 2005:223–228.

46
Long-Term Ventilation: The Taiwanese Perspective

SHIH-CHI KU and CHONG-JEN YU
Department of Internal Medicine, National Taiwan University Hospital, Taipei, Taiwan

I. Introduction

Trends in the increasing number of patients requiring long-term mechanical ventilation (LMV) are universal, with no exceptions in the Asia Pacific area. Patient characteristics and clinical outcomes are essentially the same as those in the industrialized countries (1,2). Because of the inherent diversity of cultures and socioeconomic status, the Asia Pacific area has its unique issues to address regarding health services and the medical ethics of LMV. In this chapter, we will illustrate some of these issues, as they are experienced in Taiwan and we will highlight some of the challenges that they present.

II. Epidemiology of LMV in Taiwan

A. Prevalence

Based on the LMV definition of patients requiring at least six hours per day of mechanical ventilation for a period longer than 21 consecutive days, the number of LMV patients is skyrocketing in Taiwan, increasing between 1997 and 2004 from 9000 to 30,000, more than a threefold increase in seven years (3). Approximately 20% to 23% of LMV patients in Taiwan progress to ventilator dependence (4). The prevalence of ventilator dependence in 2004 was 26 ventilator-dependent cases per 100,000 population, a figure far higher than in Europe or the United States, which have 5 to 10 cases per 100,000 population (1,2,5).

B. Patient Characteristics

A recent report from southern Taiwan noted that LMV patients transferred to a long-term acute care facility (LTACF) (6), had a mean age of 71.2 years, with a slight male predominance (53%). The average length of stay was 19 days, with 62% successfully weaned, 23% dying, and 15% being transferred to a chronic respiratory care facility. Their underlying diseases were; pneumonia and chronic lung disease (45%), postoperative (24%), postseptic (13%), oncologic (7%), cardiovascular disease (6%), and cerebrovascular accident (5%). These clinical features and outcomes are comparable to those in the West in the late 1990s (1,2).

III. Health Expenditure for LMV

A National Health Insurance program was implemented in Taiwan in March 1995. By the year 2004, the vast majority (97.6%) of the population was covered by this social insurance (7), at a cost of 18 billion US dollars, equivalent to 6.2% of the gross domestic product (GDP) (8) being spent on the national health expenditures (NHE). Because of the aging population and advances in medical care and biotechnology, health expenditure has increased dramatically. Resources allocated to chronic diseases is also growing, for example, 4.0% of NHE claims were for the medical care of LMV in 2004 (8), which includes expenses attributable to both acute care and long-term care. Within the disease category of the respiratory system, 29.5% of the expenses were used for patients with LMV. For only inpatient care, it was 15.2% of the expense spent in LMV. Medical expenditure rises with the increasing number of LMV patients, with a two-digit rate of increase annually since 2001 (8).

IV. Managed Care of LMV: The Integrated Delivery System

A. Background

To solve the problems of prolonged mechanical ventilation in the intensive care unit (ICU) and improve the effectiveness of resource allocation and quality of care in LMV, the Bureau of National Health Insurance (BNHI) initiated a program called "The Ventilator Dependents Managed Care Demonstration" in July 2000 (3). Its goal was to setup the standards of payment for LMV on a per capita basis rather than on a fee-for-service basis. With this strict form of managed care, an integrated step-down health care system was organized as follows:

a) Patients with mechanical ventilation are allowed to stay at the ICU up to 21 days;
b) If stable but still requiring LMV, they are transferred to a respiratory care center (RCC) for a weaning trial, for another 42 days; and
c) If still requiring LMV, they step down to a respiratory care ward (RCW) after the 63rd day of mechanical ventilation.

The RCC and RCW are comparable to that of the LTACF and long-term care facility (LTCF), respectively (5). The final step is home ventilator dependent (HVD), if the patients' conditions are suitable. The global budget payment is deescalated according to the level of facilities where patients stay (Fig. 1). When staying beyond the permitted limit at any level of facility, there is a penalty that reduces the reimbursements paid according to the overdue days, as long as there are no explicit reasons for the prolonged stay. In the summary report of registered patients in 2005 (4), there were 12,664 enrollees of whom 8540 (67.4%) had separated from the participant institutions, including 41.8% successfully weaned, 28.9% deaths, 15.2% discharged against medical advice, and 14.1% transferred to nonparticipant institutions. Cases not included (nonseparators) were those remaining at a participating institution and still requiring long-term ventilation.

When looking across each level of facility, the weaning rates and mortality rates were: 41.2% and 14.9% in RCC, and 6.4% and 14.0% in RCW, respectively. The details of

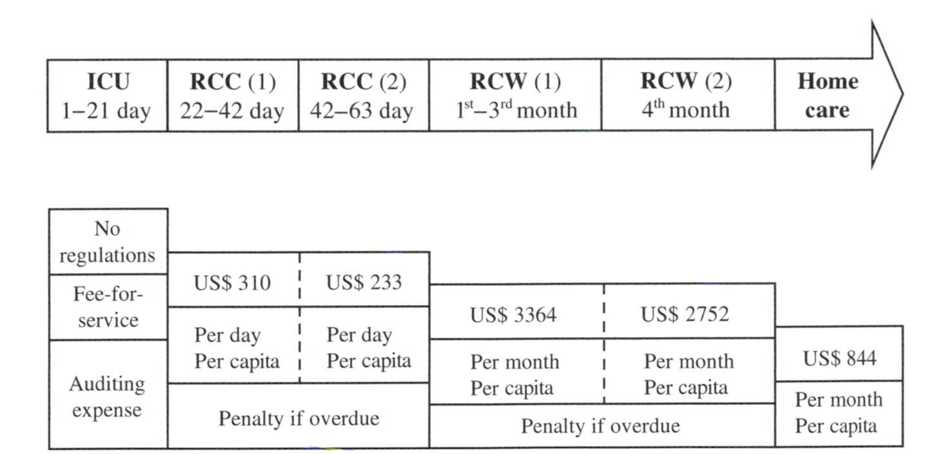

Figure 1 Global budget payment for the IDS. *Abbreviations*: IDS, integrated delivery system; ICU, intensive care unit; RCC, respiratory care center; RCW, respiratory care ward.

Table 1 Outcomes of Patients Separated[a] from the Integrated Delivery System since 2004 ($N = 8540$)

	ICU	RCC	RCW	HVD	Ward
Successfully weaned, n (%), $N = 3572$	695 (19.5)	2095 (58.6)	513 (14.3)	13 (3.0)	256 (7.1)
Discharged against medical advice[b], n (%), $N = 1299$	524 (40.3)	290 (22.3)	438 (33.7)	N/A	47 (3.6)
Transferred to nonparticipant institutions, n (%), $N = 1206$	132 (10.9)	533 (44.2)	298 (24.7)	109 (9.0)	134 (11.1)
Mortality, n (%), $N = 2463$	699 (28.3)	469 (19.0)	1124 (45.6)	45 (1.8)	126 (5.1)
Mean LOS, days	30.3	24.9	163.3	N/A	—

[a]Nonseparated LMV patients remain at participating sites.
[b]Most of these patients are discharged under critical conditions.
Abbreviations: ICU, intensive care unit; RCC, respiratory care center; RCW, respiratory care ward; HVD, home ventilator dependent; LOS, length of stay; N/A, not applicable.

events of the Integrated Delivery System (IDS) patients are displayed in Table 1. An observational study by Wu et al. (9) reported that the ICU length of stay decreased from 11.7 days to 6.2 days after the setup of an RCC in a tertiary medical center. This highlights the increasing turnover of ICU beds and the role of the RCC as the gatekeeper of more efficient resource utilization for LMV after the implementation of IDS. The above does not include those younger than 17 years. Therefore, the outcome of children and adolescents requiring LMV is not clear under the present health care system.

B. Auditing the Quality of Care

After the demonstration of IDS, the number of institutions caring for LMV increased sharply, especially the RCW. To maintain the quality of care for LMV, the BNHI audited these participating institutions, setting up quality indicators for three sectors:

1. Structure indicators, such as the qualification of the health care workers (HCWs) and the patient-to-nurse ratios per shift;
2. Process indicators, such as patient sources and patient admission criteria; and
3. Outcome indicators, such as length of stay, ventilator days, mortality, infection rate, readmission to the upstream institutions, and ventilator weaning rate.

Furthermore, the BNHI plans to operate the IDS on a compulsory basis nationwide to enroll all LMV patients. The reimbursement and the intensity of auditing will depend on the rating of these institutions after a standardized evaluation by the academic society of pulmonary and critical care medicine.

V. Special Issues of LMV in Taiwan

A. Infection Control

Because the patient flows in the IDS come from the acute care facility to the LTCF, there is an increasing awareness that patterns of drug-resistant microorganisms vary according to the disease severity of patients and the ecologies in these facilities. A surveillance from all culture samples showed that 19.9% of ICU isolates are *Acinetobacter baumannii*, 17.3% of RCC isolates are *Pseudomonas aeruginosa*, and 30.0% of RCW isolates are *Klebsiella pneumonae*, (unpublished data, 2006, with the courtesy of Dr. Chien, JY). Multidrug-resistant pathogens in the main are *Acinetobacter baumannii* in the RCC and *Pseudomonas aeruginosa* in the RCW. All of these suggest that the LTCF will become the reservoir of antimicrobial resistance. At present, there are few guidelines regarding infection control in these facilities and work is required in this area to avoid widespread antimicrobial resistance as LMV patients are transferred between these facilities and acute care hospitals.

Tuberculosis (TB) is endemic to Taiwan. The combination of chronic conditions in an environment where a history of TB infection is prevalent, ventilator-dependent patients are at risk for TB reactivation. Their airways are also prone to colonization with nontuberculous mycobacteria. In a report describing nosocomial transmission of *Mycobacterium tuberculosis* among HCWs in Taipei (10), the source of hospital transmission was believed to have been derived from an index case of an LMV patient. Subsequent hospital-wide TB screening identified 2% of HCWs as having TB. This emphasizes the urgency of setting up effective TB screening infrastructures and adequate education in health care facilities.

B. Shortage of HCWs

Since 2002 respiratory care professionals have been required to take the national examinations for licensing. There are 1300 respiratory therapists who have qualified, since then, of which one-fifth are now working in the RCW (4). Considering the number of LMV patients in the RCW, it is estimated that they take care of 21 patients per shift. Although the goals of patient care in the RCW are focused on quality of life rather than aggressive weaning from ventilators, this high workload will have an effect on the quality of respiratory care for these patients.

With the marked increase in GDP, the health human resources shortage has worsened in Taiwan over the last decade (11), as has the category of paramedical personnel in the LTCF. Although recently, immigrant HCWs have temporarily filled the need, to ensure patient safety and quality of medical care, they require regulations and standardized training programs.

C. Economic Impact on the Family with LMV

Under the influence of Chinese culture, the family bond is tight and beliefs and responsibilities are shared. Once one of the family members develops LMV and the condition progresses to ventilator dependence, the subsequent expenses will have a great impact on the family, in terms of the psychosocial stress and economical burdens. With the present IDS payment, medical expenditure directly related to the LMV is fully covered under the global budget. However, while patients stay at the RCW, the family needs to pay out-of-pocket expenses, which is on average US $1000 per month, not to mention the indirect cost that the family has to pay for the illness and its treatment. The financial burden is quite high, compared to the average annual family income per household of US $30,000 in 2004 (12).

D. Controversy in Medical Ethics

Clinicians are always confronted with challenges of how to reconcile the priorities of resource allocation and the equity of medical care. Most Chinese people want to save their loved ones at any cost during the stage of acute illness, without considering what will be the consequences on the patients' quality of life once they are in the convalescence stage. Fewer cases with terminal and catastrophic illness undergo end-of-life or palliative care in the ICU. Accordingly, some of the LMV patients at the RCW have no chance of being weaned from their ventilator, due to their debilitating comorbid conditions. Because of the growing expenditure in the LMV, as the stakeholders and policymakers regulate resource utilization, the clinicians will be forced to prioritize the limited budgets. The societal expectations remain for aggressive and comprehensive medical care for the chronically and critically ill, even under the present social insurance program.

VI. Conclusion

We have described the epidemiology and health economic issues of LMV in Taiwan. Many challenges remain for the stakeholders and clinicians in designing and implementing a cost-effective health care system for LMV. Controversies continue regarding medical ethical considerations and the need to prioritize resource allocation. It is important to address these issues for the welfare of LMV patients to be fully achieved.

References

1. Scheinhorn DJ, Chao DC, Stearn-Hassenpflug M, et al. Post-ICU mechanical ventilation: Treatment of 1,123 patients at a regional weaning center. Chest 1997; 111(6):1654–1659.
2. Votto J, Brancifort JM, Scalise PJ, et al. COPD and other diseases in chronically ventilated patients in a prolonged respiratory care unit: a retrospective 20-year survival study. Chest 1998; 113(1):86–90.
3. The Ventilator Dependents Managed Care Demonstration, Bureau of National Health Insurance. Available at: http://www.nhi.gov.tw/webdata/webdata.asp?menu=1&menu_id=26&webdata_id=942 Accessed May 20, 2006.
4. Summary report of IDS-registered patients in 2004, Bureau of National Health Insurance.
5. MacIntyre NR, Epstein SK, Carson S, et al. Management of patients requiring prolonged mechanical ventilation: Report of a NAMDRC Consensus Conference. Chest 2005; 128(6): 3937–3954.
6. Chen CH, Lin WC, Lee CH, et al. Determining factors for successful weaning of patients in a respiratory care center—a one-year experience. Thorac Med 2004; 19(4):236–242.
7. National Health Insurance Profile, Bureau of National Health Insurance. Available at: http://www.nhi.gov.tw/english/e_05pro.asp. Accessed May 25, 2006.
8. National Health Insurance Annual Statistical Report 2004, Bureau of National Health Insurance, R.O.C.
9. Wu CP, Yang PT, Tsai PI. The outcome of patients with mechanical ventilation in respiratory care center of a medical center in one year. Taiwan Crit Care Med 2000; 1:1–14.
10. Nosocomial transmission of mycobacterium tuberculosis found through screening for severe acute respiratory syndrome-Taipei, Taiwan, 2003. MMWR Morb Mortal Wkly Rep 2004, 53(15): 321–322.
11. Manpower Survey Results in May 2006, Directorate-General of Budget, Accounting and Statistics, Executive Yuan, R.O.C. Available at: http://eng.stat.gov.tw/public/Data/662216302.doc. Accessed May 15, 2006.
12. The Survey of Family Income and Expenditure, National Statistics 2004, Directorate-General of Budget, Accounting and Statistics, Executive Yuan, R.O.C.

Index